Medical Neurology

GW00792976

To our wives, Vivienne, Margaret and Linda.

Medical Neurology

David Chadwick
DM FRCP
Consultant Neurologist, Department of Medical and Surgical Neurology, Walton Hospital, Liverpool

Niall Cartlidge
MB BS FRCP
Consultant Neurologist, Royal Victoria Infirmary, Newcastle-upon-Tyne;
Senior Lecturer in Neurology, University of Newcastle-upon-Tyne;

David Bates
MA MB BChir FRCP
Consultant Neurologist, Royal Victoria Infirmary, Newcastle-upon-Tyne;
Senior Lecturer in Neurology, University of Newcastle-upon-Tyne

CHURCHILL LIVINGSTONE
EDINBURGH LONDON MELBOURNE AND NEW YORK 1989

CHURCHILL LIVINGSTONE
Medical Division of Longman Group UK Limited

Distributed in the United States of America by Churchill Livingstone Inc., 1560 Broadway, New York, N.Y. 10036, and by associated companies, branches and representatives throughout the world.

© Longman Group UK Limited 1989

All rights reserved. No part of this publication may be reproduced, stored in a retrieval system, or transmitted in any form or by any means, electronic, mechanical, photocopying, recording or otherwise, without either the prior written permission of the publishers (Churchill Livingstone, Robert Stevenson House, 1–3 Baxter's Place, Leith Walk, Edinburgh EH1 3AF), or a licence permitting restricted copying in the United Kingdom issued by the Copyright Licensing Agency Ltd, 33–34 Alfred Place, London, WC1E 7DP.

First published 1989

ISBN 0-443-03051-0

British Library Cataloguing in Publication Data
Chadwick, David
Medical neurology
1. Man. nervous system. Diagnosis
I. Title II. Cartlidge, N.E.F. (Niall Edward Foster) III. Bates, David
616.8′0475

Library of Congress Cataloging in Publication Data
Chadwick, D.
Medical neurology/David Chadwick, N.E.F. Cartlidge, David Bates.
p. cm.
Includes index.
1. Neurology. 2. Nervous system—Diseases.
I. Cartlidge, N.E.F. II. Bates, David. III. Title.
[DNLM: 1. Nervous System Diseases. WL 100 B329t]
RC346.B39 1989
616.8—dc 19
DNLM/DLC 88–23742
for Library of Congress CIP

Produced by Longman Singapore Publishers (Pte) Ltd.
Printed in Singapore

Preface

If this book has one aim above others it is to emphasise the importance of neurology in the practice of general or internal medicine. Much of general medical practice involves the management of symptoms directly or indirectly relating to the nervous system, and much of neurological practice involves patients with general medical disorders. Neurology was one of the first medical specialities to separate itself from mainstream internal medicine, and few neurologists would regard themselves as competent general physicians. As subspecialities develop in their own right within general medicine, we sense that younger generations of physicians are less confident about their practice of neurology, even though, in many parts of the world they remain responsible for the care of the majority of patients with neurological disorders. Increasingly general physicians have come to regard neurology as a rather esoteric and difficult speciality, a view heightened by the introduction of more sophisticated neurological imaging and physiological investigation.

This book aims to provide a practical approach to the diagnosis and management of patients with disorders of the nervous system that will be of value to both general physicians and neurologists in training. We hope in particular that it will be helpful to those approaching MRCP examinations who are often particularly uncertain and lacking in confidence about their approach to the neurological patient. It should update general physicians about neurological practice, as we recognise that many neurological disorders will be looked after by general physicians and not by specialist neurologists.

The overall approach of the book is a simple one: namely, that neurology is a clinically based subject in which history-taking and examination are of supreme importance in the diagnostic process. In neurological diagnosis two questions must be asked. Firstly, are a patient's symptoms and signs compatible with a single lesion, multiple lesions or diffuse pathology, and where can such pathology be localised? This basic question demands an understanding of the functional organisation of the nervous system and the significance and interpretation of neurological signs. Secondly, what is the nature of the pathology at the site to which the disease has been localised? Interpretation of the history given by the patient is of crucial importance here in directing attention to specific pathological processes and most particularly the temporal pattern of the evolution of symptoms is crucial.

It is difficult to adopt a single uniform classification of neurological disease and we have divided the book into three sections. The first section considers neurological symptoms and signs in relationship to the anatomical organisation of systems within the nervous system. In chapters 1–4 we discuss neurological symptoms and signs related to the motor and sensory systems, the autonomic nervous system and the special sensations and cranial nerves. We also consider the uses and abuses of neurological investigation (chapter 5). The second section (chapters 6–10) deals with symptom complexes relating to disease at differing levels in the nervous system which cut across longitudinal systems of organisation. These include coma, epilepsy and other paroxysmal disorders, headache and pain syndromes, spinal cord syndromes, peripheral nerve and muscle disease. In the first two sections particular attention is paid to the interpretation of symptoms and signs, their causes and the symptomatic management of neurological disorders where this is relevant. The third section (chapters 11–18) describes specific pathological processes, their clinical presentation and their management and prognosis. Chapter 19 deals with psychiatric disorders and their relationship to neurology.

In writing the book we have made the assumption that readers will be familiar with the basic neurosciences and will in particular have a background knowledge of neuroanatomy and neurophysiology. These subjects are only discussed where they have particular relevance to clinical problems. We have not dealt in any comprehensive way with paediatric neurology as this lies outside the scope of our aims. Paediatric conditions are touched upon where they are relevant to adult neurology, recognising the fact that some conditions may arise in childhood and continue into the adult age range, requiring neurologists and general physicians to have some understanding and skills in managing these conditions. The book is not referenced within chapters but each chapter has a concluding bibliography for further reading upon the subject.

This book has been written by three successive occupants of the First Assistant post in Neurology at the University of Newcastle-Upon-Tyne. We occupied this post in turn between the years of 1970 and 1979. We would wish to acknowledge our gratitude to the large number of individuals who contributed to our education during our respective tenure of this post. These include most particularly the late Professor Henry Miller and Professor David Shaw, but also their neurological and neurosurgical colleagues at the Newcastle General Hospital, some of whom are distinguished former First Assistants (Professor Sir John Walton, Dr J. B. Foster, Dr P. Hudgson), and a large number of general physicians both in Newcastle and throughout the Northern region (as far afield as Whitehaven, Carlisle, Durham and Ashington) who have passed on some of their knowledge and expertise to us. We are also grateful to our current colleagues in the neurosciences in Liverpool and Newcastle who have helped in the preparation of this book, particularly to Dr L. Brock and Dr M. Hayward for their help with radiological and neurophysiological illustrations respectively. As First Assistants in neurology we acquired the majority of our neurological training within a general provincial teaching hospital and have also been responsible for teaching neurology to both undergraduates and candidates for the MRCP. We hope that these facts are reflected in the book.

While every attempt has been made to trace owners of copyright, this has not always been possible. We will, of course, be happy to include any such acknowledgement in subsequent editions.

Liverpool and Newcastle, 1989

D.C.
N.E.F.C.
D.B.

Contents

1

Disorders of motor function

INTRODUCTION

The role of the physician when faced with the description of symptoms of motor disturbance is to attempt to identify the site and pathophysiological reason for their occurrence. Such diagnosis may require the use of appropriate investigations before the relevant treatment can be instituted. In order to identify the site of the nervous system involved it is essential to have a knowledge of the basic anatomical pathways involved in the motor system and to recognise the sites at which this system tends to be compromised. There is at present considerable debate about the functional anatomy of the motor system, a debate which complicates rather than explains the clinical syndromes and symptoms which the physician encounters. Therefore, rather than entering into the present controversies regarding motor system organisation, the following practical anatomical description will provide a guide for the physician working in the clinical situation.

ANATOMY AND PHYSIOLOGY

VOLUNTARY MOVEMENTS

The performance of voluntary movements depends upon the integration of several different descending systems from the brain to the brain stem and the spinal cord, acting ultimately on the motor cells in the anterior horn and thereby stimulating the muscle fibres of the motor unit. Such voluntary movements are achieved predominantly by the activity of the voluntary upper motor neurone cell discharging the lower motor neurone in the anterior horn of the spinal cord or brain-stem nuclei. However, this essentially two-neurone system is modified and modulated by other components of the motor system, most notably the basal ganglia whose reflex activity through the cortex and via the extrapyramidal system is responsible for resting tone in the muscles, and the cerebellum whose reflex arcs provide for co-ordination with other neurones and muscle cells in the body. There are thus four important series of structures involved in the transmission of voluntary impulses from the cortex to the muscle.

The upper motor neurone

Cells in the precentral gyrus of the frontal lobe (area 4 of Brodman) (Fig. 1.1) give rise to fibres

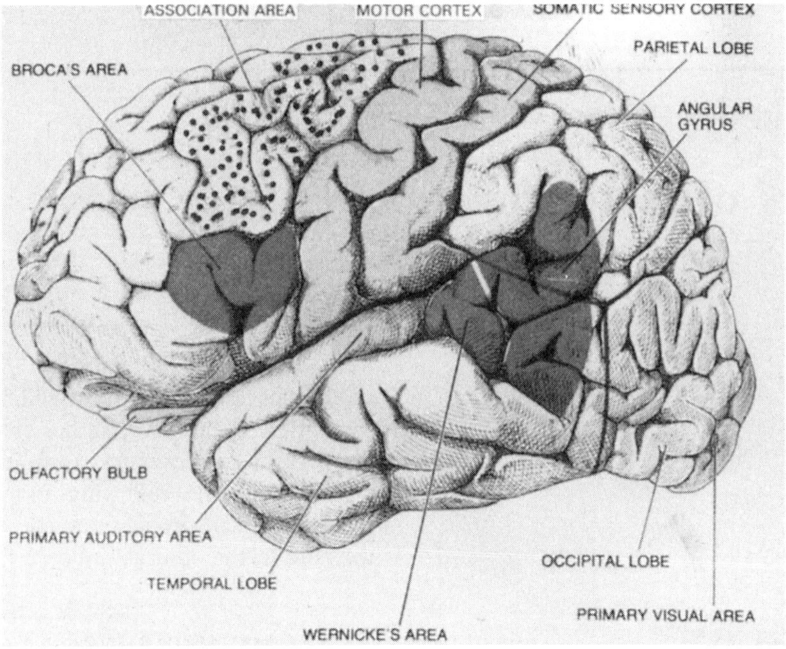

Fig. 1.1 The primary and association motor cortex.

which activate muscles on the opposite side of the body. Chief among these cells are the Betz cells in the fifth layer of the cortex which have synaptic connections with the anterior horn cells of the spinal cord and with cells in the immediately adjacent gyrus. This adjacent cortical area is referred to as the association cortex (Brodman area 6) and interconnections between groups of cells at this level are responsible for the integration of activity in the precentral gyrus and the linking of the primary motor cortex to other neurones in both hemispheres. The role of the association motor cortex is to organise agonist actions into a variety of graded and differential patterns and is probably related to the phenomenon of learned skills. Damage to these cells in the association cortex results in the phenomenon of apraxia.

The cells in the motor cortex are arranged from the foot, which lies in the parafalcine region, to the tongue in the lowest part of the convexity (Fig. 1.2) and the amount of cortex dedicated to each part of the body is proportional not to its size but to its importance in terms of movement. Thus, the areas such as the fingers, lips and tongue where great precision is required have a larger represen-

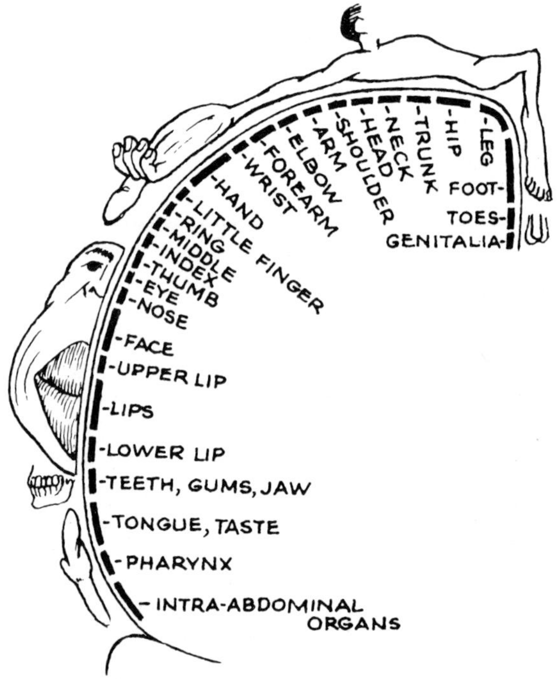

Fig. 1.2 The motor homunculus in the primary motor cortex. After Penfield W, Rassmussen T 1950 *The Cerebral Cortex of Man*. Macmillan, New York

tation than the thigh, trunk and shoulder. The cells in the cortex are concerned predominantly with movements rather than with the activity of individual muscles.

The main axons from the cortical neurones converge in the corona radiata and then pass through the posterior limb of the internal capsule and the cerebral peduncle into the base of the pons (Fig. 1.3). There are many more descending fibres in the pyramidal tracts than can be accounted for by the Betz cells in the primary motor cortex and many other cells in the motor cortex must therefore contribute towards these tracts. The fibres continue to the medulla at the lower end of which the corticospinal tracts decussate as the medullary pyramids. The proportion of fibres which cross in these tracts varies, but approximately 75% do travel to the contralateral lateral corticospinal tract; the others remain uncrossed in the ipsilateral lateral corticospinal tract or travel in the ventral corticospinal tract. The importance of the uncrossed fibres is probably significant in the degree of recovery that may be seen after hemispheric stroke and also accounts for the increased weakness which may be seen on a side contralateral to an original stroke when a second stroke occurs on the ipsilateral side. These fibres travel in the cord to the level of their destination and then synapse either with the anterior horn cell or with internuncial neurones in the spinal grey matter.

During the course of these tracts through the brain stem the fibres destined for the nuclei of the cranial nerves leave as discrete fibre bundles to form the corticopontine or corticobulbar tracts supplying the contralateral and sometimes ipsilateral cranial nerve nuclei. Thus, in the pons that portion of the facial nerve nucleus supplying frontalis is bilaterally innervated (Fig. 1.4) and in the medulla the motor nuclei of glossopharyngeal, vagus and hypoglossal nerves are bilaterally innervated. There is lamination of fibres in the descending pathways such that the fibres destined for the muscles of the lower limbs are stretched most widely around the posterior horn of the lateral ventricles and those destined for the upper limbs lie most medially in the brain stem. This explains why hydrocephalus may result in the development of a paraparesis due to stretching of these particular descending fibres and why crural paresis, or weakness of the arms, is most common with lesions in the brain stem. There are three descending fibre pathways identifiable by their terminal distribution which are important in the control of voluntary movement. The ventromedial pathway arises from brain stem nuclei and terminates on the internuncial cells of the ventromedial part of the spinal grey matter; it is concerned with axial movements and gross limb movements. The lateral pathway, originating in the red nucleus and terminating in the dorsal and lateral parts of the internuncial region, allows for independent use of the extremities. The corticospinal pathway arises from the cortex and terminates in the nucleus proprius of the dorsal horn and allows fine control of hand movements.

There remains some uncertainty about the neurotransmitters involved in the upper motor neurone systems in man. Acetylcholine, gamma-amino butyric acid, 5-hydroxytryptamine and the encephalins may all be involved. The role of these transmitters in facilitating or inhibiting neuromuscular conduction appears to vary at different sites.

Lower motor neurone

Lower motor neurones, whether in the cranial nerve nuclei of the brain stem or the anterior horn of the spinal cord, are the final common pathway for nervous impulses to the muscles. In the spinal cord their organisation is illustrated in Figure 1.5. They are acted upon by several afferent neurones and it is the summation of the effects of all these negative and positive stimuli which determines the ultimate activity of the anterior horn cell. There are two types of motor cell in the anterior horn: the α motor neurone which innervates a group of 50–200 muscle fibres forming the motor unit, and the γ motor neurone which innervates the intrafusal muscle fibres of the spindle organ within the muscle and is responsible for setting the level of tone in that muscle (Fig. 1.6).

In the spinal cord the anterior horn cells are arranged segmentally and their axons leave in the ventral root to join the dorsal root as they pass through the intervertebral foramina. These mixed roots then join to form plexuses which give rise

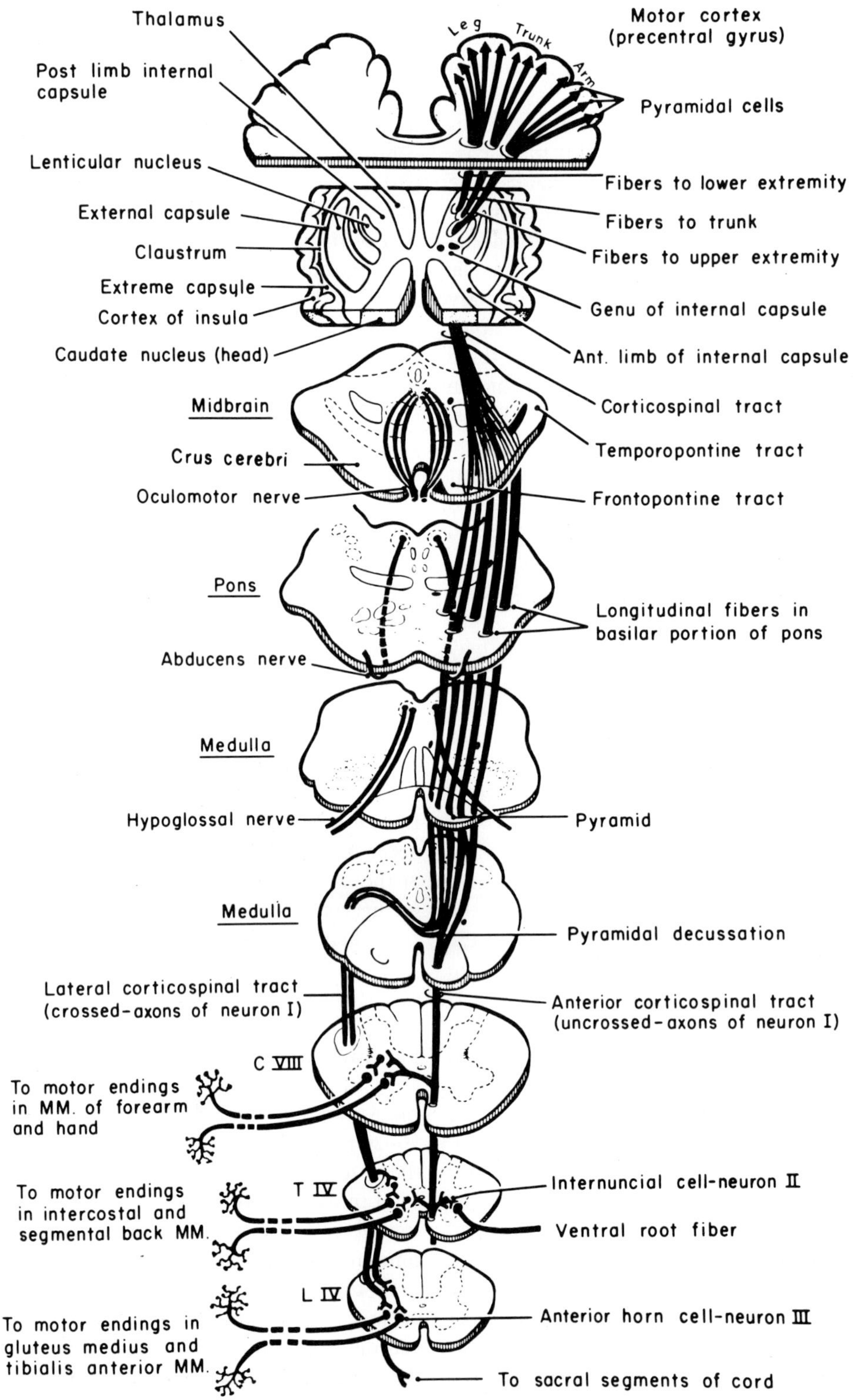

Fig. 1.3 The motor pathway from the cortex via the posterior limb of the internal capsule, the crus cerebri and the medullary pyramid to the lateral and anterior corticospinal tracts and thence to the anterior horn cells. (Reproduced from Carpenter M B, Sutin J 1983 *Human Neuroanatomy*, 8th edn. Williams and Wilkins, Baltimore, with permission.)

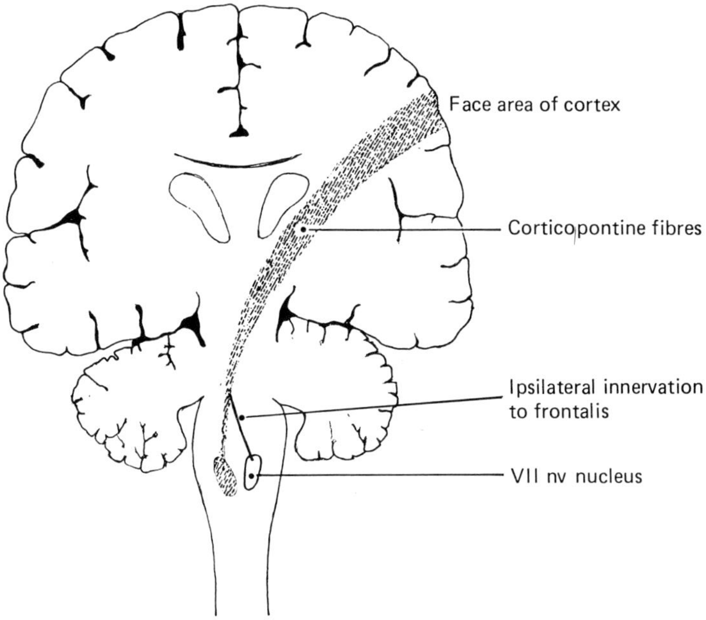

Fig. 1.4 The bilateral innervation of the facial nerve nucleus.

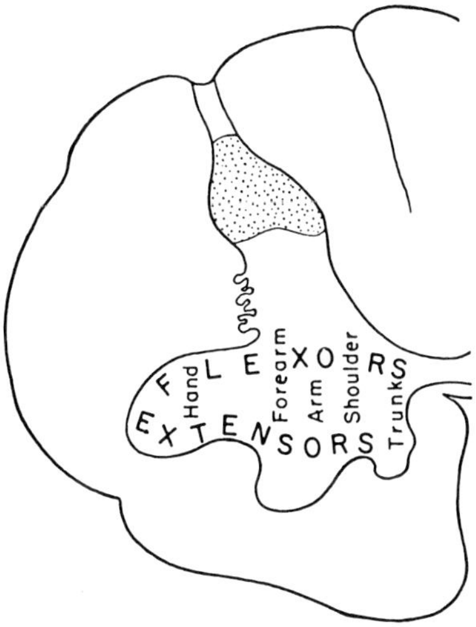

Fig. 1.5 The organisation of cells in the anterior horn at the cervical region.

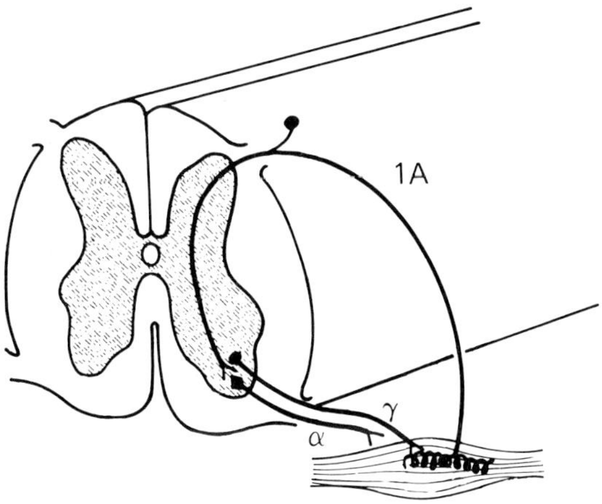

Fig. 1.6 The α and γ motor neurones and their relationships with the 1A afferent fibres in the monosynaptic stretch reflex.

to the peripheral nerves ultimately supplying the muscles. The integration of the plexus means that each individual muscle receives a supply from more than one nerve root. The innervation of the muscle by the lower motor neurone appears to be necessary for its function. The stimuli transmitted by acetylcholine to the muscle receptors in part sustains the size and function of the muscle and also alters the character of the individual muscle fibre and its chemical composition.

The major neurotransmitter of the lower motor neurone at the neuromuscular junction is acetylcholine. Its activity is influenced by inhibitory (gamma-amino butyric acid and glycine) and excitatory (glutamate and aspartate) neurotransmitters (Fig. 1.7).

The role of the α and γ motor neurones is best understood by reference to the stretch reflex. The γ motor neurone sets the length of the muscle spindle, the tendon hammer then stretches the muscle and with it the spindle and this causes stimuli in the 1A afferents which generate activity in the α motor neurone bringing about contraction of the muscle. Voluntary movements are almost certainly performed by direct activation of the α motor neurone and the cerebellum, basal ganglia, extrapyramidal tracts and spinal interneurones are responsible for the relaxation of antagonist muscles and fixation of the agonists to allow the movement to be performed.

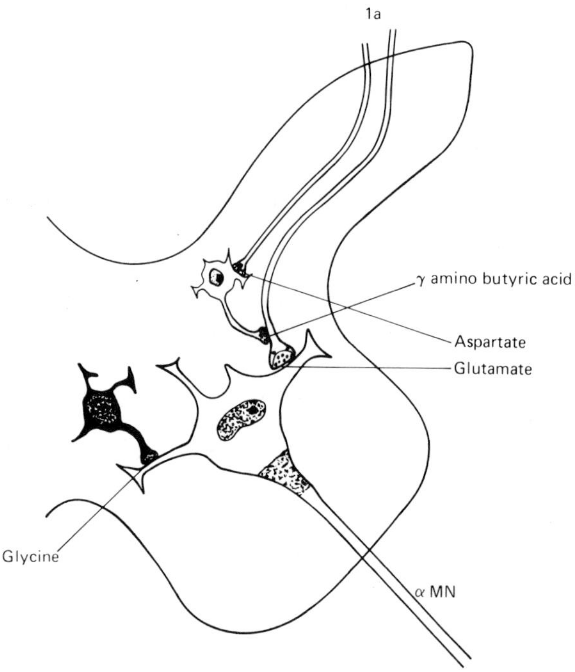

Fig. 1.7 Neurotransmitters of the monosynaptic reflex arc.

The basal ganglia

Deep in the structure of the cerebral hemispheres are grey matter structures including the caudate nucleus, the putamen and globus pallidus, the claustrum and subthalamic nucleus. These, together with the substantia nigra in the rostral end of the brain stem, make up the structures termed the basal ganglia (Fig. 1.8). The main afferent fibres to the basal ganglia appear to be from the cerebral cortex to the putamen and from the substantia nigra to the putamen. After interconnections within the basal ganglia, the main efferent pathway is to the ventrolateral nucleus of

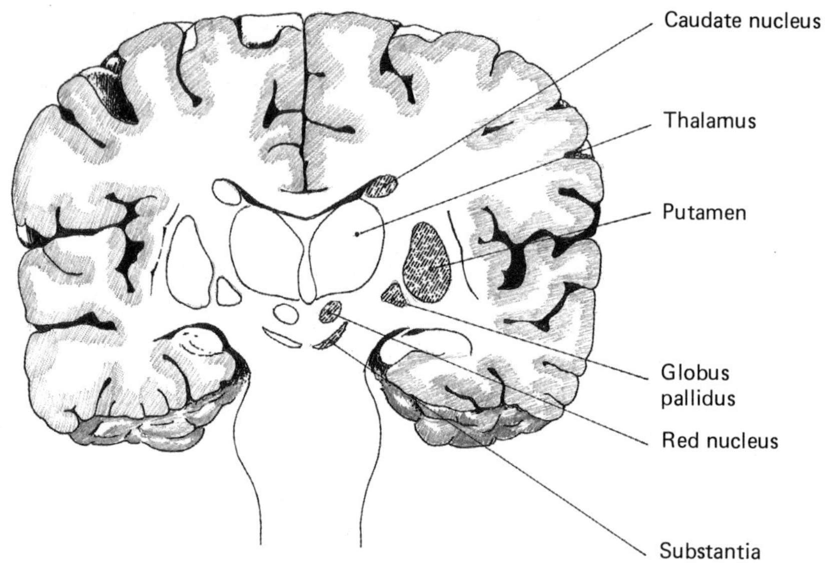

Fig. 1.8 The nuclei of the basal ganglia.

the thalamus and thence to the cortex. There are some nigrostriatal connections to the reticular nuclei in the brain stem and to the red nucleus but these are not believed to be particularly significant. The brain stem nuclei appear to exert their effect as a reciprocal governor on the activities of the cortical neurones. They are frequently termed part of the extrapyramidal system, though they do not appear to have a significant efferent tract to the spinal cord and lower centres.

The neurotransmitters involved in the organisation of the basal ganglia are among the most well-identified of the central nervous system. Figure 1.9 depicts a putative mode of action of many of the neurotransmitters, showing the important dopaminergic pathway from the substantia-nigra to the striatum and the involvement of other transmitters, including glutamate, acetylcholine, gamma-amino butyric acid and substance P, within the striatum (Ch. 8).

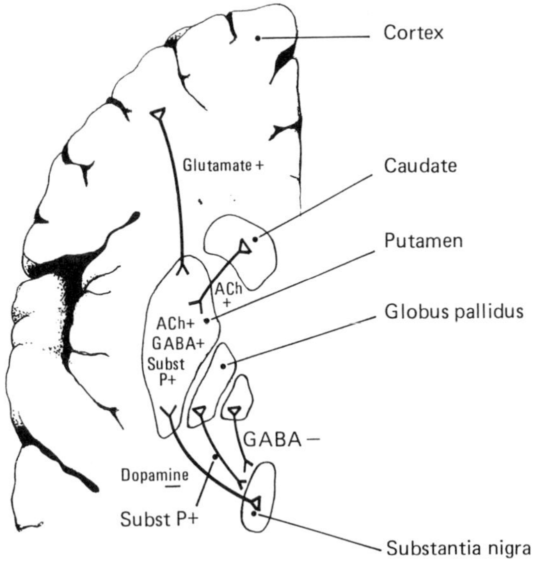

Fig. 1.9 Neurotransmitter relationships in the basal ganglia. Excitatory neurotransmitters (+), inhibitory neurotransmitters (–).

Cerebellum

The cerebellum is concerned with co-ordination of movement and the maintenance of posture. It is divisible phylogenetically into the oldest part, the flocculonodular lobe, which receives its afferents from vestibular nuclei responsible for central equilibrium; the anterior lobe, which is common to the lower animals but relatively small in man and receives the spinal input predominantly concerned with postural reflexes; and the posterior lobe, or neocerebellum, which receives afferent fibres from the cerebral cortex via the pontine nuclei and superior cerebellar peduncle and is predominantly concerned with co-ordination of voluntary movement. It is also possible to identify three sagittal zones in the cerebellum: the mid-line or vermis zone which is concerned with posture and tone in the axial part of the body; the paravermis, concerned with movements of ipsilateral limbs; and the lateral zone which is involved in fine co-ordination of the ipsilateral limbs (Fig. 1.10).

The efferent fibres from the Purkinje cells in the cerebellum project to the deep cerebellar nuclei: the fastigial, which in turn projects to the vestibular nuclei, and the globose, emboliform and

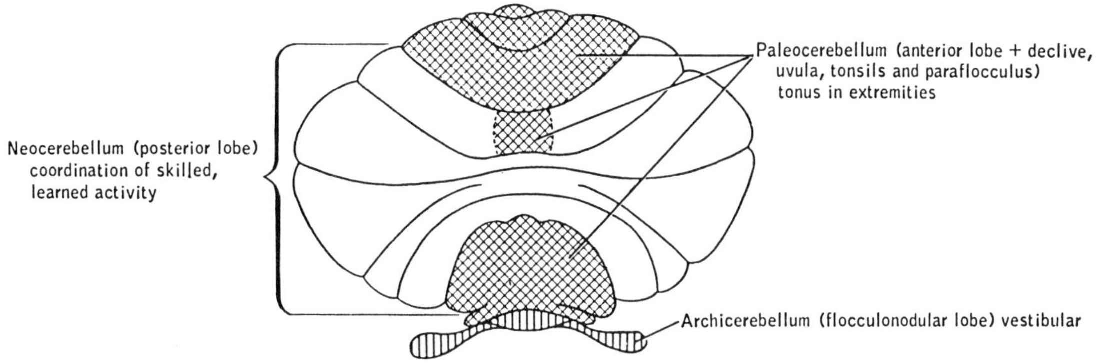

Fig. 1.10 The cerebellum: functional relationships of the cerebellar lobes.

dentate which project via the superior cerebellar peduncle to the contralateral cerebral cortex with some fibres synapsing in the red nucleus. Most of these fibres travel via the ventrolateral nucleus of the thalamus where they also have synapses. There are also fibres which relay in the reticular formation and re-enter the cerebellum forming a cerebello–reticulo–cerebellar feedback loop. Although there are no direct connections from the cerebellum to the spinal cord, movements are effected both via the cerebral cortex and the reticular nuclei. In practice the important aspects of the cerebellar anatomy are that midline lesions tend to affect axial function and lateral or hemispheric lesions affect control of the ipsilateral limbs.

Acetylcholine is recognised to be an important neurotransmitter within the cerebellar system, but little is known of the other neurotransmitters involved.

The extrapyramidal system

The definition of the extrapyramidal system varies considerably. Some authors use the term as synonymous with the basal ganglia and others include all the upper motor neurones of the motor system except those whose axons pass through the pyramids. As has been described above, both the basal ganglia and the cerebellum appear to act primarily as long-loop reflex arcs for cortex-to-cortex reflexes via the thalamus. Both structures do, however, have connections with brain stem nuclei and these nuclei, which are also supplied by corticospinal tract collaterals, do give rise to descending tracts, namely the rubrospinal, vestibulospinal and reticulospinal tracts which make up the extrapyramidal descending tracts in the lateral part of the medulla and spinal cord and they affect posture and tone in the limbs via the anterior horn cell. These pathways are also involved in long-loop reflexes from the lower limbs.

Integration

The integration of the motor system is extremely complex but may be simplified if one recognises that the production of a voluntary movement necessarily occurs against a background of normal posture and tone and must involve not only the prime muscles involved in movement but also the simultaneous reduction in resting tone in the antagonist muscles and alteration in tone in agonist groups. Thus the signal to make a voluntary movement is conducted from the cortex to the anterior horn cell, but is modified in part by the basal ganglia and in part by the cerebellum via thalamic pathways back to the cortex and via descending tracts to the level of the anterior horn cells. The summation of all of these impulses at the spinal level results in the sequence of anterior horn cell firing or inhibition which brings about the desired movement.

REFLEX MOVEMENTS

There are a variety of reflex movements which are organised through the cerebral cortex, the brain stem or at a segmental level and which are most important early in life or to indicate the results of damage at some level in the nervous system. Cortical reflexes, such as the pout reflex, the palmomental reflex and the grasp reflex, are present in small children, disappear by the end of the first year, but may recur when there is bilateral forebrain damage or lesions affecting one or other frontal lobe. The pout reflex is elicited by gently striking the closed lips, the palmomental reflex by presenting a noxious stimulus to the palm and observing movement in the ipsilateral inferior lip and the grasp reflex by drawing an object across the open palm of the individual.

Multisynaptic reflexes at the level of the brain stem are essentially nocioceptive in origin and those most commonly used are the abdominal reflex and the plantar response. The abdominal response is elicited by drawing a noxious stimulus over the anterior abdominal wall and observing movement of the anterior spinal muscles. Lesions within the dorsal or cervical spinal cord cause the reflex to be lost. The plantar response is elicited by a noxious stimulus to the sole which, in the presence of an upper motor neurone lesion, causes extension of the great toe instead of the normal flexion.

There are other reflex pathways which govern movement, such as the reticulospinal reflexes which may be revealed in cortical damage and result in turning towards sound or flexing a limb on yawning.

Monosynaptic reflexes which can be elicited physiologically in the normal person appear pathologically brisk in the presence of damage to the upper motor neurones with consequent increased activity of the anterior horn cells involved.

Damage to the motor pathways above the brain stem may result in flexion in response to pain and lesions at the level of the brain stem may result in extension in response to the same stimulus. These reactions are sometimes called, respectively, decorticate and decerebrate posturing.

DAMAGE TO THE MOTOR SYSTEM

Motor symptoms including weakness, paralysis, stiffness, unsteadiness, or involuntary movements may occur with damage to any part of the motor system. There are four major identifiable groups of symptoms which tend to affect aspects of motor control, tone and posture, as detailed below.

LOWER MOTOR NEURONE WEAKNESS

Damage to the lower motor neurones results in flaccid weakness with loss of reflexes and ultimately muscle wasting (Table 1.1). Whether the damage is to the anterior horn cell, the nerve root, plexus, nerve, neuromuscular junction or muscle, the basic findings of weak and hypotonic limbs, absent deep tendon reflexes together with wasting of muscles is common to all. There may be visible fasciculation in the muscles due to the spontaneous firing of motor units and this is particularly common with lesions in the anterior horn cell or proximal axonal lesions. Electromyographically the presence of fibrillation potentials may be seen due to the spontaneous firing of single motor fibres (p. 110). Deep tendon reflexes are lost because the monosynaptic reflex arc depends upon the integrity of the 1A afferents and the α efferents and a lesion of the lower motor neurone blocks the efferent limb of this reflex. Usually the loss of function with a lower motor neurone lesion is complete and commonly irrecoverable. There may be the development of synkinesis due to aberrant regeneration of peripheral nerves but this form of synkinesis is local, resulting in movements of muscles within the weakened areas.

Table 1.1 Differences between UMN and LMN lesions

	UMN	LMN
Pattern of weakness	Extensors of upper limb, flexors of lower limb	Individual muscles affected May affect multiple muscles (see Tables 1.2, 1.3)
Atrophy/wasting	Little—where present due to disuse.	Marked loss of bulk
Tone	Spastic	Flaccid
Reflexes	Hyperactive and extensor plantar response	Loss of reflexes
Fasciculation	Absent	Present (in anterior horn cell and proximal lesions)
EMG	No denervation, normal nerve conduction	Denervation potentials Abnormal nerve conduction

UPPER MOTOR NEURONE WEAKNESS

Damage to the upper motor neurone between the cortex and the anterior horn cell, most commonly involving a mixture of so-called pyramidal and extrapyramidal fibres, results in the syndrome of spasticity. Power is lost due to lack of voluntary control, but as a result of the loss of cortical inhibition some of the α motor neurones become hyperactive and the resting tone is increased. In addition, the tendon reflexes become more brisk due to the increased excitability of the α motor neurone. Tone is increased predominantly at the beginning of passive movement and then tends to give way, the so-called clasp knife or spastic form of hypertonia (Table 1.2).

An important feature of upper motor neurone lesions is the preferential involvement of certain muscles in the limb. In the upper limb the weakness is most marked in the extensor muscles and the limb therefore adopts a postion of flexion and may even develop contractures in flexion. In the lower limb the flexors are most weak and the limb tends therefore to be held in extension. In the milder forms of upper motor neurone lesions weakness may only be minimal and detectable on examination in the extensor muscles of the upper limb, most markedly in triceps, or the flexors of the lower limb, most markedly in the hip flexors. This pattern of extensor weakness in the upper limb and flexor weakness in the lower limb is strongly suggestive of an upper motor neurone lesion.

A further feature of upper motor neurone damage is that, although the monosynaptic reflexes are increased and the limb is hypertonic, a fact which may be reflected by the presence of clonus at the ankle, the nociceptive multisynaptic reflexes such as the plantar and abdominal reflexes undergo more complex changes. The plantar response in an upper motor neurone lesion becomes extensor, the so-called Babinski response, and the abdominal reflexes are lost. In acute lesions of the upper motor neurone there may be a period of flaccidity before the increased tone and spasticity develops. This is most commonly seen with transverse lesions in the spinal cord where it is part of the syndrome termed spinal shock (p. 216).

It is uncommon for all the muscles on one side of the body to be affected by an upper motor neurone lesion since the muscles of the bulb, thorax and abdomen are bilaterally innervated and therefore little affected.

Synkinesis may also occur with upper motor neurone lesions, but is usually complex, as with flexion of a paretic limb on yawning or stretching. In addition, an attempt to move the limbs affected may result in unusual posturing of the limb due to stimulation of numerous efferents, probably at a brainstem level.

Damage to the cortex in the region of the association motor cortex or in the parietal lobes may result in the loss of learned skills and the phenomenon of apraxia. This implies that there is no evident motor weakness, but a command or task which is well understood by the patient cannot be adequately performed either to command or by copying. The terms ideational, ideokinetic and kinetic apraxia, which are sometimes used, are of little use in the differentiation of the different forms of apraxia, all of which should be regarded as indicating either a premotor or a parietal lobe cortical disturbance.

BASAL GANGLIA DISTURBANCE

These grey matter substances are most concerned with resting tone and posture of the trunk and limbs. Disturbances in this system result in reduced movement, akinesia or bradykinesia, disorders of posture, alterations in muscle tone and involuntary movements.

Akinesia occurs without significant loss in strength and results simply in underactivity or poverty of movement. Thus the face is expressionless, voluntary and associated movements are reduced and gestures are infrequent. The patient does not blink and may show reduced swallowing and slow monotonous speech. This akinesia or bradykinesia is not simply the result of rigidity since it may be seen in the absence of the latter change in tone.

Disorders of posture are most commonly seen in Parkinson's disease as a dorsal kyphosis with flexion of the head on the trunk and reduced ability to make correcting reflexes if tilted or when falling. In some conditions, such as progressive supranuclear palsy, the postural abnormality may be extension of the spine or neck on the trunk, but the same problem with postural reflexes exists.

The typical alteration in *muscle tone* is of rigidity. This form of hypertonicity differs from spasticity in being present throughout the movement and it is likened to lead-pipe rigidity. Occasionally there are intermittent cog wheel-like resistances to moving the affected limb and this form of rigidity probably represents the tremor associated with the hypertonicity.

Involuntary movements may also be seen in basal ganglia disease, the *resting tremor* of Parkinson's disease being virtually pathognomonic of that illness, but more complex involuntary movements also occur. *Chorea* is the term used to describe involuntary movements of rapid jerky type which may be complex or turned into an almost volitional act by the patient to make them less obvious. They may involve the face, neck and trunk as well as the limbs. *Athetosis* is a slower, more writhing and dystonic movement of the arm; the two forms of involuntary movement may occur together and merge into each other. *Dystonia* or *torsion spasms* are gross movements of the limbs and trunk and also indicate disease in the basal ganglia.

CEREBELLUM

Damage to the cerebellum or its communications results in the symptom of ataxia and disturbance of balance and co-ordination. Characteristically, limbs are slightly *hypotonic* and reflexes may be *pendular*, but the most prominent abnormalities relate to *co-ordination*. Thus in cranial nerve territory there may be the presence of *nystagmus*, though this is rare in pure cerebellar disease, and there may frequently be a *dysmetria* of eye movements (the eyes tending to over-shoot the target on testing following movements). The speech will be slurred with a characteristic difficulty in repeating syllables regularly (an *ataxic dysarthria*) and rapid alternating movements of the tongue will be poorly performed. In the upper limbs there will be *rebound* or *over-shoot*, the outstretched arms not returning quickly to their resting position when displaced and rapid alternating movements will be hesitant and incoordinate. The *finger–nose test* will be poorly performed revealing a prominent *intention tremor*, the cardinal feature of cerebellar limb disturbance. In the lower limbs the *heel–knee–shin test* will be poorly performed and the ability to perform rapid alternating movements with the feet will be lost, the *gait becoming ataxic* and unsteady. The gait problem may often be best demonstrated by asking the patient to walk heel-to-toe or to turn rapidly.

These features may occur with damage to the cerebellum or its connections and, in general, the phenomena relating to the cranial nerves, speech and gait will reflect a midline disturbance whereas those most evident in the limbs will suggest a hemispheric problem. On occasions the tremulousness will be seen in the body at rest and the head may show a classic *titubation*. Rarely, with severely damaging lesions, there will be a wing-beating or *dentatorubral tremor* of the arm so as to prevent any useful movement.

CLINICAL ASSESSMENT

HISTORY

Disturbances of motor function are among the most common symptoms which cause patients to seek help from their doctors. The symptoms of disturbed motor function are varied and range from obvious weakness or paralysis of the limb through lesser grades of weakness to rarer complaints of involuntary movement, tremor and fatigue. On occasion patients may notice the presence of wasting of muscles or fasciculation. More complex complaints may include unsteadiness, clumsiness, stiffness, slowness and hesitancy. Where the muscles of the face, tongue and throat are involved, the symptoms of dysarthria, dysphonia and dysphagia are prominent. Pain can occasionally be due to motor disturbance, since spastic muscles are liable to cramps, weak muscles are likely to allow the development of arthropathy and the increased tone of Parkinson's disease can present with uncomfortable or frankly painful limbs. Muscle spasm may be associated with cramp particularly at night.

Symptoms almost always precede signs in disorders of the motor system. Perhaps the only exception to this is where disorders are very long-standing and only very slowly progressive. Thus patients with hereditary sensorimotor neuropathy may walk with a pronounced foot-drop and have marked wasting of leg muscles with very few complaints. Alternatively, patients with a markedly asymmetric paraparesis or parkinsonian syndrome may deny symptoms on the less affected side, which may nevertheless show unequivocal signs.

EXAMINATION

The examination of the motor system is arguably the most objective part of the neurological examination and consequently a part which weighs heavily in the physician's assessment of the patient and evaluation of the nature of the symptoms. Whilst it is true that some neurological conditions result in no motor disturbance, the great majority do cause disturbances of movement, which, though easy to simulate, are usually associated with unequivocal neurological signs.

Gait

After examining the skull and spine to exclude local abnormalities or deformities of the skull and to confirm a normal cervical and lumbar lordosis with a mild dorsal kyphosis and full spinal movements, the physician should then examine the patient's gait. Neurologically it is important to be able to identify the *spastic gait*, in which the lower limb is held in extension, the walking is rather jerky and if only one leg is involved then that tends to be swung to the side in a form of circumduction to enable movement to continue. It is frequently associated with hemiplegia, in which the ipsilateral arm is also held flexed. If spasticity is bilateral in the legs then the gait tends to be rather scissored with prominent spasm of the adductors and bilateral spastic foot drop, the toes being pressed firmly to the ground.

A second common gait is the *ataxic gait*, which may be most apparent when the patient walks with wide-based gait, or may be less evident and only demonstrable by asking the patient to walk heel-to-toe or to turn rapidly to one side or the other. Patients may be asked to walk round a tendon hammer placed on the floor when they will tend to veer towards the side of the cerebellar lesion. The *festinant gait* of Parkinson's disease involves not only the slow, shuffling, small-stepped gait characteristic of the illness but also the exaggerated dorsal kyphosis frequently with flexion of the head and usually with lack of associated movements of the arms. The problem of the patient with Parkinson's disease lies in both the initiation of movement and in the stopping of that particular movement; this is revealed in the phenomenon of retropulsion when the patient staggers backwards after a gentle push.

In the elderly patient an abnormal gait, which may relate to frontal lobe disturbance, is commonly associated with a slightly flexed posture, slowness and stiffness of walking and a shortened step. This is sometimes called *marche à petit pas* and it is probably related to a disturbance of frontal lobe function. Another disturbance of gait which may be seen with disease of the frontal lobe or with the development of normal-pressure hydrocephalus is the so-called *apraxic gait*. In this there is no difficulty in manipulating the limbs when sitting or when lying on a couch, but when attempting to walk the patient has difficulty in placing the feet in the right position. He may frequently respond well to triggering of the gait with pieces of paper placed on the floor where he is expected to walk and this may result in almost normal walking. The disability is a high-level motor disturbance and is usually associated with forebrain disease.

Patients showing peripheral weakness of the lower limbs will tend to walk with a *foot drop*. If present on one side, this may be due to a common peroneal nerve palsy and if present bilaterally, to a peripheral neuropathy. It gives rise to the high-steppage gait with the hip and knee flexed excessively to keep the toe from the ground. Patients with proprioceptive loss will be unsteady, their unsteadiness will be worse when in the dark and they will show a positive Romberg's test (p. 34). The gait in this condition is frequently *stamping* with the patient's foot occasionally missing the floor and on other occasions being slammed down hard against the floor.

Patients with muscle disease tend to have weakness of the proximal muscles, as a result of which they develop a considerable lordosis and bend their pelvis forwards as they attempt to walk causing the appearance of a *waddle*.

These six neurological gaits are the most typical and most commonly seen. Antalgic gait or limping may be seen with neurological conditions but is more commonly seen with painful arthropathies or muscular problems.

Cranial nerves (Ch. 3)

Somatic muscle function in the cranial nerves is tested with reference to the trigeminal nerve, the facial nerve, the glossopharyngeal and vagus nerve, the spinal accessory and the hypoglossal nerve. The trigeminal nerve motor function is tested by observing the activity of masseter in closing the jaw and assessing the strength of pterygoids in opening the jaw and moving it from side to side. In testing facial muscle function it is important to attempt to make a distinction between weakness which is reflected in voluntary movement and that which appears most evident in involuntary movement. Voluntary movement impairment usually reflects damage to the upper or lower motor neurone whereas involvement of involuntary movement is more commonly seen with basal ganglia disturbance. It is important to remember that the frontalis muscle is bilaterally innervated at the level of the pons and that therefore this part of the facial nerve is spared in unilateral upper motor neurone lesions but involved in lesions of the lower motor neurone. The facial muscle is tested by the simple expedient of assessing the strength of eye closure, eyebrow elevation, circumoral muscles and the appearance of the patient's smile.

The bulbar muscles are examined by observation of the soft palate to assess that it moves in the mid-line and freely, assessment of the strength of the tongue in its pressure against the cheek bilaterally and its protrusion from the mouth, together with co-ordination in terms of the speed that it can be waggled from side to side. An assessment of dysarthria should be made to differentiate the *flaccid dysarthria* of the lower motor neurone problems from the *spastic and high-pitched dysarthria* (p. 79) and *dysphonia* of the upper motor neurone lesions, the flat and monotonous speech of the *basal ganglia* disturbance and the *ataxic dysarthria* seen with cerebellar lesions.

The strength in sternocleidomastoid and trapezius may be tested to assess the motor function of the spinal accessory nerves.

Limbs

In testing motor function in the limbs it is first necessary to observe the size of the muscles, to note whether *fasciculation* is present and to identify any *trophic change* such as contractures or alteration in the skin. A useful test is then to ask the patient to hold the upper limbs extended with the eyes closed and to observe the phenomena of drift suggesting a pyramidal weakness, rebound identifying a cerebellar problem, pseudoathetosis indicating the possibility of proprioceptive loss or tremor. During the period of observation any involuntary movements or resting tremor may of course also be identified.

One then asks the patient to relax and assesses *tone* at each of the joints in the upper limb, trying to identify *hypotonia* suggestive of a lower motor neurone lesion or *hypertonia* suggesting an upper motor neurone lesion or an extrapyramidal disturbance. In testing tone one looks for induced or spontaneous *clonus* at the wrist or fingers. *Power* is tested next in each of the muscle groups and the individual muscles. In general it is adequate to test abduction and adduction of the shoulder, flexion and extension of the elbow and wrist, flexion and extension of the fingers and then abduction and adduction of the fingers. If there is any suggestion of a particular pattern of weakness then individual muscles need to be tested always comparing one side with the other. In the lower limbs, after observation, it is important to test tone and in particular to look for the presence of clonus at knee or ankle. Power is then tested with hip flexion and extension, knee flexion and extension, dorsiflexion and plantar flexion of the ankle and with inversion and eversion of the foot. Once again, if there is suspicion of individual muscle disturbances it is important to test each muscle and to compare from one side to the other.

Cerebellar function is tested in the upper limbs by asking the patient to perform rapid alternating movements and by the 'finger-to-nose' test in which the patient is asked to place their index finger on their nose and then to stretch to touch the finger of the examiner held some 2–3 feet away. This test should be performed relatively slowly and observation made as to whether or not a tremor is present and, if present, whether it is throughout the whole of the action or simply on intention. Intention tremor is strongly suggestive of a cerebellar lesion. Patients with lesions affecting the dentatorubral pathway will have wild wing-beating tremors on any movement, rendering much of the assessment impossible. It should always be remembered that the presence of significant muscle weakness or hypertonia will interfere with the assessment of co-ordination and ultimately may make this assessment impossible.

For patients in whom there are evident motor difficulties despite the finding of normal strength and tone, tests for *apraxia* should be undertaken by asking the patient to perform precise voluntary tasks or to copy movements made by the examiner. The distinction between a voluntary movement such as putting out the tongue and an automatic one as in licking the lips is important and should be carefully documented.

Reflexes

The most objective aspect of the nervous system examination is testing of the reflexes. There are two major types of reflex, the first *monosynaptic* or stretch reflexes and the second nociceptive which reflexes are *multisynaptic*. It was originally thought that the increased stretch reflexes seen in the spastic state were the result of interruption of descending inhibitory pathways to the monosynaptic reflex arc. But it seems that there is an active increase in facilitation of the monosynaptic reflex partly through increased activity in spindle afferents and partly through increased excitability of the α motor neurones.

The monosynaptic reflexes which may commonly be elicited include the *jaw jerk*, which is normally present but not usually very brisk. If it is exaggerated or clonic it suggests that there is a lesion above the level of the trigeminal motor nucleus which will usually be bilateral. In the upper limb the reflexes which are routinely tested are the *biceps* and *brachioradialis reflexes* both innervated by the C5/6 routes, the *triceps* innervated by C7 and the *finger jerk* reflexes innervated by C8. They should always be tested alternately from right to left and each pair of reflexes compared for briskness and ease of elicitation. Increased reflexes indicate the presence of upper motor neurone damage above that level in the cervical spinal cord and reduced or absent reflexes imply damage to the lower motor or sensory neurones. A particularly important sign in reflex testing in the upper limbs is the phenomenon of inversion or radiation of a reflex from one segment to another. The term inversion refers to the phenomenon of eliciting finger flexion by striking the biceps tendon and is usually indicative of a lesion at the C5/6 level and a hyperactive motor neurone pool at C8. It is particularly common in a mixed cervical myeloradiculopathy such as that seen in cervical spondylosis.

In the lower limbs the reflexes which are most commonly tested include the *knee* and *ankle reflexes*, the former indicative of the lumbar 3/4 roots and the latter of the first sacral root. The *medial hamstring* reflex may also be tested illustrating the presence of a lesion at the L4/5 root.

The *plantar response* is a nociceptive reflex which is elicited by stroking the outer aspect of the sole of the foot and a normal reflex involves flexion of the toes and adduction. If the toes abduct and the great toe extends, the reflex is said to be extensor or a Babinski sign and indicates an upper motor neurone lesion above the conus medullaris.

Abdominal reflexes are routinely tested above and below the umbilicus bilaterally and again are nociceptive and multisynaptic reflexes, the absence of which implies a lesion somewhere high in the cervical or dorsal spine.

In addition, there are a variety of release reflexes which indicate bilateral frontal lobe disturbance. These are particularly important in the identification of degenerative or atrophic disorders and lesions in the frontal lobes which might otherwise have been overlooked. The *pout reflex* is elicited by tapping the closed lips, the *palmomental* reflex by stroking the heel of the palm with a noxious stimulus and observing movement of the inferior mental region and a grasp reflex is elicited by stroking the palm and observing grasping of the fingers. These lesions imply frontal lobe disturbance and may indicate lateralisation.

INVESTIGATIONS (Ch. 5)

The neurological examination of the motor system can be complemented by a series of investigations. The most specific of these are related to electromyography, motor nerve conduction and central motor conduction times.

PATTERNS OF WEAKNESS

The terms paresis and plegia are frequently used to describe degrees of motor loss or paralysis. Though they are commonly used interchangeably, it seems reasonable to use the word paresis to imply a mild or partial loss of motor function or paralysis and to reserve the term plegia for severe or complete loss of motor function.

HEMIPARESIS

Hemiparesis is defined as loss of motor function in an arm and a leg. The involvement of one arm and the ipsilateral leg is usually indicative of an upper motor neurone lesion. Rarely, a high cervical lesion may result in a similar hemiplegia, the distinction frequently being made on whether or not the face is involved. If the face on one side is weakened together with a hemiparesis on the opposite side then the lesion is likely to lie within the brain stem at the level of the pons.

The picture of hemiplegia with involvement of the lower part of the face, the arm held in the position of flexion, the leg in extension with spasticity, typical upper motor neurone patterns of weakness and brisk reflexes, is usually indicative of a contralateral hemispheric lesion.

MONOPARESIS

Monoparesis is defined as the loss of motor power involving a single limb. An upper motor neurone lesion affecting one limb may occur due to pathology in a cerebral hemisphere but is more commonly seen with a lesion in the spinal cord. Classically the upper motor neurone lesion will result in spasticity with wasting with marked weakness and with brisk reflexes. The pattern of weakness will be most apparent in the extensors of the upper limb or the flexors of the lower limb, clonus may be elicited and contractures can develop.

Very rarely a flaccid monoplegia will occur with a multiple radiculopathy or plexopathy usually following trauma but occasionally with long lesions inside the spine. Motor neurone disease not uncommonly causes a mixture of both upper and lower motor neurone lesions within the same limb and may begin as a monoparesis.

PARAPARESIS

Paraparesis is defined as loss of motor power in both lower limbs. Lesions within the spinal canal in the dorsal region are liable to cause bilateral upper motor neurone problems affecting the lower limbs. Acute transection or an acute myelitis may result in an acute flaccid paralysis of the lower limbs and the pattern of spasticity may develop only days or weeks later. The reason for the development of spasticity is uncertain but some patients, particularly those with more extensive lesions in the spinal cord, will have lower limbs that remain flaccid.

In the majority after the period of spinal shock there will be the development of bilateral spasticity of the lower limbs in the condition of paraparesis or paraplegia. The muscles, particularly the extensors, are weak but there is no loss of bulk, the reflexes are brisk and the plantars extensor. Frequently knee and ankle clonus will be elicited and this particular pattern is strongly suggestive of a spinal lesion above the level of the first lumbar vertebra. Lesions below this particular region are too low to cause upper motor neurone problems because they occur at the level of the conus (p. 216).

Rarely the picture of a paraparesis with bilateral upper motor neurone involvement can result from a lesion in the parasagittal region within the cranium due to meningiomas of the falx and this possibility should always be considered in patients presenting with paraparesis.

TRIPARESIS

Involvement of three limbs in a process causing weakness may be termed triparesis. The pattern of involvement of two legs and an arm or two arms and a leg is strongly suggestive of a lesion at the high cervical cord level or multiple lesions. The weakness is of upper motor neurone type with spasticity, typical upper motor neurone patterns of weakness and brisk reflexes.

TETRAPARESIS

When all four limbs are involved in a process resulting in loss of motor function the term tetraparesis may be used. The involvement of all four limbs in an upper motor neurone weakness implies a lesion in the high cervical region, brain stem or hemispheres. Tetraparesis may also be seen of lower motor neurone nature in the presence of acute peripheral neuropathy or radiculopathy, as in the Guillain–Barré syndrome or with myopathic disturbances such as periodic paralysis.

Lesions in the high cervical region tend not be associated with a brisk jaw jerk, but those in the high brain stem or cerebrum will cause a brisk jaw jerk and cerebral rather than spinal investigations should then be considered. Motor neurone disease may cause a mixed upper and lower motor neurone lesion affecting all four limbs with evident wasting and fasciculation but often with increased reflexes.

FORAMEN MAGNUM LESION (p. 215)

Lesions arising at the foramen magnum are notoriously difficult to diagnose and are frequently associated with pain in and around the occipital region and the upper limbs. Weakness of one shoulder or arm may then progress to involve the ipsilateral leg, the opposite leg and finally the opposite arm in a pattern which is sometimes called developing a weakness 'round the clock'. Whether these particular developments are due to growth of a tumour around the foramen magnum or to vascular lesions at that site is uncertain but the pattern of evolution from either arm to the ipsilateral leg, the contralateral leg and arm should always raise this possibility.

CONUS LESIONS (p. 216)

Lesions within the spinal cord at the dorsolumbar junction will affect the conus of the spinal cord causing a mixture of upper and lower motor neurone lesions affecting the lower limbs, together with disturbance of sphincter function and usually with sensory loss. This picture is diagnostic of a lesion at this site and again makes radiology imperative and myelography obligatory.

CAUDA EQUINA LESIONS (p. 216)

Lesions in the lumbar or sacral spine which damage the lower motor neurones of the cauda equina result in disturbances of bladder and bowel function, usually preceding flaccid weakness of the lower limbs. Though this form of disturbance may occasionally be due to pathology outside the spine in the pelvis it is usually indicative of a spinal lesion and makes myelography obligatory.

CORTICAL WEAKNESS

Occasionally a condition will be seen in which the peripheral muscles in a limb, commonly the hand, are flaccid and paralysed yet with brisk reflexes. Though the possibility of motor neurone disease should be considered, this situation can arise with a true cortical lesion where damage is in the precentral gyrus.

APRAXIA

Lesions in the frontal or parietal lobe can result in the syndrome of apraxia where, although there is no overt muscle weakness, the limb is not able to perform adequately and accurately the required function. This represents the highest level of motor disturbance. Common forms of apraxia are the gait apraxia referred to earlier, constructional apraxia, in which the patient is unable to assemble objects in three dimensions or to draw them normally in two dimensions, and dressing apraxia, in which the patient is unable to put on clothes in a logical and consistent manner. An apraxia of gait is frequently an indication of bifrontal lobe disturbances whereas constructional and dressing apraxia together with topographical agnosia are frequently symptoms of non-dominant parietal lobe disease.

PERIPHERAL NEUROPATHY (Ch. 10)

When the motor fibres are involved in a peripheral neuropathy, the longest fibres are affected earliest and most severely, resulting in weakness of lower motor neurone type in the peripheral muscles of the limbs. The muscles of the feet, ankles and calves are affected before the hands and in long-standing neuropathies this weakness may result in pes cavus followed by foot drop and a high step-page gait. The patient will tend to trip easily and may suffer severe damage to weak ankles in falls.

In many instances there will be a symmetrical glove-and-stocking sensory anaesthesia indicative of damage to the peripheral nerves. There may, however, be a purely motor peripheral neuropathy and occasionally the sensory component is evident only as pain.

MONONEUROPATHY (p. 246–248)

In conditions in which a single nerve or several nerves are damaged the pattern of weakness will be confined to muscles supplied by that nerve and will frequently be associated with sensory loss and often with the symptom of pain. The commonest forms of such lower motor neurone weakness are in the compression syndromes of the median nerve, the ulnar nerve, the radial nerve or the common peroneal nerve. It may also be seen in inflammatory or vascular conditions such as polyarteritis where a mixture of similar nerve lesions may occur in the syndrome of mononeuritis multiplex. More than one nerve may also be involved in a pattern of muscle weakness of lower motor neurone type where there is a lesion of a plexus. The nerves innervating the various muscles are shown in Table 1.2. There will usually be an associated sensory disturbance in the distribution of the peripheral nerve involved.

RADICULOPATHY

Another lower motor neurone weakness with wasting, flaccidity and areflexia may follow the pattern of a single root, commonly the cervical 5, 6 or 7 in the upper limb or the lumbar 4, 5 or S1 in the lower limb due to a lateral intervertebral disc prolapse. Multiple root lesions may occur as with avulsion injuries to the cervical spine where the pattern of lower motor neurone damage will affect the muscles supplied by more than one root. Root innervation of muscles is shown in Table 1.3. Root symptoms will frequently be associated with sensory loss within the distribution of a single dermatome or pain radiating into that dermatome.

Table 1.2 Motor peripheral nerve innervation

Nerve	Muscle	Reflex
Upper limb		
Axillary	Deltoid	
Long thoracic	Serratus anterior	
Suprascapular	Supra- and infraspinatus	
Musculocutaneous	Biceps	Biceps reflex (C5/6)
Radial	Brachioradialis Wrist extensors Finger extensors Supinator Triceps	Brachioradialis (C5/6) Triceps (C7)
Median	Wrist flexion Finger flexion (except FDP 4 & 5) Pronator Abductor pollicis brevis Opponens	Finger jerk (C8)
Ulnar	FDP (4,5) Flexor carpi ulnaris Abductor digiti minimi Interossei	
Lower limb		
Femoral	Quadriceps	Knee jerk (L3/4)
Obturator	Adductors of hip	Adductor jerk (L3)
Sciatic	Hip extension Abductor of hip Knee flexion	
Common peroneal	Dorsiflexion of foot Eversion of foot	
Post-tibial	Plantar flexion of foot	Ankle jerk (S1)

FDP = flexor digitorum profundus.

MYOPATHIC WEAKNESS (p. 251)

Weakness of muscles can affect almost any group of muscles in the body and a pattern of weakness

Table 1.3 Spinal root lesions

Root	Muscle	Reflex
Upper limbs		
C5	Deltoid Rhomboids Biceps	Biceps (C5/6)
C6	Brachioradialis Biceps Pronator/supinator Extensor carpi radialis	Brachioradialis (C5/6) Biceps (C5/6)
C7	Triceps Extensor carpi ulnaris	Triceps (C7)
C8	Finger flexion	Finger jerk (C8)
T1	Intrinsic hand muscles	
Lower limbs		
L3	Iliopsoas Quadriceps Hip adduction	Knee jerks (L3/4) Adductor reflex (L3)
L4	Quadriceps Tibialis anterior	Knee jerk (L3/4)
L5	Hip abduction Hamstrings Peronei Extensor hallucis longus	Medial hamstring (L4/5)
S1	Plantar flexion of foot	Ankle jerk (S1)
S2	Intrinsic foot muscles	

which fits none of the above-mentioned descriptions should always be considered as being due to muscle disease. Usually weakness due to muscle disease will be manifest by changes in the muscle, either of swelling, of wasting or of pain together with reduced reflexes and in most cases the largest muscles are most significantly affected giving rise to a proximal weakness. The cardinal feature of myopathy is weakness of proximal muscles of the shoulders and pelvis, though in uncommon forms of dystrophy and inflammatory myopathy there may be involvement of facial muscles and peripheral limb muscles.

FATIGUE (p. 248)

The syndrome of fatigue is important and, though common in both organic and non-organic illnesses, is of particular importance in the motor system. If genuine fatigue, of lower motor neurone type, can be identified, then the probability of a neuromuscular junction abnormality such as myasthenia gravis is high and needs to be formally investigated.

MOTOR DISTURBANCES DUE TO SENSORY PROBLEMS (p. 33)

Perhaps the most common motor symptom resulting from a sensory disturbance is clumsiness or unsteadiness due to deafferentation. The problem is not uncommon with deafferentation of the upper limbs, when the hands become clumsy; with deafferentation of the lower limbs there is frequently unsteadiness particularly in dark environments or with the eyes shut (Rombergism). The possibility of motor symptoms being due to sensory disturbances should always be considered in patients whose symptoms are not explained by the evident motor signs. Careful testing of proprioception should leave the examiner in no doubt as to the cause of the disability.

SIMULATED WEAKNESS (p. 481)

The problems of patients with hysteria or malingering complaining of motor weakness are considerable. A total weakness is usually apparent as being not genuine in that the muscles show no signs of wasting or contractures and the reflexes are normal. More subtle weaknesses, however, can be very difficult to identify and one reasonable method is to assess the power of the patient against the examiner's own strength which can be varied at will by the examiner. In a genuinely weak limb there will be a constant weakness in the muscles affected, whereas in hysteria or malingering there are often fluctuations in the strength of the limb during the variable testing. None the less, the problem of factitious weakness is a very considerable one and cannot always adequately be excluded.

INVOLUNTARY MOVEMENTS

TREMOR

Tremor can be defined as a regular, rhythmic movement of part of the body within a single plane. The rhythmic quality is the aspect of tremor which distinguishes it from other involuntary movements. Tremor is perhaps the commonest of all involuntary movements and it is usually possible to distinguish resting tremor from action tremor, which is present throughout movement, and intention tremor, which is present only at the extremes of movement (Table 1.4) The *resting tremor* is diagnostic of an extrapyramidal disturbance, usually Parkinson's disease (p. 386), although it can occasionally be seen as one of the manifestations of benign familial tremor (p. 396). The *intention tremor* is classically related to disturbances of the cerebellum or its connections. The *action tremor* may be physiological or pathological. When physiological, it can be seen in some families where it is recorded as benign familial tremor, or in the aged where it is termed senile tremor. It is present in the majority of people at moments of acute anxiety and it may be a manifestation of chronic anxiety or stress (p. 481). Pathologically, it is seen in thyrotoxicosis, alcohol withdrawal, heavy metal poisoning, particularly mercury, and drugs, particularly the bronchodilators. It is believed to be related to the peripheral action of adrenergic agents.

Asterixis is often confused with true tremor. It is a movement caused, however, by simultaneous electrical silence in both flexor and extensor antagonists when a sustained posture of the outstretched hands is maintained against gravity. It is characteristically more jerky than tremor and develops after a latent period of several seconds. Whilst it is often described as 'liver flap', it will be seen, if carefully looked for, in many other encephalopathies, including those of renal and respiratory failure and drug-induced encephalopathies.

MYOCLONUS

The sudden sharp jerking movement seen in a muscle or group of muscles, often induced by action, by loud noises or by sudden movements, is termed myoclonus. There are many different causes of myoclonus as shown in Table 1.5. It can be a reflection of cortical or brain stem abnormalities or can arise at a spinal level. It is physiological as one is falling asleep, but it can become pathological and markedly disabling in patients with myoclonic epilepsy, or in those with significant anoxic injury to the brain.

EPILEPSIA PARTIALIS CONTINUA

(p. 157)

A continuing focal twitching movement, often beginning after a stroke and confined to one part of an arm or a leg, may be due to epilepsia partialis continuans which is a focal status epilepticus. It is often refractory to treatment and may cause very considerable distress and disability to the patient.

Table 1.4 Classification of tremor

Clinical type	Frequency	Association	Occurrence *Rest*	 *Posture/action*	 *Intention*	Therapy	
Resting	3–7 Hz	Parkinson's disease	+++	+	–	Anticholinergics Dopaminergics Stereotactic surgery	
Intention	2–3 Hz	Cerebellar Dentatorubral	– –	+ +++	+++ +++	Choline chloride Isoniazid Stereotaxis Weighting	poor results
Action	8–13 HZ	Physiological Anxiety Toxic (thyroid, lithium)	–	++	–	Correction of underlying cause beta-blockers	
	6–8 Hz	Essential (familial)	–	+++	+	β blockers Primidone	

Table 1.5 Classification of myoclonus

Physiological		
Sleep myoclonus (hypnic jerks)		
Anxiety		
Exercise		
Hiccough		
Essential		
Familial		
Sporadic		
Nocturnal myoclonus		
Epileptic		
Fragments of epilepsy	Isolated myoclonic jerks	
	Epilepsia partialis continuans	
	Stimulus-sensitive myoclonus	
Childhood myoclonic epilepsies	Benign myoclonus of infancy	
	Infantile astatic epilepsy	
	Cryptogenic myoclonic epilepsy	
Juvenile myoclonic epilepsy		
Symptomatic		
Degenerative:	Storage disease (Lafora, Tay–Sachs, Batten's)	
	Spinocerebellar degeneration (Ramsay Hunt, Baltic myoclonus, Ataxia telegectasia)	
	Basal ganglia (Wilson's)	
	Dementias (Creutzfeld–Jakob, Alzheimer's)	
Acquired:	Viral (SSPE, togavirus encephalitis)	
	Metabolic (hepatic, renal, etc.)	
	Toxic (heavy metals)	
	Physical (postanoxia, post-traumatic)	
	Focal damage (post-CVA, tumour)	

Table 1.6 Causes of chorea

Generalised		
Inherited:	Huntington's disease	
Acquired:	Rheumatic (Sydenham's chorea)	
	Pregnancy (chorea gravidarum)	
	Drugs—	contraceptive pill
		L-dopa
		dopamine agonists
		phenothiazines
		anticonvulsants
	Symptomatic—	thyrotoxicosis
		hypoparathyroidism
		SLE
	Postanoxic	
Hemichorea (hemiballismus)		
Infarct—in subthalamic nucleus		
Post-traumatic		
Postanoxia		

PAROXYSMAL CHOREOATHETOSIS

This term, or alternatively the term kinesogenic dyskinesia, is used to describe the syndrome seen in patients who develop sudden and sometimes painful posturing of a limb as they begin to initiate a movement. The disability is usually temporary and may occur in the context of multiple sclerosis where it is believed to be due to ephaptic transmission of nerve impulses. It can be treated with agents such as carbamazepine or phenytoin.

CHOREA

The relatively rapid jerk-like movements of chorea are often transformed into semipurposive movements by the patient and are indicative of disturbance of the basal ganglia, particularly of lesions in the caudate nucleus. They are seen most commonly with degenerative conditions such as Huntington's chorea (p. 383), occasionally with inflammatory conditions such as Sydenham's chorea and also in iatrogenic conditions such as pill chorea (p. 429) and physiological conditions such as chorea gravidarum (p. 474) (Table 1.6).

HEMIBALLISMUS

The presence of severe chorea in an arm and leg occurring quite suddenly frequently in the elderly and often diabetic patient is diagnostic of hemiballismus or hemichorea, which is due to a lesion in the subthalamic nucleus. This is usually seen in the context of vascular disease and is frequently self-limiting. The lesions which cause damage to the subthalamic nucleus are usually vascular in nature and the most frequent association of this particular condition is in diabetes mellitus.

ATHETOSIS

Athetosis is most commonly seen in the upper limbs rather than the lower limbs and almost invariably due to ischaemic disturbances, either due to birth injury and occasionally to injury and anoxia later in life.

DYSTONIA (Ch. 15)

The abnormal posturing seen with some forms of basal ganglia disturbance has already been described. Patients may often suffer considerable pain from the deformed muscles and the posturing can cause a very considerable disability.

TORTICOLLIS (p. 395)

Intermittent or continuous spasms of contraction of the neck muscles causing twisting of the head to one side or posteriorly is termed torticollis or retrocollis. There is no known cause for this syndrome which can begin at any age and tends to worsen slowly though occasionally showing periods of remission and even complete recovery. There is considerable discussion as to whether the torticollis is a genuine organic disturbance or whether it is part of a habit spasm. It has recently been suggested that, in some patients, loops of blood vessels pressing upon the spinal accessory nerves may be responsible for this particular condition.

BLEPHAROSPASM (p. 395)

Intermittent forced eye closure is a syndrome which appears to be related to spasmodic torticollis and may even occur in the same patient. No structural cause has been shown.

MYOTONIA (p. 255)

Some patients may notice that muscles, once contracted, are very slow to relax. This can occur in young people as a benign condition, Thompson's myotonia, or may develop in the second and third decades of life as part of the syndrome of myotonic dystrophy in which the more prominent abnormalities are those of frontal baldness, cataract, endocrine disturbance and gross muscle weakness.

WRITER'S CRAMP (p. 395)

The occurrence of painful spasms or cramps in any limb usually indicates an upper motor neurone lesion affecting the particular muscles. There is a particular syndrome of painful spasms of cramps within the dominant hand and forearm induced by writing, which is believed by some to be due to basal ganglia disturbance and by others to be a manifestation of psychiatric disease.

MYOKYMIA

The continuing movement of muscles of the face, often described as like a bag of worms under the skin, is believed to be due to irritative lesions at the level of the facial nerve nucleus. It can occur elsewhere in the body when it is often associated with muscle cramps (Isaacson's syndrome).

HEMIFACIAL SPASM (p. 71)

This syndrome, usually seen in patients over the age of 50 and frequently beginning as twitching around the eye, may develop to become distressing and embarrassing spasms of one half of the face.

TICS AND HABIT SPASM (p. 397, 481)

Habitual movements of the face, shoulders or a limb are not uncommon and may become stereotyped and persistent. They are most frequently seen in young children and usually resolve. In some patients the tics become more pronounced and associated with the uttering of occasional words and gestures in the syndrome of Gilles de la Tourette, in which there are multiple tics, sniffing, snorting, vocalisation and aggressive impulses.

COMMON CLINICAL PROBLEMS

There are some syndromes which involve disturbances of motor function but which cannot be adequately described as due to simple weakness or the presence of involuntary movements. The two most important of these are the clumsy hand and disturbances of gait (described below). Other common syndromes and their differential diagnoses are summarised in Table 1.7.

THE CLUMSY HAND

The patient who presents with a disability affecting a hand calls for the most careful assessment on the part of the clinician. The causes of clumsiness of the hand are many and can easily be overlooked. When the patient describes the symptom of clumsiness, most physicians look for a *cerebellar* disturbance affecting the hand, but any form of *motor disability* can result in clumsiness ranging from a minor degree of weakness of either *upper* or *lower motor neurone* type, a *basal ganglia* disturbance affecting the hand as in early Parkinson's disease, to *dyspraxia* of hand movement. It is important not to overlook the difficulties which may occur with hand movement in patients who have suffered *deafferentation* of the hand, due either to large fibre peripheral neuropathy affecting the limb or, more commonly, to a lesion affecting the lateral part of the dorsal column, which may occur with a cervical spondylotic myelopathy but is most commonly seen in the young in multiple sclerosis where the term 'the useless hand of Oppenheim' is used.

It is important in this situation that the physician undertakes a careful sensory examination of the hand as well as assessing motor disturbances in terms of weakness, tone, co-ordination and makes a formal assessment of apraxia.

DIFFICULTY IN WALKING

The classic forms of gait disturbance have already been identified in the section on clinical assessment. When patients present with symptoms of disturbed gait it is important initially to identify whether or not weakness of the lower limbs is present; if so, whether the weakness is of *upper* or *lower motor neurone* type and whether there may be additional disturbances of tone indicating *basal ganglia disease*, or of co-ordination suggesting damage to the *cerebellum* or its pathways. There must then be a formal assessment of *sensory function* in the lower limbs, in particular the asssessment of proprioception and vibration sensation to identify disturbances of the posterior column which may manifest as gait disturbances.

A gait disturbance which appears inexplicable on all of these assessments should raise the possi-

Table 1.7 Weakness in the hand or leg

Symptoms	Differential diagnosis	Weakness	Sensory loss	Reflex loss
Weak hand +/− pins & needles in hand	C8 T1 root	Interossei, APB finger flexors	Medial forearm and finger	Finger jerk
	C6 root	Brachioradialis	Lateral forearm	Brachialis
	Medial n. at wrist	APB	Lateral 3.5 fingers (palmar)	
	Ulnar n. at elbow	Interossei and ADM	Medial 1.5 fingers	—
Wrist drop	C7 root	Triceps, FCR	Middle finger	Triceps
	Radial n.	Triceps, brachioradialis	Snuff box area (dorsum of hand)	Brachioradialis
Quadriceps weakness	L3/4	Quadriceps, foot inversion	Ant. thigh and medial shin	Knee
	Femoral n.	Quadriceps	Ant. thigh and medial shin	Knee
Foot drop	L5	Hip abductn, hamstrings Foot drop, eversion	Lateral shin Dorsum of foot	Ankle jerk
	Common peroneal n.	Foot drop, eversion	Dorsum of foot	—

APB = abductor pollicis brevis, ADM = abductor digiti minimi, FCR = flexor carpi radialis, FCU = flexor carpi ulnaris.

bility of an *apraxia* of gait, which may be seen in patients with bilateral frontal lobe disease due to atrophy, tumour or to the syndrome of hydrocephalus, either obstructive or normal pressure in type. Finally it must always be remembered that some disturbances of gait do not have an organic basis, and gait problems, particularly occurring in the context of injury, which are disproportionate to the objective neurological signs that are apparent must always raise the possibility of *conscious* or *unconscious elaboration* of the walking difficulty: *hysteria* or *malingering*.

MANAGEMENT OF MOTOR DISORDERS

Although in many cases the identification of a particular cause of a motor disturbance will lead to the institution of specific therapy for the causative pathology, there are several factors common to problems affecting the motor system whether they are due to parenchymal disease of the central nervous system, peripheral nerve and root disturbances, or muscle disease.

PHARMACOLOGICAL TREATMENT

As one of the most common of all motor disturbances relates to damage to the upper motor neurone, resulting in spasticity and consequent reflex spasms, the use of *spasmolytic agents* is of considerable importance. The most commonly used agents are *benzodiazepines*, which are believed to act predominantly at the brain stem level, *gabaergic agents* such as baclofen, which are believed to act at the spinal level and peripherally acting drugs such as *dantrolene sodium*, which affect the muscle contraction itself. There are benefits and disadvantages to each of these particular therapies and in each case the dose used must be tailored to the individual patient. One of the major advantages is that, because these drugs act at different sites, they can be additive in their effect and it is therefore reasonable to introduce one spasmolytic agent and gradually supplement it with others when its dose of maximal effectiveness has been determined. It should always be remembered that, in using spasmolytic preparations, the reduction of tone in a spastic muscle may exacerbate underlying weakness and may therefore prove deleterious to function. The best example of this is the patient who has a significant paraparesis but who is able to stand on his spastic legs to enable him to transfer from bed to chair and from chair to commode. The use of a spasmolytic agent may reduce the spasticity and consequent pain in the legs, but may make his legs useless as props and therefore reduce his independence.

If spasms become more troublesome and resistant to ordinary pharmacological therapies, local nerve or root, or even intrathecal blocks by injection of local anaesthetics or phenol should be considered. If spasms and contractures become more troublesome then *surgical therapy* may have to be considered in the form of tenotomy.

The pharmacological management of extrapyramidal disease is discussed in Chapter 15.

In terms of more symptomatic treatment for motor system disorders, the problems relating to pain will occasionally call for the use of analgesics, but is should be remembered that most codeine-based analgesics have a spastic effect upon muscle tone. It is thus possible to worsen muscle spasms by the use of such agents.

In some muscle disturbances, particularly those which are paroxysmal (tonic spasms), the use of *carbamazepine* or *phenytoin* should be considered.

SURGERY

The possibility of surgery in the management of intractable muscle spasms leading to contractures has already been considered. Tenotomy is a technique which has been used less during the past few decades but which still has a part to play in the management of patients in whom contractures have added to the motor disability. It is undoubtedly better to prevent contractures than to treat them once they have occurred, but this counsel of the ideal is not always practicable and surgery is still sometimes called for.

Surgery may also have a part to play in the fixation of unstable joints particularly in conditions in which there is lower motor neurone weakness of the ankle and more rarely in upper limb disability. In patients who have significant upper limb disability following root avulsion and a consequent flail arm, amputation may be considered.

The use of stereotactic surgery in the treatment of certain movement disorders is established and particularly appropriate in patients with Parkinson's disease who have tremor as their main functional symptom. Radiofrequency or cryothalamotomy lesions in the nucleus ventralis posterior lateralis of the thalamus may frequently give considerable relief from this problem. Surgery should be considered in patients with other tremors, such as the dentatorubral tremor, though in the most common cause of this syndrome, multiple sclerosis, the results are unpredictable.

PHYSICAL THERAPY

The physiotherapist has an important role to play in the management of the patient with a motor disturbance. This role in the initial phase is to maintain movement of joints, prevent contracture of muscles and begin to retrain the patient to use those muscles which regain function. As the illness stabilises it is reasonable to expect the physiotherapist to help in retraining the patient and to prevent the development of tricks and habits which may become detrimental. Local heat, massage and occasional infrared therapy will certainly make the patient more comfortable and may retain mobility in joints and muscles. The use of faradism, which was so common in the past, now has little to recommend it though new physiological evidence suggests that there may be some point in continuing stimulation of damaged nerves when one can expect a degree of recovery to occur.

An important supplement to the physiotherapy care is that provided by nurses looking after the patient with motor disability. They should be able to undertake many of the simple physiotherapeutic tasks and in addition have the responsibility to protect the skin of patients who are immobilised and to ensure adequate care of bladder and bowel in patients who are paraplegic.

REHABILITATION

It can be argued that the whole process of therapy in patients is in fact a form of rehabilitation, but it is widely accepted now that there are specific elements to rehabilitation which are particularly important for the patient who has sustained damage to the motor system. In this respect the involvement of ancillary services such as speech therapy, occupational therapy and social work may become important, and decisions as to the use of various aids ranging from the simple walking stick to the provision of wheelchairs and ultimately the fitting of environmental control systems to the home need to be considered. There is now general awareness of the fact that physicians specialising in rehabilitation are of particular importance in the sphere of neurology and their role is most important in aspects of motor and cognitive retraining.

The long-term management of the patient with motor disabilities is of course enormously variable depending upon the underlying nature of the disease. The form of rehabilitation employed in patients who have suffered a single insult following a stroke, a head or spinal injury or an episode of isolated transverse myelitis is necessarily different from that employed in a patient with a progressive disease. None the less, patients with recurring illnesses, such as multiple sclerosis who are liable to have increasing problems, and those with more progressive diseases, such as muscular dystrophy, motor neurone disease and some of the more severe and progressive inherited neuropathies, do require rehabilitation to be provided which can be amended, modified and increased as the disability becomes more apparent.

FURTHER READING

Brodal A 1981 Neurological anatomy in relation to clinical medicine, 3rd edn. Oxford University Press. New York

Mayo Clinic and Mayo Foundation 1976 Clinical examinations in neurology, 4th edn. Saunders, Philadelphia

Medical Research Council 1981 Aids to the investigation of peripheral nerve injury. HMSO, London

2

Disorders of somatic sensation

INTRODUCTION

Sensory disorders are among the most difficult clinical syndromes to unravel, for many reasons. Not only do patients use a variety of terms to describe sensory symptoms, but different patients mean different things by these terms. Sensory symptoms are by their nature subjective and sensory tests for the same reason are difficult to assess. In general, the history of a sensory disturbance is of greater significance and help than sensory examination, while sensory signs without symptoms can usually be ignored. Finally, sensory symptoms are common and are experienced by most of us from time to time. Who, for example, has not woken up during the night with numbness of a leg, or who has not experienced paraesthesia in the fingers after a sharp tap on the olecranon process (the 'funny bone')?

Insight into the significance of sensory symptoms therefore requires a knowledge of the anatomy of the sensory pathways, an understanding of the variety of sensory symptoms that can occur, and an ability to appreciate what the patient is attempting to describe. Furthermore, as with other symptoms, it is perhaps not what the patient says but how he says it that gives significance to the symptom.

ANATOMY AND PHYSIOLOGY

This chapter will not concern itself with the special senses or with visceral sensation, which does not reach consciousness; these are dealt with in Chapters 3 and 4. The four common cutaneous sensations—touch, pain, heat and cold—together with the deep sensations of pressure and proprioception are referred to as the somatic sensations. These are consciously appreciated in all parts of the body and have a common pathway within the nervous system. An appropriate stimulus generates an impulse at the periphery which passes into the central nervous system, is relayed by the thalamus and thence, by a final relay, is passed to the appropriate part of the cerebral cortex. In simple terms, the pathway for somatic sensation is subserved by three orders of neurones: the first-order neurone is concerned with transmitting information from the periphery to the spinal cord; the second-order neurone transmits information from the spinal cord to the thalamus, and the third-order neurone transmits information from the thalamus to the cerebral cortex.

RECEPTORS

Information to the first-order neurones comes from a variety of receptors. Every sensation depends on impulses excited by the adequate stimulation of these receptors, which comprise two main groups—those in skin and those in the deeper somatic structures. Many morphological variants have been described, although with a few exceptions it has not been possible to ascribe specific functions to each.

Although individual cutaneous sensory receptors are 'most' sensitive to a particular form of natural stimulation, this specificity is not absolute and other forms of stimulation may also excite the ending. Table 2.1 lists some cutaneous receptors and their sensory function.

TRANSMISSION OF INFORMATION FROM RECEPTORS

Stimulation of a sensory ending gives rise to a receptor potential, which appears at the specialised end of an afferent nerve fibre. This is not an all-or-none phenomenon, but varies in amplitude and time course and may be rapidly dissipated even though the stimulus continues, with resulting falling away of the firing frequency in the nerve fibre. Impulses from the receptors travel centrally through the first-order neurones, the perikarya of which are are in the dorsal root ganglia. The fibres are of varying calibre and are classified into groups A, B and C. Group C comprises unmyelinated axons, with diameters ranging from less than 1 μm up to 2 μm, and with conduction velocities of from 0.7 to 2 m/s. A and B fibres are myelinated, those in the B group being the preganglionic neurones of the autonomic nervous system of mammals. The (myelinated) axons of the A group have been subdivided into groups α, β, γ and δ, with αA fibres having the fastest conduction velocity and δA fibres the slowest.

Different types of fibres transmit different sensory modalities. α and β fibres transmit information from tactile receptors, whereas γ and δ fibres transmit heat, cold and certain information concerned with pain. The ratio between receptors and neurones varies: pacinian corpuscles have a one-to-one ratio with primary afferent fibres; that is to say, the peripheral end of a single fibre branches to supply one receptor.

Table 2.1 Correlation of cutaneous receptors and their sensory function

Receptor	Elementary sensation
Meissner corpuscle, or hair follicle receptor	Tapping
Pacinian corpuscle	Vibration or tickle
Merkel cell	Pressure
Ruffini corpuscle	No sensation
Fine C-terminals	Pain

THE AFFERENT PATHWAYS TO THE SPINAL CORD

The afferent sensory fibres from the various receptors pass up the differing peripheral nerves and enter the spinal cord via the dorsal roots. To understand the variety of peripheral nerve disturbances that may occur requires knowledge of the anatomy of the distribution of peripheral sensory nerves and sensory roots which is illustrated in Figures 2.1 and 2.2. It should be emphasised that there is considerable overlap in the peripheral nerve distributions and in the dermatome distributions.

There is some evidence to suggest that a number of afferent fibres enter the cord in the ventral roots. The significance of these is uncertain but their presence may be responsible for the persistence of pain in some patients after dorsal rhizotomy.

SOMATIC SENSORY PATHWAYS (Fig. 2.3)

All the somatic sensory pathways are crossed and terminate in the opposite sensory cortex in the cerebral hemisphere. Three anatomically separate pathways may be recognised.

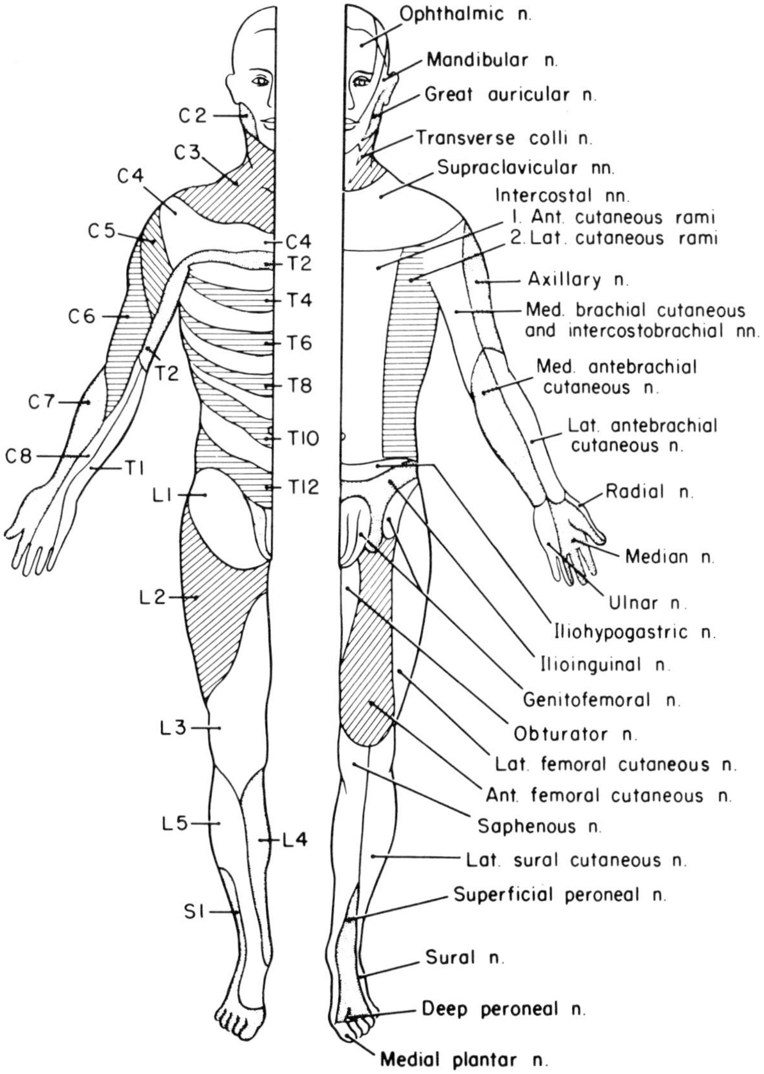

Fig. 2.1 The sensory distribution of peripheral nerves and dermatomes (anterior view). (Reproduced from Carpenter M B, Sutin J 1983 *Human Neuroanatomy*, 8th edn, Williams and Wilkins, Baltimore, with permission.)

Dorsal column medial lemniscus pathway

Input to this pathway within the spinal cord is via large thickly myelinated fibres which pass through the medial division of the dorsal spinal nerve root to enter the dorsal white column of their own side, dividing into ascending and descending branches. The descending branches establish reflex connections by sending collateral branches into the dorsal grey column; the ascending branches are the first link in the sensory pathway. At their entrance these ascending fibres are situated immediately medial to the dorsal horn, but during their course up the spinal cord they are steadily pushed in a more medial direction because the fibres entering at succeeding rostral levels intrude between the ascending fibres and the dorsal horn. As a consequence of this, the fibres occupying the most medial part of the dorsal column in the upper cervical region will belong to the sacral roots, whilst the fibres from the upper extremity are found most laterally. The fibres terminate at the

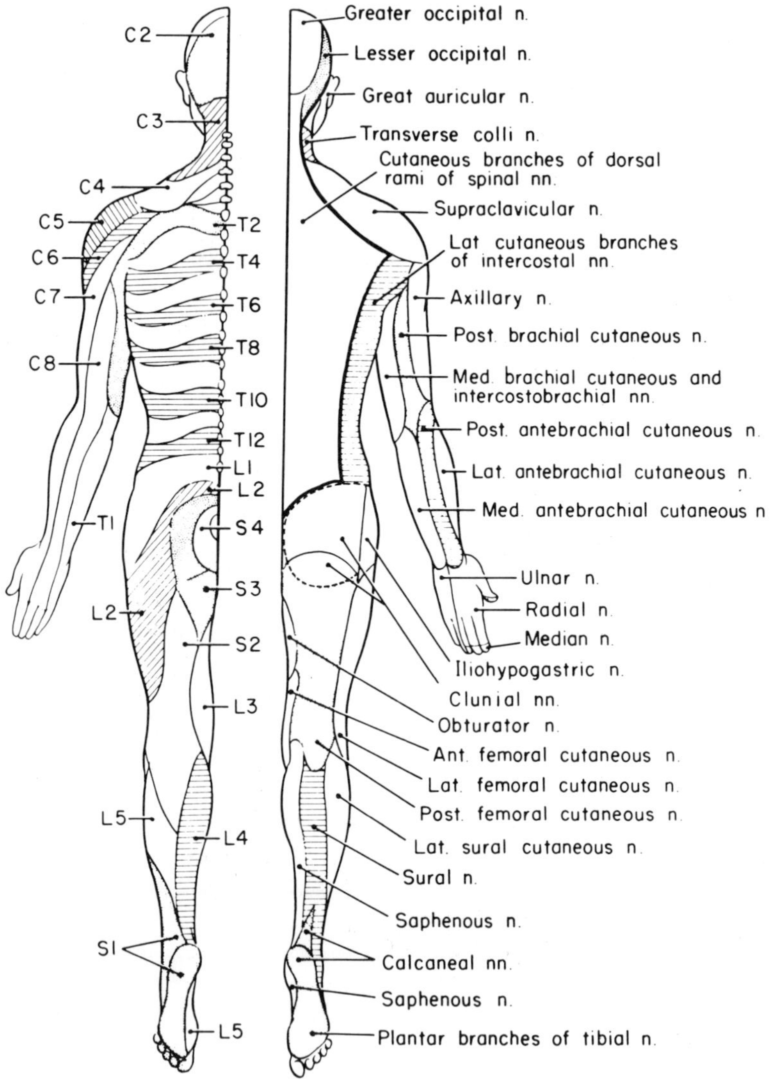

Fig. 2.2 The sensory distribution of peripheral nerves and dermatomes (posterior view). Reproduced from Carpenter M B, Sutin J 1983 *Human Neuroanatomy*, 8th edn, Williams and Wilkins, Baltimore, with permission.

cervicomedullary junction in the nucleus gracilis and nucleus cuneatus. Figure 2.4 shows, in simplified form, the somatotopic representation of the sensory pathways in the spinal cord. The fibres terminate synaptically on to the second-order neurones in the gracile and cuneate nuclei and the axons of these neurones curve ventrally and medially and then turn upwards to form a prominent bundle of fibres, the medial lemniscus.

The classic view is that the impulses ascending in the fibres of the dorsal columns mediate the sensations of touch, deep pressure, vibratory sense and sense of position of joints and are particularly important for sensory discrimination. During the past few years this view has been seriously challenged and, although the matter is far from certain, it appears clear that the dorsal columns mediate sensory signals necessary for complex discriminative tasks.

The segmental somatotopic organisation present in the dorsal columns and their nuclei is maintained in the medial lemniscus as it ascends to the

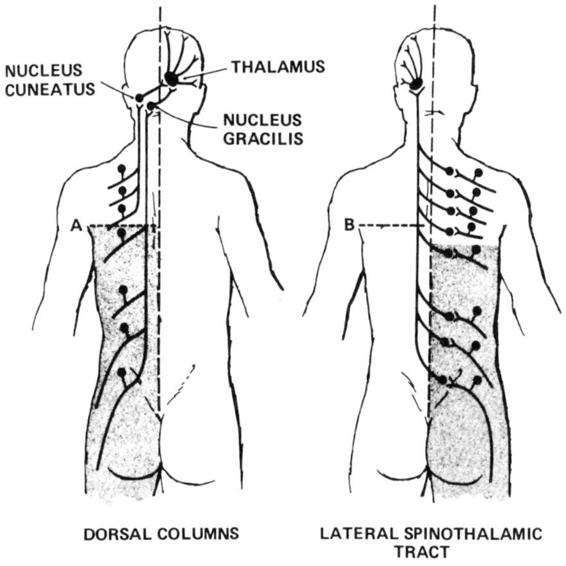

Fig. 2.3 The ascending sensory pathways.

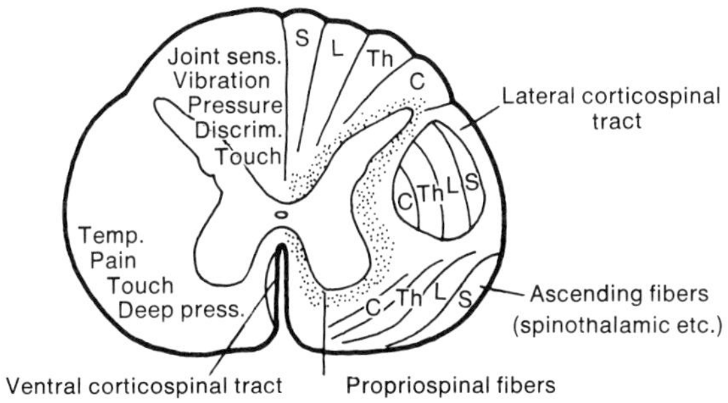

Fig. 2.4 The somatotopic representation of the sensory pathways of the spinal cord (S = sacral, L = lumbar, Th = thoracic, C = cervical).

thalamus where the fibres enter the ventroposterior lateral nucleus which contains the cell bodies of the third-order sensory neurones.

Spinothalamic pathway

This transmits impulses which are concerned with the appreciation of heat, cold and pain. It also provides an alternative pathway for touch sensibility—so-called crude or coarse touch. The first-order neurones have their cell bodies in the dorsal root ganglia and their fibres are thinner than those of the dorsal column medial lemniscus pathway; some, indeed (the C fibres), have no myelin at all. They enter the spinal cord in the lateral part of the dorsal root and divide into short descending and ascending branches. The ascending branches run for one or two segments in the posterolateral column before synapsing with second-order sensory neurones which lie deep in the dorsal column. The axons then cross the midline, in the so-called ventral white commissure and ascend in the ventrolateral white column as the spinothalamic tract. Some authors recommend that the spinothalamic tract be divided into a lateral and a ventral portion, but this is probably an unnecessary subdivision. Some of the spinothalamic fibres give off collaterals to certain nuclear regions such as the reticular formation. The somatotopic representation of the spinothalamic tract is shown in Figure 2.4.

In the brain stem the spinothalamic tract lies lateral to the medial lemniscus which it accompanies to terminate in the thalamus in the ventroposterior lateral nucleus. Important features of the spinothalamic pathway include the following:

1. The second-order neurone fibres cross the midline only one or two segments above the level of entry of the dorsal root fibres.
2. The site of decussation of the fibres in the cord exposes these to damage by expanding central cord lesions.
3. Fibres concerned with pain and temperature sensibility are situated dorsally to those involved with touch and pressure.
4. The spinothalamic tract is less compactly organised than the medial lemniscus, being intermingled with other ascending pathways giving off collaterals to the brain stem reticular formation.

The trigeminothalamic pathway (p. 65)

This pathway carries information from the distribution of the trigeminal nerve which serves such structures as most of the skin of the face, the forehead as far as the vertex, the mucous membranes of the nasal cavities, paranasal sinuses, mouth, tongue and parts of the pharynx, the teeth and gums, and from part of the dura mater.

About half of the entering fibres in the trigeminal nerve divide into a branch which terminates in the chief nucleus of the trigeminal nerve and the other half descends in the spinal tract to end in the spinal nucleus. The chief nucleus, which is in the lateral part of the pons, contains the second-order neurones concerned with tactile and postural sensibility; it gives rise to fibres which cross the midline to ascend near the medial lemniscus. The nucleus of the spinal tract, which extends downwards in the lateral part of the medulla to about the level of C2, contains the second-order neurones concerned with pain and temperature sensibility. The ophthalmic division of the trigeminal nerve terminates in the more caudal part

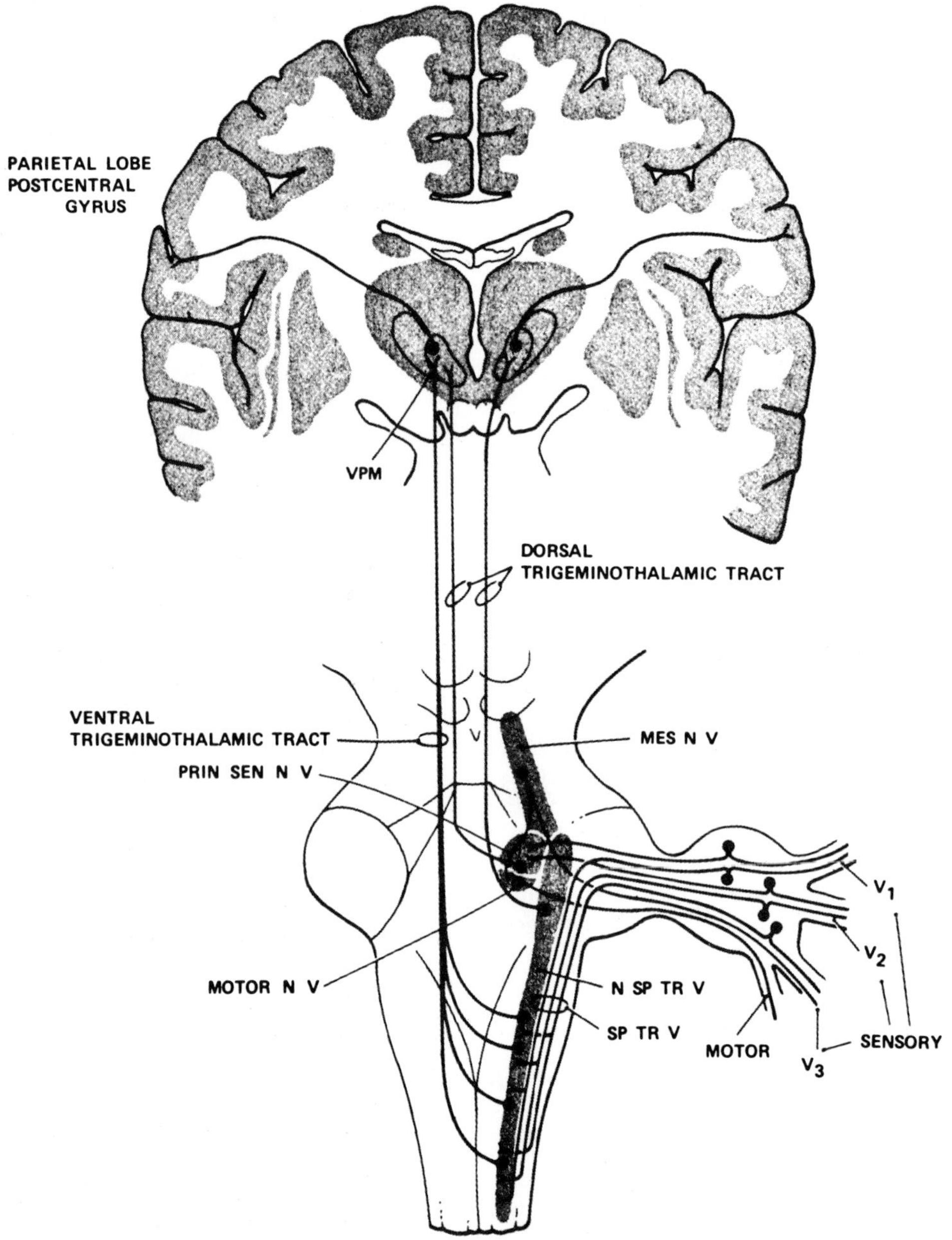

Fig. 2.5 The somatotopic representation of the trigeminothalamic pathways. VPM = nucleus ventralis posterior medialis, MES N V = mencephalic nucleus, PRIN SEN N V = principal sensory nucleus, MOTOR N V = motor nucleus, N SP TR V = spinal nucleus, SP TR V = spinal tract.

and the mandibular division terminates in the most cephalic part of the nucleus. Second-order neurones cross to the quintothalamic tract which ascends close to the spinothalamic tract. Both sets of second-order neurone fibres terminate in the ventroposterior medial nucleus of the thalamus.

A small group of trigeminal first-order sensory fibres terminate in the mesencephalic nucleus and are thought to be important in proprioceptive reflexes concerned with chewing and regulating the strength of the bite. The trigeminothalamic pathway is illustrated in Figure 2.5.

THE THALAMUS AND THALAMOCORTICAL PROJECTIONS

The third neuronal link in the ascending somatic sensory fibre system is made up of neurones, the nuclei of which are in the thalamus. The axons of these neurones transmit impulses to the central cortex.

As previously mentioned, the ventrolateral posterior nucleus of the thalamus receives fibres from the medial lemniscus: the fibres from the gracile nucleus end most laterally and those from the cuneate nucleus most medially. The exact area of termination of the spinothalmic fibres has been the subject of much controversy, although many believe that these terminate in the ventroposterior lateral nucleus. There is now a considerable amount of information to suggest that the medial part of the posterior complex of the thalamus represents a terminal area of spinothalamic fibres and the available physiological evidence suggests that this nucleus has a role in central pain mechanisms.

THE SOMATOSENSORY CORTICAL AREAS

From clinical and physiological observations it has been known for many years that the postcentral gyrus in man is the main (primary) somatosensory area. Another area beneath the lower end of the postcentral gyrus is known as the second somatosensory area. Since the work of Penfield, it has been known that there is a clear somatotopic representation in the sensory cortex (Fig. 2.6).

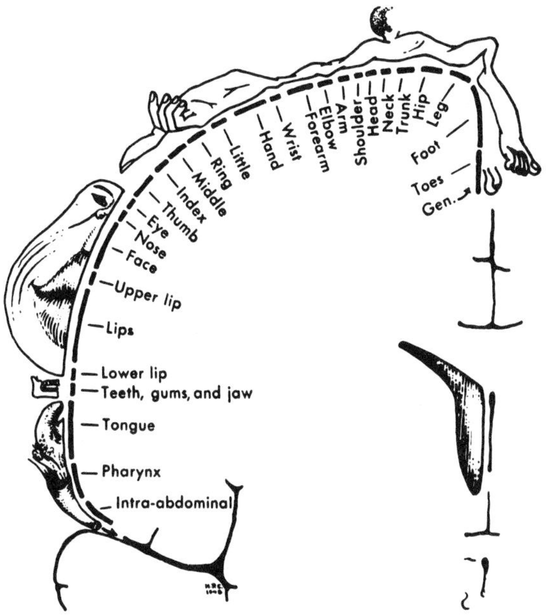

Fig. 2.6 The somatotopic representation of the sensory cortex. After Penfield W, Rassmussen T, 1950 *The Cerebral Cortex of Man*, MacMillan, New York, with permission.

The first sensory area appears principally to reflect activity in the dorsal column medial lemniscus system and also in the associated trigeminal system. The thalamic relay for these impulses passes through the internal capsule.

There is still debate as to whether thermal and painful stimuli are related to the first cortical somatosensory area. Some evidence suggests that there is such a relay to the second somatosensory cortical area, although our understanding of the sensory cortex is hindered by its complexity. What is known so far of the somatosensory cortical areas is that they are not functionally equivalent and each has specific tasks.

However inadequate our understanding of the sensory cortex, one thing is clear: provided that the subcortical structures—especially the thalamus—are intact, certain sensations such as pain, touch, pressure and extremes of temperature can reach consciousness. Their accurate localisation, however, as well as the patient's ability to make sensory discriminations, depends on the integrity of the sensory cortex. This is a fundamental distinction and will be discussed further when considering individual sensory syndromes.

CLINICAL ASSESSMENT

HISTORY

When attempting to assess sensory symptoms, the following three questions should be asked.

Is it a sensory symptom? Patients often have difficulty in describing disorders of sensation and they may use the words 'numb' or 'dead' when in fact they are describing weakness. Patients need to be asked specifically if the disorder they are experiencing is a loss of sensitivity.

Is it a significant sensory symptom? The significance of a sensory symptom depends on whether it is normal or abnormal. Many sensory symptoms occur in normal individuals and their description by patients may not necessarily indicate any disease process. Common symptoms that all of us may at one time or other experience are numbness in the finger tips when our hands are cold, numbness of an extremity after inadvertent pressure on a peripheral nerve while asleep, or tingling in the lips and mouth induced by hyperventilation. Many neurotic individuals may describe sensory symptoms to their physician, mistakenly believing that these may indicate a pathological state; the interpretation of such symptoms requires a knowledge of what is normal and abnormal.

What anatomical pathways are involved and at what level? The level at which a sensory disturbance is occurring may occasionally be deduced from the symptoms described (see below), but usually it is the sensory examination which enables the precise anatomical diagnosis to be made. The pattern of sensory symptoms, however, may be helpful.

Sensory symptoms may be divided into 'negative' or 'postive' sensory symptoms.

'Negative' sensory symptoms

By this we mean symptoms due to loss of a particular sensory modality. Total anaesthesia is rare and implies loss of all sensory modalities from the particular area involved. This may be described as a loss of feeling, but patients often use the term 'loss of feeling' as a description of what is, in fact, a partial sensory loss. *Total* inability to feel touch as a sensory symptom is uncommon. Loss of proprioception in the hands is often described as 'clumsiness', in that manipulative skills are affected. Patients often state that the skin feels thick and they may be unable to recognise by touch a coin in a pocket or in a purse. The patient may be unaware of loss of pain and thermal sensation and may suffer multiple burns or injuries without distress or alarm (trophic ulcers) (p. 234). Observant patients in this circumstance may notice, however, that they cannot feel the temperature of the bath water with the affected limb.

'Positive' sensory symptoms

These often mimic the sensory modality in the particular pathway involved. Tingling, or 'pins and needles' have no localising value and may be present in a sensory disturbance at virtually any level in the sensory pathway. However, burning feelings and pain usually result from a disorder affecting the sensory pathways concerned with the transmission of impulses for pain and temperature. Feelings of tightness or drawing, or more specifically a feeling of a tight band or girdle around the limb or trunk, are common symptoms in disorders affecting the proprioceptive fibres: a limb may feel swollen or about to burst. All such abnormal sensations are termed paraesthesias or dysaesthesias.

EXAMINATION

It cannot be emphasised too strongly that the examination of sensory functions relies very much on what the patient himself experiences. The symptoms that the patient feels during examination are the result not only of the stimulation of one or more receptors but also of the cerebral analysis and integration of the impressions perceived.

The detail of the sensory examination will be determined by the clinical situation. At a routine examination, if a patient has no sensory symptoms then it is probably sufficient to test vibration and position sense in the fingers and toes and the appreciation of a pin prick over the face, trunk and extremities. This quick examination will usually detect any sensory defects of which the patient is unaware. In a patient with specific sensory symptoms a more detailed examination will be required. In the presence of weakness, trophic ulcers, or neurogenic joints, a similarly detailed examination will be necessary. A complete examination of sensation is a tiresome and lengthy procedure for the patient as well as the examiner and may require several sessions. Without friendly co-operation from a patient the sensory examination is a waste of time: accordingly, it should not be performed in a patient who is tired, or in one who has a low IQ, is demented, or is dysphasic.

Touch sensibility

This is best tested with a wisp of cotton, although the examiner's finger tip can be used. The patient should be asked to say 'Yes' every time he feels the touch. Areas of thickened skin, such as on the soles of the feet, will require a heavier stimulus than elsewhere. Often the patient's own finger tips can be used to map out an area of tactile loss. Von Frey hairs have been used as a more precise method of testing the sense of touch, but in practice these are not essential.

Pain sensibility

This is most easily tested using a sharp, sterile pin. The patient should be asked to report whether he feels a sharp sensation and it is often helpful to compare his reactions to the blunt and to the sharp end of a hat pin. The risk of transmitting hepatitis has led some physicians to forbid the traditional use of hat pins for this purpose by their staff and they suggest that a fresh sterile pin should be used for each patient. Unfortunately, the venesection needles which are often used are too sharp for sensory testing.

In practice, more than one pinprick should be made, each stimulus being of equal intensity, as far as possible. To achieve this, special devices have been designed to enable precise intensities of pinprick to be applied; however, in practice these are of little clinical value. If an area of impaired pinprick sensation is detected it is best demarcated by proceeding from the area of impaired sensation towards the normal.

Deep pressure sense

This modality may be simply estimated by pinching or pressing firmly over the tendons or muscles. Pain can often be elicited by pressure even when superficial sensation is diminished, whereas in some diseases, such as tabes dorsalis, loss of deep pressure pain may be a prominent feature, without superficial loss.

Temperature sensibility

Careful assessment of this sense requires a large object to be applied to the skin, and an unhurried examination. The perception of thermal stimuli is relatively delayed and the objects should be applied firmly and maintained in a single position for a few seconds. Under normal circumstances, it is possible to detect a difference of 1°C or less between successive objects within the range of temperature of 28–42°C and, for those who have the time, the procedure should be as follows:

The patient should be examined in a warm room and the areas to be tested exposed. Glass tubes should be used, one containing warm water (45°C) and one cold water (10°C). If areas of impaired temperature sensation are found the borders can usually be mapped accurately by drawing the tube along the skin from the insensitive to the normal region. In practice such detailed sensory testing will rarely yield valuable clinical information that cannot be obtained by the simple technique of applying a cold tuning fork to the area in question and asking whether or not the patient feels that it is cold.

Position sense

Loss of this particular sensory modality may be revealed in a variety of ways. If the patient stretches out his arms and closes his eyes, the affected arm may wander from its original position and if the fingers are spread apart they may undergo a series of changing postures (so-called piano-playing movements or pseudoathetosis).

Lack of a similar sense in the legs may be demonstrated by moving the patient's leg when his eyes are closed and he is seated, and asking him to point at his large toe. If position sense is defective in both legs, then the patient will be unable to maintain his balance with feet together and eyes closed (Romberg's sign). This sign, however, should be interpreted with caution. The patient should be asked to stand with feet together and eyes open and then be asked to close his eyes. If he sways only when the eyes are closed, then this can be regarded as positive. However, even a normal person will sway a little with eyes closed and a patient with cerebellar ataxia will sway, not only with eyes closed, but with eyes open.

Loss of position sense in the limbs is often most obvious in the fingers and toes. The digit should be firmly grasped at the sides opposite to the plane of movement and it may be worth moving the toe and asking the patient with his eyes open to describe the direction of movement. The patient should then close his eyes and be asked to describe whether the movement is up or down. It is said that as little as one degree of movement may be appreciated, although in practice it is not possible to move a digit such a small amount. What the observer is looking for is an asymmetry of appreciation of movement, or impairment to a degree that is clearly abnormal. Slight impairment may be inferred from a slow response.

Vibration sense

This sensation is a mixture of touch and rapid alterations of deep pressure sense. Its conduction depends on cutaneous and deep afferent fibres which traditionally are believed to ascend in the dorsal columns of the spinal cord. It is disturbed in cases of polyneuritis and in disease of the dorsal columns, medial lemniscus and thalamus. With increasing age, loss of vibration sense in the feet is common. It is tested by placing a tuning fork with a low rate (128), over the bony prominences. Patients must be informed that it is the vibration or buzzing that they are expected to feel: more subtle degrees of vibration loss may be delineated by allowing a vibrating fork to run down until the patient can no longer feel it and then this may be applied for comparison to the same part of the examiner's anatomy.

Discriminative sensory function

A special type of sensory disturbance results from damage to the sensory cortex or to the sensory fibres linking thalamus to cortex. Lesions in these areas may disturb position sense but leave the primary modalities of touch, pain, temperature and vibration sense relatively unaffected. In such a situation, or when a cerebral lesion is suspected, the following tests may be of value.

Two-point discrimination. The ability to distinguish two points from one may be tested by using a special instrument (a two-point discriminator) or a compass. The instrument should have blunt points, each of which is applied simultaneously. Such testing is usually only of value on the finger tips where a normal person should be able to recognise 3–5 mm of difference between the two points. A cortical lesion will often result in the patient mistaking two points for one.

Number writing (graphaesthesia). The ability to recognise numbers or letters on the palm of the hand depends on discriminative skills and is a useful test of these. Loss of this skill is called dysgraphaesthesia.

Cutaneous localisation. It is sometimes useful to test the patient's ability to localise a cutaneous stimulus with eyes closed. The patient may be simply asked to point to the part that was touched.

Appreciation of texture, size and shape (stereognosis). The ability to recognise texture of an object, for example the milled edge of a coin, and the ability to recognise the shape of an object, for example to differentiate between a 5 p piece and a 2 p piece, depends on cutaneous impressions and those from deeper receptors. Impairment of these may occur with lesions of the spinal cord and brain stem and in this instance will be associated with loss of the primary sensations of touch, pain, temperature and vibration. This type of sensory defect is called stereoanaesthesia. This should be distinguished from astereognosis, which refers to a similar inability when the primary sensations are intact and is due to a cortical lesion. Astereognosis in turn should be distinguished from tactile agnosia, which is an inability to recognise an object by touch or handling in both hands. This is a disorder of perception of symbols and results from a lesion of the dominant parietal lobe (p. 149).

PATTERNS OF SENSORY DISTURBANCE

MONONEUROPATHY (p. 245)

Changes in this instance will vary, depending on whether the nerve involved is predominantly motor, sensory or mixed. In sensory nerves the area of touch loss is usually more extensive than the area of pain loss. Because of overlap from adjacent nerves the area of sensory loss following damage to a cutaneous nerve is always less than its anatomical distribution. Deep pressure and joint position senses remain intact, because they are mediated by nerve fibres from the subcutaneous structures and joints. Particular types of pathological lesion may differentially affect the fibres in a sensory nerve. Compression typically disturbs large touch and pressure fibres and leaves intact small pain, thermal and autonomic fibres. Lesions of the brachial or lumbar sacral plexus may be differentiated from multiple peripheral nerve involvement by the distribution of the sensory and motor loss.

POLYNEUROPATHY (p. 238)

In most instances of polyneuropathy the longest and largest fibres tend to be involved. The sensory loss is most severe over the feet and legs and less severe over the hands, and the trunk and face are usually spared except in the most severe cases. Typically, the sensory loss involves all the modalities, although this varies depending on the type of neuropathy. The term 'glove and stocking' sensory loss draws attention to the distal pattern of involvement. However, it is an inaccurate term as the border between normal and abnormal sensation is not sharp and the sensory loss shades off gradually. In hysteria (see p. 480) the border between normal and abnormal sensation is usually sharp.

RADICULOPATHY

Irritative symptoms may be present when the dorsal roots are the subject of traction or compression. This shows itself as pain which is often limited to the dermatome belonging to the affected root. In some root disorders pain is absent and paraesthesias in the dermatome distribution are present. Damage to a dorsal root will result in loss of sensory modalities of all types within the distribution of the dermatome. Because of overlap between dermatomes, interruption of one single dorsal root will often give no definite sensory loss. When two or more roots have been completely divided, the zone of sensory loss is usually greater for pain than for touch; surrounding the area of complete loss will be a zone of partial loss.

SPINAL CORD SYNDROMES (Ch. 9)

Lesions of the dorsal horn (the tabetic syndrome) (Fig. 2.7(1))

Lesions of the dorsal horn produce syndromes similar to that seen in lesions of the dorsal roots. Depending on the number of segments involved there will be a segmental sensory loss affecting vibration and position senses in particular. Accompanying this may be pain which often is called 'lightning pain'. Such repeated pains are described as occurring at right angles to the skin and penetrating through an affected limb. Most commonly this syndrome results from neurosyphilis, although it may be seen in meningeal tumours and diabetes mellitus.

Transverse cord lesions (Fig. 2.7(2))

A complete transverse lesion of the spinal cord will be associated with loss of all forms of sensation below the segmental level which corresponds to the lesion. There may be a narrow band of hyperaesthesia at the upper margin of the level of sensory loss. Loss of pain, temperature and touch sensation is usually evident two or three segments below the level of the lesion, whereas vibratory and position sense is less easy to delimit. A progressive cord lesion is usually associated with ascending loss of sensation as the outermost fibres carrying pain and temperature sensation are from the legs. A lesion expanding from the centre of the cord, such as an intramedullary tumour, will tend to involve the innermost fibres carrying pain and temperature sensation and thus there may be relative sparing of the most superficial fibres from the sacral segments; this may lead to so-called sacral sparing.

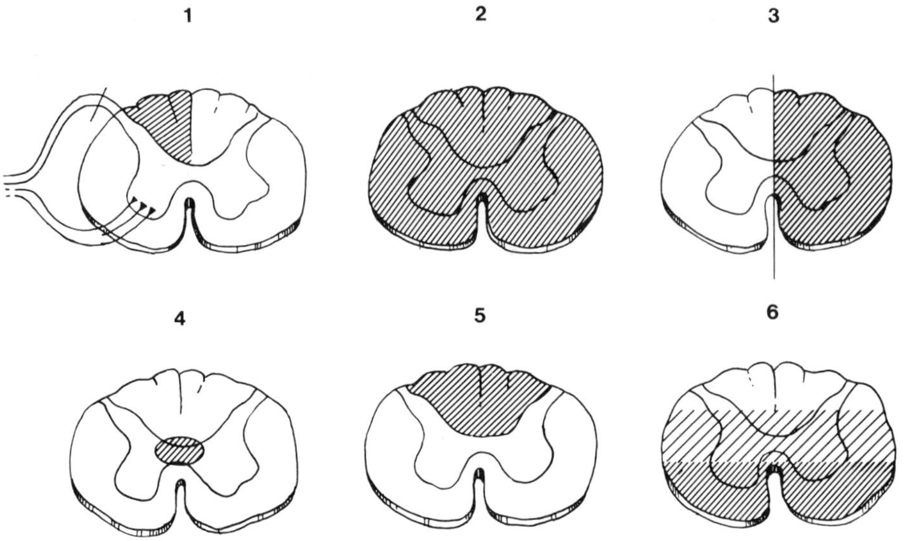

Fig. 2.7 1—The tabetic syndrome, 2—the transverse cord syndrome, 3—the hemisection of the cord syndrome, 4—the central cord syndrome, 5—the posterior column syndrome, 6—the anterior cord syndrome. (After Adams R D, Victor M 1981 *Principles of Neurology*, McGraw-Hill, New York, with permission.)

Hemisection of the spinal cord (The Brown-Sequard syndrome) (Fig. 2.7(3))

Occasionally in spinal cord disorders pathology is limited to one side of the spinal cord. Loss of pain and temperature sensation is found on the opposite side and the upper margin of this is usually two or three segments below the level of the lesion. Proprioceptive sensation is affected on the same side as the lesion and an associated motor paralysis occurs on the same side. Touch sensation is not involved, because the fibres are distributed in both posterior columns and the spinothalamic pathway on both sides of the cord. In clinical practice a complete hemisection of the spinal cord is rarely seen, although a partial syndrome occurs in multiple sclerosis.

Central spinal cord lesions (the syringomyelic syndrome) (Fig. 2.7(4))

A central spinal cord lesion characteristically will involve the pain and temperature fibres as they cross in the anterior commisure. Typically, these modalities are affected on one or both sides over a number of dermatomes, with relative preservation of tactile sensation (so-called dissociated sensory loss). Abolition of tendon reflexes in the affected segment is usually seen. The commonest cause of this is syringomyelia but intramedullary tumours, such as gliomas or ependymomas, may produce a similar picture. Dysaesthetic pain may also be seen in the affected segments or, in a progressive lesion, may precede the frank sensory loss.

The posterior column syndrome (Fig. 2.7(5))

In lesions preferentially affecting the dorsal columns there is loss of vibration and position sense below the level of the lesion, with preservation of pain, temperature and touch. When such a sensory loss affects the legs there is typically a sensory ataxia and a positive Romberg's sign. Sensory loss of this type in the hands produces clumsiness when manipulating small objects and inability to recognise shapes such as coins in a pocket. Tingling and pins-and-needles sensations are common and patients often complain that the hands and feet feel swollen or tight.

The anterior cord syndrome (Fig. 2.7(6))

In anterior cord disturbances there is typically damage to the spinothalamic tracts producing pain and temperature loss below the level of the lesion.

BRAIN STEM SYNDROMES

Because of the complex structure of the brain stem, with multiple ascending and descending tracts intermingled with a variety of cranial nerve nuclei, lesions result in far more complex clinical pictures than those which may be seen in spinal cord disorders. A characteristic feature of a medullary or lower pontine lesion is that the sensory disorder is crossed, i.e. there is loss of pain and temperature sensation on one side of the face and on the opposite side of the body. This results from involvement of the trigeminal tract or nucleus, resulting in ipsilateral facial sensory loss, and of the lateral spinothalamic tract, resulting in contralateral loss of sensation on the trunk and limbs. Higher in the brain stem the trigeminothalamic and lateral spinothalamic tracts run together and a lesion will therefore produce contralateral loss of pain and temperature sense on the whole of the opposite side of the body. In the upper brain stem the spinothalamic tract and the medial lemniscus become confluent, so that a lesion at this level may cause contralateral sensory loss of all types.

In brain stem lesions there is frequently bilateral involvement and a variety of syndromes have been described involving sensory, motor and cerebellar dysfunction accompanied by cranial nerve paresis (p. 77). Lesions, particularly vascular lesions, are rarely discrete and it requires a detailed knowledge of the anatomical structure of the brain stem to achieve accurate localisation. Another point of practical importance is that partial involvement of the sensory tracts may produce sensory impairment which may mimic lesions in the cord.

THALAMIC DISORDERS

Thalamic sensory disorders usually result from discrete cerebral infarcts. A destruction of the entire thalamic area receiving sensory fibre systems would be expected to result in an impairment or loss of somatic sensation in the whole of the opposite half of the body. In documented cases where such a lesion was identified, the perception of pain has often been found to be only slightly affected. Position sense typically is affected more profoundly than any other sensory function. Pure lesions of the ventroposterior lateral nucleus of the thalamus will be associated with contralateral sensory disorders of the limbs and trunk, whereas involvement of the ventroposterior medial nucleus will produce sensory impairment on the contralateral face.

In thalamic disorders there often is accompanying spontaneous pain or discomfort. These thalamic pains are often very intense and occur in paroxysms affecting the opposite side of the body. They typically are more pronounced in the face, hand or lower leg and are uncommon on the trunk (p. 190).

CORTICAL DISORDERS

Circumscribed lesions of the postcentral gyrus will be followed by localised sensory loss in parts of the opposite half of the body. This is typically a loss of discriminatory sensory function and includes loss of position sense, impaired ability to localise touch and pain stimuli, elevation of the two-point threshold, and astereognosis. In acute lesions of the parietal cortex there may appear to be impairment of pain sensibility, but this is rarely persistent or a prominent feature. The whole range of parietal sensory disorders is covered in Chapter 6.

Occasionally sensory seizures are seen in lesions of the sensory cortex, although these are rare. Typically, these show themselves as a wave of sensory irritative symptoms spreading over the body in accordance with the somatotopic organisation of the sensory cortex (p. 155).

SIMULATED SENSORY LOSS (p. 480)

A variety of sensory disorders may be simulated. Patients may complain of their simulated sensory loss but more commonly this is found incidentally during examination. The area of sensory loss is usually sharply demarcated and, in other than medical personnel, does not conform to a recognised anatomical distribution. Characteristically, pain loss is the most striking feature and loss of position sense is uncommon. Bearing in mind the difficulties of the sensory examination it is probably safer to ignore sensory findings that do not fit with any other neurological abnormalities that are present. Often it is possible to make a positive diagnosis of a simulated sensory loss because the individual's knowledge of anatomy is not sufficient to enable him to get it right. For example, anybody who is found to have unilateral loss of vibration sense on the skull can be confidently diagnosed as simulating this. It might be added, however, that the positive findings of a simulated sensory loss does not necessarily indicate that the whole of the individual's neurological problems are simulated. Sensory loss that is simulated is often added on to a patient's symptoms and signs as a degree of functional overlay.

FURTHER READING

Brodal A 1981 Neurological anatomy in relation to clinical medicine, 3rd edn. Oxford University Press, New York

Medical Research Council Memorandum no. 45 1976 Aids to the examination of the peripheral nervous system, HMSO London

3

Disorders of special sensation and cranial nerves

INTRODUCTION

The cranial nerves and their disorders probably cause as much confusion for non-neurologists as any other area of neurology. They do, however, provide an enormous number of neurological signs which greatly aid localisation, and their assessment has an important role in the examination of the unconscious patient. Without a good understanding of the function of cranial nerves, the clinician will have considerable difficulty with many neurological patients.

OLFACTORY NERVE AND DISORDERS OF SMELL

ANATOMY

A diagram of the anatomy of the olfactory nerve and its connections is given in Figure 3.1. Olfactory receptors in the mucous membranes of the upper part of the nasal cavity have central processes which pass through the cribiform plate to synapse with olfactory nerve cells in the olfactory bulb. First-order neurones pass centrally to make up the olfactory tract. This is related to the inferior surface of the frontal lobe and divides into medial and lateral olfactory striae. The medial striae carry fibres across the midline to the olfactory bulb at the opposite side; the lateral striae carry fibres to the medially situated uncus of the temporal lobe, the site of the primary olfactory cortex.

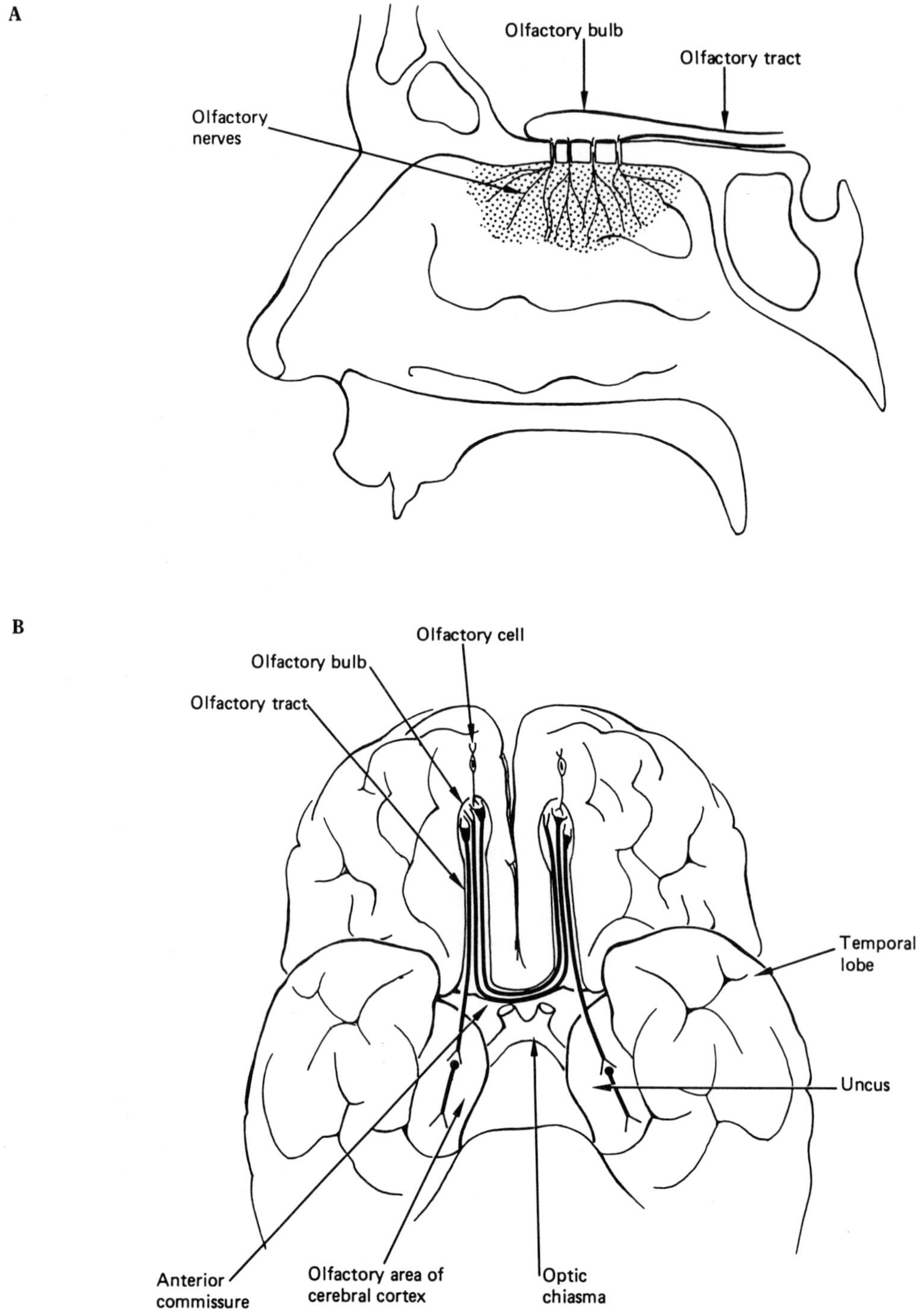

Fig. 3.1 The anatomy of the olfactory system showing: **A** the peripheral anatomy, **B** the central connections.

CLINICAL ASSESSMENT

Anosmia (absence of smell)

Patients with bilateral damage to olfactory receptors, bulb or tract, as well as complaining of loss of smell also describe loss of taste, as olfaction conveys more subtle information about aromas than does taste (which is more concerned with sweetness, bitterness, saltiness and acidity). Unilateral damage to receptors, olfactory bulb or tract will usually be asymptomatic.

Common causes of anosmia include head injury (see p. 365) and nasal infection. Anosmia is less commonly seen with olfactory groove meningiomas and other frontal tumours. Other causes of anosmia are summarised in Table 3.1. Anosmia may be temporary, but if the symptom persists for more than a few months it is likely to remain permanently.

Parosmia

Parosmia is an alteration and perversion of smell, which is characteristically unpleasant. Common causes include tumour, head injury and nasal infection, but it may also be a symptom of depressive illness.

Olfactory hallucination

Olfactory hallucinations represent a common and striking symptom of partial seizures arising in the medial aspect of the temporal lobe (uncinate seizures). These hallucinations tend to be pungent, such as burning rubber, or a smell of gas. Olfactory hallucination is not uncommon in psychosis, when unpleasant smells may be attributed to either the patient himself or to others.

The sense of smell may be tested using bottles containing coffee, oil of cloves and camphor, but exhaustive testing of this sensation is rarely necessary, the patient's description being of greater importance.

Table 3.1 Causes of olfactory symptoms

Symptom	Cause
Anosmia	Congenital/hereditary Nasal and sinus infection Nasal and sinus tumours Head injury Cranial surgery Subfrontal meningioma Hydrocephalus Frontal lobe tumours Mengingeal tumours Anterior communicating artery aneurysm
Parosmia	Nasal infection/tumour Head injury Depression
Olfactory hallucination	Uncal seizures Psychosis

TASTE AND ITS DISORDERS

The sense of taste is not invariably linked with a single cranial nerve and, because of its intimate association with sense of smell, is considered here.

ANATOMY

Taste buds are located over the surface of the tongue and pharynx and are chemoreceptors responding to four primary tastes: saltiness, sweetness, bitterness and sourness. Small non-myelinated fibres convey impulses from the anterior two-thirds of the tongue, initially via the lingual nerve by fibres which diverge after a short distance to enter the chorda tympani and the seventh cranial nerve, to run into the brain stem and synapse in the tractus solitarius of the medulla. Fibres from taste buds in the posterior third of the tongue, the soft palate and pharynx, pass with the glossopharyngeal and vagus nerves to the tractus solitarius. Second-order neurones probably pass up to the medial thalamus with synapses to third-order neurones closely associated with the tongue representation of the somatosensory cortex.

CLINICAL ASSESSMENT

Loss of taste is rarely an isolated symptom, but when present it usually indicates a disturbance of olfaction (see above). When genuine, gustatory disturbance is always peripheral and usually is dominated by other neurological symptoms such as facial weakness in Bell's palsy. Gustatory hallucinations are particularly common in seizures arising in temporoparietal regions.

OPTIC NERVE AND VISUAL DISTURBANCE

ANATOMY

A series of four neurones conduct visual information to the occipital cortex. Rods and cones, the specialised receptor cells of the retina, are connected via bipolar neurones of the retina to ganglion cells, axons of which run in the optic nerve via the chiasm and optic tract and relay mainly in the lateral geniculate body (a thalamic nucleus). The optic radiation sweeps through the temporal and parietal lobes to the visual cortex. A schematic representation of these pathways is given in Figure 3.2. Some fibres from the optic tract pass to the pretectal nucleus and superior colliculus to mediate light reflexes.

As well as being organised in relation to decussation of fibres, the optic pathway is also organised somatotopically in a precise fashion. In the optic nerve, fibres originating in the upper part of the retina (subserving the lower field of vision) are uppermost, and macular fibres are central. Following decussation at the chiasm, crossed and

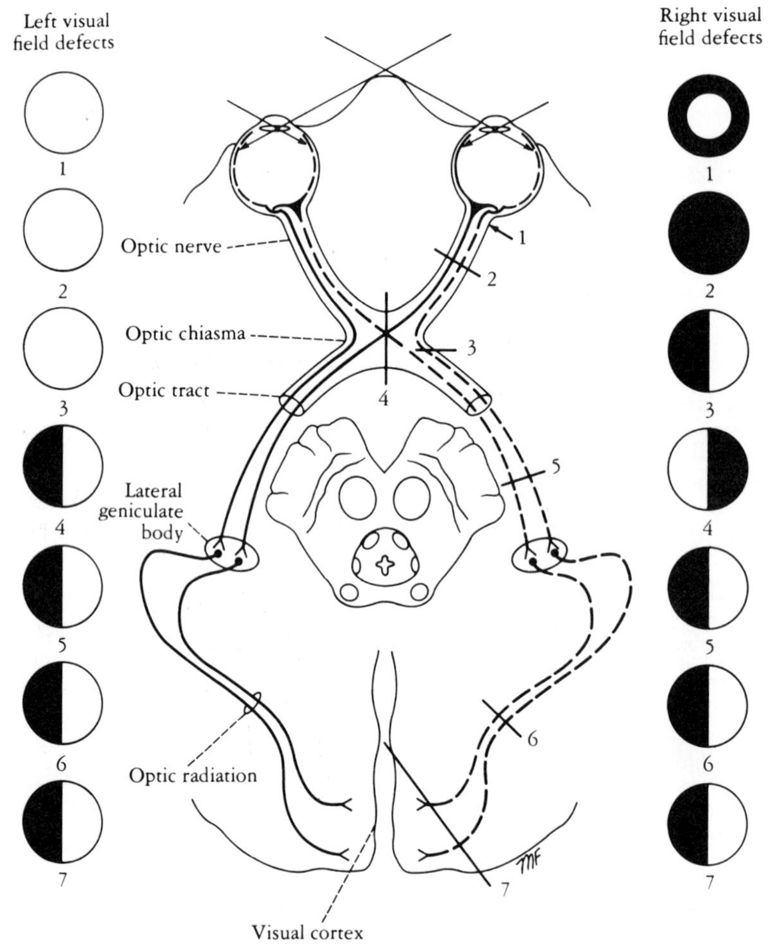

Fig. 3.2 The anatomical organisation of the visual system and visual field defects that may result from lesions at different sites. (Reproduced from Snell R S 1987 *Clinical Neuroanatomy for Medical Students*, Little, Brown & Co., Boston, with permission.)

uncrossed fibres from corresponding parts of the retina become reorganised and intermingled so that macular fibres are represented dorsolaterally, those from the upper retinal quadrants dorsomedially and those from the lower retina ventrolaterally in the optic tract. A similar distribution is found in the lateral geniculate nucleus, the larger part of this body being taken up centrally and posteriorly by the macular representation. Peripheral fibres terminate more anteriorly.

At the calcarine cortex, the largest most posterior area is concerned with macular vision, while upper retinal quadrants are represented above the calcarine fissure and lower quadrants below it. The macular area of vision is probably represented bilaterally, at the occipital pole.

CLINICAL ASSESSMENT

Symptoms

Symptoms of visual disturbance may encompass both positive and negative phenomena.

Negative visual phenomena

Impaired acuity. Patients complaining of *blurred vision* describe difficulty in reading, often because the central field of vision appears foggy or 'like looking through ground glass or water'. This symptom needs to be differentiated from patients with visual problems due to minor degrees of diplopia, whose symptoms are improved by covering one or the other eye. Impairment of visual discrimination is usually noted by patients in brightly lit conditions. Difficulties with vision in dimly lit surroundings (night blindness) are symptomatic of peripheral retinal disorders, such as retinitis pigmentosa.

The symptom of true visual blurring or visual loss, when unilateral, indicates ipsilateral disease of the orbit, retina or optic nerve; when it is bilateral it indicates pathology at or around the optic chiasm, or bilateral occipital lesions affecting the macular representation at the occipital pole (cortical blindness). Whereas pupillary responses are impaired in the former, they will be preserved in the latter, because fibres to the mid-brain will not be involved.

Blurring of vision or visual loss may be temporary and unilateral in amaurosis fugax, which is occasionally migrainous (p. 194) in younger patients but is a more important symptom in older patients with atheromatous carotid vascular disease (p. 276). The onset may be described as a curtain coming across or down the field of vision or, less commonly, as a patchy loss of vision likened to a jigsaw puzzle which gradually coalesces to result in complete loss of vision. It usually lasts for only a few minutes and vision reappears in a reverse fashion to its mode of onset.

Longer-lasting but recoverable unilateral visual disturbance lasting from hours to days or weeks is a characteristic of retrobulbar neuritis (see below). Rarely, this may affect both eyes simultaneously.

Transient bilateral impairment of vision may occur with visual obscurations in patients with raised intracranial pressure during bending, coughing and sneezing and is an important indication that vision is critically at risk.

Permanent visual loss may be very sudden, as in retinal artery occlusion, or may develop over a few days with retrobulbar neuritis. More commonly, however, it develops slowly and progressively in the syndrome of optic atrophy. The association of unilateral pain and visual loss suggests either orbital lesions (glaucoma, iritis), or optic nerve compression by tumours or aneurysm, or retrobulbar neuritis.

Symptoms of visual field loss. It is always important to differentiate between patients who attribute difficulty in seeing to one side (a true hemianopia) erroneously to a problem with one eye, and those with truly unilateral visual disturbance.

Many patients do not complain of homonymous field defects, particularly when these result from non-dominant hemisphere lesions, because these are so frequently associated with inattention. Such visual field loss may become apparent only because of patients bumping into objects in the hemianopic field or perhaps even driving motor vehicles into objects in this field. Field defects are most likely to result in symptoms when they involve the central field of vision, when the patient very often will complain of having to look round an impaired area of vision.

Visual field defects which are unilateral indicate lesions of the retina or optic nerves, but when they affect both eyes (in either a homonymous or heteronymous fashion) they are indicative of lesions at, or posterior to, the optic chiasm (Fig. 3.2). Field defects may be transient or permanent, depending on the pathology.

Positive visual disturbance

The most common positive visual disturbances are fortification spectra and scintillation during classic migraine. Such symptoms are usually perceived from both eyes and take up homonymous fields. However, on occasion anterior vascular spasm may result in unilateral scotomata. Similar primitive visual hallucinations occur more rarely, with partial seizures arising in the occipital lobe. More formed visual hallucinations may occur in both complex partial seizures and psychotic illness.

Rarer positive phenomena include movement phosphenes—a symptom of retrobulbar neuritis—in which movement of the orbit results in the perception of a glowing light by the affected eye.

Signs

Accurate assessment of visual function is essential for localisation of pathology in the visual pathways. Too often, permanent loss of vision results from the lack of adequate quantification and documentation of patients' visual function during the evolution of their symptoms. Furthermore, failure to test fully visual acuity, visual fields and pupillary reflexes will make interpretation of changes seen on ophthalmoscopy more difficult for the inexperienced observer.

Testing of visual acuity

This can be tested using a Snellen chart. The patient stands 6 m from the chart and at this distance should be able to read characters to 6/6 or better. The patient with 6/60 vision can discern at 6 metres what someone with normal acuity would discern at 60 metres. Alternatively, close vision may be tested using standard typescripts such as the Jaeger chart. It is important to correct for patients' refractive error by allowing the patients to use glasses, or by testing visual acuity through a pin-hole.

Testing of visual fields

Visual fields will usually be tested by confrontation, in which the observer's visual field is compared with that of the patient. A convenient object to use is the blunt end of a hat-pin. It is important to test both peripheral and central vision (the central 15 degrees of vision corresponding to macular vision). A red object or hat-pin is most sensitive for detecting central field defects. It must be remembered that, in patients with diminished acuity, larger-than-normal reference objects must be used to determine visual fields accurately. However, confrontation should be regarded as a screening test and any suspicion of visual field defects should be confirmed by formal perimetry in the case of peripheral visual disturbance or by Bjerrum screen in the case of central field defects.

Pupillary testing

A fuller discussion of the efferent limb of pupillary reflexes is in Chapter 4. In lesions of the anterior visual pathways including or anterior to the optic chiasm, the pupil may be larger at rest, and reacts more sluggishly to a direct light stimulus. However, the pupil will constrict on a light stimulus to the healthy eye (consensual reflex). After a light stimulus to a normal eye, some pupillary dilatation will be seen to occur after a brief period of constriction. This hippus may be more marked in the eye with an ipsilateral optic nerve lesion. Furthermore, an afferent pupillary defect may be demonstrated by swinging a light stimulus, first from one eye then to the other, and back again in a repetitive fashion. The eye on the side of an optic nerve lesion shows pupillary dilatation instead of constriction when the light is directly stimulating that eye (Marcus Gunn phenomenon).

The preservation of pupillary light reflexes in the presence of diminished or absent visual function differentiates optic nerve and chiasmal lesions from the much rarer syndrome of cortical blindness due to bilateral occipital lobe lesions, and from hysterical blindness.

Ophthalmoscopy

Ophthalmoscopy represents the most difficult aspect of visual examination. A number of differing structures must be examined.

Vessels. With increasing arteriosclerosis and hypertension, the lumina of *arteries* become narrowed and they assume a silver- or copper-wire appearance with increasing tortuosity. At sites where thickened arterioles cross veins there may be evidence of a-v nipping. In severe central retinal artery disease, occlusion may occur, resulting in pallor of the retina, gross narrowing of arterioles and a prominent reddened appearance of the fovea. Cholesterol or platelet emboli may occasionally be seen in the retinal arteries, after either amaurosis fugax or retinal artery occlusion.

Venous engorgement may be seen in papillitis and papilloedema (see below) and also in central retinal vein occlusions. Retinal vein pulsation will be lost.

Sheets of fine *capillary vessels* may be seen in severe diabetic retinopathy, but otherwise capillary disease is more likely to be manifest by haemorrhages.

Haemorrhages. Haemorrhages in the superficial layers of the retina tend to be flame-shaped because of confinement by horizontally orientated

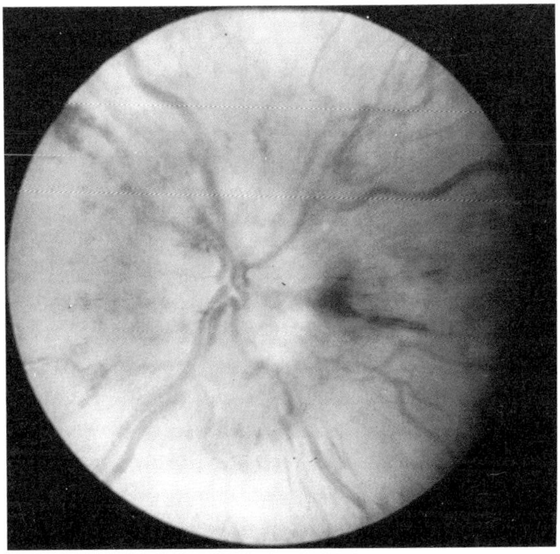

A

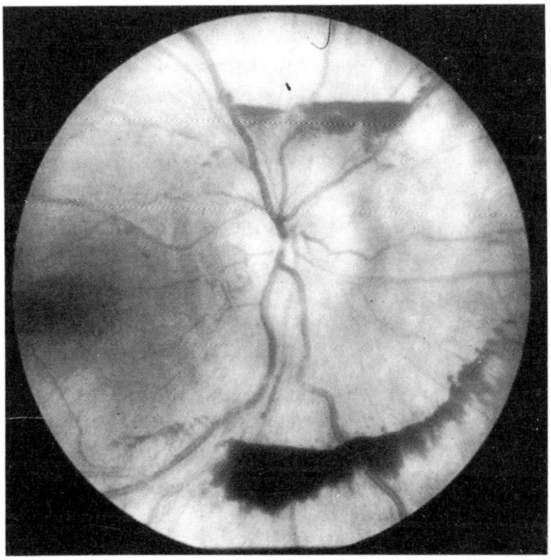

B

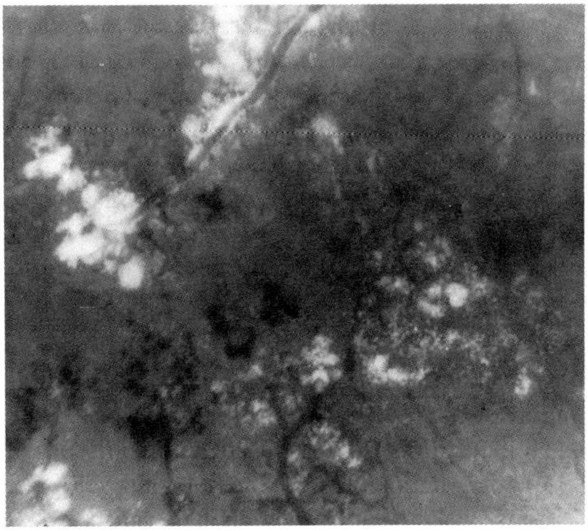

C

Fig. 3.3 Fundal appearances in: **A** acute papilloedema with venous engorgement, disc swelling, haemorrhages and exudates; **B** subhyaloid haemorrhage following subarachnoid haemorrhage associated with some disc swelling; **C** a florid vascular retinopathy with exudates and haemorrhages.

nerve fibres. Deeper haemorrhages are seen end-on as round (dot) haemorrhages (Fig. 3.3C), as these tend to be confined between radially orientated rods and cones. The rupture of arterioles caused by sudden rises in intracranial pressure in subarachnoid haemorrhage leads to accumulation of blood between the internal membrane of the retina and the vitreous (subhyaloid haemorrhage) (Fig. 3.3B). When the patient assumes an upright posture, red cells may settle because of gravity, giving a horizontal upper margin to the haemorrhage. However, this will not be the case if the patient remains recumbent! Some retinal haemorrhages may show central pallor (Roth's spots), which is said to be particularly characteristic of haemorrhages in bacterial endocarditis.

Exudates. Soft exudates occur due to infarction of the superficial retinal layers involving the nerve fibres. As such they overlie retinal blood vessels (Fig. 3.3C). Hard exudates are more commonly seen behind retinal vessels, usually in diabetes and hypertension. They sometimes may be arranged around the fovea in a macular star.

Retinal degeneration. Retinitis pigmentosa is seen peripherally as profuse black corpuscles in the hereditary trait that bears this name or, less commonly, in association with other disorders, e.g. Kearns–Sayre syndrome, Refsum's disease, Lawrence–Moon–Biedl syndrome. The choroid is often involved in inflammatory reactions in association with an iridocyclitis (e.g. in toxoplasma, syphilis, tuberculosis and sarcoidosis).

The optic nerve. Papilloedema consists of characteristic changes of varying severity: initially, retinal veins become congested and pulsation disappears; the optic disc becomes pink and the edges blurred; the optic disc becomes progressively swollen with, initially, loss of the physiological cup and, later, elevation of the optic head. Oedema around the optic head tends to obscure blood vessels and, subsequently, haemorrhages and exudates occur in a radial distribution around the optic disc. With chronic changes, the disc becomes more gliotic and optic pallor ultimately may develop because of secondary optic atrophy. The main causes of papilloedema are summarised in Table 3.2, and the appearances are displayed in Fig. 3.3A.

The most important causes of papilloedema are raised intracranial pressure and optic neuritis. The latter can be differentiated from raised intracranial pressure because of the complaints of visual loss which occur with optic and retrobulbar neuritis. The patient with raised intracranial pressure will develop visual failure only when the condition is chronic and, in this situation, increasing enlargement of the blind spot will be evident, in contrast to the centrocaecal scotoma of retrobulbar neuritis.

Table 3.2 Causes of papilloedema

Raised intracranial pressure
Optic neuritis
Retinal arterial disease
malignant hypertension
arteritis
Venous obstruction
cavernous sinus thrombosis
orbital tumour
Increased c.s.f. protein concentration
Guillain–Barré syndrome
spinal cord tumours
Miscellaneous
anaemia
hypercapnia
hypoparathyroidism

In a small proportion of patients some apparent swelling of the disc is evident without pathological significance. Such pseudopapilloedema may be seen particularly in hypermetropic patients, and in patients with drüsen of the optic head. In difficult cases fluorescein angiography may help to differentiate between true papilloedema and pseudopapilloedema. Increasing pallor of the optic disc occurs with optic atrophy (see below).

PATTERNS OF VISUAL DISTURBANCE

Visual symptoms and signs combine to produce a number of syndromes which aid localisation.

Disorders of the orbit and retina

Careful ophthalmological examination is essential to differentiate between ocular pathology and more posterior lesions in the visual pathways. Examination of the eye frequently also provides important information which aids the diagnosis of neurological disease.

The cornea

Opacification of the cornea itself is usually seen secondary to trauma or infection. However, clouding of the cornea may also occur in hypercalcaemia (e.g. in sarcoidosis, vitamin D intoxication and hyperparathyroidism). Crystal deposition may occur in cystinosis and with chronic chloroquine therapy. Polysaccharides may be deposited in Hurler's syndrome. Deposition of copper in Wilson's disease leads to the characteristic appearance of the Kayser–Fleischer ring which may be demonstrable only by slit lamp examination. Corneal ulceration and subsequent scarring may occur as a complication of herpes zoster infection in the ophthalmic division of the trigeminal nerve, as well as in Behçet's syndrome and Reiter's disease. Keratitis may be seen less commonly in congenital syphilis and tuberculosis.

The anterior chamber

Glaucoma represents an important factor in the differential diagnosis of visual disturbance. A patient with acute glaucoma may present with orbital pain, visual loss and opacification in the anterior chamber; more chronic glaucoma is associated with progressive visual failure, very often with peripheral visual field loss and characteristic cupping and pallor of the optic discs. In both instances, measurement of intraocular pressure will confirm the diagnosis.

The lens

Cataract formation may be seen in metabolic conditions such as diabetes, hypoparathyroidism and galactosaemia. It may be related to drug treatment with chlorpromazine or corticosteroids and is one of the hallmarks of myotonic dystrophy. Subluxation of the lens may occur in Marfan's syndrome and homocystinuria.

The retina

Lesions affecting the retina may give rise to symptoms of diminished visual acuity when the macular region is involved in macular degeneration. Retinal lesions such as choroiditis, haemorrhage and partial retinal artery occlusions will give rise to unilateral visual field defects, which usually reflect the topography of the lesion on the retina. However, centrally placed lesions, close to the optic head, may also disturb the conducting apparatus, causing a field defect corresponding to the fibres involved. This gives rise to nerve-bundle defects (arcuate or centrocaecal scotomas) spreading from the blind spot, which are also commonly seen with optic nerve lesions (Fig. 3.4).

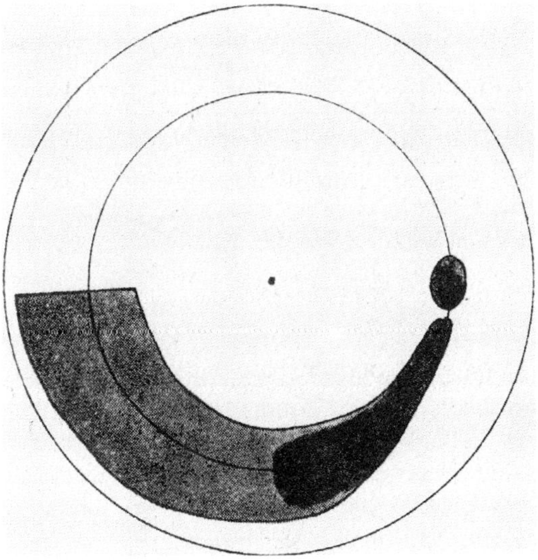

A

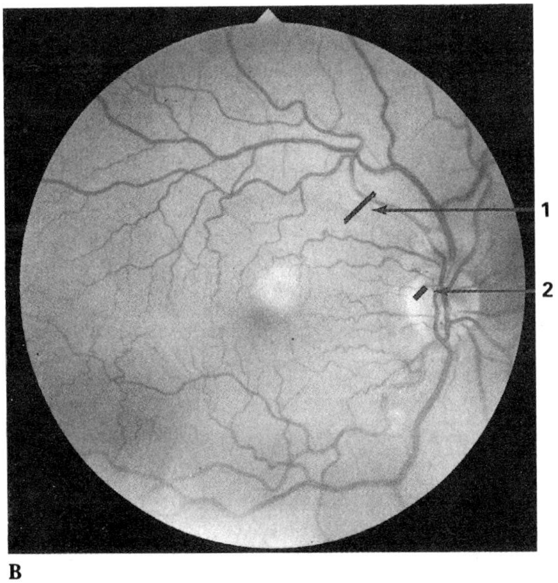

B

Fig. 3.4 The organisation of nerve fibres in the optic nerve and retina illustrating how lesions give rise to characteristic arcuate scotomas. In **A** the field defects, resulting from lesions at sites 1 and 2 in **B**, are illustrated.

Altitudinal or segmental unilateral visual field defects commonly indicate retinal pathology. These must be differentiated from bilateral altitudinal field defects attributable to occipital infarction, but ophthalmoscopic examination should avoid any confusion between anterior and posterior causes of altitudinal field defects.

Optic nerve lesions

Pathology affecting the optic nerves will present with one of three striking symptom complexes, i.e. retinal artery/venous occlusion, retrobulbar (optic) neuritis or progressive optic atrophy. Many individual pathologies are capable of causing these latter clinical syndromes.

Table 3.3 Causes of retrobulbar/optic neuritis

Demyelinating
multiple sclerosis
Devic's disease
Schilder's adrenoleukodystrophy
acute disseminated encephalomyelitis
Infections
orbital cellulitis/sinusitis
meningitis
viral encephalitis
postviral demyelination
neurosyphilis
Toxic/metabolic
tobacco–alcohol amblyopia
B_{12} deficiency
toxins (methyl alcohol, ethambutol, insecticides, etc.)
Hereditary
Leber's optic atrophy

Retinal artery/venous occlusion

In these disorders the onset of unilateral visual loss is over a period of minutes. Visual loss may be complete or partial, when segmental or altitudinal field defects may be found. Recovery is unusual.

Retinal artery occlusion may complicate any occlusive cerebrovascular disease. Retinal vein occlusion is most frequently seen with diabetes or hypertension but occasionally is symptomatic of haematological disorders such as myeloma, hyperviscosity syndromes, megaloblastic anaemias, and sickle cell disease.

Retrobulbar neuritis/optic neuritis

The syndrome presents with rapidly progressive visual failure over a period of hours or days associated with retro-orbital pain, which is frequently exacerbated by ocular movement or pressure on the orbits. Visual acuity will be markedly diminished and usually there is a dense central or centrocaecal scotoma. There is usually some visual recovery but its degree may well vary with the underlying pathology. The differentiation between retrobulbar and optic neuritis is made on the ophthalmoscopic appearances of papillitis in optic neuritis. This should readily be differentiated from papilloedema because of altered visual acuity which is a prominent feature of papillitis.

The causes of the retrobulbar neuritis syndrome are listed in Table 3.3. However, it is most common to fail to find any underlying cause for retrobulbar neuritis. A demyelinating pathology is often suspected in these instances and this may be confirmed by later neurological episodes. However, many younger patients with retrobulbar neuritis never suffer further clinical episodes. Although there may be pathological evidence at postmortem of such episodes, as shown by widespread plaques of demyelination, these can remain subclinical.

Optic atrophy

This syndrome is characterised by slowly progressive visual failure which may be unilateral or bilateral. There is evidence of diminishing visual acuity, pallor of the optic disc, and most commonly central field defects. An exception to this may be syphilitic optic atrophy, in which peripheral diminution of visual field is said to occur. The causes of optic atrophy are listed in Table 3.4. It must be remembered that any cause of retrobulbar neuritis may give rise to the fundal appearances of optic atrophy.

Investigation of optic atrophy must particularly exclude potentially reversible chronic raised intracranial pressure and local compressive optic nerve lesions. These problems will usually be associated with pressure headache or localised pain. One unusual presentation of frontal tumours is the

Table 3.4 Causes of optic atrophy

Retrobulbar neuritis (see Table 3.3)
Sequential optic atrophy (due to raised ICP)
Optic nerve/chiasmal compression
meningioma (subfrontal/tuberculum sellae)
pituitary tumour
optic nerve glioma
carcinomatous/chronic meningitis
Paget's disease of skull
arachnoiditis
Retinal disease (glaucoma/choroiditis)
Trauma
Multisystem degenerative disorders

Foster Kennedy syndrome, consisting of ipsilateral optic atrophy with contralateral papilloedema; this is, however, extremely rare.

Chiasmal lesions

Lesions of the optic chiasm present with increasing visual impairment, which may at first be unilateral, but which subsequently becomes bilateral. Unilateral or bilateral optic atrophy with, classically, bitemporal field defects are found. It must be remembered that chiasmal lesions are notorious for causing unusual field defects. These may initially affect only one eye, or affect central vision only. Temporal quadrantic field defects are not uncommon, when chiasmal compression arises predominantly from above or below. On occasions, binasal hemianopias may be seen as a result of lateral compression from atherosclerotic carotid arteries. Pituitary tumours are also capable of causing homonymous hemianopic field defects due to pressure on the optic tracts (see Fig. 3.2). In such instances the visual field defects are commonly incongruous (see below).

Early recognition of chiasmal compression is essential to prevent permanent blindness. The causes of chiasmal lesions are summarised in Table 3.5.

Table 3.5 Causes of chiasmal syndromes

Tumours
pituitary adenoma
craniopharyngioma
aneurysms of the circle of Willis
chiasmal glioma
secondary carcinoma
eosinophilic granuloma
Inflammatory
sarcoidosis
tuberculosis
basal arachnoiditis

Lesions of the geniculocalcarine pathway and visual cortex

Lesions posterior to the optic chiasm do not give rise to alterations in visual acuity (with the exception of bilateral occipital pole lesions). The anatomical basis for visual field defects of these lesions is schematically represented in Figure 3.2.

Lesions of the optic tract are rare and give rise to a contralateral homonymous hemianopia which is usually incongruous, i.e. it takes up a larger part of the field of the ipsilateral eye than the contralateral. Lesions of the temporal lobe tend to involve the lower parts of fibres in the optic radiation, thus giving rise to a contralateral upper quadrantic field defect. Parietal lesions, in contrast, involve upper fibres of the optic radiation, resulting in a lower homonymous quadrantic field defect. When either temporal or parietal lesions become extensive they are more likely to be associated with a homonymous field defect which splits the macula. Lesions of the occipital lobe in contrast give rise to contralateral homonymous hemianopic field defects which tend to spare macular vision.

In some instances parieto-occipital lesions give rise to inattention defects. The patient recognises an individual visual stimulus, e.g. a moving finger on the contralateral side, but when simultaneous stimuli are presented bilaterally he or she consistently ignores the stimulus in one visual field. Depending on the extent of the lesion, this may be associated with somatosensory inattention on the same side.

When they are bilateral, occipital lobe lesions may give rise to altitudinal field defects, bilateral tunnel vision or (even more rarely) bilateral central scotomata with reduced visual acuity. These possibilities arise because of the spatial representation of the field of vision over the visual cortex, peripheral vision being represented more anteriorly in the occipital lobes than macular vision. More complex disorders of the interpretation of visual material due to parietal and occipital lesions are discussed in Chapter 6.

THE INVESTIGATION OF PROGRESSIVE VISUAL FAILURE

Progressive visual failure demands full and active investigation to exclude a treatable neurological cause. Acute visual failure will usually be due to vascular causes (e.g. bioccipital infarction), or bilateral retrobulbar neuritis (see Table 3.3). Subacute or slowly progressive visual failure is more likely to be due to structural disease at or anterior to the optic chiasm (Tables 3.4 and 3.5).

Whilst it is essential to exclude toxic causes and deficiency states (Table 3.3), the main investigations required will be neurological imaging. CT scanning will display causes of raised intracranial pressure and most compressive lesions. However, small lesions may only be detected by air or positive contrast cisternography. Magnetic resonance imaging may prove a very useful tool. C.s.f. examination is necessary to exclude meningitic infection, tumour or arachnoiditis. In the last resort, surgical exploration may be necessary.

DISORDERS OF EYE MOVEMENTS

A full and conjugate range of eye movement is essential for normal visual function. Examination of eye movement conveys considerable information, allowing accurate localisation particularly of brain stem lesions. Unfortunately, the subject is poorly understood by those without specific neurological training.

ANATOMY

Figure 3.5 gives a schematic representation of the importance of anatomical structures controlling eye movements. The final common pathways are via the oculomotor cranial nerves (III, IV, VI), but superimposed upon these are higher levels of organisation, i.e. supranuclear and internuclear mechanisms.

Supranuclear centres and pathways

Frontal gaze centres are located anterior to the motor strip in the frontal lobe (area 8). They subserve voluntary eye movement which results in rapid jerky (saccadic) eye movements mediating the voluntary switching of the visual target from one object to another, and the fast phase of optokinetic or vestibular reflex nystagmus. Pathways from these centres pass in the anterior part of the internal capsule closely associated with corticobulbar tract fibres to connect with vertical and lateral gaze centres in midbrain and pons respectively.

At the hemispheric level there is also a parieto-occipital gaze centre which is responsible for coordinating the conjugate eye movement that mediates visual tracking of a moving object passing in front of the subject, in order to maintain its fixation in the macular field of vision. Such pursuit eye movements are slower and smoother than saccades. The pathways connecting this parieto-occipital centre to brain stem conjugate gaze centres are less clearly defined than those from frontal gaze centres.

Similar slow-velocity eye movements can be induced by vestibular stimulation via the vestibulo-ocular reflex; however, these persist in the dark, thus differentiating them from true pursuit movements.

At a brain stem level there are poorly defined centres controlling vertical gaze (anatomically related to the superior and inferior colliculi and third nerve nuclei in the mesencephalon), and lateral (pontine) gaze centres closely related to the sixth nerve nuclei. In addition to receiving inputs from cortical conjugate gaze centres, these brain stem centres also receive important vestibular, proprioceptive, tonic neck and somatosensory stimuli. They may also (to a lesser degree) be influenced by basal ganglia and cerebellar inputs.

Internuclear organisation

The vertical and horizontal brain stem gaze centres and the oculomotor nuclei are interconnected by the important medial longitudinal bundle which runs close to the midline between the mesencephalon and pons.

A

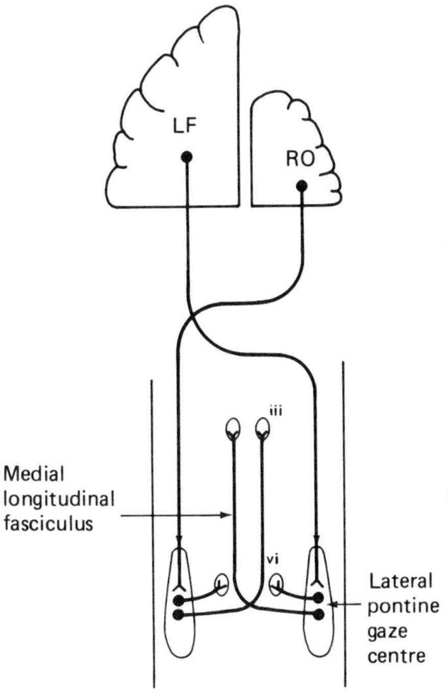

B

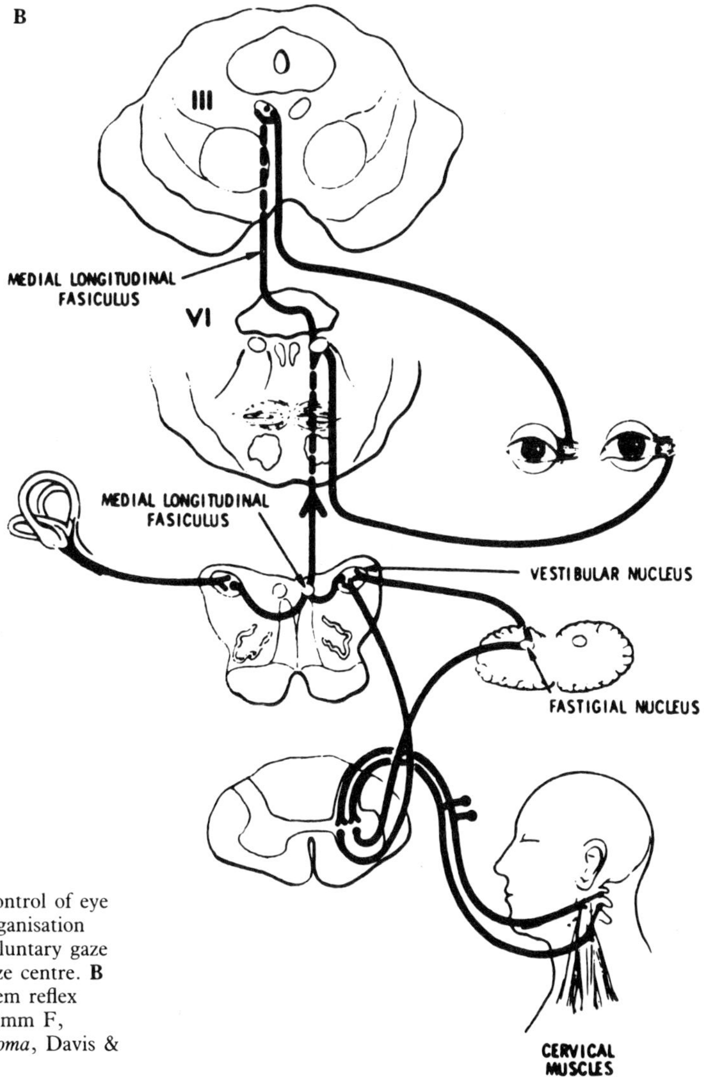

Fig. 3.5 The anatomical organisation of the control of eye movement. **A** Supranuclear and internuclear organisation represented schematically. LF = left frontal voluntary gaze centre, RO = right parieto-occipital pursuit gaze centre. **B** Vestibular and proprioceptive input to brain stem reflex control of eye movement. (Reproduced from Pimm F, Posner J B 1972 *The Diagnosis of Stupor and Coma*, Davis & Co., Philadelphia, with permission.)

Nuclear organisation

The third nerve nuclei are groups of paired nuclei close to the midline and ventral to the aqueduct of Sylvius. They consist of an autonomic nucleus (Edinger–Westphal) with, ventral to this, a nucleus mediating elevation of the lid, and innervating superior and inferior recti, inferior oblique and medial rectus, in this order from dorsal to ventral (Fig. 3.6). It appears that, whereas medial and inferior recti and inferior oblique are represented in a homolateral fashion in the oculomotor nuclei, superior rectus receives only crossed fibres; this can lead to a relative sparing of superior rectus in nuclear third nerve lesions. Levator palpebrei superioris has bilateral innervation at a nuclear level.

The efferent fibres from the third nerve nuclei pass ventrally through the brain stem through the median longitudinal bundle (Fig. 3.7A). The nerve emerges from the brain stem close to the posterior cerebral artery and tentorial hiatus. It passes anteriorly and crosses the internal carotid artery at the junction with the posterior communicating

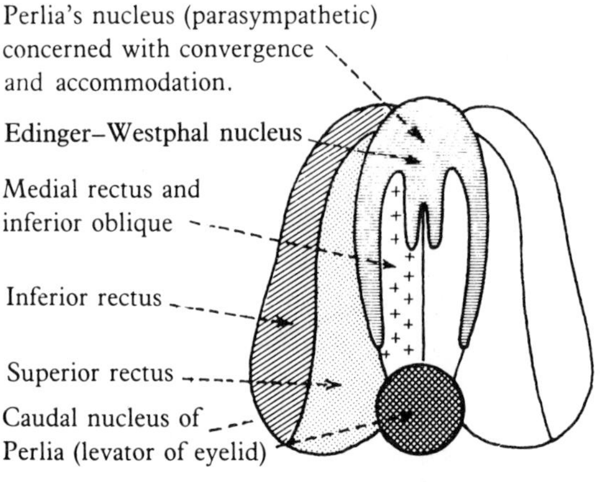

Fig. 3.6 The anatomy of the third nerve nucleus. (Reproduced from Lindsay K W, Bone I, Callander, R 1986 *Neurology and Neurosurgery Illustrated*, Churchill Livingstone, Edinburgh, with permission.)

artery. It then enters the cavernous sinus and passes via the superior orbital fissure into the orbit (Fig. 3.8).

The third nerve innervates the medial, superior and inferior recti, and inferior oblique muscles.

The nucleus of the trochlea nerve which innervates the superior oblique muscle is found immediately caudal to the nuclei of the third cranial nerve. Unlike the third and sixth nerves, the fourth nerve decussates and emerges after a short intramedullary passage from the dorsal surface of the brain stem caudal to the inferior colliculi (Fig. 3.7B). The nerve then passes anteriorly to enter the cavernous sinus (Fig. 3.8) with the third and sixth cranial nerves.

The fourth nerve innervates the superior oblique muscle.

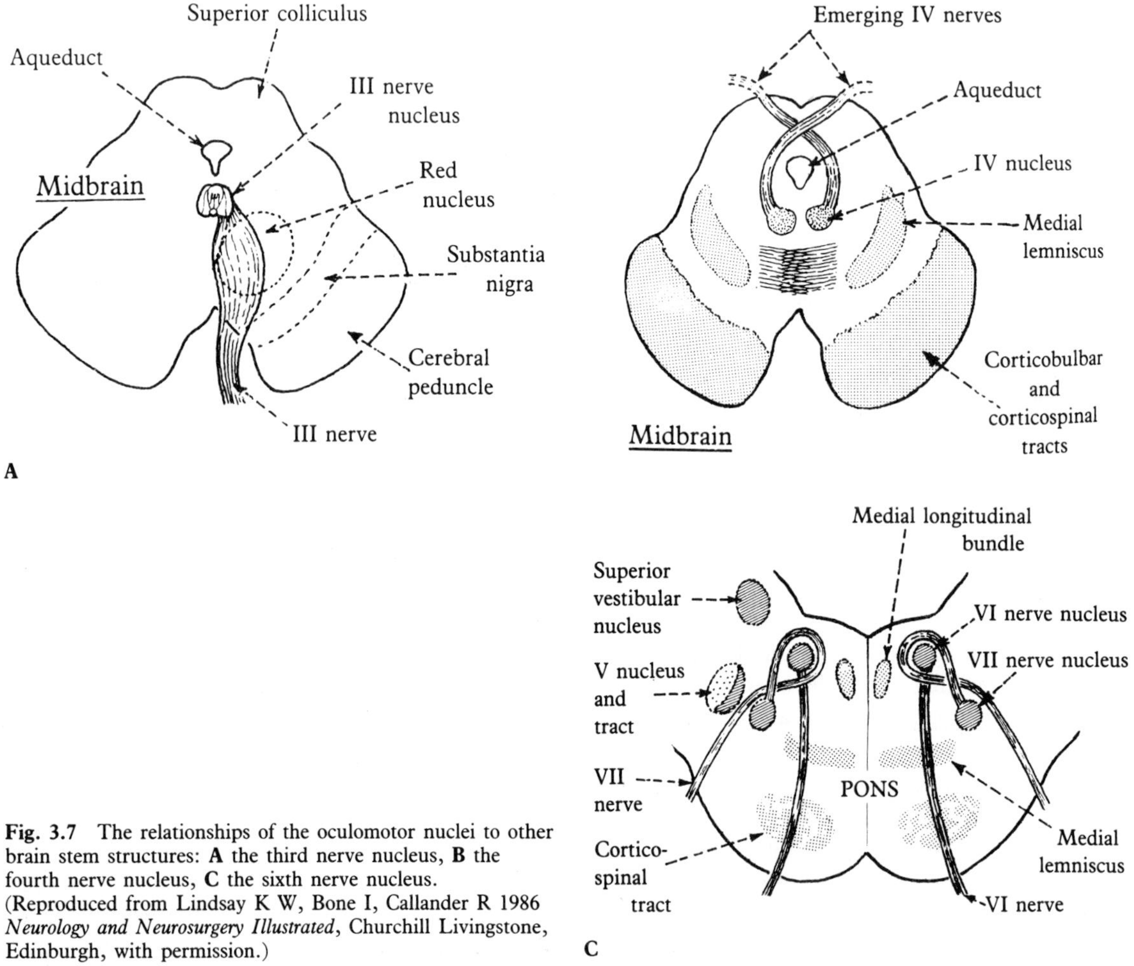

Fig. 3.7 The relationships of the oculomotor nuclei to other brain stem structures: **A** the third nerve nucleus, **B** the fourth nerve nucleus, **C** the sixth nerve nucleus. (Reproduced from Lindsay K W, Bone I, Callander R 1986 *Neurology and Neurosurgery Illustrated*, Churchill Livingstone, Edinburgh, with permission.)

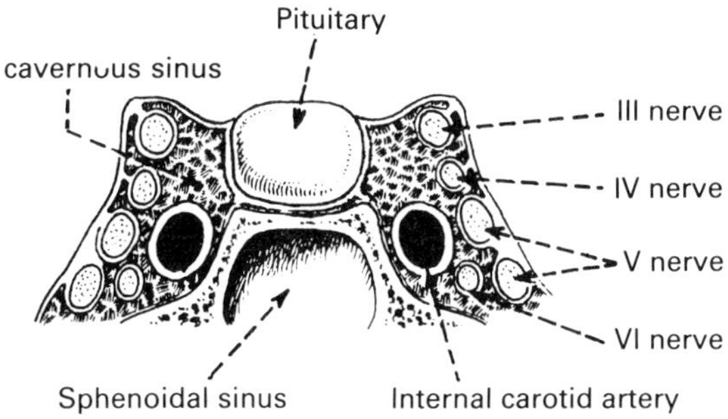

Fig. 3.8 The relationships of the cranial nerves within the cavernous sinus. (Reproduced from Lindsay K W, Bone I, Callander R 1986 *Neurology and Neurosurgery Illustrated*, Churchill Livingstone, Edinburgh, with permission.)

The sixth nerve nucleus is found at a pontine level close to the midline and ventral to the fourth ventricle. It is closely associated with the median longitudinal bundle and seventh nerve nucleus as well as the lateral gaze centres. Fibres pass anteriorly through the pons and pyramidal tracts (Fig. 3.7C) before leaving the brain stem and sweeping upwards to enter the cavernous sinus (Fig. 3.8).

The sixth nerve innervates the lateral rectus muscle.

EXAMINATION OF EYE MOVEMENTS

Examination of eye movements gives important information of localising value in both the conscious and unconscious patient. The position of the eyes at rest and eye movement during spontaneous activity should initially be noted, followed by formal testing of eye movements, not only in response to command, but also in response to visual and vestibular stimulation.

Eye movements to command

In testing eye movement it must be emphasised that it is *movements* that are tested, not individual extraocular muscles. This is best illustrated by considering the actions of the superior oblique muscle (Fig. 3.9). When in the central position the isolated action of superior oblique would be to cause intorsion of the eye because of the site of its insertion. However, when the eye is adducted by medial rectus it becomes a pure depressor of the orbit.

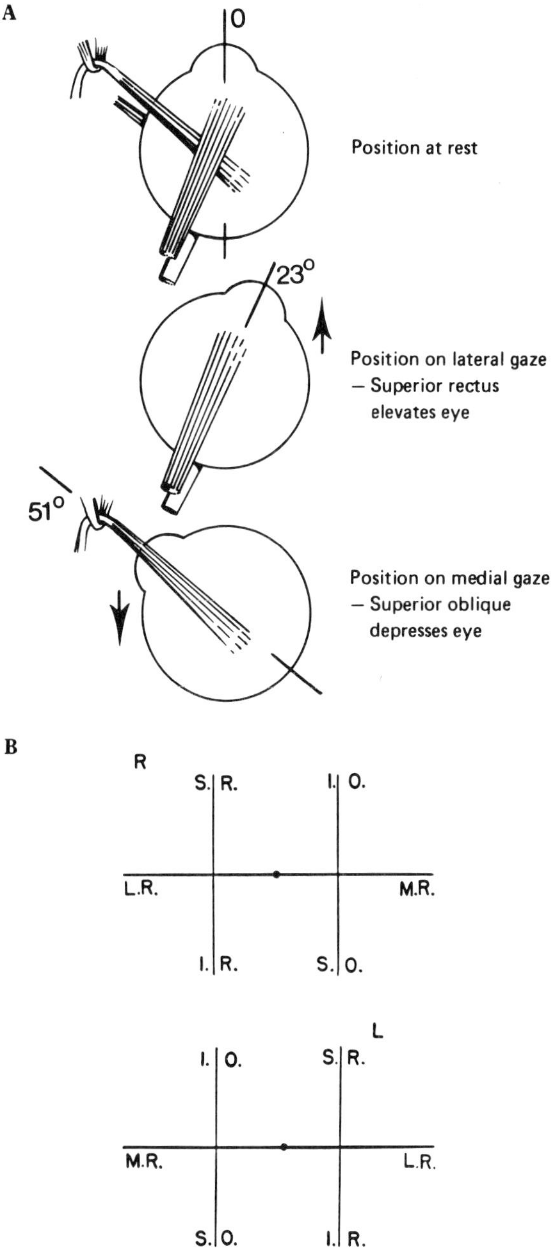

Fig. 3.9 **A** and **B** The planes of action of the extraocular muscles. S.R. = superior rectus, L.R. = lateral rectus, M.R. = medial rectus, I.R. = inferior rectus, S.O. = superior oblique, I.O. = inferior oblique.

When testing eye movement the patient should be requested to look to each side, to look up and

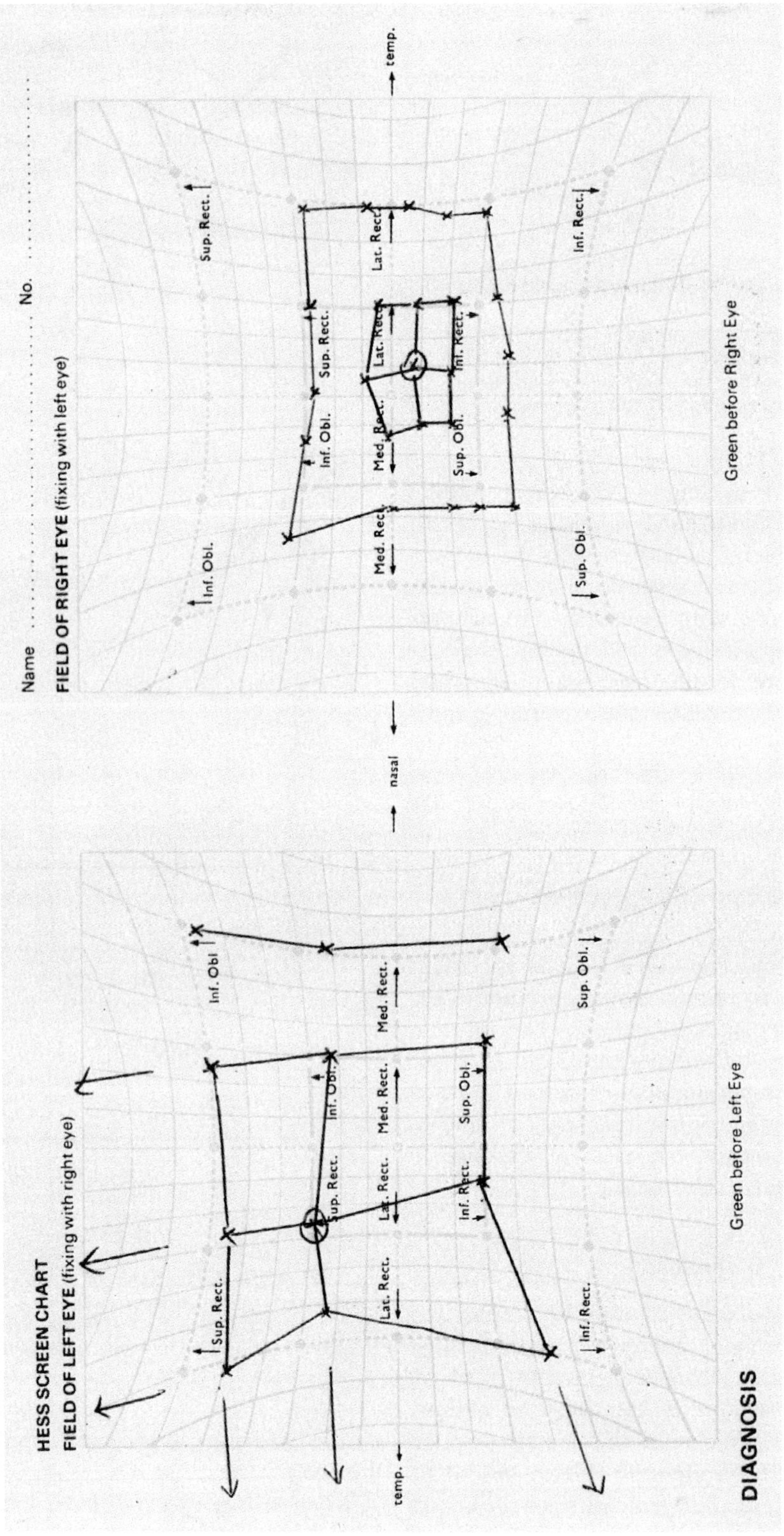
HESS SCREEN CHART
FIELD OF LEFT EYE (fixing with right eye)
Sup. Rect.
Lat. Rect.
Inf. Rect.
Sup. Rect.
Lat. Rect.
Inf. Rect.
Inf. Obl.
Med. Rect.
Sup. Obl.
Inf. Obl
Med. Rect.
Sup. Obl.
temp.
nasal
Green before Left Eye
DIAGNOSIS
Name
No.
FIELD OF RIGHT EYE (fixing with left eye)
Inf. Obl.
Med. Rect.
Sup. Obl.
Inf. Obl.
Med. Rect.
Sup. Obl.
Sup. Rect.
Lat. Rect.
Inf. Rect.
Sup. Rect.
Lat. Rect.
Inf. Rect.
temp.
Green before Right Eye

A

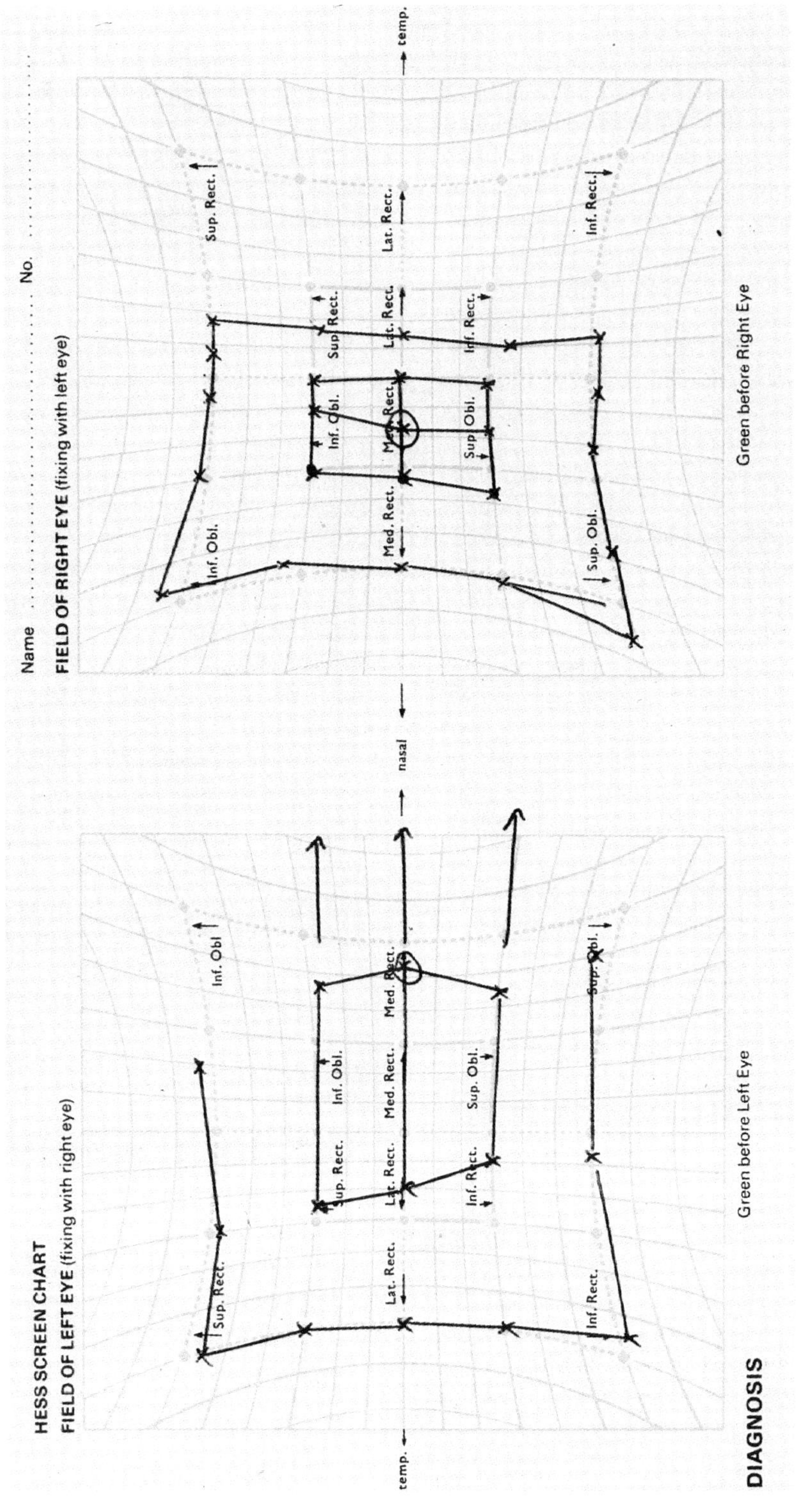

B

Fig. 3.10 Hess charts from patients with **A** a right third nerve palsy, **B** a right sixth nerve palsy.

to look down, as well as following the examiner's finger through a full range of abduction and adduction of the eyes with elevation and depression in full abduction and adduction. Such testing should detect major degrees of conjugate gaze paresis as well as dysconjugate abnormalities due to individual extraocular paresis and internuclear ophthalmoplegia. Figure 3.9B shows the major plane of action of the six extraocular muscles used for a full range of eye movement. With partial extraocular paresis, deviation of the eyes from parallel axes may not be apparent to the examiner and the patient will have to be questioned about the presence or absence of diplopia in varying directions of gaze. The following rules should be applied:

1. The plane of separation of images will correspond to the plane of action of the weak muscle or muscles. Thus, in lateral rectus weakness, images are separated horizontally, whereas in a superior rectus weakness, images will be separated vertically and horizontally.

2. The maximal separation of images will be when gaze is in the direction of action of the affected muscle.

Using these first two rules, all that will then be necessary will be to determine from which eye the false image is perceived. If a patient describes horizontal displacement of images which is maximal on gaze to the right, this might indicate either a right lateral rectus weakness, or a left medial rectus weakness.

3. Each eye is covered in turn and the patient is asked to decide whether the innermost or outermost image has disappeared. The peripheral image is always perceived by the eye associated with the weak muscle. Therefore in the case of a right lateral rectus weakness, when the right eye is covered the innermost image would persist, whereas when the left eye was covered, the outermost image would persist.

Although this scheme of examination will allow accurate identification of most extraocular palsies, in some more complicated instances doubts may persist. The Hess test may then be helpful.

The patient sits in front of a red Hess grid with his head immobilised. He is asked to point in turn to the points on the grid (Fig. 3.10) (the inner points are most commonly used, outer points may be used for minor disturbances) with a green light rod. One eye is covered with a green glass, the other with a red glass, and then the glasses are reversed. The positions at which the pointer appears to coincide with the dots on the grid are marked on a chart. The red covered eye will see the grid and dots, the green covered eye the green pointer.

The rules of interpretation are:

1. If the Hess field is not distorted, but merely displaced, this indicates a concomitant strabismus.

2. Muscle paresis produces shrinkage of the Hess field; relative overactivity produces expansion.

3. The eye with the paretic muscle is the one in which the field is diminished when covered by the green glass.

4. The paretic muscle corresponds to the most displaced point of the field, and can simply be read off from the chart (Fig. 3.10).

Complaints of diplopia from a single eye (monocular diplopia) are either hysterical or rarely indicative of disease of the retina, iris or lens of the affected eye.

Eye movement responses to visual stimuli

The connections between the parieto-occipital gaze centre and brain stem conjugate gaze centres can be tested by rotating a striped drum in vertical and horizontal directions in order to induce a following response and consequent optokinetic nystagmus (OKN). Such clinical testing should be sufficient to detect gross asymmetry in the slow pursuit phase of OKN, but electronystagmographic recording may be undertaken for more sophisticated analysis.

Eye movements induced by vestibular stimulation

Labyrinthine stimulation by rapid head movement causes the eyes to deviate in an opposite direction to the head movement in order to maintain the point of fixation (Fig. 3.11A). This response forms the basis of the oculocephalic reflex (doll's head reflex). The patient is asked to fixate on a stationary object (such as the examiner's brow) while the patient's head is rotated vertically and then horizontally. While this reflex can be voluntarily suppressed in the conscious patient, its presence in patients with impaired conscious states is helpful in indicating intact brain stem pathways connecting the peripheral vestibular apparatus with the brain stem vestibular nuclei, pontine and midbrain conjugate gaze centres. The relative preservation of a doll's head movement compared with voluntary or pursuit movement is also a hallmark of supranuclear gaze palsy (see below).

An alternative means of testing the vestibular influence of pontine gaze centres is by caloric stimuli. The instillation of cold water into the ear will result in a tonic deviation of both eyes towards the side of the stimulated ear (Fig. 3.11B). In a fully conscious patient this slow drift is opposed by rapid correcting movements to pull the eyes back to a central position, resulting in nystagmus. In patients with impaired consciousness this nystagmoid response is diminished or abolished, and only a tonic deviation of the eyes may be seen. Failure to see such deviation indicates impairment of the peripheral labyrinthine apparatus or, more importantly, its central brain stem connections. This represents a valuable means of assessing patients in coma (see p. 132).

A

B

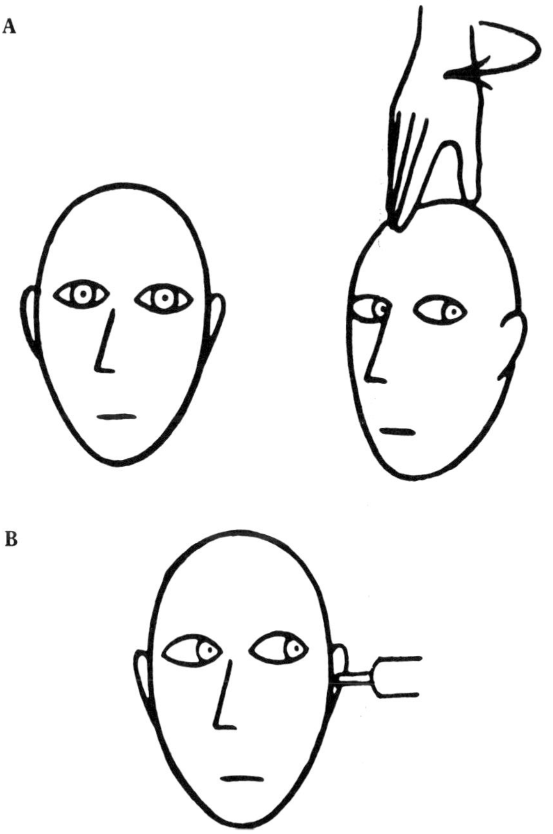

Fig. 3.11 Vestibular stimulation of reflex eye movements: **A** the oculocephalic reflex, **B** the caloric reflex to instillation of cold water. (Reproduced from Pimm F, Posner J B 1972 *The Diagnosis of Stupor and Coma*, Davis & Co., Philadelphia, with permission.)

SUPRANUCLEAR AND NUCLEAR DISORDERS OF CONJUGATE EYE MOVEMENT

Disorders of conjugate gaze are rarely a source of major symptoms in themselves. However, they give rise to important neurological signs.

Clinical disorders related to frontal gaze centres

Frontal gaze centres are located anterior to the motor strip in the frontal lobe. Tracts pass from this centre closely associated with corticobulbar tracts to vertical and lateral gaze centres in midbrain and pons respectively.

Unilateral disorders of the frontal gaze centres are common. Epileptic activity of this area results in forced deviation of the eyes and head to the opposite side and forms an important part of the adversive frontal lobe seizure.

Acute infarction of the frontal gaze centre leads to a failure of conjugate gaze away from the side of the lesion. Indeed, in the acute phase of such infarction the eyes and head may be tonicly deviated towards the side of the lesion, because of the unopposed action from the contralateral gaze centre. This is a feature of acute hemisphere stroke but compensation for this occurs usually within a period of a few days.

It is rarer to see bilateral lesions of frontal gaze centres. This condition may be congenital or acquired and results in a syndrome of oculomotor apraxia. The patient loses the ability to make voluntary eye movements and changes his direction of gaze by moving his head as a whole.

Commonly, impairment of voluntary eye movements may be seen in lesions of the internal capsule where bilateral infarction of the tracts connecting frontal and brain stem gaze centres and the closely associated corticobulbar tracts cause an association between impaired voluntary eye movement and pseudobulbar palsy.

Disorders of parieto-occipital gaze centre and connections

Integrity of the relationship between the parietal gaze centre and brain stem gaze centres can be tested using a rotating striped drum to induce optokinetic nystagmus.

Epileptic discharge in parietal regions may lead to deviation of the eyes, but these symptoms will usually be dominated by the presence of positive somatosensory and visual disturbance. Unilateral parietal lesions, e.g. infarction or tumour, lead to loss of optokinetic nystagmus in a horizontal plane.

Progressive supranuclear palsy (Steele–Richardson–Olszewski syndrome)

In this degenerative disorder (see p. 392) there is a progressive impairment, first of vertical and then of lateral eye movements. It can be shown that both voluntary and optokinetic movements become grossly impaired, but some residual eye movements can be elicited by brain-stem reflexes (e.g. doll's head eye movements and caloric stimulation). This constellation of findings forms the clinical syndrome of supranuclear gaze palsy, which is caused by damage to connections between the frontal and parietal cortical centres and brain stem gaze centres. It is associated with extrapyramidal and pyramidal features and a mild dementia.

Disorders due to basal ganglia disturbance

The basal ganglia play an important role in influencing vertical eye movements. They may mediate compensatory vertical eye movements to maintain the direction of gaze during walking.

Overactivity of basal ganglia input to brain stem gaze centres causes oculogyric crisis which is now most commonly seen in idiosyncratic reactions to phenothiazines and other dopamine receptor antagonists such as metoclopramide. Historically, they were a prominent feature of postencephalitic parkinsonism.

More commonly, impairment of basal ganglia input to vertical gaze centres is responsible for the mild to moderate impairment of vertical gaze which is commonly seen in both Parkinson's disease and ageing.

Lesions directly affecting the vertical gaze centre

Lesions of the pretectal region of the midbrain result in a paralysis of gaze in a vertical plane, giving rise to Parinaud's syndrome. Upward gaze is usually more affected than downward gaze and there is frequently some pupillary dilatation with loss of convergence and accommodatory pupillary reflexes. Very rarely, retractory nystagmus may be seen. The syndrome is most commonly seen with tumours of the pineal region, but elements of the syndrome will also be seen with symmetrical bilateral uncal herniation causing a diencephalic cone through the tentorial hiatus.

Lesions of the pontine lateral gaze centres

In contrast to lesions affecting the frontal gaze centres, which cause a failure of conjugate gaze to the opposite side, lesions of the pontine lateral gaze centre (receiving fibres crossing from the contralateral corticobulbar tract at a pontine level) result in ipsilateral paresis of lateral conjugate gaze. Thus, in acute pontine lesions the eyes are deviated towards the side of a hemiparesis, in contrast to acute frontal lesions where they are deviated away from the hemiparesis.

Such pontine lateral gaze palsies are not infrequently associated with ipsilateral facial weakness, contralateral sixth nerve palsy, or contralateral internuclear ophthalmoplegia (one-and-a-half syndrome).

INTERNUCLEAR EYE-MOVEMENT DISORDERS

Lesions affecting the centrally placed median longitudinal bundle, which runs the length of the

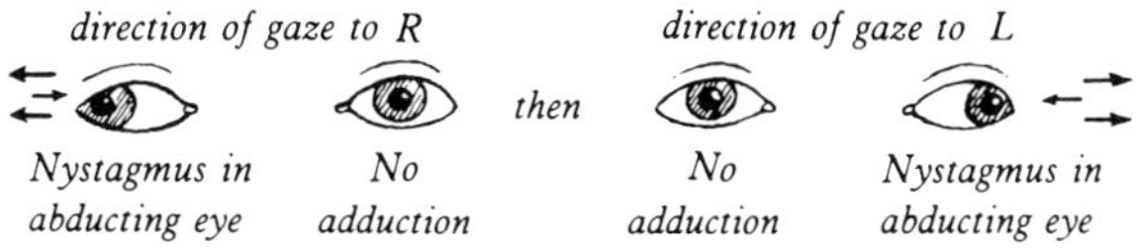

Fig. 3.12 Eye movements in internuclear ophthalmoplegia (ataxic nystagmus), resulting from lesions of the median longitudinal bundle.

brain stem joining the oculomotor nuclei in the midbrain and pons (Fig. 3.5) lead to a characteristic pattern of eye movement abnormality. Patients with this syndrome often have symptoms of associated ataxia, but rarely have ocular symptoms other than transient diplopia with lateral gaze.

On testing lateral gaze there is a failure of full movement of the adducting eye, while the abducting eye moves laterally and shows a coarse nystagmus (Fig. 3.12). In partial lesions all that may be seen is a slightly delayed movement of the adducting eye with the development of a nystagmus which is of greater amplitude in the abducting eye (ataxic nystagmus). Internuclear ophthalmoplegia can be differentiated from medial rectus nerve weakness, as convergence will usually improve the range of medial movement of the eye in internuclear ophthalmoplegia. Less commonly, posterior lesions of the median longitudinal bundle may give rise to failure of abduction during lateral gaze.

Although any lesion of the central mid-brain or pons may cause internuclear ophthalmoplegia, the syndrome is most commonly associated with demyelinating plaques in multiple sclerosis.

Skew deviation causes separation of the axis of the eyes in a vertical direction, with consequent vertical diplopia in the absence of oculomotor nerve or muscle disorder. The sign does not have major localising value and can be seen in lesions of both the midbrain and cerebellum.

NUCLEAR AND CRANIAL NERVE EYE-MOVEMENT DISORDERS

As soon as eye movements become dysconjugate, i.e. visual axes cease to be parallel, patients immediately experience diplopia. This symptom is most severe initially but with the passage of time suppression of one image may occur.

Third cranial nerve (oculomotor)

The relationship of the third nerve nucleus to other midbrain structures is illustrated in Figure 3.7. The third cranial nerve comprises an external oculomotor supply innervating superior rectus, inferior oblique, medial and inferior rectus; it also supplies levator palpebrae superioris and parasympathetic pupillary constrictor fibres to the pupil. Thus, in a complete third nerve palsy there is unilateral external ophthalmoplegia with the eye deviated laterally and slightly downwards; the pupil is dilated and there is a complete ptosis. With more minor degrees of involvement the ptosis may be less severe and the patient may then experience diplopia.

This clinical syndrome will vary in its associations, depending on whether the lesion responsible is sited in the brain stem or along the course of the cranial nerve itself. These syndromes are summarised in Table 3.6 and the anatomical basis of brain lesions is shown in Figure 3.7.

Lesions in the brain stem more commonly show dissociation between internal ophthalmoplegia (pupillary dilatation) and external ophthalmo-

Table 3.6 Clinical syndromes of the oculomotor nucleus and nerve

Site	Associated and distinguishing signs	Pathology
Dorsal midbrain	Contralateral tremor and ataxia	Vascular Tumour
Ventral midbrain	Contralateral hemiparesis	Vascular Tumour
Other localised midbrain lesions	Pupillary sparing	Diabetes Vascular
Tentorial hiatus	Ipsi- or contralateral hemiparesis and depressed consious level	Raised ICP
Carotid artery	Retro-orbital pain	Posterior communicating artery aneurysm
Cavernous sinus	Pain and ipsilateral IV, VI and 1st div. V	Cavernous sinus thrombosis Carotid aneurysm
Superior orbital fissure	Pain and ipsilateral IV, VI and 1st div. V	Tumours Granulomas

plegia; however, this rule is not absolute. Brain stem third nerve lesions are frequently associated with ipsilateral fourth nerve lesions and should be suspected whenever there is bilateral involvement of muscles innervated by the third nerve. Because of its anatomical organisation (see above) superior rectus may be relatively spared in nuclear lesions.

The fibres of the third nerve pass ventrally through the brain stem. More dorsal lesions are associated with contralateral red nucleus tremor (Benedict's syndrome), whereas more ventral brain stem lesions give an association between a third nerve palsy and contralateral hemiparesis (Weber's syndrome).

On leaving the brain stem the third nerves are closely related to the tentorial hiatus where they may be damaged in uncal herniation. They then pass forward in close association with the carotid artery where they may be damaged by posterior communicating artery aneurysms. The third cranial nerve then enters the carotid sinus where it is initially associated with fourth and sixth cranial nerves, as well as all three divisions of the fifth cranial nerve: tumours, cavernous sinus thrombosis, and aneurysms of the internal carotid may all give rise to third nerve lesions at this site. The third nerve gains access to the back of the orbit via the superior orbital fissure where it is associated with the fourth and sixth cranial nerves and the ophthalmic division of five: here these cranial nerves may be involved by invasive tumours and by granulomatous infiltration (Tolosa–Hunt syndrome).

When associated with pain, an isolated third nerve palsy must always be suspected as being due to a posterior communicating artery aneurysm, until proved otherwise. In many instances the cause of an isolated third nerve palsy will remain obscure, but vascular disease consequent on diabetes probably represents the most common cause. Brain stem demyelinating lesions rarely cause isolated third nerve lesions and more commonly give rise to internuclear ophthalmoplegia (see above).

Fourth cranial nerve (trochlear)

The trochlear nerve innervates the superior obligue muscle; this primarily depresses the orbit in adduction. Frank diplopia occurs when the patient looks downwards and away from the side of the affected eye. This very often presents particular problems to patients descending stairs, or reading. Often, compensatory head tilt is developed towards the opposite shoulder.

However, the picture of an isolated fourth nerve palsy is rare and nerve involvement usually accompanies and is dominated by the occurrence of third nerve lesions. In the presence of a third nerve lesion, testing of fourth cranial nerve function becomes more difficult. As the eye adopts a position of abduction under these circumstances, intact fourth nerve function is demonstrated by intorsion, rather than depression, of the eye.

It may be impossible to differentiate between nuclear and peripheral fourth nerve lesions. A nuclear lesion is indicated usually by involvement of the third nuclei leading to appropriate signs on the side opposite to the fourth nerve palsy (because of the decussation of the latter).

In peripheral lesions of the fourth nerve there is frequently involvement of third and fourth nerves because of the shared course in the cavernous sinus and superior orbital fissure. Trauma and vascular disease are perhaps the commonest cause of fourth nerve palsies.

Sixth cranial nerve

As the sixth cranial nerve supplies only the lateral rectus muscle, lesions result in diplopia with horizontal displacement of images. When complete, the visual axes converge at rest because of the unopposed action of the medial rectus muscle. Often, patients with sixth nerve palsies may either show unilateral eye closure or head turning towards the side of the lesion in order to reduce the degree of diplopia.

Sixth nerve dysfunction may result either from brain stem disorders or from more peripheral lesions. The anatomical basis of brain stem disturbance is shown in Figure 3.7 and the syndromes are summarised in Table 3.7.

More dorsal pontine brain-stem lesions cause lateral rectus palsy associated with seventh nerve palsy and varying degrees of nystagmus and paresis of conjugate gaze to the side of the lesion (Fig. 3.7). More ventral lesions involve the pyram-

Table 3.7 Clinical syndromes of the abducens nerve

Site	Associated and distinguishing signs	Pathology
Dorsal midbrain	Ipsilateral V and VII Conjugate gaze paresis	Vascular Tumour Demyelination
Ventral midbrain	Contralateral hemiparesis	Vascular Tumour
Petrous temporal bone	Ipsilateral V	Middle ear disease and Tumours
Cavernous sinus	Pain and ipsilateral III, IV and 1st div. V	Cavernous sinus thrombosis Carotid aneurysm
Superior orbital fissure	Pain and ipsilateral III, IV and 1st div. V	Tumours Granulomas

idal tract, giving rise to unilateral sixth nerve paresis with a crossed hemiplegia (Fig. 3.7). Isolated sixth nerve palsies may result from vascular disorders, tumours or nutritional disturbances (Wernicke's encephalopathy). Diabetes is again a common cause of an isolated sixth nerve palsy.

The sixth nerve emerges from the front of the brain stem at the pontomedullary junction and ascends on the front of the brain stem. It angles sharply forward over the petrous bone and it may be associated with fifth nerve lesions due to tumours of the petrous bone (Gradenigo's syndrome). It then enters the cavernous sinus to be associated with the other oculomotor nerves. The long intracranial course of the sixth cranial nerve is responsible for the fact that raised intracranial pressure with brain stem displacement commonly causes false localising sixth nerve palsies.

DISORDERS OF THE ORBIT LEADING TO EYE-MOVEMENT DISORDERS

Orbital tumour

Orbital mass lesions displace the globe of the eye, interfering with the normal plane of action of the extraocular muscles. They thus cause diplopia early in their development, but the symptom is usually associated with pain in or behind the eye, visual disturbance and proptosis.

On examination the most striking feature is proptosis and diplopia, usually at rest associated with non-axial displacement of the globe. Often the diplopia increases with eye movement, particularly upward gaze. Papilloedema can occur because of obstruction of venous drainage as well as optic atrophy. Ptosis is commonly present, but lid retraction may occur with thyroid disease.

A variety of pathologies may occur within the orbit (Table 3.8). Bilateral proptosis, chemosis, impaired upward gaze (particularly affecting superior rectus) and lid retraction are indicative of dysthyroid eye disease, although on occasion unilateral abnormalities are seen with this condition. Characteristic swelling of extraocular muscles with increased radiodensity is seen on CT scanning (Fig. 3.13). Very rarely tumours such as neurofibromas can result in bilateral proptosis.

OCULAR MUSCLE DISEASE

Dysconjugate eye movements and diplopia will also be seen in a number of conditions affecting the extraocular muscle themselves. Such disorders are characterised by diffuse involvement of extraocular muscles, with sparing of the pupil (Table 3.9).

Table 3.8 Causes of proptosis

Neoplastic
a. primary
- rhabdomyosarcoma
- optic nerve glioma
- neuroblastoma
- tumours of lacrimal glands

b. secondary
- carcinoma (metastases, spread from nasopharynx)
- lymphoma, leukaemia

Endrocrine
- dysthyroid eye disease

Vascular
- cavernous fistula
- cavernous sinus thrombosis
- orbital varices

Infective
- orbital cellulitis

Idiopathic
- orbital pseudotumour

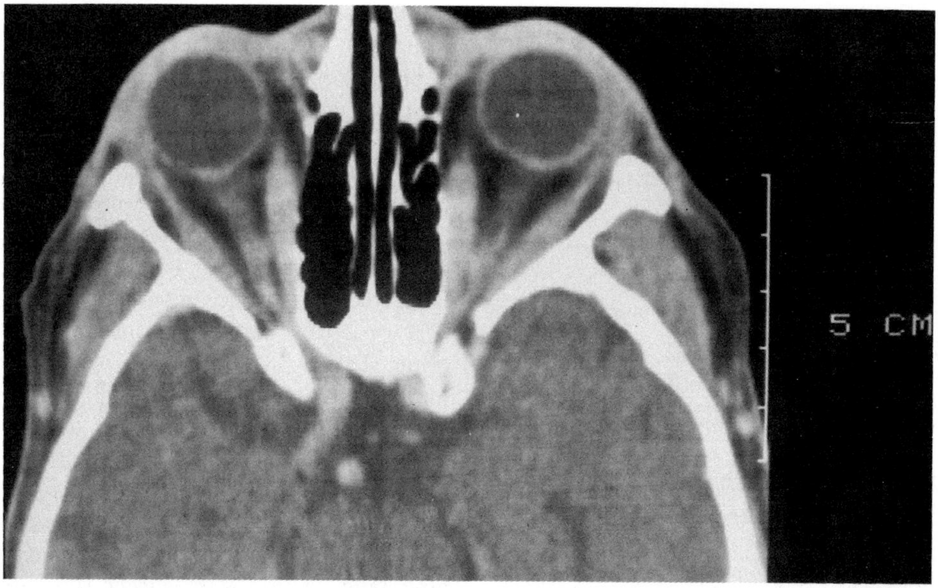

Fig. 3.13 CT scan in dysthyroid eye disease showing swelling and increased radiodensity of extraocular muscles, particularly the medial recti.

Perhaps the most common of such conditions is myasthenia gravis in which the diplopia and ptosis exhibit fatiguability and variability through the day; muscles mediating upward gaze are most frequently involved. Diplopia is also seen in dysthyroid eye disease where the diplopia and ophthalmoplegia are most commonly associated with exophthalmos, lid retraction and lid lag. The superior rectus muscle is often the first and most severely affected in dysthyroid eye disease.

Table 3.9 Disorders of extraocular muscles

Disorder	Associated signs
Neuromuscular transmission	
Myasthenia gravis	Fatiguability Bulbar weakness
Primary extraocular muscle disease	
Oculopharyngeal myopathy	Bulbar weakness
Progressive external ophthalmoplegia	
Ophthalmoplegia plus (mitochondrial cytopathy)	Proximal myopathy Retinitis pigmentosa Cardiac conduction defects Other c.n.s. disorders
Secondary extraocular muscle disease	
Dysthyroid eye disease	Proptosis Lid-lag and retraction

A variety of primary muscle diseases have been described under the term of progressive external ophthalmoplegia. Cases are often familial and there is a progressive impairment of all ocular movement, usually associated with ptosis and variably associated with other evidence of myopathy (e.g. oculopharyngeal dystrophy) or other central nervous system involvement with retinitis pigmentosa and heart block (ophthalmoplegia plus, or the Kearns–Sayre syndrome) (see p. 258).

Perhaps the most common cause of dysconjugate eye movements is long-standing congenital squint. One eye becomes partly amblyopic and the squint is concomitant, i.e. covering one eye allows correct fixation of the other eye, but both eyes will not be fixated correctly at the same time.

Ptosis

Whilst ptosis almost always accompanies weakness of the extraocular muscles it may also occur independently. The major causes of ptosis are summarised in Table 3.10.

Table 3.10 Causes of ptosis

Aetiology	Distinguishing factors
Congenital	Unilateral Occasionally bilateral No other neurology
Central Brain stem	Bilateral Impaired upward eye movement Coma is common
Third nerve and nucleus	Unilateral and may be complete External ophthalmoplegia Dilated pupil
Horner's syndrome	Unilateral and partial ptosis Small pupil Enophthalmos
Myasthenia gravis	Unilateral or bilateral ptosis + fatiguability + extraocular muscle paresis —
Ocular myopathy	See Table 3.9

NYSTAGMUS

Nystagmus may be defined as an involuntary rhythmic oscillation of the eyes. As in disorders of conjugate gaze, nystagmus may arise from lesions which impair brain stem vertical and horizontal gaze centres, or the vestibular, cortical or cerebellar inputs to these centres.

Nystagmus is rarely symptomatic, except in oscillopsia, in which patients with nystagmus experience movement of their visual field, either with their nystagmus or on walking. However, correct interpretation of nystagmus is of great localising value. Full evaluation of nystagmus may require study of its changes with changes in position of the eyes, changes in position of the head and, occasionally, changes in fixation.

Nystagmus of pathological significance must be differentiated from end-point nystagmoid jerks at extreme deviation of gaze or from the few unsustained nystagmoid jerks observed at the completion of a lateral or vertical eye movement. It must be remembered that some subjects can produce rapid oscillations of the eyes at will, which can be mistaken for nystagmus. These tend to be of high frequency and cannot be maintained for long periods.

Nystagmus may be spontaneous or induced physiologically by caloric or rotatory stimuli to the labyrinth or by opto-kinetic stimuli (see above). Pathological nystagmus may be of three types: pendular, phasic or dysconjugate (Table 3.11).

Dysconjugate or ataxic nystagmus is pathognomic of brain-stem disease and is discussed above (internuclear ophthalmoplegia).

Table 3.11 Classification of nystagmus

Physiological
optokinetic
vestibular (caloric/rotational)
Pathological
pendular
phasic
horizontal
rotatory
vertical
dysconjugate

Pendular nystagmus

Pendular nystagmus is characterised by oscillations of equal velocity and results from long-standing ocular disorders, with impaired macular vision from early in life. A similar syndrome has been described in miners (miner's nystagmus), although this phenomenon remains rare. Congenital nystagmus is a very dramatic eye movement disorder present from birth: movements are non-stop and pendular or phasic and usually present at the position of rest but usually are abolished by eye-closure. The movements are horizontal, rarely (if ever) vertical. The mechanisms giving rise to this kind of nystagmus are obscure.

Phasic nystagmus

Phasic nystagmus has fast and slow components alternating in opposite directions and, by convention, the direction of nystagmus is that of the fast component. The plane of nystagmus may be horizontal or vertical, or compound giving rise to rotatory nystagmus. A variety of types of phasic nystagmus may be seen.

Vestibular nystagmus. Acute labyrinthine, vestibular nerve or nuclear lesions cause an impairment of the vestibular drive which normally helps to maintain conjugate gaze away from the affected side. Thus, when the patient attempts to look away from the side of the vestibular lesion there tends to be a slow drift back towards the midline with a brisk correcting movement. This generates a nystagmus which is maximally seen on looking away from the side of the lesion, with the fast phase directed away from the side of the lesion. The nystagmus remains unidirectional, no matter what the direction of gaze, and is horizontal or rotatory.

Although this kind of nystagmus most commonly occurs with peripheral lesions of the labyrinth or eighth nerve, it is seen in brain stem lesions of the vestibular nuclei. Removing fixation may enhance this form of nystagmus when it has a peripheral origin but inhibit it when the nystagmus is of central origin.

Positional nystagmus. This form of nystagmus is elicited by positional testing (Fig. 3.14). The patient from sitting is pulled backwards so that the head hangs at an angle of approximately 45° over the end of the couch with rotation of the head and eyes to one side.

The most common kind of response to this stimulus is so-called 'benign paroxysmal positional nystagmus', with associated symptoms of vertigo. The nystagmus is rotatory and develops after a latency of 3–10 seconds and lasts for between 10 and 40 seconds. The nystagmus is specific for one particular head position and a burst of nystagmus in the reverse direction is sometimes seen as the patient sits up again. The response fatigues with repeated positional testing.

This type of response is particularly associated with labyrinthine disease and may be associated with other signs of vestibular disease, such as vestibular nystagmus or canal paresis. It is commonly seen following head injury, viral labyrinthitis and vascular disorders of the ear. However, positional nystagmus can be associated with brain stem or cerebellar lesions close to the fourth ventricle but here the nystagmus is usually purely horizontal or vertical. In this instance the onset of nystagmus is immediate, longer lasting, and the head posture which produces it less predictable. The response is less likely to fatigue with repeated testing and may not be associated with vertigo.

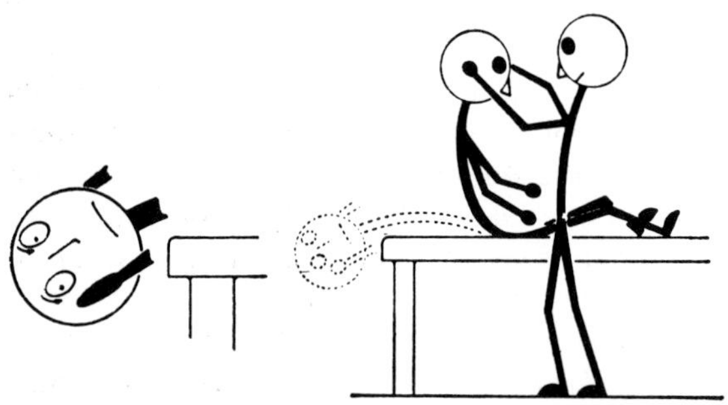

Fig. 3.14 Technique for exhibiting positional nystagmus. (Reproduced from Cawthorne T, Dix M R, Hallpike C S, Hood J D 1956 *British Medical Bulletin* 12: 131–142, with permission.)

Gaze paretic nystagmus. The hallmark of this form of nystagmus is that the direction of nystagmus varies with the direction of gaze. Fast phase is always in the direction of gaze.

This type of nystagmus indicates disorder of brain-stem centres controlling conjugate gaze. It is seen with drugs such as anticonvulsants, alcohol and sedatives; it is most commonly horizontal. Horizontal and rotatory gaze paretic nystagmus is of poor localising value. Vertical gaze paretic nystagmus is most commonly seen in patients who also have horizontal nystagmus. When occurring in isolation, vertical nystagmus is a useful localising sign. Upbeat nystagmus most commonly occurs with lesions of the midbrain at or around the superior colliculus, whereas downbeat nystagmus is a rare phenomenon that is most frequently associated with disorders at or around the foramen magnum (meningioma, Arnold Chiari malformation).

Cerebellar nystagmus. Pure cerebellar disorders are rarely associated with nystagmus in spite of a popular misconception to the contrary. Cerebellar lesions will most commonly cause nystagmus when they produce secondary brain stem disturbances. Occasionally, however, involvement of the flocculus of the cerebellum appears to result in nystagmus: in this situation there is a loss of drive towards the side of the lesion, resulting in a nystagmus with a fast phase towards the side of the unilateral cerebellar lesion (in contrast to vestibular nystagmus).

Convergence or retractory nystagmus. This unusual disorder causes rhythmic retraction and convergence of the eyes when the patient attempts to look upwards, or to converge. It is usually associated with other phenomena in Parinaud's

Table 3.12 Differentiation between peripheral and central phasic nystagmus

	Peripheral	Central
Direction of fast phase	Horizontal/rotatory	Any
	Unidirectional	Direction-changing
Fixation	Suppresses nystagmus	Little effect
Time course	Present days/weeks after acute lesion	May be permanent
Associated symptoms and signs	Deafness/tinnitus Vertigo	Brain-stem

syndrome (see above), resulting from pretectal mid-brain lesions.

See-saw nystagmus. This is rare; while one eye elevates, the other drops. There may be a degree of intorsion and extorsion associated with these movements. It is most commonly seen in patients with bitemporal hemianopia and visual impairment, but can also occur following basilar occlusion.

Differentiating peripheral from central nystagmus. The major problem in the interpretation of nystagmus is the differentiation between phasic nystagmus of peripheral origin and that arising from central disease. Although this differentiation can be difficult, a number of criteria summarised in Table 3.12 may be useful.

OTHER EYE MOVEMENT DISORDERS

Ocular dysmetria is a conjugate overshoot and undershoot of the eyes during voluntary saccadic movements to fixate on an object. It is analogous to intention tremor and is seen in cerebellar lesions.

Opsoclonus is a rare eye movement disorder with random rapid frequency conjugate movements; it is sometimes called the 'dancing eyes syndrome'. It may be associated with limb myoclonus in conditions such as brain stem encephalitis and as a remote effect of systemic carcinoma and neuroblastoma.

Ocular bobbing consists of abrupt conjugate downward jerks of the eyes followed by a slow return to mid position; it may be seen in massive pontine infarction or brain stem compression. Recovery is unusual.

Ocular myoclonus. A rhythmic oscillation of the eyes, this is seen very occasionally in association with the syndrome of palatal myoclonus (see below), when the eye movements are said to be synchronous with that of the palate.

FIFTH CRANIAL (TRIGEMINAL) NERVE DISORDERS

ANATOMY

The anatomy of the central connections of the trigeminal nerve and its area of cutaneous distribution of sensation in the three divisions are displayed in Figure 3.15. Sensory function is also discussed in Chapter 2.

The sensations of facial pain, temperature, touch and pressure are subserved by axons with cell bodies situated in the trigeminal sensory (Gasserian or semilunar) ganglion. The central processes enter the brain stem and either ascend or descend. Ascending branches terminate in the main sensory nucleus, subserving touch and pressure. Fibres subserving pain and temperature pass to the spinal nucleus, those of the ophthalmic division being represented most caudally and those of the mandibular division most rostrally. Proprioceptive impulses from facial and extraocular muscles are conveyed in fibres bypassing the trigeminal ganglion and have cell bodies situated in the mesencephalic nucleus of the trigeminal nerve. Axons of neurones of the main and spinal nuclei cross the midline to become closely associated with the medial lemniscus and ascend the thalamus, and thence project to the cortex.

The motor nucleus supplies axons to the muscles of mastication (masseters, medial and lateral pterygoids) as well as tensor tympani, the anterior belly of the digastric and the myelohyoid muscle.

The *ophthalmic division* of the trigeminal nerve runs through the cavernous sinus (with third, fourth and sixth nerves) (Fig.3.8) and enters the orbit through the superior orbital fissure. The *maxillary division* of the trigeminal nerve passes through the inferior part of the cavernous sinus

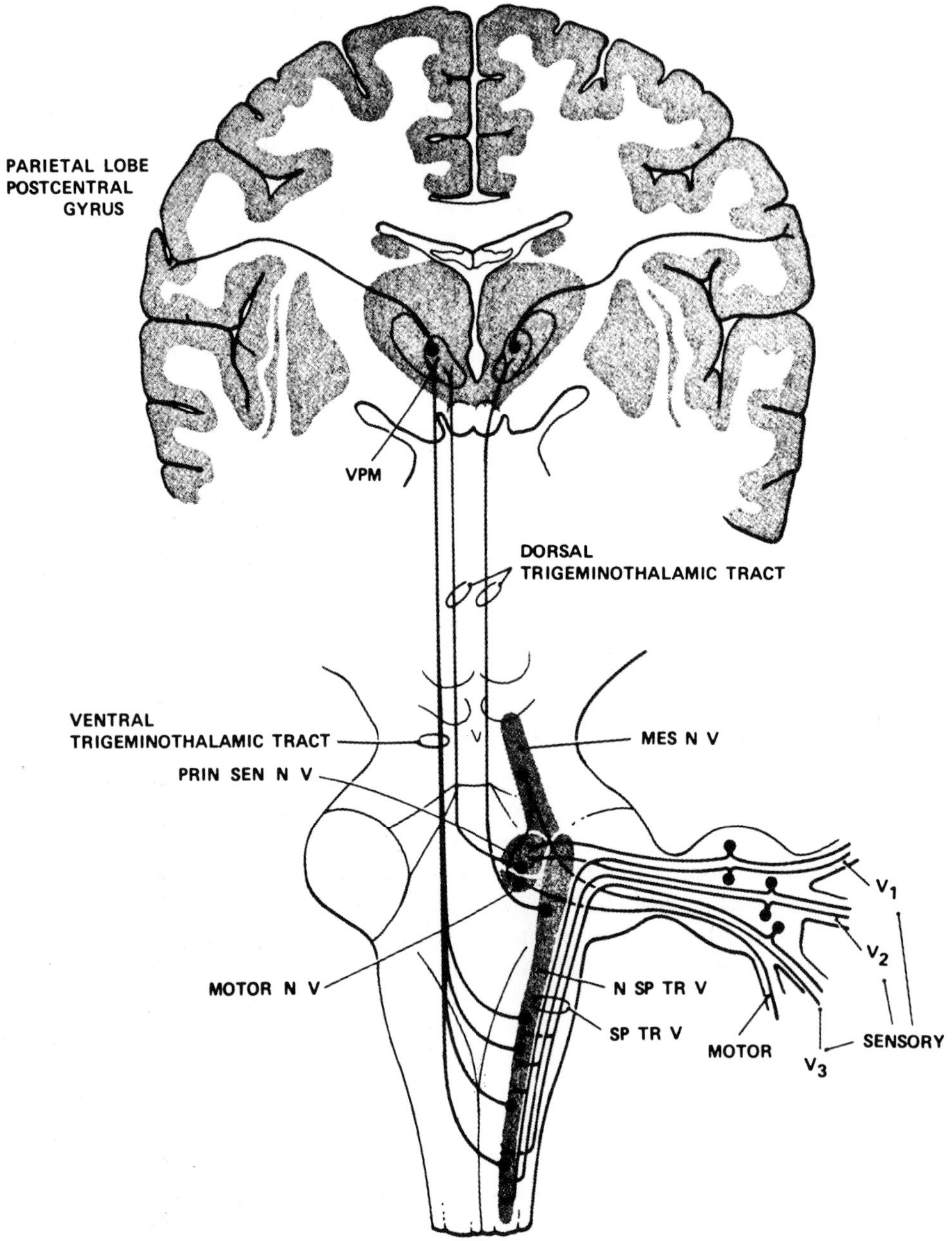

Fig. 3.15 Anatomical connections of the fifth cranial nerve. VPM = nucleus ventralis posterior medialis, MES N V = mesencephalic nucleus, PRIN SEN N V = principal sensory nucleus, MOTOR N V = motor nucleus, N SP TR V = spinal nucleus, SP TR V = spinal tract.

and via the foramen rotundum into the spheno-palatine fossa. It is joined by parasympathetic fibres here which are secretory to the lacrimal glands. It enters the orbit through the inferior orbital fissure and subsequently passes to the face via the infra-orbital foramen. The *mandibular division* of the trigeminal nerve is formed by the third division of the trigeminal ganglion and the motor root; these leave the skull through the foramen ovale.

CLINICAL ASSESSMENT

Symptoms

The commonest symptom of trigeminal nerve disturbance is pain. Detailed descriptions of specific trigeminal pain syndromes are given in Chapter 8. It must be remembered that facial pain is often referred from other structures innervated by the fifth nerve: the dura, sinuses and teeth. Numbness or paraesthesiae are less common symptoms, but when present greatly aid localisation of the lesion responsible (see below).

Complaints of weakness of the muscles of mastication are rare, but most commonly occur in myasthenia gravis (Ch. 10), when there is usually evidence of more extensive facial weakness.

Signs

Examination of facial sensation by classic methods is straightforward but invaluable for the accurate localisation of lesions. An early sign of sensory disturbance is often impairment of the corneal reflex, which is dependent on the ophthalmic division. Difficulties may arise in interpreting this reflex in the presence of an ipsilateral facial palsy, but it should be remembered that the reflex is bilateral in its expression so that an intact reflex is demonstrated by a contralateral response.

Wasting of temporalis and masseter muscles may be evident, and weakness of pterygoids is shown by impaired jaw opening or deviation of the jaw towards the side of the weak muscle. The jaw jerk which depends on the trigeminal nerve for both its afferent and efferent limbs is exaggerated in supranuclear lesions. It may not be elicitable in the normal subject.

PATTERNS OF TRIGEMINAL NERVE DYSFUNCTION (Table 3.13)

Brain-stem lesions

Lesions in the tegmentum of the pons may affect sensory and motor components of the trigeminal nerve commonly associated with sixth and seventh nerve palsies.

In other brain stem lesions, dissociation of sensory loss commonly occurs because of the widespread anatomical distribution of the trigeminal sensory nerve nuclei. Pontine lesions predominantly cause alteration of light touch with preservation of pain and temperature sensitivity. Lateral lesions of the medulla in contrast cause disturbances of pain and temperature sensation (commonly associated with disturbance of similar modalities in the contralateral arm and leg and ipsilateral facial weakness, Horner's syndrome, nystagmus and vertigo, as part of the lateral medullary syndrome) whereas light touch tends to be preserved. In central medullary lesions, such as syringomyelia, there is a characteristic advance of the border of analgesia towards the nose and mouth, giving rise to a 'balaclava' pattern of sensory loss. More rostral central lesions, such as syringobulbia, are more likely to be associated with circumoral paraesthesia and numbness, which advances in the opposite direction, i.e. from within outwards—so-called 'onion-skinning'. Lesions of the upper cervical cord and foramen magnum commonly cause disturbance in the ophthalmic distribution (with impaired corneal reflex) before mandibular and maxillary divisions are involved.

Table 3.13 Clinical syndromes of the trigeminal nerve

Site	Associated and distinguishing signs	Pathology
Dorsal pons	Ipsilateral VI and VII	Vascular Tumour
Lateral medulla	Pain and temp. V loss Contralateral pain and temp loss (arm and leg) Ipsilateral VII, Horner's vertigo and nystagmus	Posterior inferior cerebellar artery occlusion
High central medulla	Onion-skin analgesia	Syringobulbia
Low central medulla or high cervical cord	Balaclava analgesia	Syringomyelia
Cerebellopontine angle	Ipsilateral VII and VIII Nystagmus	Acoustic neuroma Meningioma AVM
Petrous temporal bone	Ipsilateral VI	Middle ear disease and tumours

Peripheral lesions of the trigeminal nerve

The trigeminal nerve may be involved between the pons and trigeminal ganglion by basal meningitic processes or tumours. The trigeminal ganglion lying in the cerebellar pontine angle may be compressed by acoustic neuromas or meningiomas at this site, where it is closely associated with the seventh and eighth cranial nerves. Autonomic fibres to the eye, lacrimal and salivary glands travel with the proximal divisions of the fifth nerve. Proximal lesions of the ophthalmic division may therefore be associated with Horner's syndrome and suppression of tearing (Raeder's syndrome).

More anteriorly, tumours of the petrous temporal bone can cause fifth nerve lesions associated with sixth nerve palsy (Gradenigro's syndrome). Ophthalmic and maxillary divisions of the trigeminal nerve enter the cavernous sinus but pathological damage in the anterior part will affect only the first division of the trigeminal nerve in association with the oculomotor nerves; the same is true for pathological changes at the superior orbital fissure.

Other syndromes of the trigeminal nerve

Syndromes of facial pain are discussed in Chapter 8.

Progressive unexplained facial sensory loss (idiopathic trigeminal neuropathy) is occasionally seen; this may lead to facial anaesthesia with trophic changes. Such cases are unusual and there is little information regarding their pathology. Facial sensory loss may occur with collagen vascular disorders.

Neuromas of the trigeminal nerve occur much less commonly than acoustic neuroma.

SEVENTH CRANIAL (FACIAL) NERVE DISORDERS

ANATOMY

A schematic representation of the relationships of the seventh cranial nerve in the brain stem and its course thereafter are given in Figure 3.16. The facial nerve supplies motor innervation to all the facial muscles with the exception of the levator

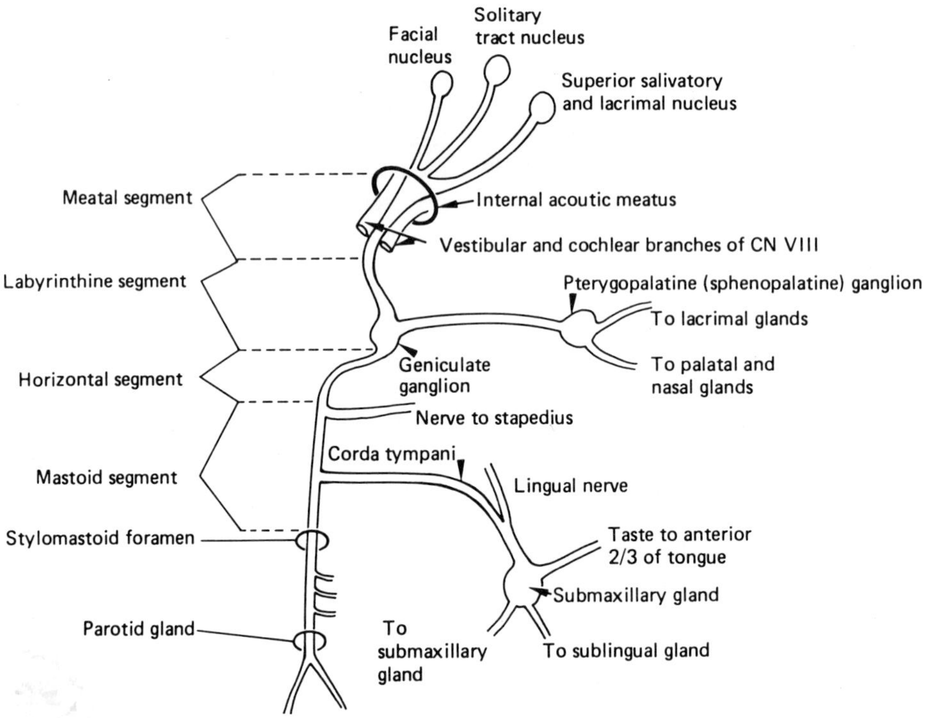

Fig. 3.16 Anatomy and course of the facial nerve.

palpebrae superioris. It also carries the corda tympani conveying taste sensation from the anterior two-thirds of the tongue and carries parasympathetic fibres to the lacrimal glands.

CLINICAL ASSESSMENT

Symptoms

Seventh nerve lesions cause facial weakness with variable weakness of eye closure, but never ptosis. Loss of taste sensation may be noted by the patient and symptoms of hyperacusis may occur due to involvement of the nerve to stapedius.

Signs

Facial appearance and movement should be examined at rest, during speech and normal patterns of movement, and more formally by comparing strength of eye closure on each side and the ability to smile and whistle.

A degree of facial asymmetry at rest is of no significance, whereas unilateral delay in blinking, or asymmetry during talking or smiling, may be. Patients with incomplete recovery from a facial palsy often show a marked degree of asymmetry, with facial contracture (synkinesis).

A variety of abnormal facial movements may be seen: these include hemifacial spasm, blepharospasm, myokymia and facial tics. Inappropriate movements may be seen in facial synkinesis when blinking may be associated with a twitch of the corner of the mouth, and smiling with partial eye closure. Florid orofacial movements are seen in choreic syndromes, particularly drug-induced disorders (tardive dyskinesias related to phenothiazines, or L-dopa-induced dyskinesias in Parkinson's disease) (p. 428).

Particular problems may arise with bilateral facial weakness. This is often missed by the inexperienced observer, or mistaken for the facial akinesia of extrapyramidal disorders. The problem should not arise if eye closure is formally tested.

Other seventh nerve functions rarely require clinical testing. Taste may be tested on the anterior two-thirds of the tongue, but assessing the stapedius reflex by measuring acoustic impedance is rarely necessary. Facial nerve palsies may be associated with abnormalities of tearing and salivation. Watering of the eye is common in severe upper facial weakness due to mechanical disruption of the lacrimal sac and duct; 'crocodile tears' can occur after recovery. Severe lower facial weakness is often associated with salivation from the corner of the mouth on the affected side.

PATTERNS OF FACIAL WEAKNESS (Table 3.14)

Supranuclear lesions

Because of the bilateral cortical representation of the upper facial muscles, unilateral supranuclear facial involvement is characterised by a more severe weakness of the lower face than upper face. Inability to close the eye is unusual in these circumstances, in contrast to facial weakness seen in lower motor neurone seventh nerve palsies. In some instances of supranuclear facial weakness there may be dissociation between voluntary and emotional facial movement, indicating slightly different pathways from the frontal lobe subserving these functions.

Bilateral supranuclear weakness may accompany pseudobulbar palsy. Extrapyramidal disorders are

Table 3.14 Clinical syndromes of the facial nerve

Site	Associated and distinguishing signs	Pathology
Supranuclear	Preservation of eye closure Ipsilateral hemiparesis	Vascular Tumour
Dorsal pons	Ipsilateral V and VII	Vascular Tumour
Ventral pons	Contralateral hemiparesis	Vascular Tumour
Cerebellopontine angle	Ipsilateral V and VIII Nystagmus	Acoustic neuroma Meningioma AVM
Basal meningitis	Often bilateral	Sarcoidosis Malignant meningitis
Temporal bone	No alteration in taste	Fracture middle fossa Middle ear disease

characterised by a poverty of facial expression in the absence of true weakness.

Pontine syndromes

Pontine lesions of the facial nerve are most commonly associated with sixth nerve palsies, and often with paralysis of the motor components of the fifth cranial nerve. Facial weakness may form a part of the lateral medullary syndrome (see below) and more central infarction may be associated with contralateral hemiparesis.

Posterior fossa syndromes

In the cerebellar pontine angle the facial nerve is involved by acoustic neuromas or meningiomas. In this instance, lower motor neurone facial weakness will be associated with loss of taste in the anterior two-thirds of the tongue, trigeminal and eighth nerve palsies. Facial palsy may also occur with meningeal infiltration, when it may be bilateral. Other causes of bilateral facial palsy include infective polyneuropathy and muscle disease, when more extensive cranial nerve involvement is usually evident, and sarcoidosis, infectious mononucleosis, Lyme disease and syphilis.

Syndromes of the temporal bone

Fibres from the corda tympani join the facial nerve proximal to the entry of the facial nerve into the facial canal: thus, more distal lesions are not usually associated with altered sensation of taste. Within the temporal bone the facial nerve can be involved in chronic middle ear disease, fractures involving the middle fossa and tumours in this area.

Extracranial

Inflammatory and malignant processes of the parotid glands may cause facial weakness, but often some parts of the face may be spared.

Primary muscle and neuromuscular end-plate disorders

Bilateral symmetrical weakness of facial muscles is most often seen in myasthenia gravis where there may be evident weakness of eye closure as well as ptosis and a myasthenic 'snarl' with attempts to smile. Facial muscle involvement may also occur in facioscapulohumeral dystrophies, polymyositis and dystrophia myotonica.

Other specific disorders of the facial nerve

Bell's palsy. Although the aetiology of Bell's palsy remains obscure, it is commonly believed to be related to swelling of the facial nerve within the facial canal, possibly as a result of viral infection. It can occur at any age, but is more common in young adults; it is rarely, if ever, bilateral. The development of facial weakness is acute over a period of a few hours and it is frequently associated with pain and discomfort in the mastoid region. Hyperacusis and, occasionally, loss of taste in the anterior two-thirds of the tongue may occur if the inflammatory process extends proximally. For reasons that are not clear, patients with Bell's palsy may complain occasionally of minor subjective facial sensory disturbance; however, this is never marked and the presence of objective sensory signs excludes the diagnosis of Bell's palsy.

The diagnosis of Bell's palsy should rarely present major problems. The association of other neurological signs rules out the diagnosis, as does bilateral facial weakness. An isolated lower motor neurone facial weakness is sometimes seen in multiple sclerosis but here it is more likely to be associated with significant sensory disturbance. Involvement of the facial nerve and its connections with herpes zoster (Ramsey Hunt syndrome—geniculate herpes) may be difficult to differentiate unless a careful search for vesicles, either on the tonsils or at the external auditory meatus, is made. Very rarely, lower motor neurone facial weakness may occur in association with migrainous headache (facioplegic migraine).

Complete recovery from Bell's palsy will occur in 80–90% of cases. Treatment with steroids, e.g. prednisone or ACTH, within the first day or two of onset may slightly improve the prognosis. Decompression of the facial nerve is not indicated. The eye must be protected with an eye patch while eye closure is weak, or, if prolonged, by tarsorrhaphy. There is little evidence that facial nerve stimulation affects the outcome.

In those cases in which complete recovery does not occur, there may be development of a facial synkinesis; this is due to aberrant reinnervation of facial muscles. The face appears asymmetric because of an apparent chronic spasm of the muscles at the angle of the mouth and around the eye. When the cheeks are blown out or the lips pursed, very frequently the eye on the same side will close. Blinking may be associated with movement of the corner of the mouth. More rarely, for similar reasons, eating may cause profuse tearing—'crocodile tears', instead of evoking salivation.

Hemifacial spasm. This is a disorder most commonly seen in middle or later life. It is characterised by spasms of varying speed and frequency, which are irregular but most frequently affect the musculature around the eye, and less commonly synchronously involve the muscles at the angle of the mouth and platysma. The syndrome is unilateral and no clear aetiology is usually found. The condition should be distinguished from facial tics (occurring in a younger age group), blepharospasm (which is usually bilateral) and myokymia (which is a more chaotic and unsynchronised muscular rippling seen around the eyes).

Hemifacial spasm is difficult to treat and tends to persist over many years. On occasion diazepam, phenytoin or carbamazepine may be helpful. Some success has been claimed for posterior fossa exploration. In some instances, aberrant vessels are found lying over the course of the facial nerve and geniculate ganglion: if these are pulled away, relief of symptoms may ensue.

Melkersson–Rosenthal syndrome. This consists of a rare triad of recurrent facial paralysis, facial and labial oedema and hypertrophy and fissuring of the tongue. The cause is obscure.

Facial hemiatrophy of Romberg. This is an unusual disorder which occurs mainly in females. There is loss of subcutaneous tissue on one side of the face and the skin appears wrinkled. Muscles and bones are not involved but on occasions localised hair loss may occur. Loss of retro-orbital tissue may result in enophthalmos. The condition is self-limiting but, on rare occasions, has been associated with atrophy of the contralateral cerebral hemisphere and occasionally with focal seizures.

Facial myokymia. This is a rippling movement of muscles around the eye, which may sometimes be confused with hemifacial spasm. It is most commonly seen with demyelinating brain-stem lesions, but very occasionally with brain-stem tumours.

DISORDERS OF BALANCE AND HEARING (EIGHTH CRANIAL NERVE AND CONNECTIONS)

ANATOMY

The eighth cranial nerve is composed of two divisions: the vestibular nerve and the cochlear nerve, subserving balance and hearing respectively. The central connections of these divisions are illustrated in Figure 3.17.

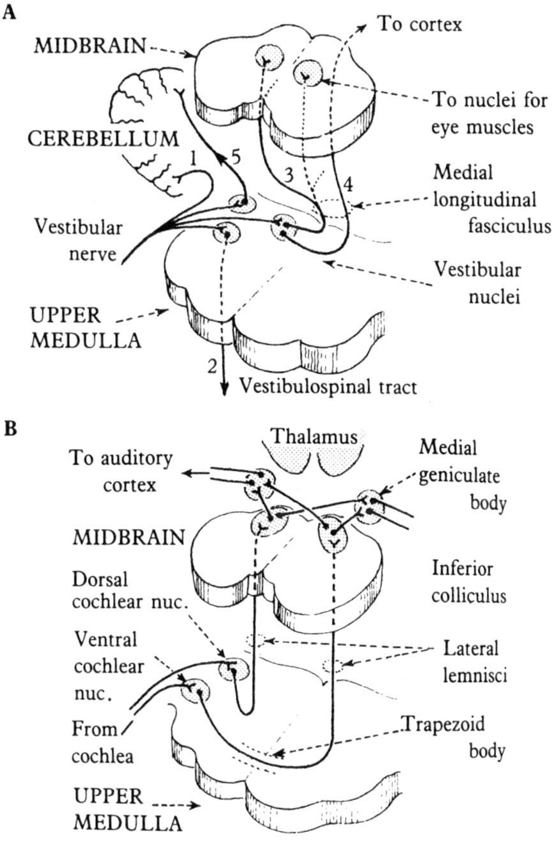

Fig. 3.17 The connections of **A** the vestibular component and **B** the cochlear component of the eighth cranial nerve. (Reproduced from Lindsay K W, Bone I, Callander R 1986 *Neurology and Neurosurgery Illustrated*, Churchill Livingstone, Edinburgh, with permission.)

CLINICAL ASSESSMENT

Symptoms

Dizziness. The patient with a complaint of dizziness makes up a large part of neurological practice. The term will continue to present difficulties to clinicians as long as there is uncertainty as to what each individual patient means by it. Although associated symptoms may be helpful in localising the cause of dizziness, the patient must always be asked initially to give a careful description of his symptoms without the use of the terms 'dizziness' or 'giddiness'.

Dizziness may be defined as a sensation of altered orientation in space. As visual and proprioceptive inputs as well as vestibular input provide information about the position of the head and body in space, the symptom of dizziness can arise from lesions affecting any of these systems.

The primary symptom of vestibular disorder is vertigo—an illusion of rotation due to imbalance between the sensory input from the labyrinthine canals. It may comprise a sensation of rotation in either the horizontal or (less commonly) the vertical plane: the environment may appear to rotate about the patient, or the patient rotate within the environment; the differentiation between these two is not clinically important.

Vestibular vertigo usually has an abrupt onset, with decreasing intensity as compensation occurs over a matter of hours or days. More chronic vestibular disorders are characterised by brief paroxysms of vertigo related to sudden head movement, turning over in bed being a prime precipitating factor. Continuous 'dizziness' without fluctuation over long periods is atypical of vestibular disease. Although unsteadiness and faintness due to cerebral hypoperfusion or vertebrobasilar insufficiency may occasionally be related to changes in posture, this is more commonly caused by the patient rising to a standing position after sitting or bending, than by changes of head position in the horizontal plane.

Symptoms associated with dizziness may be helpful in localising lesions. Nausea and vomiting commonly accompany vestibular vertigo but are uncommon with other types of dizziness. Pallor and sweating may be common with very acute and severe symptoms and in some instances vertigo may be so severe as to be associated with prostration, incontinence and occasionally with loss of consciousness. Vertigo due to labyrinthine disease is commonly associated with auditory symptoms (see below) such as deafness, tinnitus and a feeling of pressure in the ear. It is more often longer-lasting and more severe than centrally induced vertigo. More central vestibular lesions will not be associated with auditory symptoms, but may be associated with diplopia, dysarthria, ataxia and other signs of brain stem disturbance.

Very occasionally symptoms of true vertigo may arise from a cortical level, vertigo representing a very unusual form of epileptic aura. Almost as rare is cerebellar vertigo, which may result from damage to the flocculonodular lobe of the cerebellum.

Non-vestibular dizziness. The specific symptom of vestibular vertigo must be differentiated from non-specific feelings of giddiness, light-headedness, depersonalisation, drunkenness and faintness.

Many patients with systemic disorders, e.g. septicaemia, complain of a non-specific dizziness. Drugs, particularly aminoglycosides and salicylates, sometimes cause vestibular vertigo, but antihypertensive medication tends to produce a non-specific dizziness related to postural hypotension. Sedative drugs including alcohol, benzodiazepines and anticonvulsant drugs may lead to a feeling of unsteadiness.

Diplopia, or the correction of a long-standing refractory visual problem with glasses, can lead to a feeling of disorientation. Patients with peripheral neuropathy involving proprioceptive input, paraparesis, or cerebellar disturbance, may all complain of unsteadiness which initially may be described in terms of a dizzy feeling.

Non-specific light-headedness is usually a symptom of chronic anxiety, with or without hyperventilation. Patients with agoraphobia may, similarly, describe their fear of leaving the house as 'a dizzy feeling'. The typical presyncopal aura may be described as dizziness.

Tinnitus. Tinnitus usually arises from disorders of the ossicles, inner ear or eighth nerve. Under these circumstances it is almost invariably associated with a degree of deafness and very often can be lateralised to one or other ear. Tinnitus from conductive disorders tends to be of lower frequency that that accompanying sensorineural loss.

Other noises in the head may occur: it is quite common to be aware of, and to hear, flow of blood close to the ear when the head is placed on the pillow; both patient and examiner may be able to hear bruits related to arteriosclerotic stenoses or large arteriovenous malformations or fistulas; the rare syndrome of palatal myoclonus may give rise to repetitive clicking.

Deafness. Deafness represents a major cause of disability. It may result from disturbances affecting the external ear, tympanic membrane and ossicles (i.e. conductive deafness) or of the cochlea, auditory nerve and central connections (sensorineural deafness). Either type of deafness can be associated with tinnitus. Sensorineural deafness is most likely to be associated with symptoms of vertigo or other vestibular disturbance. Causes of deafness are grouped in Table 3.15.

Sometimes, slowly progressive unilateral deafness may be ignored by a patient until the disability declares itself when using the telephone.

Signs

Sensory information from the vestibular apparatus is particularly important in the control of posture and eye movement, and it is in these areas that most of the useful information from physical examination can be obtained.

Patients with vestibular lesions have subjective and objective sensations of unsteadiness; these are particularly likely to be increased if compensation by visual information is prevented, in a dark room or with the eyes closed. With acute vestibular lesions there is a tendency to fall towards the side of the lesion.

Patients should be examined with the eyes in the primary position as well as during the full range of movement. The particular characteristic features of spontaneous vestibular nystagmus have already been discussed: they include unidirectional nystagmus with the fast phase away from the side of a vestibular lesion, whether this is peripheral or central.

It is important also to examine reflexly induced nystagmus. This should involve testing (see Fig. 3.11) to elicit the oculovestibular reflex and detection of positional nystagmus. These functions have already been discussed in the section on eye movements.

A number of more specific tests of vestibular function may be helpful.

Caloric testing. In this technique water 7°C below normal body temperature is used to irrigate the external auditory meatus with the patient lying on a couch with the head elevated to an angle of approximately 30 degrees. Irrigation causes movement of fluid within (predominantly) the horizontal semicircular canal, leading to an appropriate vestibular response and nystagmus. Irrigation with cold water causes a tonic deviation towards the side being irrigated, whereas irrigation with warm water induces tonic deviation away from the stimulus. In both instances there will be a rapid corrective phase so that the fast phase of the nystagmoid response is away from the side of the cold-water stimulus and towards the side of the warm-water stimulus.

Some confusion may arise if both sides are stimulated in rapid succession. In such instances, cold stimulus given bilaterally will tend to cause an upbeat nystagmus whereas a warm stimulus will tend to cause a downbeat nystagmus.

Conventionally, the stimulus is applied for 40 s and the duration of the evoked nystagmus is then recorded. Two major patterns of abnormality can

Table 3.15 Causes of deafness

Conductive
otosclerosis
chronic serous otitis media
suppurative otitis media/cholesteatoma
head injury
Sensorineural
a. cochlear
hereditary deafness
viral infection (rubella/mumps)
industrial noise
drugs (aminoglycosides)
Ménière's disease
b. neural
cerebellopontine angle tumours
basal meningitis (TB, malignant, sarcoid)
c. brain stem connections
demyelination
infarction
multisystem degenerations

be recognised: canal paresis describes a significant reduction in the length of responses to cold and hot water from one side and indicates an abnormality confined to one side of the vestibular system, usually the end organ on that side. In contrast, directional preponderance is an abnormality in which the nystagmus in one direction tends to be greater and longer-lasting, irrespective of whether this is produced by cold irrigation in one ear or warm irrigation of the other. Although each of these patterns of abnormality sometimes may be seen independently, it is perhaps more common to see a combination of both types of abnormality.

Canal paresis is indicative of a lesion of the vestibular apparatus, eighth nerve or vestibular nucleus. Directional preponderance is less specific and may be found in both peripheral labyrinthine and nerve disorders, as well as with brain stem lesions.

Electronystagmography makes use of the electrical field changes that can be induced by eye movement. Although these artefacts may be troublesome when interpreting the EEG, they nevertheless offer a satisfactory means of providing a record of eye movements and, in particular, of nystagmus. As well as providing a permanent record, they also allow quantification of the effects of fixation on nystagmus, whether this is spontaneous or reflexly induced. Allowing the patient to fixate during testing will generally have an inhibitory effect on nystagmus due to peripheral vestibular lesions (which effect becomes more marked when fixation is removed either by eye closure, performing the tests in darkness, or by using Frenzel's glasses); on the other hand, central brain stem or cerebellar lesions characteristically show that nystagmus is uninhibited by fixation.

Tests of cochlear function

Rinne's test. A vibrating tuning fork (512 or 256 cycles per second) is placed on the mastoid and then held close to the ear. The patient is asked to determine which sound is loudest. In patients with conductive deafness, bone conduction is superior to air conduction.

Weber's test. A vibrating tuning fork is applied to the forehead in the midline. The patient is asked to localise the sound to one side or the other. In patients with conductive deafness it is located to the side of the deaf ear, whereas in patients with sensorineural deafness it is lateralised to the normal ear.

More objective assessment of hearing can be undertaken using pure tone audiometry. Thresholds for the detection of tones ranging from 0.75 to 8 Hz are determined for both air and bone conduction.

A number of other tests are available to help to differentiate cochlear deafness from neural deafness. Auditory recruitment is a test in which the intensity of sound applied to each ear is adjusted so as to appear equally loud to the patient. In lesions of the nerve trunk the difference in hearing persists as the reference sound is increased in intensity; in lesions of the cochlea, the difference between the two ears may finally disappear with increasing intensity (recruiting deafness).

Speech discrimination consists of a test in which a number of phonetically similar words are presented to a patient and the number correctly perceived is recorded. Marked reduction in speech discrimination relative to pure-tone audiometry is a characteristic of eighth nerve lesions.

Tone decay is a phenomenon in which sound presented slightly above threshold levels is heard for only a limited period. In the normal individual, sounds 5–10 decibels above the threshold at any frequency will normally be heard for a full minute; similar absence of marked tone decay is also seen in patients with cochlear deafness. However, in nerve fibre deafness many patients require increments in sound intensity to 15 decibels or more above threshold in order for a sound to be heard for a full minute. Brain-stem lesions associated with deafness may show this abnormal pattern of tone decay.

Auditory evoked potentials. The application of averaging techniques to EEG recording has led to the identification of a series of potential changes related to click stimuli. These are much more complicated than visual evoked potentials and consist of a number of waves recorded for up to 400 ms after a click stimulus. The first five waves are probably related to activity in the eighth cranial nerve, cochlear nuclei, superior olivary complex and inferior colliculus. The origin of middle and later responses is less certain, although some may be related to activity at cortical structures (p. 106).

Auditory evoked potentials have been studied mainly in multiple sclerosis where abnormalities in the latency and amplitude of early components appear to accompany clinical brain stem disease. Abnormalities may also be found in patients in whom the diagnosis is clinically suspected but who have no clinical evidence of brain stem disorder.

PATTERNS OF EIGHTH NERVE LESIONS

Localisation of eighth nerve lesions should not present major difficulty. Peripheral lesions of the semicircular canals and cochlea and eighth nerve are characterised by the association of vestibular and auditory symptomatology. In the cerebellopontine angle lesions these are usually associated with involvement of the trigeminal and facial nerves. In brain stem lesions there is most commonly a dissociation between vestibular and auditory symptoms and signs, perhaps with involvement of long tracts. Characterisation of any nystagmus may be of particular help in differentiating between central and peripheral lesions affecting the eighth nerve (see p. 65).

Other disorders of eighth nerve function

Ménière's disease

This syndrome is characterised by the association of paroxysmal attacks of vertigo with tinnitus and deafness. The vertigo is of abrupt onset and lasts from several minutes up to a few hours; this is associated with nausea and vomiting, tinnitus and quite frequently a feeling of fullness of the ear. The patient will be unable to walk and any head movement is avoided because of the exacerbation of vertigo. Looking away from the side of the lesion also tends to make the vertigo worse. The frequency of attacks is very variable but over a period of years more persistant deafness and tinnitus are likely to develop. Caloric testing usually shows evidence of a canal paresis. Audiometry shows evidence of a sensorineural type of deafness with higher frequencies particularly involved. Loudness recruitment is usually preserved.

Ménière's syndrome can occur at any age and is rarely bilateral. The attacks of vertigo may well cease when a marked degree of deafness is present.

The disorder is characterised by a rise in endolymphatic pressure which results in progressive distension of the scala media. The underlying mechanism for this is uncertain; one suggestion is that it is membrane rupture that may lead to attacks.

Vestibular sedatives may be helpful in treatment (prochlorperazine, cinnarizine). In unilateral and disabling disease, ablation of the labyrinth may be considered.

Benign positional vertigo

The onset of symptoms is usually quite abrupt and the frequency of attacks of vertigo decreases over a period of weeks to months; occasionally, recurrence is seen. The patient becomes aware that particular head postures, usually when turning over in bed, provoke a brief episode of vertigo. It is possible to demonstrate vestibular positional nystagmus using conventional testing (see above). This disorder is frequently attributed to labyrinthine viral infection and symptoms complicate recovery from head injury. In up to half the cases no cause is apparent.

Vestibular neuronitis

This symptom is complex, characterised by attacks of intense vertigo in the absence of tinnitus or deafness. It usually affects young adults and vertigo is of abrupt onset with nausea and vomiting. There is evidence of vestibular paresis on one side with nystagmus to the other side. Complete recovery is the rule within a period of weeks, although in some cases recurrences are seen.

There is little reason to consider this a single pathological entity, although when originally described it was attributed to viral infection. Identical syndromes may be seen with vascular causes and drugs and the term acute vestibular failure may serve as a more appropriate description.

Other causes of vertigo

Vertigo not infrequently accompanies head injury and intercurrent illness. Viral illness, particularly mumps, may involve the labyrinth and cochlea, and similar disturbances can complicate otitis media. Rarely, occlusion of the internal auditory artery can cause acute vertigo and unilateral deafness. Drugs may be ototoxic, e.g. streptomycin, gentamycin (p. 431).

DISORDERS OF THE BULBAR CRANIAL NERVES

THE NINTH CRANIAL (GLOSSOPHARYNGEAL) NERVE

The ninth nerve has motor, sensory and parasympathetic efferent fibres. It emerges from the lateral surface of the medulla by a number of small roots rostral to those of the vagus nerves. Its somatic sensory functions probably subserve sensation from the tonsils, posterior wall of the pharynx and soft palate and mediate taste from the posterior one-third of the tongue; however, some of these functions may be subserved by the tenth cranial nerve. It also receives fibres from the carotid sinus and may have a role in the reflex control of circulation. Motor fibres supply stylopharyngeus muscle only. Parasympathetic fibres from the inferior salivatory nucleus supply the glands of the pharyngeal mucosa and parotid.

The ninth cranial nerve is of limited clinical importance. Its only component that is readily tested is pharyngeal sensation, supplying the afferent limb of the gag reflex.

Isolated ninth nerve lesions are virtually unknown and function is most commonly disturbed by lesions at or around the jugular foramen, when the tenth and eleventh cranial nerves are also involved. The patient presents with hoarseness and dysphagia with nasal regurgitation. The syndrome is most commonly seen with glomus jugulare tumours, but may more rarely result from trauma, neuromas of the lower cranial nerves and meningeal infiltration.

Glossopharyngeal neuralgia is described on p. 200.

TENTH CRANIAL (VAGUS) NERVE

The vagus nerve has three major nuclei situated in the medulla: the motor nucleus supplies the muscles of the larynx, pharynx, and palate; the sensory nucleus is the lower part of the nucleus of the tractus solitarius and receives sensory information from the external ear, pharynx, larynx, trachea, oesophagus, thoracic and abdominal viscera; the parasympathetic nucleus located beneath the floor of the fourth ventricle has a wide distribution of efferent fibres supplying involuntary muscle in the bronchi, heart, oesophagus, stomach, small intestine and large intestine. These aspects of vagal function are considered in Chapter 4.

Unilateral tenth nerve paresis causes palatal weakness with nasal speech and nasal regurgitation of fluids, with deviation of the palate to the opposite side. There is difficulty in swallowing, because of pharyngeal weakness, and paresis of the vocal cords leads to hoarseness with a bovine cough. Indirect laryngoscopy shows an immobile, abducted vocal cord on the side of the lesion; the gag reflex is lost.

Isolated tenth nerve lesions are rare and, when present, are usually distal, constituting a recurrent laryngeal nerve palsy. Associated neurological signs may be helpful in localising the site of tenth nerve lesions. Medullary tenth lesions are usually associated with ipsilateral cerebellar disturbance, Horner's syndrome and dissociated sensory impairment on the ipsilateral face and contralateral side of the body. Tenth nerve lesions in the posterior fossa usually comprise a part of the jugular foramen syndrome (ninth and eleventh nerves are also involved at this site). Meningeal infiltration may involve the tenth nerve, but more distally the recurrent laryngeal nerve on the left may be involved as a result of thoracic disease due to tumours of the bronchi and mediastinum. Under these circumstances, palatal movement is preserved but vocal cord paresis occurs.

Palatal myoclonus is a rare disorder in which there is rhythmic contraction of the palate and pharynx at rates up to 60/minute, which persists during sleep. The patient may be aware of a clicking noise. The syndrome may be caused by lesions of the inferior olives, dentate nucleus or red nucleus connections. Similar repetitive pharyngeal movements may affect the hyoid.

ELEVENTH CRANIAL (ACCESSORY) NERVE

This nerve is purely motor. It derives fibres from the anterior horn cells of the upper five cervical cord segments; these pass up through the foramen magnum and travel with a part of the tenth nerve for a short course. The nerve then leaves the skull through the jugular foramen.

Lesions of the eleventh nerve result in weakness of trapezius and sternomastoid muscles. Trapezius can be tested by asking the patient to shrug his shoulders. There may be delay in elevation of the shoulder, and weakness of this movement. Very often a degree of atrophy is present. Sternomastoid may be tested by asking the patient to look away from the side of the lesion, while one palpates the muscle. This movement may be overcome by force exerted to the opposite side of the head, and wasting of the body of sternomastoid may be evident.

Overactivity of sternomastoid may be involved in spasmodic torticollis (p. 395).

TWELFTH CRANIAL (HYPOGLOSSAL) NERVE

This motor nerve arises from the medulla and leaves the skull through the hypoglossal foramen. It supplies the muscles of the tongue, which act to protrude the tongue (genioglossi), the hyoglossus, which retracts and elevates the root of the tongue and the hypoglossus muscle, which causes the upper surface to become convex. Interruption of the nerve results in paralysis of the tongue on one side with curving of the tongue to the affected side when it is protruded. The wasted tongue becomes wrinkled and atrophied and shows fibrillation and fasciculation.

The nerve is rarely involved with structural lesions but may be involved in more generalised processes such as infiltration of the basal meninges, and as part of the syndrome of bulbar palsy. Occasionally trauma and vertebral aneurysm may cause isolated twelfth nerve lesions.

LOCALISATION OF CRANIAL NERVE PALSIES

The combination of cranial nerve palsies with other neurological signs are of major value in localising lesions in the brain stem and cranial cavity.

BRAIN STEM SYNDROMES

Brain stem lesions are likely to cause cranial nerve palsies associated with long tract signs. These will result in motor or sensory disturbance usually affecting the side contralateral to the cranial nerve palsy, because of the anatomical fact that both motor and sensory pathways cross at a lower

Table 3.16 Cranial nerve palsies and crossed brain stem syndromes

Cranial nerve	Site	Associated signs	Usual cause
III (Weber's)	Midbrain	Crossed hemiplegia	Infarction/tumour
III (Benedikt's)	Midbrain	Crossed ataxia and tremor	Infarction/tumour
VII ± VI (Millard–Gubler)	Pons	Crossed hemiplegia	Infarction/tumour
V, IX, X, XI	Lateral medulla	Ipsilateral Horner's Crossed ataxia and loss of pain and temperature sensation in limbs.	Posterior-inferior cerebellar artery occlusion

medullary level, whereas individual cranial nerve nuclei receive connections individually at the specific nuclear level of the cranial nerve within the brain stem. A number of such cross brain stem syndromes are described in Table 3.16.

SYNDROMES ASSOCIATED WITH LOCALISED INTRACRANIAL, EXTRAMEDULLARY LESIONS

Because of the close association of many cranial nerves during their passage through the various foramina in the skull, localised pathology in particular sites will give rise to striking neurological syndromes. The most important of these are summarised in Table 3.17.

SYNDROMES OF DIFFUSE MULTIPLE CRANIAL NERVE INVOLVEMENT

More diffuse widespread cranial nerve involvement is seen in a number of pathological conditions (Table 3.18). Meningeal infiltration, most frequently seen with carcinomatous or lymphomatous disease, is characterised by a striking number of cranial nerve palsies. The oculomotor nerves, facial nerve, eighth nerve and trigeminal nerve are most commonly involved in a patchy and asymmetric fashion. Granulomatous meningitis may cause similar syndromes but it is unusual to see as many cranial nerves involved as with malignant meningitis; in both, radicular limb signs may be present.

Table 3.17 Multiple cranial nerve syndromes

Cranial nerves	Site	Cause
III, IV, V(1), VI	Superior orbital fissure	Tumours/aneurysm
III, IV, V(1 ± 2), VI	Cavernous sinus	Aneurysm/tumour
V, VI	Apex of petrous temporal	Tumour
V, VII, VIII	Cerebellopontine angle	Accoustic neuroma Meningioma/AVM
IX, X, XI	Jugular foramen	Glomus jugulare tumour

Table 3.18 Causes of multiple cranial nerve palsies

Patchy (usually asymmetrical)
a. malignant meningitis
   carcinoma
   lymphoma
   leukaemia
   glioma
   ependymoma

b. granulomatous meningitis
   sarcoid
   TB
   syphilis

c. bone pathology
   secondary carcinoma
   Paget's disease

Diffuse (usually symmetrical)
   Acute infectious polyneuropathy (Guillain–Barré)
   Cranial polyneuropathy
   Motor neurone disease
   Myasthenia gravis
   Polymyositis

Pathology of the bones of the basal skull due to nasopharyngeal or secondary carcinoma, or Paget's disease, may also lead to multiple cranial nerve compression. A number of other conditions may cause multiple cranial nerve palsies. The Guillain–Barré syndrome frequently involves cranial as well as peripheral nerves and roots. Seventh and fifth nerve palsies are common and bulbar palsies are sometimes seen (see below). Sometimes a syndrome characterised by the subacute development of multiple cranial nerve palsies in the absence of peripheral nerve involvement is seen (cranial polyneuropathy): this syndrome may represent a disorder similar to acute infective polyneuropathy. Disorders characterised by diffuse involvement of the anterior horn cell (motor neurone disease), neuromuscular junction (myasthenia gravis) and muscle itself (polymyositis) may give rise to the syndrome of bulbar palsy.

BULBAR PALSY

This syndrome describes bilateral weakness of muscles supplied by cranial nerves with nuclei in the medulla, ninth, tenth and twelfth nerves. It may arise because of lower motor neurone disturbance or disorders of neuromuscular transmission

Table 3.19 Causes of bulbar palsy

Acute	
	Guillain–Barré syndrome
	cranial polyneuropathy
	poliomyelitis
	diphtheria
Chronic	
	motor neurone disease
	myopathy (polymyositis)
	myasthenia gravis

or primary muscle disease (Table 3.19). The patient develops dysarthria characterised by nasal escape and flaccidity of muscles associated with difficulty in swallowing, with nasal regurgitation and, sometimes, with aspiration. Wasting and fasciculation of the tongue may be evident bilaterally.

PSEUDOBULBAR PALSY

This syndrome must be differentiated from bulbar palsy: it represents bilateral upper motor neurone (supranuclear) disturbance affecting the bulbar motor function. Once again it gives rise to dysarthria and dysphagia; however, the characteristics of this are strikingly dissimilar from those of bulbar palsy. There is no wasting of the tongue, but the tongue becomes stiff and spastic and the patient has difficulty in performing rapid alternating movements of the tongue. The jaw jerk becomes very brisk, and there is frequently a degree of emotional incontinence with inappropriate laughing and crying. The dysarthria takes on a very strained tone due to the spasticity of the bulbar muscles. Nasal regurgitation is less commonly seen than in bulbar palsy, but choking attacks are frequent and distressing. A patient with pseudobulbar palsy has a striking facial expression with a mask-like facies and staring eyes. Occasionally there is some associated impairment of ocular movement of a supranuclear type which becomes very marked in the syndrome of progressive supranuclear palsy.

Pseudobulbar palsy is most commonly seen in motor neurone disease when it may also be associated with some wasting and fasciculation of the tongue because of lower motor neurone involvement. Other causes include vascular disease (most commonly in hypertensive patients with multiple lacunar strokes, and severe brain-stem multiple sclerosis and brain stem tumours). It may be symptomatic of degenerative diseases, such as progressive supranuclear palsy, or Creutzfeld–Jakob disease.

FURTHER READING

Brodal A 1981 Neurological anatomy in relation to clinical medicine, 3rd edn. Oxford University Press, New York

Mayo Clinic and Mayo Foundation 1976 Clinical examinations in neurology, 4th edn. Saunders, Philadelphia

Miller N R 1982 Walsh and Hoyt's clinical neuro-ophthalmology, vols 1 and 2, 4th edn. Williams and Wilkins, Baltimore

Rudge P 1983 Clinical neuro-otology. In: Clinical neurology and neurosurgery monographs, vol 4. Churchill Livingstone, Edinburgh

4

Disorders of the autonomic system

INTRODUCTION

Dysfunction of the autonomic nervous system is an important, but often overlooked, cause of symptoms and signs in neurological disorders. Bladder and sexual dysfunction, in particular, often contribute very significantly to the morbidity of disease. Careful and sympathetic appraisal of such problems will usually be rewarding.

ANATOMY AND PHARMACOLOGY

The peripheral anatomy of the autonomic nervous system is schematically represented in Figure 4.1. The outflow of the autonomic is divided into a thoracolumbar (*sympathetic*) system and a craniosacral (*parasympathetic*) system; the actions of these systems are largely antagonistic. Preganglionic fibres arise from cell bodies associated with cranial nerve nuclei and the intermediolateral cell column of the spinal cord grey matter (Fig. 4.2). Synapses with postganglionic fibres are found in the paravertebral, prevertebral and peripheral ganglia.

PARASYMPATHETIC EFFERENT SYSTEM

Parasympathetic nuclei are associated with the third, seventh, ninth and tenth cranial nerve nuclei. Preganglionic fibres (containing acetylcholine as neurotransmitter), synapse in four cranial parasympathetic ganglia (ciliary, sphenopalatine, submandibular and otic) giving efferent (acetylcholine) fibres to the iris and ciliary muscles of the eye, lacrimal and salivary glands. Preganglionic fibres from the tenth cranial nerve terminate in ganglia situated in the walls of the thoracic and abdominal viscera. Postganglionic fibres activate smooth muscles and glands of the pharynx, oesophagus and gastrointestinal tract as far as the proximal transverse colon as well as the heart, pancreas, liver and gall bladder. The autonomic plexuses in these organs also receive sympathetic innervation.

The sacral outflow of the parasympathetic system is derived from the second, third and fourth sacral segments. Preganglionic (acetylcholine) fibres run to the distal colon and rectum, bladder and sexual organs from autonomic plexuses in these sites. The effects of parasympathetic stimulation are described in Table 4.1.

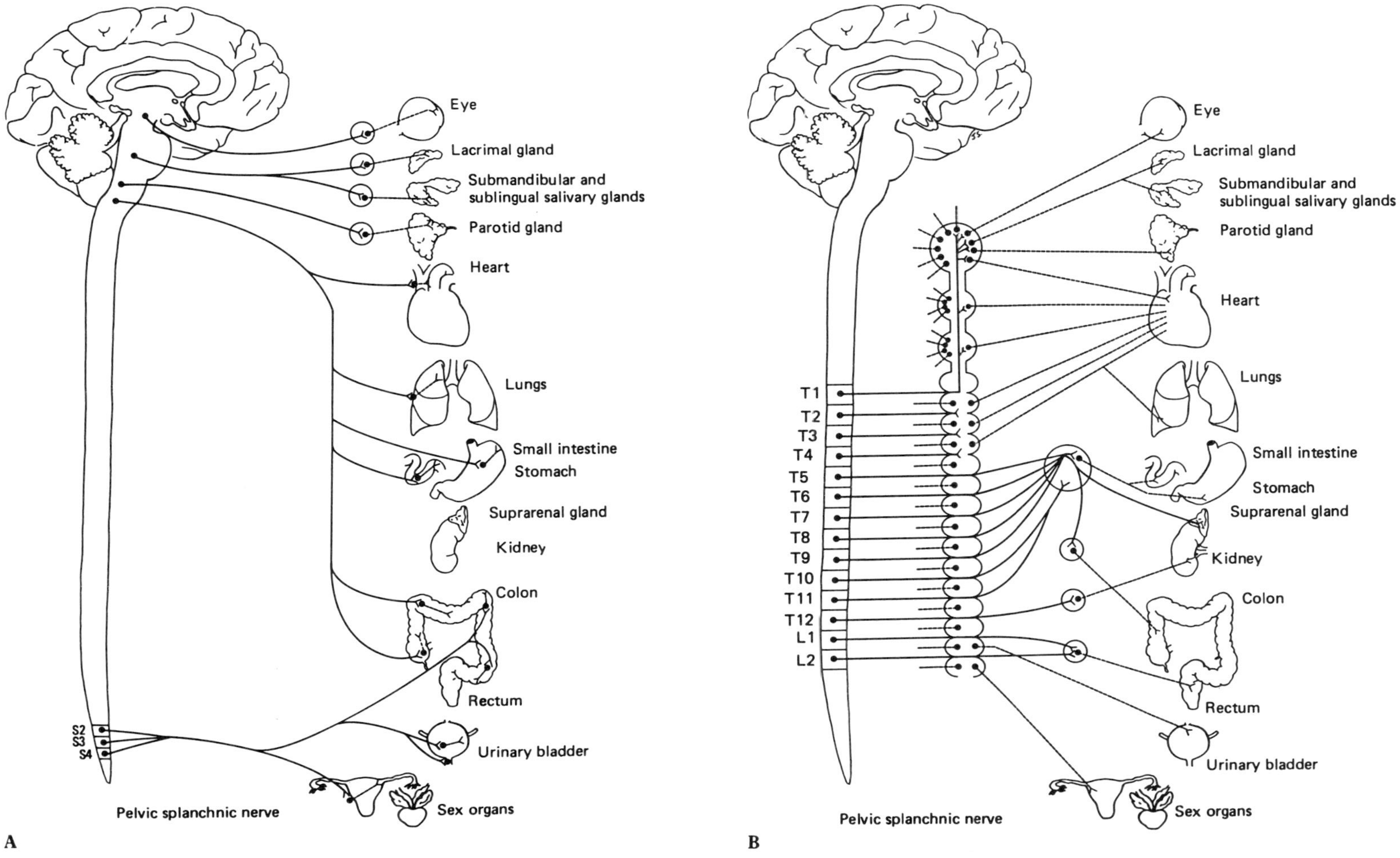

Fig. 4.1 Pathways and innervation of **A** the peripheral parasympathetic system, **B** to peripheral sympathetic system.

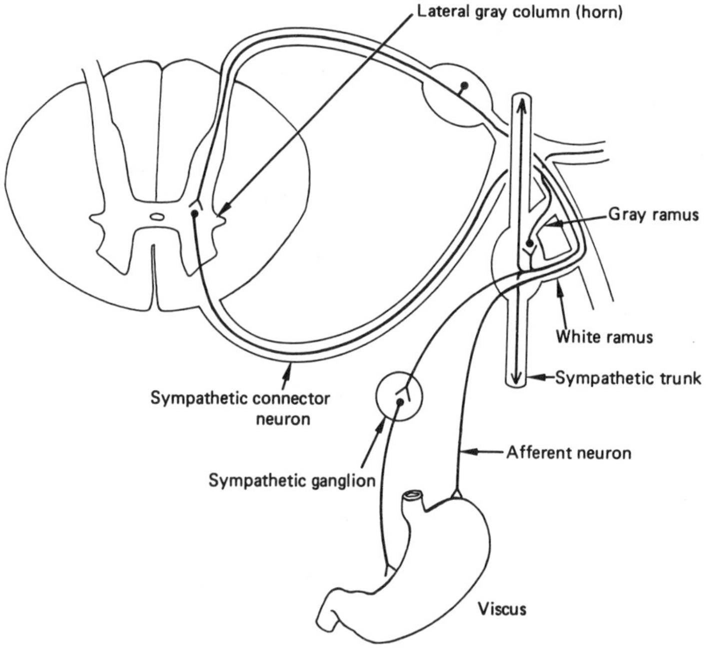

Fig. 4.2 Spinal pathways of the autonomic system.

SYMPATHETIC SYSTEM

Preganglionic fibres originate from cell bodies in the lateral horns of the first thoracic to third lumbar cord segments (with acetylcholine as neurotransmitter), and pass into the paravertebral chain of ganglia travelling up or down, sometimes for a considerable length, before finally synapsing with postganglionic neurones. Some preganglionic fibres pass through the paravertebral ganglia as splanchnic nerves to synapse in prevertebral coeliac, superior and inferior mesenteric ganglia. Postganglionic fibres form the hypogastric, splanchnic and mesenteric plexus innervating the glands and smooth muscle of blood vessels and intestines respectively. The superior and middle cervical ganglia and the inferior (or stellate) ganglia provide a postganglionic outflow to the eye, blood vessels of the head, and glands associated with the eye, nasal and oral cavities. The arm receives postganglionic innervation from the upper thoracic segments via the stellate ganglion. The cardiac and other thoracic plexuses are derived from the fifth to tenth thoracic segments. The lower three lumbar ganglia have no visceral connections and supply only the legs. The effects of sympathetic stimulation are described in Table 4.2.

Table 4.1 Parasympathetic efferent effects

Organ	Effect of activity
Eye	Accommodation Myosis
Salivary glands	Secretion
Heart	Decreased contractility Decreased rate Decreased coronary flow
Stomach, intestines, colon and rectum	Increased peristalsis Secretion Inhibition of anal tone Defaecation
Bladder	Bladder contraction Inhibition of internal sphincter Micturition
Genital organs	
male	Vasodilatation and erection
female	Vasodilatation

Table 4.2 Sympathetic efferent effects

Organ	Effect of activity
Limbs	Vasoconstriction Piloerection Sweating
Heart	Increased contractility Increased rate Increased coronary flow
Lungs	Bronchial dilatation
Intestines	Inhibition of peristalsis Inhibition of secretion Vasoconstriction Sphincter contraction
Adrenal gland	Secretion
Bladder	Inhibition of bladder tone Contraction of sphincter
Uterus	Contraction

VISCERAL SENSATION

As well as efferent connections, all visceral nerves convey sensory information from the viscera. Cell bodies of such sensory fibres lie in the posterior root ganglia; these not only subserve visceral spinal cord reflexes but also synapse with secondary afferents carrying impulses to the thalamus via the lateral spinothalamic tract.

PHARMACOLOGY OF THE PERIPHERAL AUTONOMIC SYSTEM

The pharmacological properties of the autonomic nervous system have been well studied. The transmitter substance at both sympathetic and parasympathetic ganglia is acetylcholine. Unlike the postganglionic (muscarinic) effects of acetylcholine, which are blocked by atropine, the preganglionic (nicotinic) activity of acetylcholine is blocked by drugs such as hexamethonium.

Most sympathetic postganglionic fibres have catecholamines as neurotransmitters, the exception being fibres to sweat glands, which are cholinergic. Catecholamine sympathetic postsynaptic receptor sites may be designated as *alpha* or *beta* by their affinity for noradrenalin and adrenalin respectively. The effects of sympathetic impulses on organs with alpha receptors is largely excitatory, causing dilatation of the pupil, contraction of piloerector muscles and a decrease in motility of the gastrointestinal tract with contraction of bowel and bladder sphincters; superficial blood vessels constrict. Sympathetic stimulation of organs with beta receptors (bronchial muscles and sino-atrial node) causes relaxation of bronchial smooth muscles and increased heart rate.

Parasympathetic postganglionic fibres release acetylcholine, causing constriction of the pupil, glandular secretion, slowing of heart rate, increased intestinal motility and sphincter relaxation.

In addition to these direct neural connections the autonomic nervous system has intimate connections with pituitary and adrenal glands, to mediate systemic effects via hormonal mechanisms.

CENTRAL CONNECTIONS OF THE AUTONOMIC SYSTEM

The central organisation and control of the autonomic system is less well understood than that of the peripheral system. Three major areas appear to influence and co-ordinate the central control of autonomic activity: these comprise the *frontal lobe*, the primitive *limbic system* (hippocampus, amygdaloid nuclei and olfactory cortex) and the *hypothalamus*. The frontal lobe is capable of effecting voluntary control over bladder and bowel function by fibres which pass with corticospinal fibres to the hippocampus and hypothalamus, which in turn send fibres to brain stem and spinal cord levels. The limbic system (Fig. 4.3) appears to be capable of mediating those autonomic disturbances associated with primitive feeding responses, as well as 'flight and fight' reactions; it influences aggressive behaviour.

The hypothalamus receives fibres from both frontal and limbic systems. The anterior (superoptic and paraventricular) nuclei give rise to fibres which pass through the stalk of the pituitary gland to terminate in the posterior lobe, releasing antidiuretic hormone and oxytocin. The middle group of hypothalamic nuclei are directly involved in the control of the anterior hypophysis. Cells of this

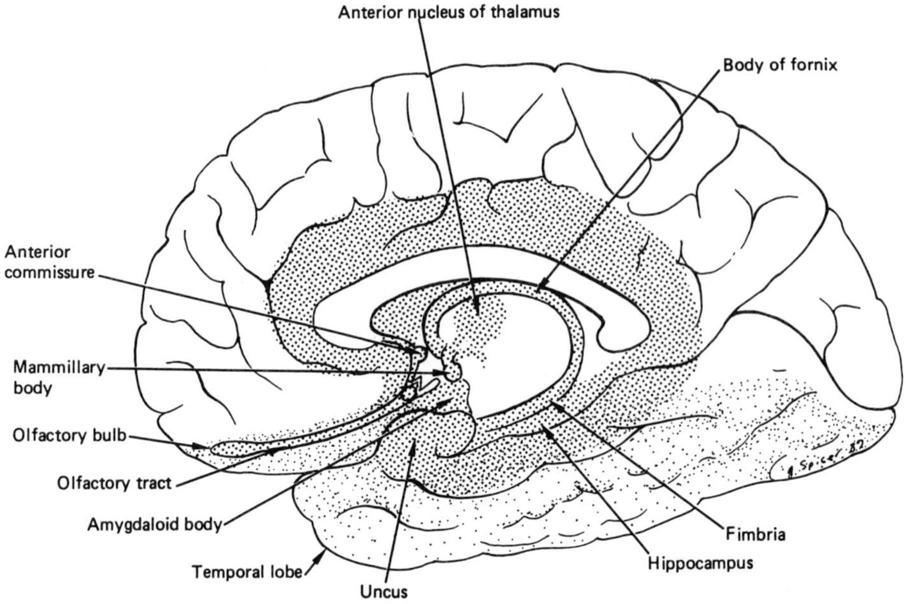

Fig. 4.3 Structure and connections of the limbic system.

system release hypothalamic releasing factors controlling the secretion of growth hormone, adrenocorticotrophic hormone, thyrotrophic stimulating hormone, luteinising hormone, follicle-stimulating hormone and prolactin. The medial part of the hypothalamus contains centres which control appetite, food intake and body weight. The hypothalamus also has important connections with the preganglionic fibres of both sympathetic and parasympathetic systems via poorly defined descending tracts. The hypothalamus is important in temperature control: anterior areas mediate responses to heat; posterior areas mediate those to cold.

Although the frontal lobes, limbic system and hypothalamus provide overall control of autonomic function, other brain-stem centres are important in the control of more basic autonomic reflexes. Afferents from the vagus, and carotid sinus baroreceptors and chemoreceptors, project to the nucleus solitarius of the medulla. Stimulation of the pontomedullary reticular formation may lead to effects on cardiac rhythm and vasomotor changes suggesting reflexes at this level which may be modulated by higher control. The major centres controlling respiration are found in the lateral reticular formation of the lower brain stem of the lower and mid pontine level. Here, expiratory and inspiratory neurones discharge alternately to produce respiratory activity. These centres respond reflexly to stimuli from the carotid sinus chemoreceptors (mediating the response to hypoxia) and are themselves directly responsive to alterations in $P\text{CO}_2$ and pH. In addition, chemical reflexes from the chest wall, intercostal and diaphragmatic muscles and lungs may affect their function.

The importance of respiratory movement to speech and communication require that higher autonomic levels of organisation interact with medullary respiratory centres.

CLINICAL ASSESSMENT

VASOMOTOR TESTS

A number of procedures which have reflex effects on blood pressure and heart rate may be studied clinically. Satisfactory results can be obtained using heart rate, recorded clinically or more satisfactorily by ECG, as well as routine recording of systolic and diastolic blood pressure.

Postural testing

Testing the effect of posture on blood pressure and heart rate is perhaps the most clinically important vasomotor investigation. On standing, the normal patient will show an increase in heart rate (maximal at about the 15th beat) without any sustained fall in blood pressure; this will be followed by an overshoot bradycardia, maximal by the 30th beat. Heart rate may be recorded before and after the patient rises from a sitting or lying position, and blood pressure can be measured both erect and supine. The heart rate response can be measured and expressed as a ratio of the longest ECG R–R interval around the 30th beat to the shortest R–R interval around the 15th beat.

More sophisticated testing can be undertaken using a tilt-table. Postural reflexes depend on an intact reflex arc involving baroreceptors and sympathetic efferents.

Valsalva's manoeuvre

The Valsalva manoeuvre, the forced expiration against a closed glottis for 10–15 s, normally causes a sharp reduction in venous return and cardiac output with a fall in blood pressure. Baroreceptors cause a reflex tachycardia and peripheral vasoconstriction via sympathetic efferents. With the release of intrathoracic pressure, venous return, stroke volume and blood pressure rebound to higher than normal levels and parasympathetic influences then predominate, causing a reflex bradycardia (Fig. 4.4).

The result of this manoeuvre can be expressed as a ratio of the longest ECG R–R interval after the manoeuvre to the shortest R–R interval during the manoeuvre.

Cold pressor test

In normal persons, immersion of the hand in iced water for 60 s will raise systolic blood pressure by 15–20 mm of mercury and diastolic pressure by 10–15 mm of mercury; there is an associated increase in heart rate. The efferent limb of this reflex is mediated by the sympathetic nervous system.

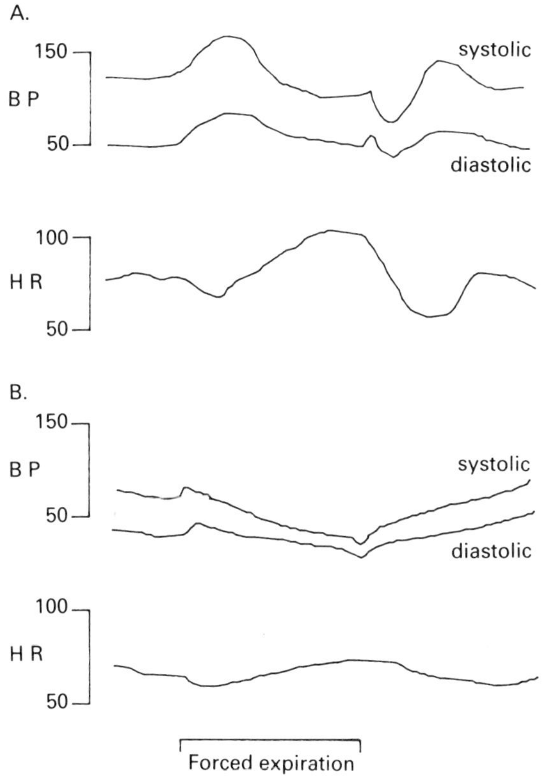

Fig. 4.4 Changes in blood pressure and heart rate during **A** Valsalva's manoeuvre in a normal subject and **B** patient with autonomic dysfunction.

Mental arithmetic

Mental arithmetic in stressful conditions will normally stimulate a small but measurable rise in heart rate and blood pressure; the efferent limb of this reflex is mediated by the sympathetic nervous system.

Sustained hand-grip

Sustained hand-grip causes a rise in blood-pressure mediated by a heart-rate dependent increase in cardiac output via the sympathetic system. The result can be presented as the difference between blood pressure before the test and the highest recorded during a 5-minute sustained test.

A battery of easily performed vasomotor tests of autonomic function with normal and abnormal values is presented in Table 4.3.

Table 4.3 Cardiovascular tests of autonomic function (after Ewing & Clarke 1982)

	Normal	Abnormal
Parasympathetic mediated		
Valsalva (heart-rate ratio)	>1.22	<1.10
standing (heart-rate ratio)	>1.05	<1.00
Sympathetic mediated		
fall in systolic BP on standing	<10 mmHg	>30 mmHg
rise in diastolic BP to handgrip	>16 mmHg	<10 mmHg

Tests and methods of calculation are described in the text.

SKIN TESTS

Sweat tests

Sweating results from stimulation of sweat glands by cholinergic sympathetic fibres; it occurs in response to thermoregulatory stimuli as well as in emotional states. Demonstration of increased or reduced sweating is rarely necessary, other than to define the topography of the disturbance: in such instances starch or a colour indicator such as quinazarin may be used.

Histamine tests

The intracutaneous injection of 0.05 ml histamine (1:1000) causes a physiological response comprising a central wheal surrounded by a narrow red areola and a further surrounding flare reaction. This outer flare reaction is dependent not on the local action of histamine but on a local axon reflex mediated via sensory fibres by antidromic transmission; this may be lost in brachial plexus lesions, but preserved in root lesions.

LACRIMATION

Lacrimation may be tested using Schirmer's test, in which one end of a thin strip of filter paper is inserted into the lower conjunctival sac, the other end hanging over the edge of the lower lid. The presence of tears is shown by wetting of the filter paper: the damp portion will normally comprise a length of over a centimetre within five minutes.

BLADDER FUNCTION

Although a satisfactory amount of information can be obtained from an adequate history, an examination of the patient and, sometimes, further investigation of bladder function, may be helpful in determining the choice of therapeutic approach. Intravenous urography (IVU) with pre- and post-micturition films may well display either a large atonic (lower motor neurone) or small spastic (upper motor neurone) bladder, with or without incomplete emptying. It is also important in the detection of developing hydronephrosis and calculus formation which may occur in patients with neurogenic bladders.

However, more sophisticated urodynamic studies are usually necessary in the assessment of patients with neurogenic bladder symptoms. These will involve the measurement and recording of urine flow, intravesicular pressure, intra-abdominal (rectal) pressure, and detrusor pressure (that due to bladder wall contraction, which is derived from intravesicular pressure less intra-abdominal pressure) during bladder filling and voiding usually simultaneously with visualisation by video-urodynamics. A variety of disturbances may be seen (Table 4.4) which will be important in determining symptomatic management (see below).

Table 4.4 Urodynamic studies: important questions in planning management

Initially
Is there residual urine present?

During filling
1. Is sphincter competent?
   a. at rest
   b. during straining or coughing
2. What is functional capacity of bladder?
   a. reduced in the spastic bladder with detrusor instability
   b. increased in the atonic, insensitive lower motor neurone bladder
3. Is there normal bladder sensation?

During voiding
1. Is detrusor–sphincter dyssynergia present (sphincter contraction before complete emptying) and if present is it causing significant urinary retention?
2. Is there residual urine?
3. In the atonic bladder can satisfactory voiding be achieved by straining etc. or is there sphincter obstruction?

GASTROINTESTINAL FUNCTION

Satisfactory evidence of autonomic disturbance related to gastrointestinal dysfunction may be obtained simply from history and examination. However, radiological procedures including barium swallow with follow-through examination may show a tonic dilatation of the oesophagus and stomach, and delayed gastric emptying with increased frequency and amplitude of peristaltic waves in the small intestine leading to rapid transit times.

PUPILLARY FUNCTION

Pupillary reactions offer a helpful and clinically important means of examining the autonomic innervation of the eye. Pupillary constriction is mediated by the parasympathetic system and opposed by the sympathetic. Direct and consensual light reflexes are easily tested, together with pupillary constriction in response to accommodation and convergence. The anatomy is summarised in Figure 4.5.

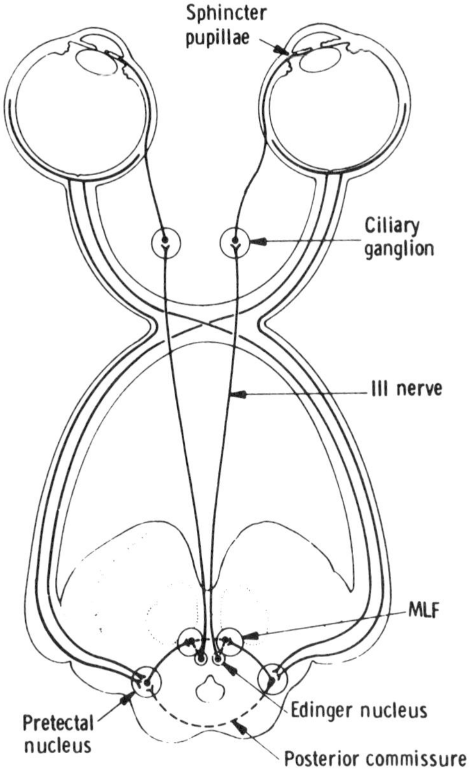

Fig. 4.5 Pathways for the pupillary light reflex (MLF = median longitudinal fasciculus).

Further pharmacological testing may be helpful in some instances. The application of adrenaline eye drops (1 in 1000) will have no effect on a normal pupil but will cause the pupil to dilate where there has been sympathetic denervation. Cocaine (4%), by potentiating the effect of endogenous adrenergic transmission, will normally cause pupillary dilatation; however, in sympathetic denervation caused by lesions of the post- or preganglionic fibres, no change in pupillary size occurs; with more centrally placed lesions, some slight pupillary dilation will be seen. The application of freshly prepared 2.5% methacholine will cause constriction of the tonically dilated pupil of the Holmes–Adie syndrome.

SYNDROMES OF LOCALISED AUTONOMIC DYSFUNCTION

DISORDERS OF THE CONTROL OF BLOOD PRESSURE

Hypertension

Hypertension is rarely seen in association with neurological disease. Phaeochromacytomas are, in essence, tumours of postganglionic sympathetic fibres. They present with paroxysmal hypertension which may be associated with headache, palpitation, pallor and sweating. Occasionally, paradoxical hypotension may occur during attacks, possibly because of the oversecretion of adrenaline rather than noradrenaline. Diagnosis is usually made by estimation of catecholamine metabolites in the urine (vinyl mandelic and homovanillic acids) and by estimation of plasma noradrenaline and adrenaline.

It is well recognised that rising systemic blood pressure may be seen as part of the syndrome of medullary cloning due to intracranial space-occupying lesions; occasionally, however, cerebellar tumours may produce paroxysmal symptoms, including headache, palpitations and sweating, associated with hypertension, which may mimic phaeochromacytoma.

Spinal cord lesions at a T6 or higher level can result in overactivity of autonomic reflexes in the isolated spinal cord. Thus, hypertension and vasoconstriction and piloerection below the level of the lesion may occur in response to a full bladder or rectum in the paraplegic patient. With high cord lesions, sufficient arterial hypertension may occur to cause headache and flushing above the level of the lesion. Hypertension may also be seen in the acute Guillain–Barré syndrome and in tetanus.

Hypotension

Hypotension may occur as a reflex phenomenon leading to syncope. Causes of such phenomena are considered in Chapter 7. Postural hypotension resulting in faintness and loss of consciousness may, however, occur in a number of other circumstances.

In complete or partial transection of the spinal cord above the level of the major splanchnic outflow, the body may be deprived of much of the sympathetic pressor control of blood vessels, leading to severe orthostatic hypotension. This is likely to present particular problems when patients begin to be mobilised after a prolonged period in bed.

Orthostatic hypotension and consequent syncope are common symptoms of disorders of generalised autonomic dysfunction (see below).

Hypotension may occur in the acute Guillain–Barré syndrome where there may be temporary loss of baroreceptor reflexes. Other chronic polyneuropathies may result in orthostatic hypertension (see below).

It must be remembered that drugs may impair circulatory reflexes: such drugs include hypotensive agents, such as α-methyldopa and, to a lesser degree, beta blockers, as well as chlorpromazine, tricyclic compounds and barbiturates (p. 431).

Management of chronic orthostatic hypotension

When orthostatic hypotension is severe it presents a difficult management problem. Perhaps the most important single measure is to block the head of the patient's bed by 20°: this results in a significant increase in extracellular fluid volume. A variety of pharmacological approaches can be used: the mineralocorticoid 9-α-fludrocortisone can help by expanding plasma volume; other drugs reported to be helpful include sympathomimetics, such as ephedrine and tyramine, dihydroergotamine and indomethacin. The number of drugs advocated indicates that none is very satisfactory.

Mechanical treatment including elasticated stockings and, occasionally, antigravity suits may be used.

DISORDERS OF RESPIRATION

A number of distinct abnormalities of respiratory pattern are seen in association with neurological disease (Fig. 4.6). Although these have some localising value, this is often obscured by changes which result from pulmonary congestion and other metabolic changes in patients with neurological disorders.

Cheyne-Stokes respiration

This is a pattern of waxing and waning respiration with intervening periods of apnoea. It is most frequently seen in patients with diffuse hemisphere disturbance, e.g. hypoxia. This results in a decreased drive from forebrain centres allowing an increased response to CO_2 stimulation: thus, as the $P\text{CO}_2$ rises, patients respond with an increasing tidal volume which diminishes as the $P\text{CO}_2$ falls in response; subsequently, apnoea occurs until the rising $P\text{CO}_2$ again results in respiratory drive. It is most commonly seen in heart failure resulting in cerebral hypoxia, but may also occur with cerebral infarction and metabolic disorders such as renal or hepatic failure.

Hyperventilation

Sustained hyperventilation is seen in patients with lesions of the paramedian reticular formation of the lower mid brain and pons. However, this syndrome is rare and more commonly tachypnoea may occur in patients with neurological disease because of reflexly induced pulmonary congestion and oedema.

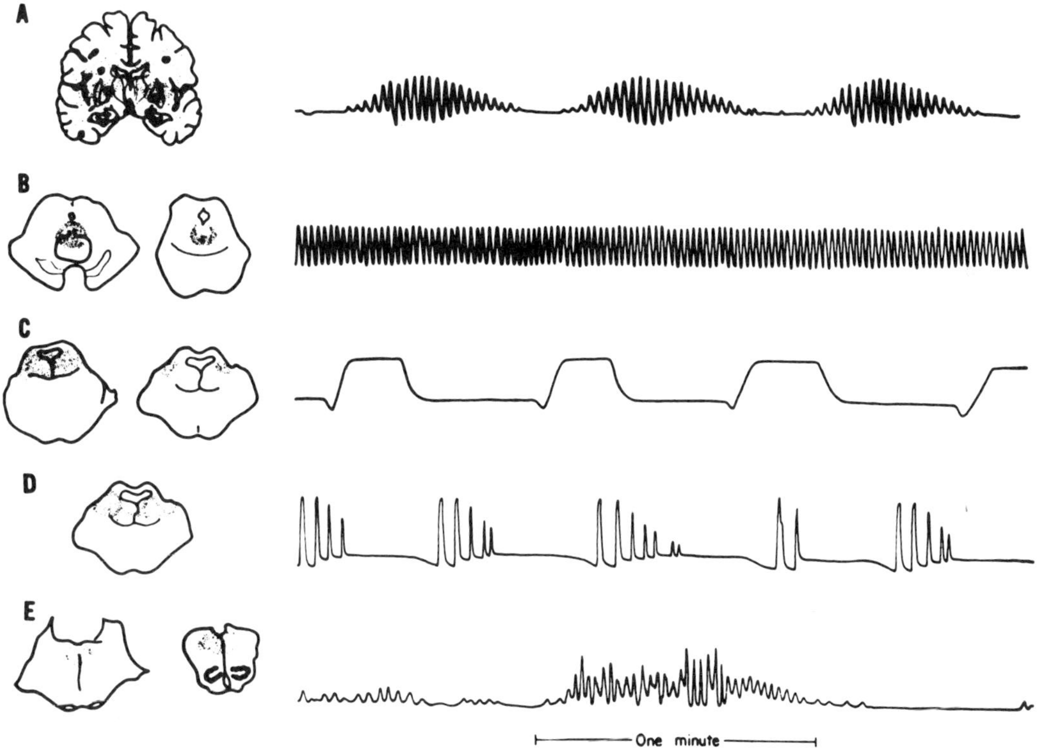

Fig. 4.6 Respiratory patterns in neurological disease at various sites. **A** Cheyne–Stokes respiration, **B** hyperventilation, **C** apneustic respiration, **D** cluster breathing, **E** ataxic respiration. (Reproduced from Plum F, Posner J B 1972 *The Diagnosis of Stupor and Coma*, 2nd edn. Davis, Philadelphia, with permission.)

Apneustic breathing

This abnormal respiratory pattern is characterised by an inspiratory pause at full inspiration. This pattern may be of greater localising value than others, indicating lesions at the level of the mid-pons. It is most often seen in basilar artery occlusion.

Ataxic breathing

Ataxic breathing is a completely irregular pattern in which deep and shallow breaths alternate unpredictably. It appears to be due to lesions at the medullary level which directly affect the respiratory centres; its occurrence may herald complete respiratory arrest. It is most commonly seen with slowly expanding posterior fossa lesions and with rare vascular lesions involving the medulla.

Neurogenic hypoventilation

This occurs in individuals whose respiratory drive is relatively insensitive to CO_2; this results in somnolence, cyanosis and, in the longer term, cor pulmonale. An unusual variation of this is 'Ondine's curse': while they are awake, patients maintain adequate ventilation, but become apnoeic during sleep. This abnormality is most often seen with medullary lesions (stroke and tumours).

Yawning

Yawning is a complex reflex response which encompasses stretching, deep inspiratory effort and vasomotor lacrimal salivary secretion. It may be partly suppressed by voluntary effort and is most commonly seen with normal and pathologically drowsy states. On occasion, repeated yawning may occur in the absence of drowsiness in patients with posterior fossa lesions and possibly also lesions of the medial temporal lobe and third ventricle.

Hiccup

This reflex phenomenon appears to represent a gastrointestinal reflex which involves the respiratory muscles. It is most commonly seen in association with thoracoabdominal disorders, when gastric dilatation may be an important stimulus. It is, however, mediated by a supraspinal reflex involving medullary centres and very occasionally hiccuping may be a symptom of structural brainstem disorders, such as syringomyelia, neoplasm or infarction; the disorder is more commonly caused by drugs. In intractable cases, chlorpromazine or metoclopramide may be of value.

DISORDERS OF THERMOREGULATION AND SWEATING

Body temperature may diverge from normal levels in a number of circumstances.

Hypothermia

Hypothermia causes a progressive decline in conscious level with confusion, drowsiness and coma before cardiopulmonary arrest occurs. It will occur in individuals with normal temperature regulation when exposed to cold. However, it is more frequently seen in patients with defective thermoregulation attributable to a number of factors. Severe hypothermia may occur in myxoedema, due to inability of patients to increase basal metabolic rate in response to ordinary degrees of cold. More commonly, hypothermia is seen in the elderly, who show a more extreme fall in rectal temperature, with an impaired ability to increase heat production and to decrease heat loss on exposure to cold. Impaired thermoregulation may also be seen in patients with more definite neurological disorders, such as Parkinson's disease.

Drugs may also increase susceptibility to hypothermia, particularly overdosage with alcohol and barbiturates. Less commonly, prazosin and chlorpromazine may produce hypothermia.

Posterior hypothalamic lesions are sometimes complicated by hypothermia, often associated with somnolence and hypotension.

Hyperthermia

Fever represents a physiological response to infection, probably attributable to the effect of pyrogens on central thermoregulatory structures.

Hyperpyrexia can cause dizziness, weakness and confusion with, ultimately, coma and seizures. Such disturbances may be seen in individuals with normal thermoregulation exposed to extremes of heat. It may also occur in patients with defective thermoregulation due to anhydrosis (see below).

Specific neurological causes of hyperpyrexia include the neuroleptic malignant syndrome and malignant hyperpyrexia (see Ch. 17), a syndrome in which there is a rapid rise of body temperature during or after anaesthesia; it is characterised by continuous muscle activity and stiffness, hyperventilation, acidosis and hyperkalaemia. The syndrome has a high mortality. A variety of anaesthetic agents have been implicated in the pathogenesis, including halothane and suxamethonium. Many patients appear to come from families in which there is a history of myotonia, or other muscle disease, and it may be that increased creatinine phosphokinase activities may be predictive of malignant hyperpyrexia in individuals from within an affected family.

The basic defect may be related to calcium effects at muscle membranes. Anaesthetic agents may release stored calcium into the cytoplasm, resulting in an increase in cellular metabolism, myofibrillary contraction with increased oxygen consumption and lactic acidosis and heat production.

Anterior hypothalamic lesions may be associated with impairment of mechanisms for lowering body temperature. Operations involving the fourth and third ventricle may be complicated by a rapid postoperative rise in temperature.

Hyperhidrosis

Generalised excessive sweating may occur in a number of conditions, including infection, disseminated lymphoma and carcinoma, and endocrinological disease (hyperthyroidism and phaeochromocytoma), as well as with anxiety, and in a number of specific neurological conditions.

Excessive sweating of the hands, feet and axilla is seen on occasion in isolation from pathological abnormality and can be a source of embarrassment. Symptoms affecting the upper limb may be treated by resection of the upper thoracic sympathetic ganglia (T2–T4).

Localised abnormalities of sweating over the face may occur following facial palsy, head injury or surgical injury to the superficial petrosal nerve. In such instances abnormal regeneration of fibres may occur: thus, previously salivary fibres may develop innervation to sweat glands or lacrimal glands so that ingestion of food leads to abnormal facial sweating (auriculotemporal syndrome of Frey) or lacrimation (crocodile tears).

Abnormal sweating may occur after spinal cord transection when autonomic reflexes through the isolated spinal cord (usually due to distention of the bladder) result in hyperhidrosis. In high cord lesions this may affect the face, head and upper limbs, but with lower lesions the lower limbs only will be affected. Sometimes pathological hyperhidrosis is seen at an upper level of a spinal cord lesion.

Anhidrosis

Thermoregulatory sweating will not be seen below the level of cord transection, although spinal reflex sweating can still occur. Tetraplegics may thus be heat intolerant and may need to be nursed in air-conditioned surroundings. Loss of sweating on the face may occur as part of Horner's syndrome (see below). In peripheral nerve lesions, areas of anhidrosis may be seen corresponding to the distribution of the nerve in question. Occasionally with severe polyneuropathy, e.g. alcoholic neuropathy or diabetic neuropathy, a loss of sweating may be seen. Anhidrosis may be seen with the rare syndrome of congenital insensitivity to pain.

PUPILLARY DISORDERS

These are illustrated in Figure 4.7.

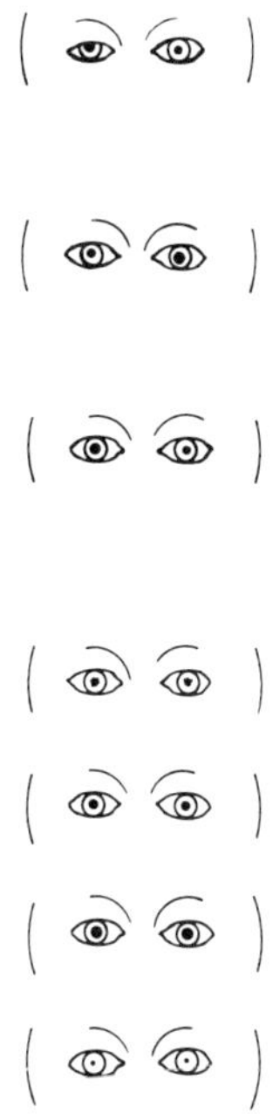

	REACTION TO LIGHT	ASSOCIATED SIGNS
UNILATERAL		
IIIrd nerve palsy	Negative	Ptosis (may be complete) External ophthalmoplegia
Horner's syndrome	Poor dilation to shade	Ptosis (always partial) Anhydrosis Enophthalmos
Holmes–Adie syndrome	Slow reaction	Constriction to methacholine
BILATERAL		
Argyll Robertson	Negative	Depigmented iris
Metabolic coma	Positive	Coma
Midbrain compression	Negative	Coma +/− lateralising signs
Pontine stroke	Negative	Coma Hyperventilation Hyperpyrexia

Fig. 4.7 Pupillary abnormalities.

Third nerve palsy (parasympathetic)

The parasympathetic innervation of the eye is related to the third cranial nerve. Third nerve palsy results in dilatation of the pupil with absence of response to both direct and consensual light stimuli and accommodation, associated with characteristic external ophthalmoplegia and ptosis. Dissociation between pupillary abnormalities and external ophthalmoplegia are most likely to occur with brain stem lesions, being particularly common with diabetic third nerve palsies; however, this rule is by no means absolute.

Horner's syndrome (sympathetic lesion)

This results from interruption of sympathetic supply to the eye, upper lid and facial sweat glands. The syndrome consists of myosis with impairment of pupillary dilatation in response to shading the eye. A mild ptosis is seen due to paresis of smooth muscle fibres of the upper eyelid (this is never complete, which differentiates this form of ptosis from ptosis due to third nerve palsy), with anhydrosis and enophthalmos.

Horner's syndrome may result from pontine and medullary brain-stem lesions interrupting the sympathetic pathway between hypothalamus and thoracic cord, e.g. as part of a lateral medullary syndrome. It may also result from central cord lesions, particularly in syringomyelia and from damage to the first thoracic root and lower brachial plexus (Pancoast's syndrome). More distally the sympathetic innervation of the eye is closely associated with the internal carotid artery and may be damaged by internal carotid artery occlusion, as well as by carotid angiography (Fig. 4.8).

Holmes–Adie syndrome

The syndrome is characterised by a tonic pupil which is dilated relative to the contralateral pupil but will constrict very slowly on accommodation. Pupillary reaction to light is usually absent, but after the patient has been in a dark room for some time, bright light may cause slow and incomplete constriction. The pupil will usually constrict in response to 2.5% methacholine, indicating a supersensitivity to acetylcholine possibly resulting from parasympathetic denervation, due to degeneration of postganglionic neurones with cell bodies in the ciliary ganglion.

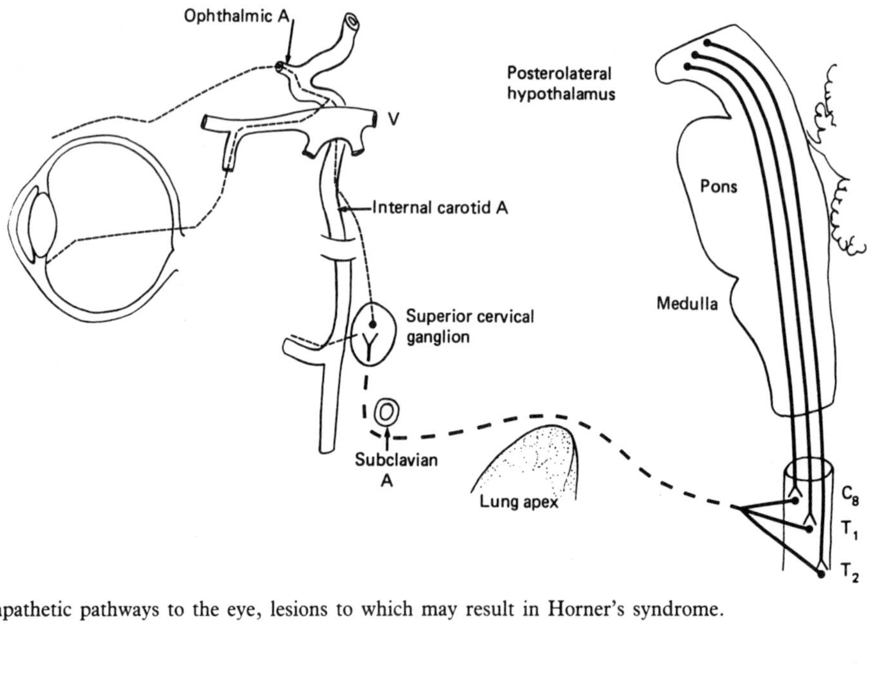

Fig. 4.8 Sympathetic pathways to the eye, lesions to which may result in Horner's syndrome.

The aetiology of the syndrome is uncertain, but it occurs almost exclusively among young women during the second and third decades of life. Often the disorder is noted by a friend, but sometimes the abnormality develops acutely and may cause subjective visual disturbance due to loss of normal accommodation. Patients complain of sensitivity to light because of the loss of normal pupillary reflexes. The pupillary syndrome is variably associated with areflexia, particularly of the lower limbs. Rarely other forms of dysautonomia may be associated, such as segmental loss of sweating (Ross's syndrome) or cardiac dysrhythmias.

Argyll Robertson pupils

This bilateral abnormality is characterised by small unequal and irregular pupils which constrict on accommodation but not on exposure to light. Very often there is depigmentation of the iris. The pupil shows little response to atropine, physostigmine or methacholine.

The anatomical basis for this abnormality remains obscure, but is probably due to a midbrain lesion. The syndrome was a classic sign of tertiary neurosyphilis but is now rarely seen. It may occasionally be seen in patients with diabetes.

Other pupillary abnormalities

A variety of pupillary abnormalities may be seen in brain-stem or tentorial herniation, and other brain-stem disorders. Abnormalities of pupillary function may also result from lesions of the afferent limb of the light reflex (afferent pupillary defect, p. 44).

BLADDER DYSFUNCTION

Disorders at various levels of the nervous system give rise to characteristic syndromes of urinary incontinence.

Confusional states are frequently associated with both urinary and faecal incontinence. More localised *bifrontal lesions* are characterised by incontinence, which occurs suddenly with the patient apparently unaware of, or inattentive to, the desire to void. Patients may often deny urinary incontinence which is obvious. This form of incontinence is usually accompanied by frontal lobe indifference and passivity: it is seen with frontal lobe and corpus callosum gliomas, and subfrontal meningioma; it may also be seen in patients with hydrocephalus.

Bladder disturbance is a common and important symptom of *spinal cord disease*. It may occur early in demyelinating cord lesions, but its development in patients with cord compression is an indication that urgent decompression is necessary to avoid permanent neurological disability. Two types of bladder disturbance are seen with spinal cord disease.

Acute severe cord lesions

After acute transection, compression or transverse myelitis, the bladder may dilate and become atonic with loss of sensation. Painless retention with overflow will develop. This usually represents a temporary phase and, over the next few days to weeks, return of reflex bladder function will occur.

Chronic or partial cord lesions

Chronic cord transection, or partial slowly progressive cord lesions, are associated with an overactivity of bladder reflexes. Patients with partial lesions become aware of the desire to void with small volumes of urine in the bladder, giving rise to frequency. The reflexes are hyperactive and less amenable to voluntary control, resulting in urgency. These problems may be exacerbated by abnormal internal sphincter function, leading to premature closure of the involuntary components of the sphincter and retention of residual urine (detrusor-sphincter dyssynergia). This causes symptoms of hesitancy, poor stream and post-micturition dribbling and also increases symptoms of frequency and urgency. In chronic complete lesions, reflex emptying of the bladder occurs without the patient's awareness.

Lesions of the conus, cauda equina and bilateral sacral roots and plexuses result in an insensitive atonic bladder with large volumes of residual urine and overflow with dribbling incontinence.

Management of the chronic neurogenic bladder

The management of the chronic neurogenic bladder is of great importance, and applies chiefly to patients with multiple sclerosis. The aim is to restore satisfactory voiding of urine by the least invasive and most socially acceptable means. Prevention of chronic retention and urinary infection is the end.

To plan management it is essential to have an accurate account of urinary symptoms, intravenous urography and cystometric studies (see above). Regular review of a patient's problems is necessary and new problems may require different management. A number of methods of management are available: these are pharmacological, mechanical, and surgical and must be tailored to the individual patient; they are summarised in Table 4.5.

Pharmacological therapy is of greatest value in detrusor instability causing urgency and urge incontinence, but is disappointing for other problems. Where retention becomes a problem, urethral dilatation and bladder neck surgery may be helpful but, if this fails, intermittent self-catheterisation, or an indwelling catheter may become necessary. In the latter instance every effort must be made to minimise urinary infection by regular antiseptic bladder washouts.

Enuresis

Although nocturnal incontinence may occur in patients with a neurogenic bladder, as well as in metabolic disturbances such as diabetes mellitus, diabetes insipidus, epilepsy and urinary tract disease, it most commonly occurs during childhood and is independent of other disorders. It appears that intravesicular pressures rise to higher than normal levels during sleep in enuretic patients who fail to show a normal arousal to this stimulus. Behavioural conditioning and imipramine may be effective in the treatment of this disorder.

Mechanical causes of disturbed micturition

Neurological causes of altered micturition must be differentiated from mechanical ones, which can of course occur in patients with neurological disease. Frequency, when it is accompanied by marked

Table 4.5 Management of the chronic neurogenic bladder

	The upper motor neurone bladder			The lower motor neurone bladder
	Detrusor instability*	Sphincter instability*	Bladder of cord transection	
Symptoms	Urgency Frequency	Hesitancy Poor stream Retention	Insensitivity Reflex emptying	Insensitivity Atonic bladder Retention with overflow
Drug therapy	Anticholinergics probanthine imipramine emepromium	Cholinergics distigmine bromide Antiadrenergics phenoxybenzamine		Cholinergics distigmine bromide
Mechanical	Male condom Female incontinence pads catheter	Intermittent self-catheter Indwelling catheter	Male condom catheter Female catheter	Bladder drill and emptying by straining Indwelling catheter
Surgical		Urethral dilatation Bladder neck surgery		Urinary diversion

* These may coexist in the same patient.

urgency of micturition, is the most striking indication of a neurological cause of disturbed bladder function. Frequency in the absence of marked urgency is more common with local bladder pathology such as prostatic hypertrophy.

Disturbed bladder function due to lower motor neurone lesions is, however, more likely to be confused with mechanical causes of incontinence. In particular, the insensitive distended bladder may give rise to dribbling incontinence during straining, stooping and coughing and therefore may be confused with stress incontinence in women.

DISORDERS OF GASTROINTESTINAL FUNCTION

Swallowing

Dysphagia of neurological origin is almost always accompanied by dysarthria and most commonly results from pseudobulbar or bulbar palsy, causing disturbance to the function of pharyngeal voluntary muscle.

In achalasia there is degeneration of Auerbach's plexus and resultant cardiospasm and oesophageal dilation. Disorders of oesophageal motility may occur with ageing, autonomic neuropathy, and parkinsonism, but these are rarely symptomatic.

Gastric motility

Vomiting may occur as a symptom of neurological disease. It is controlled by a discrete area of the dorsolateral reticular formation. Neurological vomiting is usually accompanied by vertigo, indicating the close relationship of this area to the vestibular system. However, lesions close to the floor of the fourth ventricle may sometimes give rise to positional vomiting without vertigo.

Gastroparesis, causing abdominal distension and effortless vomiting, may be seen in patients with severe diabetic autonomic neuropathy.

Intestinal motility

The intrinsic plexus of the intestine may be impaired either congenitally (Hirschsprung's disease) or because of infection with *Trypanosoma cruzi* (Chaga's disease), leading to constipation and abdominal distension. Patients with diabetic autonomic neuropathy may suffer from either constipation or diarrhoea: the latter characteristically occurs at night, persists for a few hours, and may be associated with incontinence; however, radiological abnormalities of intestinal mobility are usually absent, and abnormal gastrointestinal flora may have a role in this symptom.

Defaecation

The rectum and anal sphincters receive autonomic innervation similar to that of the bladder, and syndromes of faecal incontinence largely mimic those of bladder disturbance.

Normal defaecation occurs when the rectum fills following a colonic mass movement. It can be inhibited by voluntary control over the external anal sphincter; such control may be lost with lesions at various sites in the nervous system. Frontal lesions lead to a lack of awareness, with incontinence; spinal cord lesions, when severe, initially lead to constipation, but subsequently reflex defaecation without sensation can become established. Here defaecation may be associated with sweating and vasoconstriction below the level of a cord lesion. Partial cord lesions can lead to urgency of defaecation; the symptom is usually much less prominent than urgency of micturition. Lesions of the conus, cauda equina and bilateral sacral plexus result in loss of rectal sensation with colonic distension and constipation.

SEXUAL DYSFUNCTION

Male sexual function requires normal libido, penile erection and ejaculation. Erection is mediated by the parasympathetic outflow from the sacral roots via the pudendal nerves. Ejaculation occurs reflexly and is probably dependent on sympathetic fibres.

Psychological factors including depression most commonly cause loss of libido; however, this may also occur in frontal lobe disease and epilepsy, as well as endocrine disorders. In such conditions reflex penile erection and nocturnal emissions may still occur. Occasionally, heightened and disinhibited sexual desire may be seen with lesions of the diencephalon, frontal and temporal lobes.

Impotence (failure of erection) is usually associated with depressive states, but is also seen in patients with spinal cord disease particularly affecting the sacral segments, and it may be an important early symptom of autonomic neuropathy. However, in paraplegics with higher cord lesions, erection may occur as a reflex response to penile or perineal stimulation. In cord transection, reflexes subserving erection may become overactive and result in priapism.

Disorders of ejaculation can be associated with neurological disease. Lesions between the sixth thoracic and third lumbar cord segments abolish ejaculation, as do lesions of the sacral cord and cauda equina. However, erection and ejaculation may be possible in paraplegic patients with cord transection at other levels.

Fertility in male paraplegics may be further reduced because of reduced sperm counts, the cause of which are uncertain, and by flexor spasms of the lower limbs interfering with intercourse. On occasion, autonomic reflexes may cause reflex hypertension during intercourse, and subarachnoid haemorrhage has been reported.

Retrograde ejaculation may occur in diabetic autonomic neuropathy, cord and cauda equina lesions and, of course, in patients who have required bladder neck surgery because of micturition difficulties.

Sexual dysfunction in women is less specific and less frequently complained of than in men, and rarely requires treatment.

Management of sexual dysfunction

Treatment of sexual dysfunction in neurological disorders is of greatest importance in the male with spinal cord disease or autonomic neuropathy, but is often unsatisfactory. Erectile problems may be overcome by the use of vibrators to stimulate reflex erection. Failing this, penile protheses may be implanted. Ejaculation difficulties can in some cases be overcome by the use of vibrators. Where this is not possible, semen may be harvested, where this is important, for artificial insemination, using a technique of electrical stimulation via rectal electrodes. In cases of retrograde ejaculation semen may again be harvested from urine, or ejaculation in the presence of a full bladder may be successful.

HYPOTHALAMIC DYSFUNCTION

Hypothalamic disorders most commonly present with anterior pituitary dysfunction and visual field abnormalities. A number of specific symptoms and syndromes are more specifically associated with hypothalamic disease.

Diabetes insipidus

This results from lesions involving the supraoptic and paraventricular hypothalamic nuclei or supraopticohypophyseal tract. Failure of normal secretion of antidiuretic hormone (ADH) gives rise to an inability to concentrate urine, with symptoms of both polyuria and thirst. The syndrome may occur with hypothalamic tumours, meningitis, sarcoidosis, histiocytosis and trauma—postsurgical diabetes insipidus being most common.

Treatment consists of replacement therapy with DDAVP which can be administered via a nasal route or intramuscularly.

Inappropriate ADH secretion

Inappropriate release of ADH results in excessive retention of water and a dilutional hyponatraemia and hypo-osmolarity of serum. Sodium concentrations of less than 110 mEq/l are associated with neurological disturbance, including confusion, seizures and increasingly deep coma (p. 462).

Although the syndrome is most commonly seen complicating oat-cell carcinoma, it also occurs in a number of neurological conditions, including the Guillain–Barré syndrome, subarachnoid haemorrhage, cerebral infarction, tumour, abscess, meningitis and head injury. In such circumstances inappropriate ADH secretion is usually temporary and subsides with treatment of the underlying disorder. When neurological disorders cause inappropriate ADH secretion this is usually incidental to an already obvious neurological diagnosis: neurological investigation of patients with inappropriate ADH syndrome of uncertain aetiology is rarely, if ever, indicated.

Hypothalamic adiposity and appetite control

Lesions of the tuberal nuclei and tuberoinfundibular tracts result in a syndrome of obesity associated with arrested sexual development. No obvious pathological cause may be apparent (Froehlich's syndrome), but this syndrome may be a presenting feature of craniopharyngioma. In the Lawrence–Moon–Biedl syndrome obesity, hypogonadism, mental retardation, polydactyly and retinitis pigmentosa are associated.

SYNDROMES OF GENERALISED AUTONOMIC DISTURBANCE

A number of uncommon conditions are seen which primarily affect the autonomic system with a multiplicity of symptoms. Patients' main complaints are usually related to orthostatic hypotension, which occurs in the absence of pallor and sweating. There may be associated symptoms of bladder and bowel dysfunction, impotence and anhydrosis. Such generalised autonomic disturbance may be seen in conditions primarily affecting the peripheral or central nervous system.

PERIPHERAL DISORDERS

Chronic progressive autonomic disturbance may occur in a variety of peripheral neuropathies due to diabetes, alcohol, porphyria, paraneoplastic neuropathy and primary amyloidosis. Autonomic changes may also complicate the Guillain-Barré syndrome. These conditions are discussed in more detail in Chapter 10.

Acute autonomic neuropathy has been observed in a small number of adults developing complete autonomic paralysis over a period of a week or so, with subsequent gradual recovery over a few months. The pathogenesis of the disorder is not understood.

Autonomic paresis also occurs in the Riley–Day syndrome which affects Jewish children. This presents at birth with failure to thrive, unexplained fever and episodes of pneumonia. There is hyporeflexia and impairment or loss of pain and temperature sensation. It is an autosomal recessive condition which seems largely due to a neuropathic disturbance particularly affecting small myelinated and unmyelinated fibres. The condition is not compatible with prolonged survival.

CENTRAL DISORDERS

Progressive autonomic failure (idiopathic orthostatic hypotension) is a rare syndrome occurring in isolation from other c.n.s. disease. It is characterised by degeneration of preganglionic autonomic neurones of the brain stem and spinal cord. More commonly, although still rarely, a similar pattern of autonomic disturbance is seen in association with multisystem degenerative disease in the Shy–Drager syndrome and olivopontine cerebellar degeneration; it is seen to milder degrees in Parkinson's disease (see p. 386).

FURTHER READING

Bannister R 1983 Autonomic failure. Oxford University Press, Oxford

Ewing D J, Clarke B F 1985 Diagnosis and management of diabetic autonomic neuropathy. British Medical Journal 285: 916–918

Johnson R H, Spalding J M K 1974 Disorders of the autonomic nervous system. Blackwell Scientific Publications, Oxford

5

Neurological investigations

INTRODUCTION

The use and value of neurological investigations are frequently misunderstood by non-neurologists. It must be recognised that, in almost all cases, the results of specialised neurological investigations cannot be interpreted in the absence of adequate clinical appraisal of the patient: their major value is in supporting and confirming clinical opinion; they rarely stand alone in offering a satisfactory diagnosis. Thus the CT appearances of cerebral infarction and cerebral tumour may be impossible to differentiate without knowing whether the patient's neurological problems developed suddenly or progressively. Similarly, EEGs recorded shortly after a generalised seizure may show generalised slow activity which could not be differentiated from a metabolic encephalopathy in the absence of adequate clinical information.

NEUROPHYSIOLOGY

THE ELECTROENCEPHALOGRAM (EEG)

The EEG may be the most abused neurological investigation: there is considerable ignorance of the significance of abnormalities that it shows, and a great tendency to overinterpret the results in defining specific pathologies. It must be emphasised that abnormalities seen in the EEG are never specific for any one individual pathological condition.

Methods

The electrical activity of the brain is recorded via electrodes placed over the scalp. Standard electrode placements are usually employed (10–20 system). Most commonly, bipolar recordings are made in varying montages which allow localisation of abnormal potentials on the basis of the distribution of phase shifts. Occasionally, monopolar recordings are made using a common reference point. Electrical activity is subsequently amplified, filtered and written out on a continuous paper record.

Recordings must be made in a quiet environment with the patient relaxed. Detailed observations by skilled technicians are necessary to correlate changes in the record with any movement or disturbance. Recordings are usually undertaken at rest, with the eyes open, closed, following a period of hyperventilation, and on stroboscopic stimulation. Recording during sleep may be a further helpful provocative procedure in patients with epilepsy.

EEG activity

Normal EEG activity

Alpha rhythm is the most striking component of the normal EEG. It is of regular and moderate amplitude with a frequency of between 8 and 13 Hz. It occurs during wakefulness with the eyes closed, is attenuated by eye opening and disappears during sleep, and is most clearly demonstrated in posterior leads (Fig. 5.1).

Beta activity is defined as any rhythmic activity with a frequency of more than 13 Hz. It is usually generalised and may be seen in normal subjects who are tense or anxious about the procedure and also as a drug-induced effect in patients receiving sedative or tranquillising drugs.

Theta activity has a frequency of 4–7 Hz. It is a normal component of the EEG of children and adolescents, particularly over the temporal regions, but becomes more sparse with maturation. The finding of temporal theta activity represents a non-specific abnormality in adult patients with a variety of neurological disorders.

Artefactual changes

Numerous physiological and technical artefacts may be seen during EEG recording. These include large-amplitude frontal potentials due to eye movements, activity of very short duration due to muscle activity, ECG and electrode artefacts. The limitation of these problems demands a high level of technical expertise.

Abnormal EEG activity

Delta activity is defined as activity with a frequency of less than 4 Hz. Although delta activity may occur in normal individuals during sleep and in children, its presence in the waking state in adults is abnormal. Generalised delta

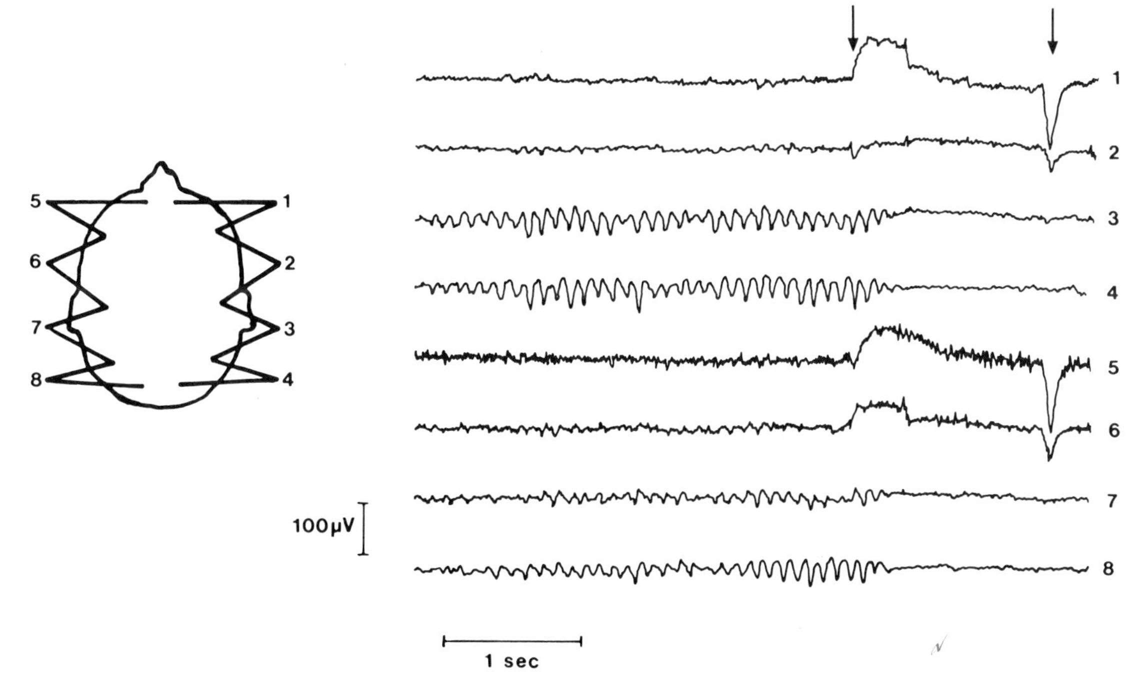

Fig. 5.1 A normal EEG showing a posterior alpha rhythm which is attenuated by eye opening (the first arrow). The first and second arrows indicate eye-movement artefact seen in the anterior leads.

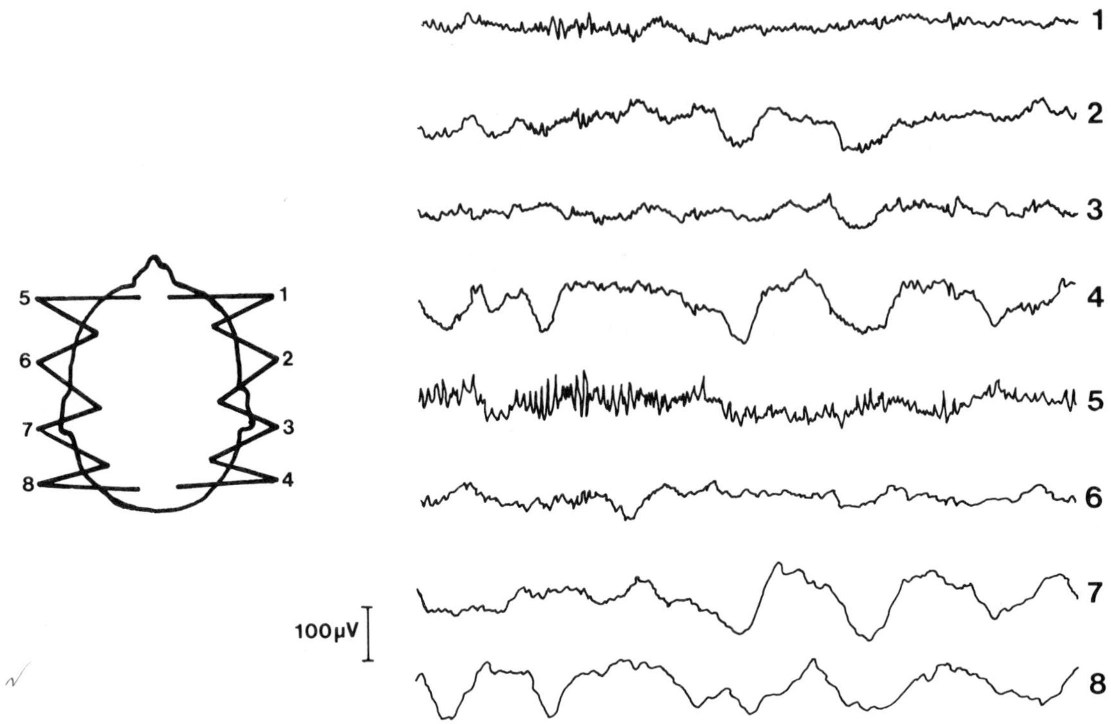

Fig. 5.2 Generalised slow (delta) activity of high amplitude, maximal in posterior leads in a patient in coma due to a viral encephalitis.

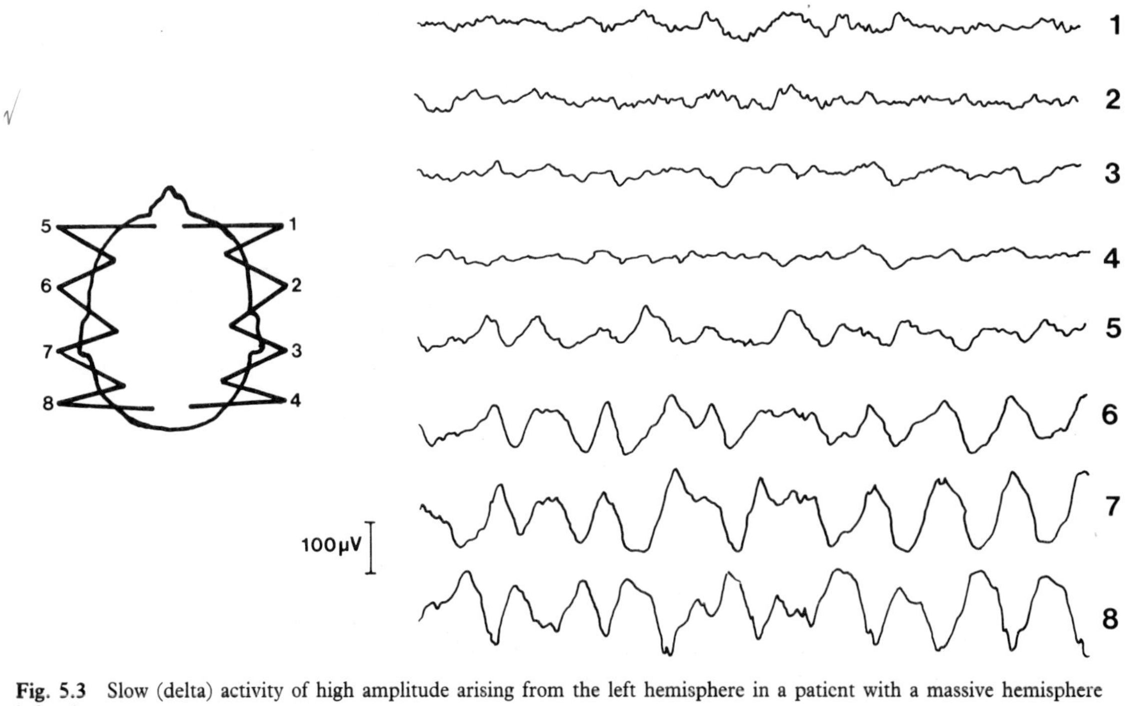

Fig. 5.3 Slow (delta) activity of high amplitude arising from the left hemisphere in a patient with a massive hemisphere infarction.

activity is seen postictally, in patients with metabolic encephalopathy, and in patients with a diffuse encephalitis (Fig. 5.2). When it is localised to one area of the hemisphere it is usually indicative of some form of structural pathology (Fig. 5.3). However, it is impossible to differentiate between tumour and infarction on the basis of localised delta activity.

Spike discharges or sharp waves of a duration of up to 200 ms are the characteristic interictal abnormality found in epileptic patients. When they are generalised, interictal spikes are most commonly associated with following slow waves. When they are localised, although spikes and sharp waves may be associated with slow activity, they are more likely to occur independently. Sharp waves may be induced by drugs and alcohol withdrawal.

Paroxysmal activity may be defined as activity of very sudden onset and termination. This obviously includes spike wave activity, but also describes bursts of faster theta activity, seen as part of an epileptic process, and periodic complexes (see below).

EEG responses to activation

Hyperventilation leads to a general slowing of activity often with the development of paroxysmal high voltage delta activity. These changes are most evident in younger patients and diminish with increasing age. Hyperventilation may provoke spike wave discharges in patients with absence and other forms of idiopathic generalised epilepsy. Occasionally hyperventilation may enhance local abnormalities in the EEG.

Photic stimulation is performed with a stroboscopic stimulus usually with the eyes closed and open. This generates some posterior rhythmic activity that is time-locked to the rate of stroboscopic stimulation. In some instances photomyoclonic responses may be generated with muscle activity most commonly localised around the eyelids, occurring at the rate of stimulation. However, in patients with photosensitive epilepsy, a photoconvulsive response occurs: this consists of bursts of spike-slow wave activity which are usually bilateral and synchronous and which persist briefly after the termination of the stroboscopic stimulus. This abnormality is seen in patients with idiopathic and symptomatic generalised epilepsies.

Historically drugs have been used to 'activate' the EEG. This is now rarely performed, though sodium methohexitone may be used in the specialised investigation of patients being assessed for temporal lobectomy.

Recordings during natural sleep show a significant modification of EEG activity: there tends to be a generalised slowing of activity, with loss of alpha rhythm and quite dramatic activity with K complexes and bursts of sleep spindles may occur; however, a full description of these is beyond the scope of this chapter. The main value of sleep recording is in the detection of abnormalities in patients with suspected partial seizures, and in the investigation of sleep apnoea.

Indications for the EEG

Epilepsy

The major indication for EEG recording is in the diagnosis and classification of epilepsy. The value is related to the occurrence of interictal paroxysmal activity in a significant number of patients with epilepsy. Seizure activity during standard EEG recordings remains uncommon.

It must be emphasised that some patients without a history of seizures may have EEG abnormalities and that a significant proportion of patients with epilepsy have normal interictal records: thus the diagnosis of epilepsy can neither be proved nor disproved from EEG recording. Different types of interictal abnormalities are seen in various epileptic syndromes.

Idiopathic generalised epilepsy (p. 158). The characteristic interictal abnormality in primary generalised epilepsy is paroxysmal bursts of bilateral synchronised spike or poly spike and wave activity which is regular and well organised at a rate of 0.5–6 Hz (Fig. 5.4). Short bursts of such activity may occur without symptoms, but longer bursts may be associated with absence (petit mal): 3 Hz generalised spike wave activity must be demonstrated in the EEG before a diagnosis of petit mal epilepsy can be accepted. Sometimes myoclonic jerking may be time-locked to the spike wave discharges.

Symptomatic generalised epilepsy (e.g. Lennox-Gastaut syndrome) (p. 159). In these syndromes,

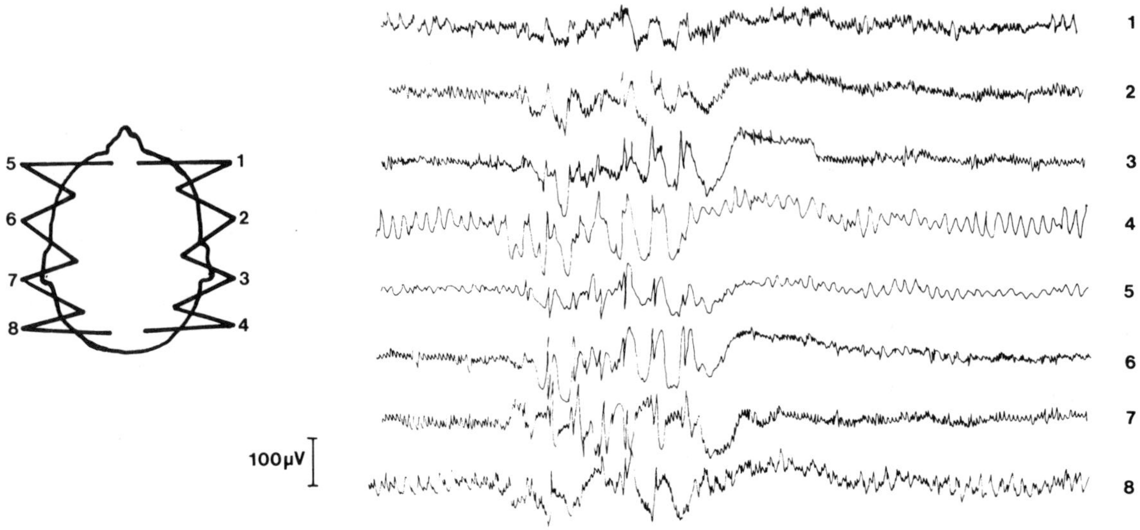

Fig. 5.4 A short burst of generalised 3–4 Hz spike wave activity in a patient with benign myoclonic epilepsy of adolescence (see Ch. 7).

background activity is usually abnormal and generalised spike wave discharges are much more irregular and less well formed than in primary generalised epilepsy (Fig. 5.5). A pathognomonic EEG abnormality hypsarrhythmia is seen in patients with the infantile spasm syndrome.

Partial epilepsy (p. 160). In patients with partial epilepsies the most striking diagnostic feature is of localised spike, sharp wave or spike wave disturbances (Fig. 5.6). Some patients show paroxysmal bursts of localised theta activity. However, it is not uncommon for interictal recordings to be unremarkable in partial epilepsies.

It must always be remembered that localised epileptiform abnormalities may occur in areas remote from recording electrodes. In some instances, recording from nasopharyngeal or sphenoidal leads may be necessary to detect medial temporal disturbances. In partial epilepsies, associated structural abnormalities, such as tumours, may also declare themselves as localised delta wave disturbance.

C.n.s. infection

The other major indication for EEG recording is in the diagnosis of c.n.s. infections. In most meningitic and encephalitic illnesses a generalised disturbance of background activity is seen, with generalised slowing and the occurrence of moderate-amplitude slow activity (Fig. 5.2). However, in a number of infections more specific abnormal activity is seen.

In generalised *periodic activity* the background tends to be isoelectric. Superimposed on this are periodic slow waves moderate to high amplitude of occurring 1–4 s apart (Fig. 5.7). This form of activity can be diagnostic of subacute sclerosing panencephalitis (SSPE) when present in children, and of Creutzfeldt–Jakob disease when found in older patients with subacute or chronic dementing illnesses. These periodic complexes are not, however, wholly pathology-specific: they may also occur in patients with severe post-hypoxic damage, and similar periodic triphasic activity may be seen in hepatic encephalopathy. Localised periodic activity is seen over one or other temporal lobes in herpes simplex encephalitis.

Diagnosis of brain death (p. 138)

Whereas an isoelectric EEG is a requirement for the diagnosis of brain death in some countries, this is not the case in the UK where clinical

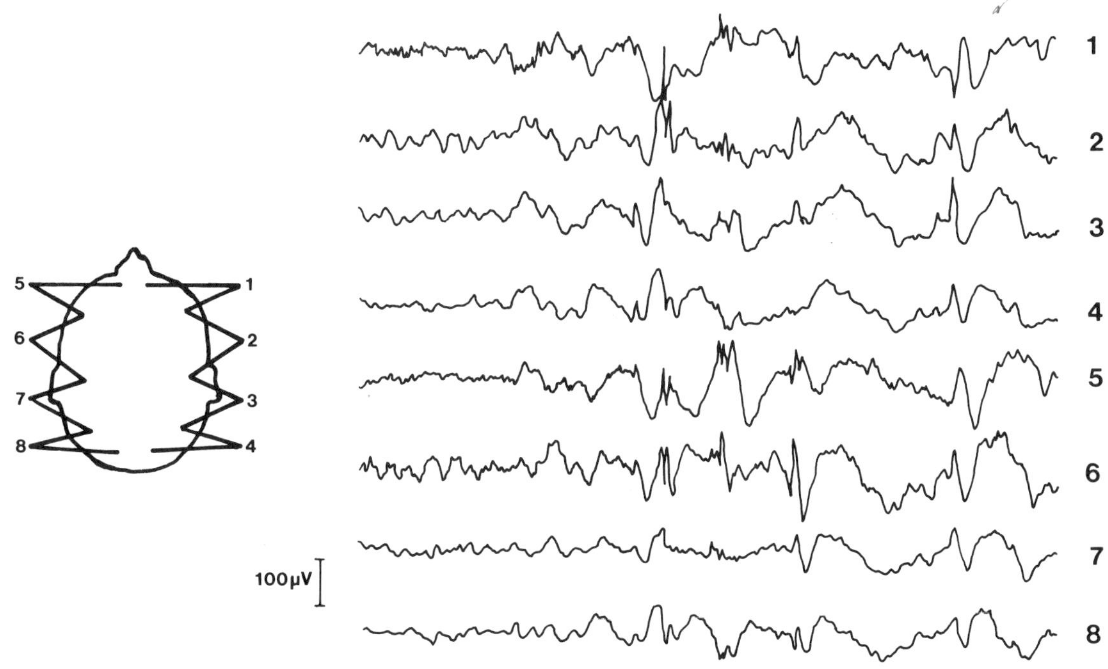

Fig. 5.5 Irregular generalised slow spike wave activity in a child with Lennox–Gastaut syndrome (see Ch. 7).

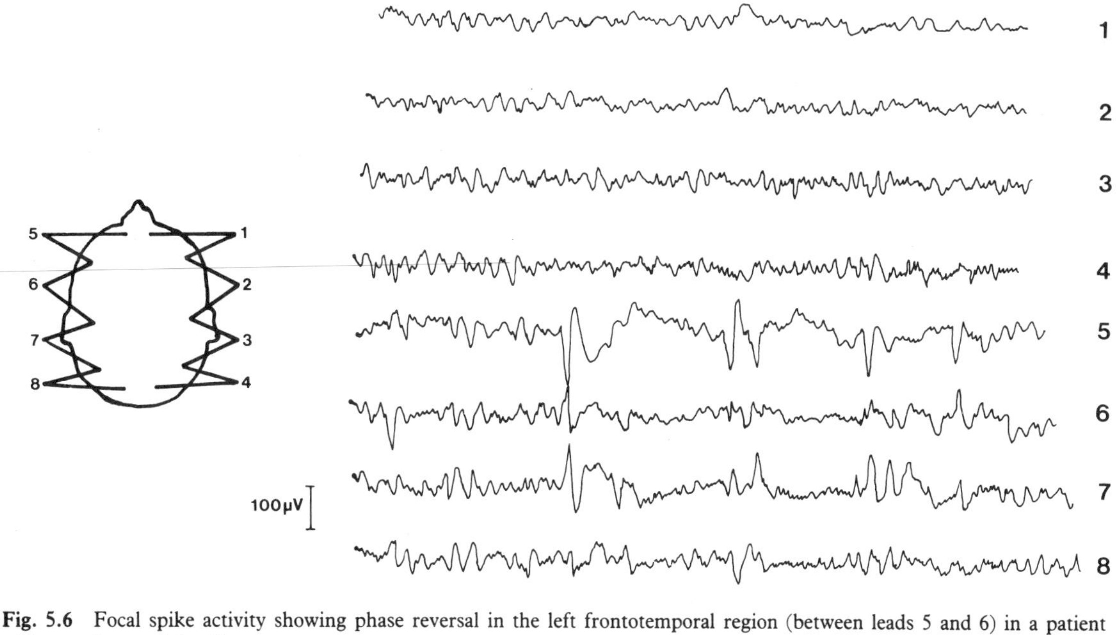

Fig. 5.6 Focal spike activity showing phase reversal in the left frontotemporal region (between leads 5 and 6) in a patient with complex partial epilepsy.

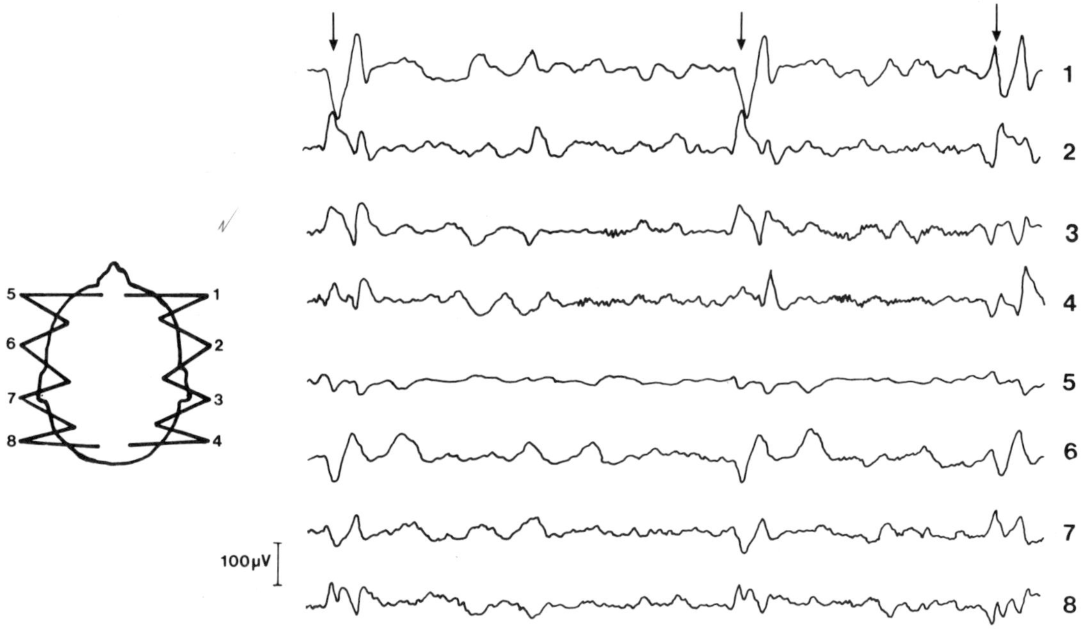

Fig. 5.7 Periodic activity (marked by arrows) separated by periods of relatively featureless EEG in a patient with subacute sclerosing panencephalitis.

criteria of brain-stem death are held to be adequate.

Diagnosis of coma and states of altered awareness (Ch. 6)

The EEG may be of some use in the investigation of coma. In particular, it may demonstrate a normal EEG in simulated coma and epileptiform activity in non-convulsive status.

The advent of sophisticated non-invasive means of brain imaging has greatly reduced the need for EEG recording in the localisation of structural disease. It should therefore rarely be necessary to record EEGs in patients being investigated for c.n.s. tumour or vascular disorders.

Prolonged EEG monitoring

In recent years, technological advances have allowed more prolonged EEG recording. Initially, this took the form of telemetry in which the patient to be studied was confined to a restricted area in which the EEG could be recorded from a limited array of electrodes, either by radio link or by direct connection, and behavioural changes in the patient could be monitored on video tape. This technique has advantages in allowing recording from large numbers of EEG electrodes, but is expensive in its demand for appropriate hospital inpatient facilities. Recent miniaturisation has allowed monitoring with 4- and 8-channel recorders with which the patient can be fully ambulant, with recording to a cassette tape; thus, records can be undertaken in outpatients. A visual record cannot be obtained and detection of symptomatic events is dependent on the subject pressing a 'panic' button. The major value of prolonged EEG monitoring is in the capture of symptomatic events to differentiate between true seizures, pseudoseizures and other causes of episodic loss of consciousness, diagnosis of which in a limited number of cases continues to present difficulty. The use of an ECG channel may help to elucidate whether dysrhythmias are primarily cardiac or cerebral.

EVOKED POTENTIAL RECORDINGS

The availability of computerised averaging techniques has enabled the detection of potential changes recorded at scalp electrodes to a variety of sensory stimuli. The principle involves the application of a specific sensory stimulus with an electrode potential being recorded and averaged for a specific period after each stimulus. Averaging thereby eliminates unrelated potential changes, leaving only a record of a potential change generated by the application of the stimulus (Fig. 5.8).

Visual evoked potentials (VEPs)

Early experiments with simple stroboscopic flash produced a complex evoked potential, the clinical interpretation of which presented considerable difficulties. The use of a patterned stimulus of uniform intensity produces a simpler wave form

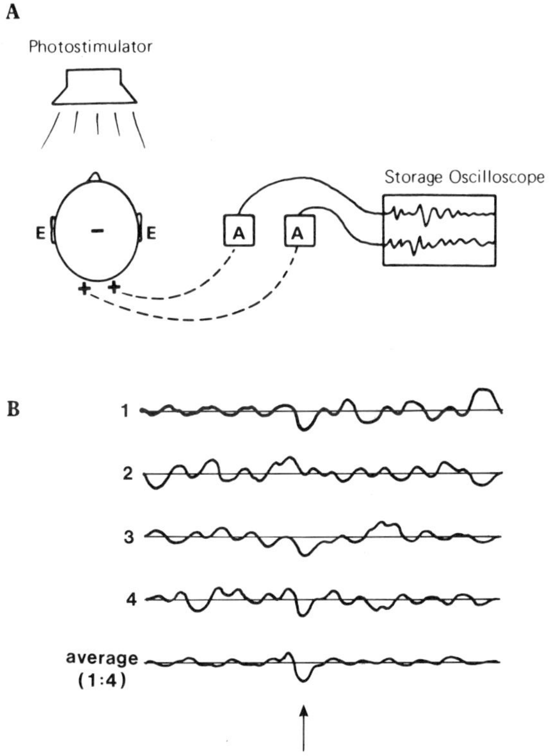

Fig. 5.8 **A** Techniques in recording visual evoked potentials. The photostimulator is usually a pattern generator. **B** The effects of averaging repeated sweeps.

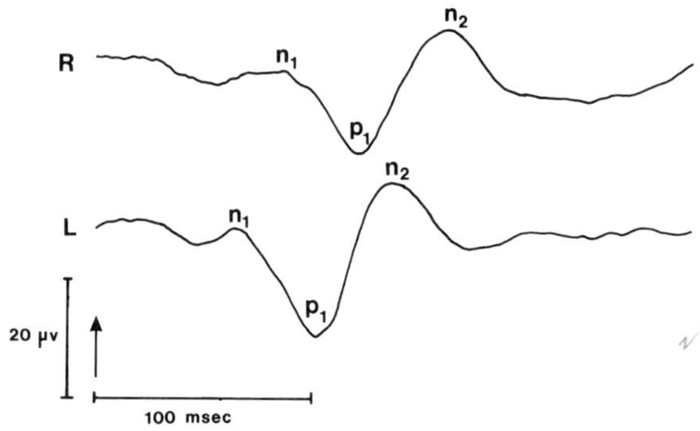

Fig. 5.9 Visual evoked potentials from the right and left eyes. The response from the left (lower trace) is of normal latency. The response from the right is delayed due to a recent retrobulbar neuritis.

that can be more readily analysed (Fig. 5.9). The most commonly used stimulus is a chequer-board pattern in which the stimulus is a change of each black square to white and vice versa. Pattern change can be presented on a cathode ray tube to one eye at a time and the EEG recorded from contralateral occipital electrodes averaged with respect to each pattern change. In normal individuals this generates a potential of variable amplitude but with a latency of 95–120 msec to peak following the stimulus change. The range of normal varies somewhat from laboratory to laboratory, as it does for all types of evoked potentials.

Indications

The clinical value of visual evoked potentials is in the detection of subclinical optic nerve lesions in patients with suspected multiple sclerosis (MS) (p. 419). Delay in the pattern-evoked potential may occur in the absence of previous symptoms of retrobulbar neuritis and in the absence of visual signs. Thus, where patients present with a history of one or more lesions affecting the brain stem or spinal cord, VEP evaluation may provide adequate evidence of further disseminated lesions. A high proportion of patients with clinically definite MS (approximately 90%) have abnormally delayed evoked potentials. However, in patients with clinically possible or probable MS, or with evidence only of isolated brain stem or spinal cord lesions, the percentage of detected abnormalities decreases greatly, so that only 20–30% of patients with such 'possible' MS have abnormal VEPs which facilitate a diagnosis. VEPs are of more occasional use in investigation of hysterical visual loss, and can also be used as a sophisticated means of visual field assessment.

It must be remembered that abnormalities in the visual evoked potential have no diagnostic pathological significance: they may be seen with pathology anywhere in the visual pathways. Before they can be satisfactorily interpreted, a full ophthalmological examination must be undertaken to exclude disorders of the eye and retina. Abnormalities will be present in compressive lesions of the optic nerve and pituitary chiasm, and in lesions of the optic radiation.

Auditory evoked potentials (BAEP)

In a similar manner to that for visual evoked potentials, a series of potentials from click stimuli can be recorded with averaging techniques from bipolar electrodes from vertex and mastoid. These result in a complex of five successive potentials related to activity in the auditory pathway firstly in peripheral, pontomedullary, pontine and midbrain portions of the pathway. These successive waves are conventionally described as I–V (Fig. 5.10).

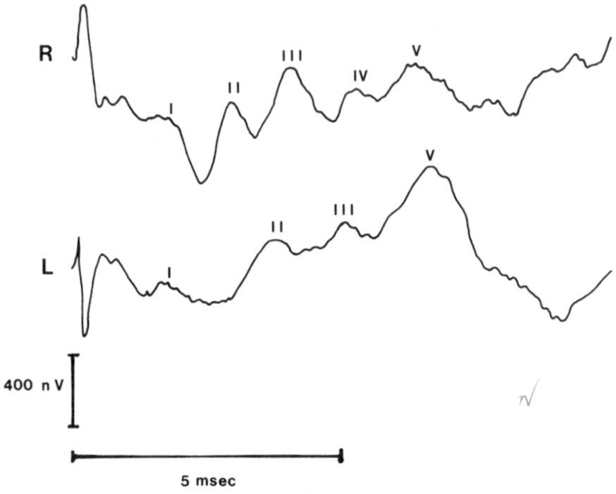

Fig. 5.10 Brain-stem auditory evoked potentials (BAEPs) from right and left ears. The response from the right (upper trace) is normal. That on the left shows delay of components II and III due to an acoustic neuroma.

Indications

The main clinical use for brain-stem evoked potentials has been in the diagnosis of MS, though it is less helpful and widely used than VEP. Abnormalities or abolition of the later brain-stem generated potentials may be sufficient to identify subclinical brain-stem lesions in patients with a history of retrobulbar neuritis or spinal cord disease. This evidence of disseminated disease may allow a more confident clinical diagnosis to be made. Again it must be emphasised that abnormalities of the brain-stem evoked potential are not pathologically specific and abnormal recordings will be obtained with posterior fossa tumours, vascular lesions and other causes of brain-stem demyelination, e.g. central pontine myelinolysis.

The other use suggested for auditory evoked potentials is in the assessment of patients in coma. Impairment of brain-stem generated potentials may indicate an adverse prognosis to coma. This may be particularly helpful as auditory evoked potentials seem relatively resistant to metabolic disturbance and depressant drugs. This use has been limited in the United Kingdom where clinical methods of assessing brain-stem function are more commonly used (p. 138).

Somatosensory evoked potentials (SSEPs)

Evoked potentials can be recorded from areas over the somatosensory cortex by averaging, following square-wave electrical pulses applied either to the electrodes on the fingers or over peripheral nerves. Delay, or disturbance in the wave form, may result from lesions anywhere in the sensory pathway from a peripheral nerve to the cortical level.

Abnormalities have no pathological specificity and SSEPs have only limited value in the detection of subclinical lesions in patients suspected of having MS. They are being used as a means of monitoring function during surgery.

PERIPHERAL NERVE CONDUCTION

Studies of nerve conduction are complementary to EMG recording in the investigation of neuromuscular disorders.

Motor nerve conduction studies

Motor nerves can be stimulated by electrodes placed over motor or mixed nerves and by recording the generated compound muscle action potential from a muscle innervated by that nerve (Fig. 5.11). In many instances a nerve may be stimulated at different points along its anatomical pathway so that by comparing latencies of response from different sites and by making appropriate measurements it is possible to calculate conduction velocities in various sections of motor nerves. Normal conduction velocities range from 40 to 55 m/s in the lower limbs and from 50 to 70 m/s in the upper limbs. Conduction velocities vary according to age and recording technique: in addition, terminal conduction tends to be slower than conduction in the main trunk of nerves. The amplitude of the muscle response will be the same from different stimulation sites unless there is conduction block (e.g. in segmental demyelination).

In addition to the direct (M) wave at supramaximal stimulation, later F waves may be recorded (Fig 5.12). These are probably due to antidromic activation of the motor nerve, firing anterior horn cells and generating a subsequent orthodromic discharge of some nerve axons. The latency of F waves is variable, but gives some indication of conduction in proximal segments of motor nerves which are otherwise difficult to study.

Sensory nerve conduction

Sensory conduction velocities and amplitudes can be determined either by stimulating sensory nerves distally, e.g. with digital electrodes, and recording proximally over cutaneous or mixed nerves, or by stimulating mixed nerves and recording antidromically over a cutaneous nerve (Fig. 5.13). Surface recording is usually satisfactory. Recording at differing sites allows calculation of conduction velocity, and changes in sensory nerve action potential amplitude are often the most sensitive means of detecting early peripheral neuropathy. Sensory conduction velocities are generally faster than motor conduction but there is a greater dispersal of recorded potential because

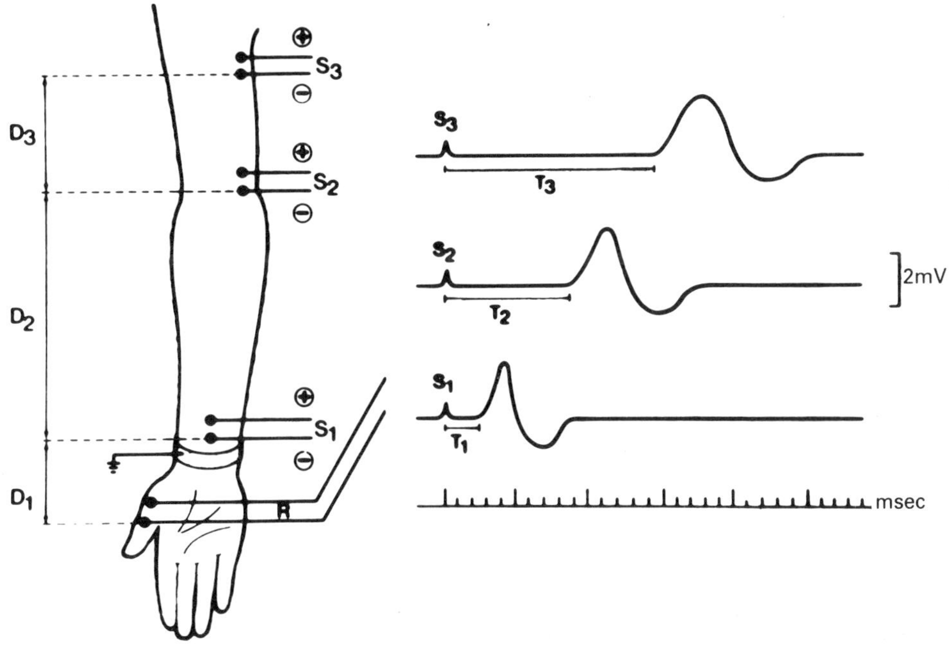

Fig. 5.11 The techniques of motor conduction recording. Surface evoked potentials are recorded at R, following stimulation at S1, S2 and S3. With measurement of distances D1, D2, D3, velocity can be calculated.

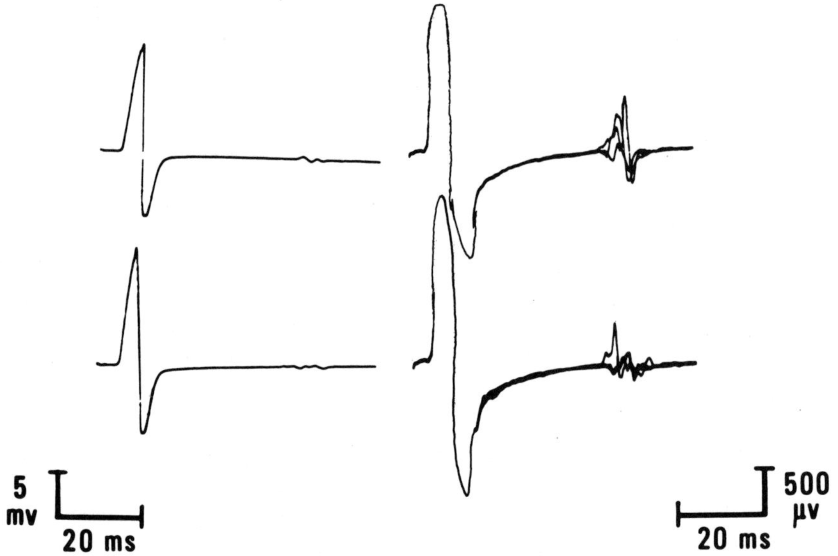

Fig. 5.12 Surface recordings of normal muscle responses from abductor hallucis brevis on tibial nerve stimulation at standard (left) and high amplification (right). A direct 'M' response is followed by a much smaller more variable 'F' wave. (Reproduced from Aminoff M J 1980 *Electrodiagnosis in Clinical Neurology*, Churchill Livingstone, Edinburgh, with permission.)

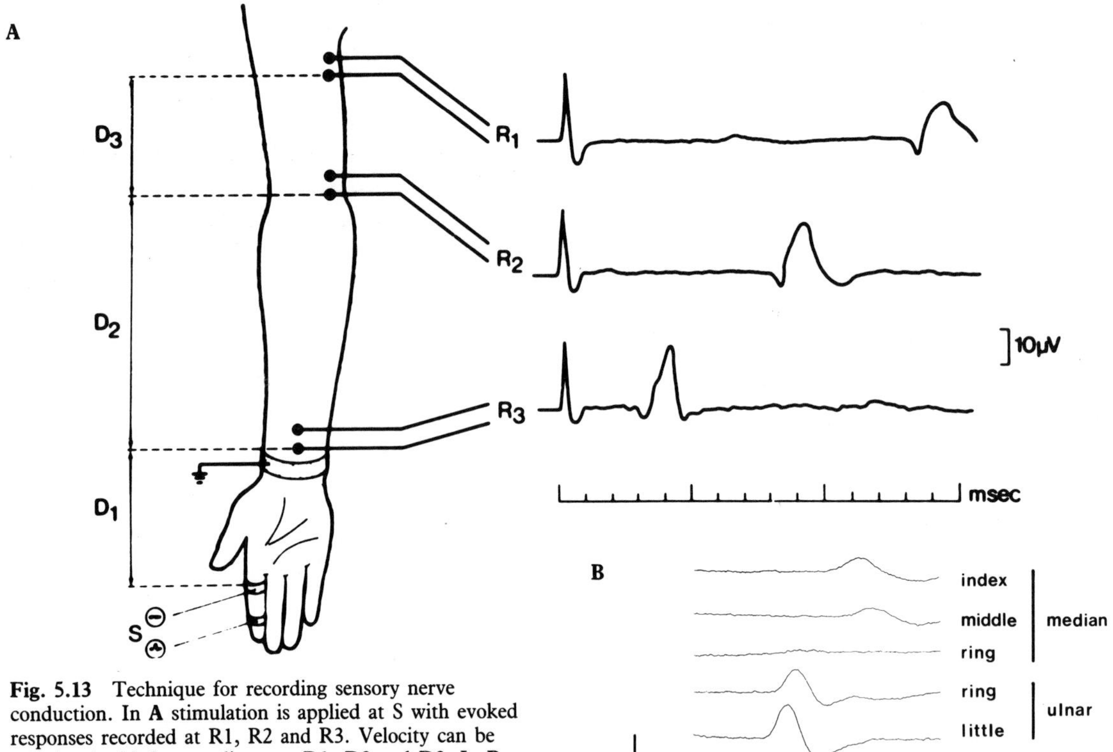

Fig. 5.13 Technique for recording sensory nerve conduction. In **A** stimulation is applied at S with evoked responses recorded at R1, R2 and R3. Velocity can be calculated with known distances D1, D2 and D3. In **B** response of reduced amplitude and delayed latency (relative to ulnar nerve) is illustrated in a patient with carpal tunnel syndrome.

of the wide variation in conduction in sensory nerve fibres. Sensory nerve action potentials range from a few microvolts to 100 microvolts in amplitude.

A variety of abnormalities of nerve conduction may be seen:

Conduction block occurs in local lesions of nerves and in segmental demyelination. In these conditions there may be major attenuation of an evoked motor or sensory response across an affected segment of nerve.

Slowing of conduction, with dispersion and widening of evoked nerve action potential, is most marked in segmental demyelinating neuropathies and is seen to a lesser degree in severe axonal neuropathies.

Reduced or absent responses are seen in severe demyelinating and axonal neuropathies. Thus, characteristic patterns of abnormality of motor and sensory nerve conduction are seen in axonal and demyelinating neuropathies and compressive mononeuropathies (Table 5.1). This emphasises the great value of conduction studies in the localisation of peripheral nerve lesions, and the differentiation between axonal and demyelinating neuropathies, which tend to have very different aetiologies (p. 236).

ELECTROMYOGRAPGHY

The electrical activity of muscle may be recorded in a number of ways: most commonly, concentric needle electrodes are used for routine diagnostic procedures, surface recording, and microelectrode needles are sometimes employed in the study of neuromuscular transmission.

Normal muscle

The electrical activity recorded from normal muscle varies depending on the state of the muscle.

Unless a needle electrode is placed close to an end-plate region, normal muscle is electrically silent when fully relaxed. However, following insertion or movement of a needle electrode a short burst of activity lasting 2–3 seconds may occur.

Concentric needle electrode recording during muscle activity displays motor unit potentials. The activity recorded from each single motor unit (i.e. a motor neurone and all the muscle fibres it innervates) is the sum of from that of those muscle fibres within the unit that are close to the needle. Normal motor unit potentials are usually bi- or triphasic with a duration of up to 15 ms and an amplitude of up to 3 μV. For a given needle electrode position various motor unit potentials that can be studied will have distinct wave forms which identify that individual motor unit.

When a muscle is contracted weakly a few motor units will be seen firing irregularly at a low rate. Increasing the force of contraction increases the rate of firing of these initial units and, as the force increases, additional units of higher amplitude are recruited (Fig. 5.14). As force is further increased, many units may be firing so frequently that it is no longer possible to identify the activity of individual units and a complex interference pattern is seen.

Table 5.1 Abnormalities of nerve conduction

	Motor conduction			Sensory conduction		
	Velocity	*Amplitude*	*Duration*	*Velocity*	*Amplitude*	*Duration*
Axonal neuropathy		–			– –	
Demyelinating neuropathy	– –	–	+	– –	–	+
Mononeuropathy	–	–	+	–	– –	+
Motor neurone disease		–				
Myopathy						

+ = increased – = reduced – – = greatly reduced no entry = normal

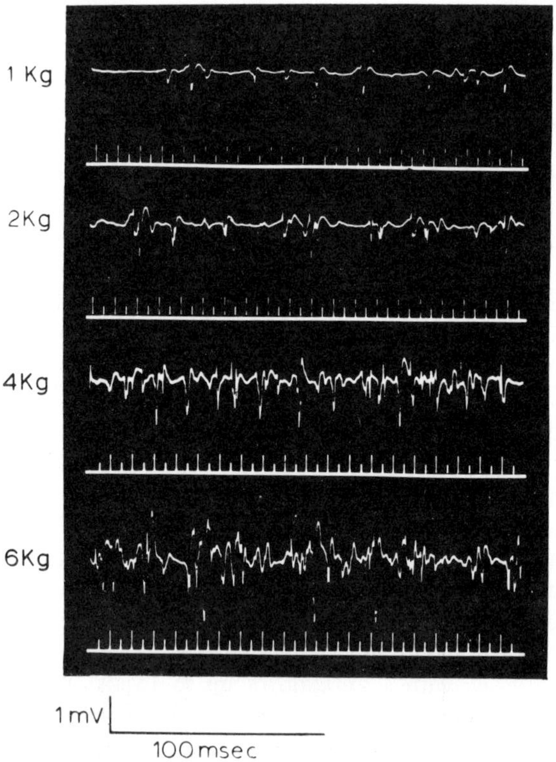

Fig. 5.14 EMG activity during voluntary muscle contraction against increasing loads. A normal pattern of recruitment is seen with an increasing number of motor units firing at increasing rates with increasing loads. (Reproduced from Hayward M 1977 *Journal of Neurological Sciences* 33: 397–413, with permission).

EMG activity in neuromuscular disease (Fig. 5.15).

At rest, a variety of abnormalities may be apparent in diseased muscle. Insertional activity can be unusually prolonged in denervated muscle, myotonic disorders and some myopathies (particularly polymyositis). In addition various types of spontaneous activity may be seen.

Fibrillation potentials are action potentials arising spontaneously from single muscle fibres. They are thus of very short duration (less than 3–5 ms) and relatively low amplitude (100 μV to 1 μV). They are found in acutely denervated muscle and also in acute polymyositis.

Positive sharp waves are often found in association with fibrillation potentials: they consist of an initial positive deflection followed by a slow potential change. Their duration is usually approximately 1 ms or more with similar amplitude to fibrillation potentials. Positive sharp waves are found in denervated muscle particularly following acute nerve injuries.

Fasciculation potentials are found in chronic partial denervation, particularly that of anterior horn cell disease, but occasionally with root lesions. These potentials are similar in dimension to motor unit potentials and are due to spontaneous activity in motor units of denervated muscle.

Myotonic discharges are high-frequency trains of action potential which can be produced by needle movement, percussion or contraction of muscle. They are enhanced by cold and resemble trains of fibrillation or positive sharp waves. They give rise to a characteristic 'dive-bomber' noise when played through a loudspeaker, and are particularly characteristic of myotonic disorders. These abnormalities in resting muscle are illustrated in Fig. 5.15.

Abnormalities of diseased muscle during activity can best be considered in terms of the morphology of motor units and changes in recruitment pattern. The shape, amplitude and duration of motor unit potentials are determined by the compound activity of muscle fibres within that unit. In myopathic disorders, fibres are usually lost from motor units: this results in smaller-amplitude shorter-duration potentials and also in low amplitude polyphasic rather than bi- or triphasic potentials. In contrast, the amplitude and duration of remaining functioning motor units in chronically denervated muscle is often increased. This may be because surviving motor axons sprout to reinnervate muscle fibres whose motor axon has died. Thus surviving motor units tend to be larger, of longer duration, and are polyphasic. In neuropathic disorders, recruitment patterns are markedly abnormal. The number of functioning motor units will be reduced and in severe neurogenic weakness it may be possible to recognise individual motor unit potentials during maximum contractions.

The diagnosis of neuromuscular disease

From the above description it can be seen that electromyography is a qualitative rather than a

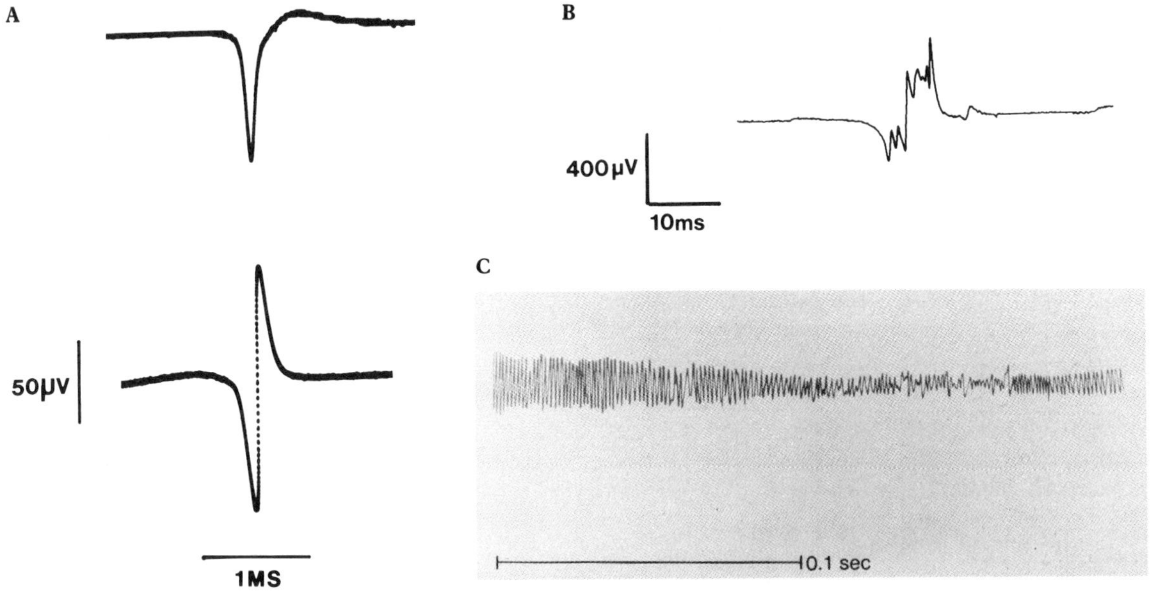

Fig. 5.15 EMG activity at rest recorded by needle electrode in abnormal muscle showing: **A** positive sharp wave (upper trace) and fibrillation potential (lower trace), **B** fasciculation, **C** myotonia.

quantitative assessment of neuromuscular activity and demands considerable experience and expertise in interpretation. Although in early mild cases it may be difficult to differentiate between primary neurogenic or myopathic disorders on the basis of EMG alone, such differentiation is the major value of these techniques. The EMG in myopathies is characterised by increased insertional activity (and myotonia in certain myotonic disorders). Motor unit potentials are of small amplitude and short duration and frequently polyphasic, producing a characteristic crackle over the loudspeaker.

In patients with early acute neurogenic lesions, recording reveals only a reduction in the number of motor unit potentials under voluntary control. If denervation occurs, however, the amount of insertional activity will increase and fibrillation and positive sharp waves will soon be seen. In patients with chronic partial denervation, insertional activity will again be increased, with spontaneous fibrillation, positive sharp waves and fasciculation potentials. Motor units are of larger amplitude, longer duration and are polyphasic.

The patterns of changes in both neuropathies and myopathies of varying kinds are summarised in Table 5.2.

In addition, EMG may allow accurate topographical identification of denervated muscles, which may aid the localisation of neurogenic lesions.

STUDIES OF NEUROMUSCULAR CONDUCTION

In patients with myasthenia gravis or the myasthenic syndrome, minor abnormalities in electromyography may be present. Motor unit potentials may be variable in amplitude and configuration and, sometimes, frankly myopathic features may be present in patients with myasthenia of long standing. However, these changes may be subtle and difficult to detect, and confirmation of the clinical diagnosis of myasthenia will demand specialised techniques.

Neuromuscular stimulation

A record of muscular activity can be obtained by stimulating a motor nerve and recording the evoked potential. This is relatively easily done by

Table 5.2 Abnormalities of electromyography

	Insertional activity	Resting activity	Active contraction motor unit potentials: *numbers*	Active contraction motor unit potentials: *morphology*	Active contraction: recruitment
Axonal neuropathy	prolonged	fibrillation	–	large polyphasic	abnormal
Demyelinating neuropathy					loss of voluntary firing
Mononeuropathy		fibrillation +ve sharp waves			loss of voluntary firing
Motor neurone disease	prolonged	fibrillation	–	large amplitude long duration	abnormal
Myopathy	prolonged (myotonia + polymyositis)	fibrillation +ve sharp waves		short duration polyphasic	

– = reduced
no entry = normal

stimulating the ulnar nerve and recording from abductor digiti minimi. Short tetanic trains of 1–10 Hz will not lead to significant decrement in the size of evoked potentials in normal individuals. However, immediate decrement may be present in patients with myasthenia (Fig. 5.16). Although it may be possible to obtain confirmatory evidence of neuromuscular block by observing such decrements, their absence does not exclude the diagnosis of myasthenia: this is because peripheral muscles such as abductor digiti minimi are often relatively spared by the myasthenic process.

Stimulation at other sites (e.g. Erb's point and recording over deltoid) may show a higher incidence of decremental changes, but this technique is more unpleasant for the patient than the administration of short tetanic trains to the ulnar nerve.

Single-fibre studies

Single-fibre electromyography is a more sophisticated technique for detecting abnormalities of neuromuscular conductions. If a needle with one or more small recording electrodes along its length is inserted into muscle, it may be possible to so position it that recordings can be made from two or more single muscle fibres within a motor unit. If the muscle is then activated, individual fibres will be activated in close temporal association. The

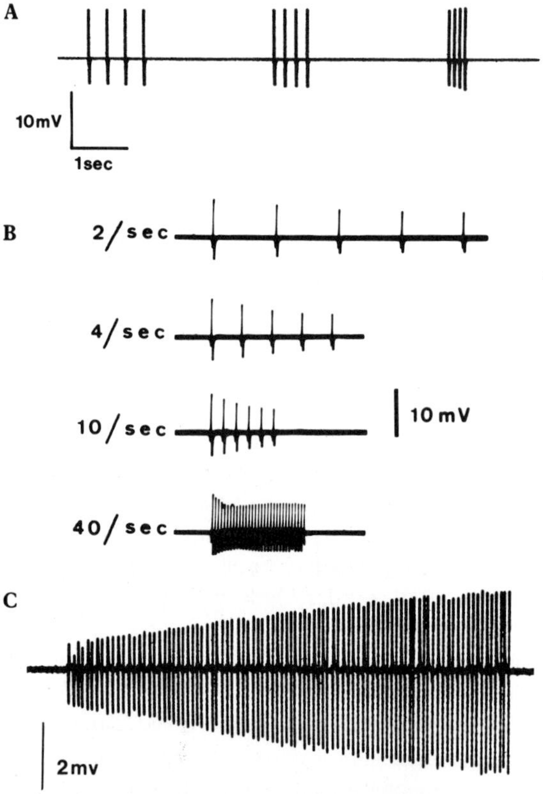

Fig. 5.16 Responses to tetanic stimuli of surface recordings from abductor digiti minimi following ulnar stimulation. **A** Normal response, **B** decremental responses in myasthenia gravis at different rates of stimulation, **C** incremental response in the myasthenia syndrome during stimulation at 50 Hz.

activation of fibres should have a relatively fixed temporal relationship with little jitter (i.e. little variation in latency of activation of fibres) and no blocking (i.e. no absence of individual fibre activity). In disorders of neuromuscular transmission such recording techniques reveal a greatly increased amount of jitter, evidence of neuromuscular block (Fig. 5.17).

Two major clinical and neurophysiological disorders of neuromuscular transmission are recognised. In myasthenia gravis there is evidence of decrement in evoked potentials to tetanic trains, an increased jitter, and blocking with single-fibre techniques. In the myasthenic syndrome, motor unit potentials are initially abnormally small, but rapid rates of tetanic stimulation produce a progressive increment in the size of evoked potentials.

NEUROLOGICAL IMAGING

THE SKULL X-RAY

Plain radiographs of the skull may be taken from a variety of angles with or without tomographic techniques. The necessity for varying views will be determined by the individual patient and circumstances, as well as by the availability of other neuroradiological techniques. A wide variety of abnormalities may be detected on plain films.

Calcification

Calcification may occur normally at a number of sites, and its presence may be helpful when such calcified structures are displaced: thus, displacement of a calcified pineal (Fig. 5.18) or choroid

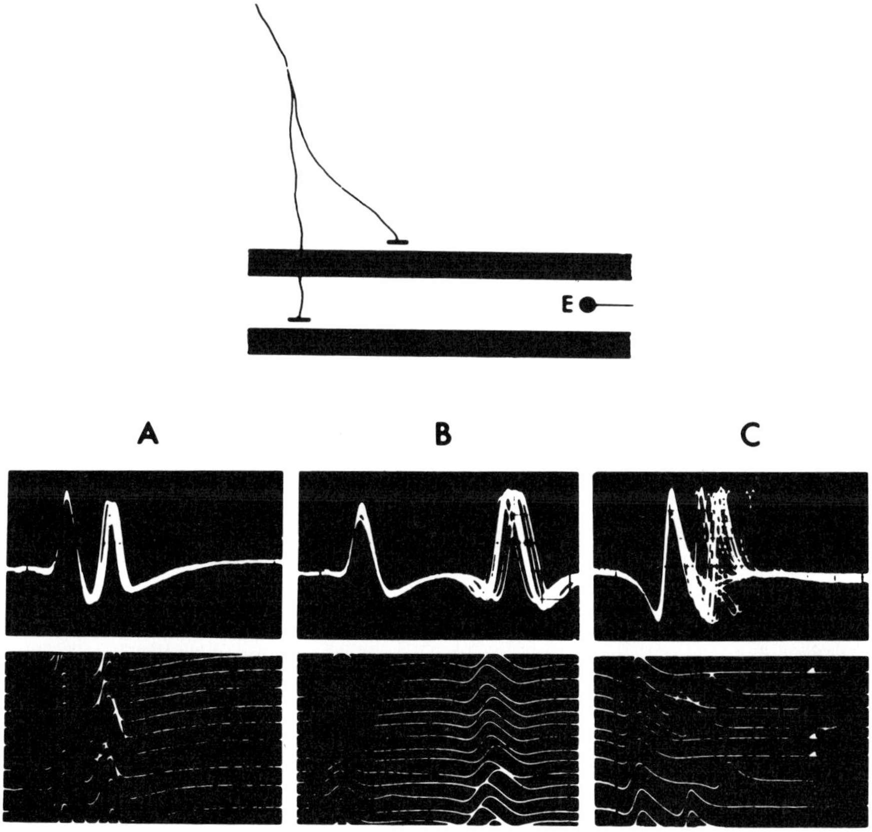

Fig. 5.17 Single fibre recordings from two fibres of a single motor unit, the sweeps being triggered by the first action potential. **A** Normal subject—note uniformity of relationship between first and second action potential; **B** a myasthenic subject showing increased jitter, i.e. varying latency between first and second action potentials; **C** a myasthenic subject showing increasing jitter and also blocking, i.e. failure of the second action potential to occur. (From Stålberg E 1974 *Single fibre electromyography*, Disa electronics.)

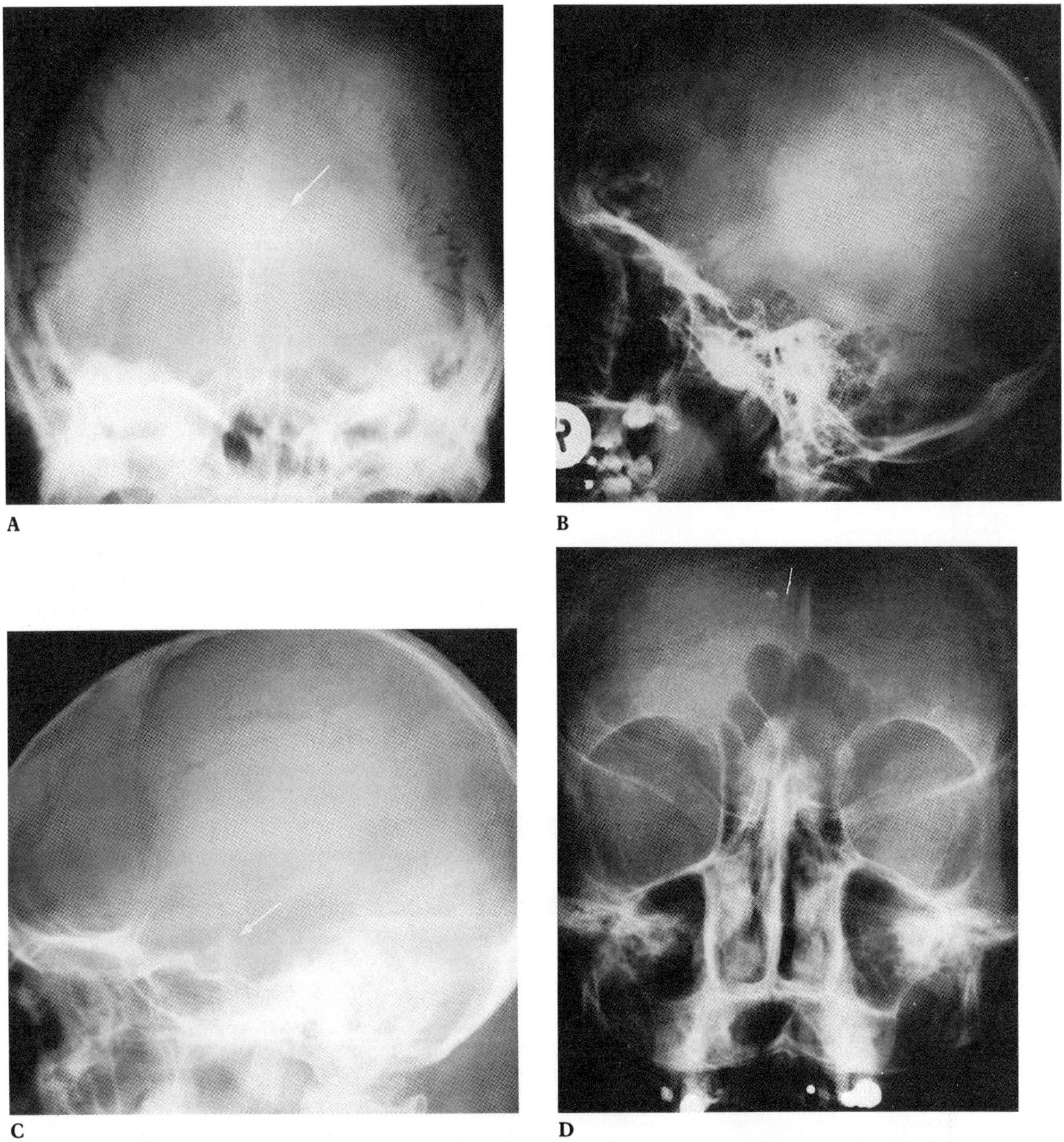

Fig. 5.18 Abnormal calcification on skull X-rays. **A** Displacement of a calcified pineal gland (marked by arrow) in PA view, **B** serpiginous calcification in a frontal arteriovenous malformation, **C** suprasellar calcification (marked by arrow) in a craniopharyngioma, **D** calcification in a subfrontal meningioma shown in an AP view.

plexus may indicate the presence of a mass lesion. Alternatively, some degree of basal ganglia or falx calcification may be evident on the skull X-ray without any pathological significance.

Abnormal calcification may occur in a number of intracranial tumours (Fig. 5.18): these include meningiomas (15% calcify), oligodendrogliomas (50% calcify) and craniopharyngiomas (75% calcify). Abnormal vasculature, e.g. aneurysm and arteriovenous malformations as well as atheromatous arteries and chronic subdural haematomas, may also exhibit calcification. More rarely, infectious processes such as tuberculoma, toxoplasma or cystercercosis may cause intracranial calcification. Intracranial calcification may be seen in tuberose sclerosis.

Biplanar views are essential in localising abnormal calcification. This will usually allow differentiation between the surface calcification of a meningioma and that more diffuse calcification, not necessarily of pathological significance, that is seen affecting the falx cerebri in some patients.

Bone density (Fig. 5.19)

A variety of changes in bone density affecting the skull may be seen. Thus, loss of calcification of the posterior clinoid processes of the pituitary fossa may indicate raised intracranial pressure (or advancing age), whereas generalised changes in bone density may occur in Paget's disease of the skull, and myeloma or carcinoma. More localised erosion of the skull may occur with carcinoma of the nasopharynx, cordoma and with some meningiomas. Erosion and enlargement of the internal auditory meatus may be seen in plain tomographic views in patients with acoustic neuroma. Alternatively, increased sclerosis may be seen with some secondary deposits and with meningiomas.

Vascular markings

While it is by no means uncommon to detect some degree of vascular marking of the normal skull from meningeal vessels, large feeding vessels of either meningiomas or arteriovenous malforma-

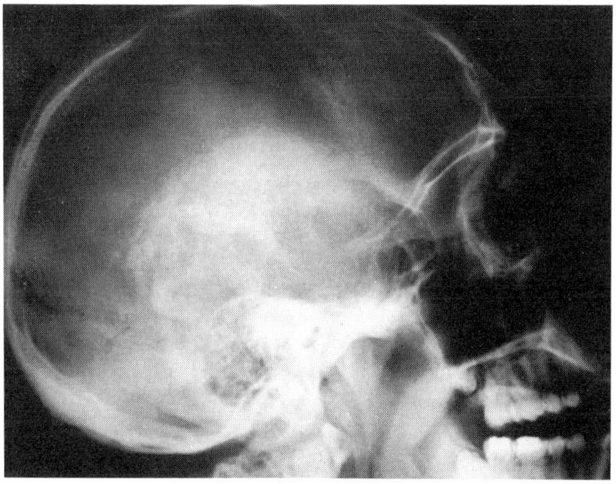

A

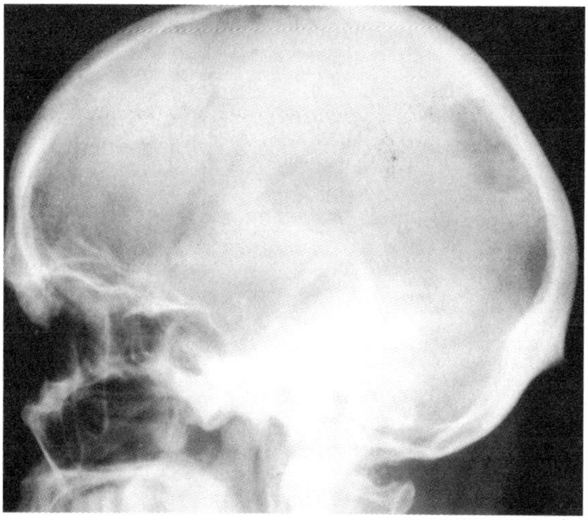

B

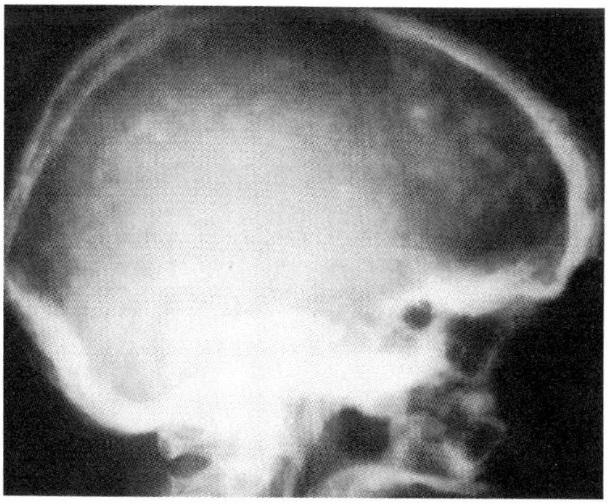

C

Fig. 5.19 Abnormal bony erosion in the skull X-ray. **A** Erosion of posterior clinoid processes (there is also diffuse intracranial calcification in an oligodendroglioma), **B** two large translucencies due to myeloma, **C** Paget's disease of the skull.

tions may cause unusually prominent vascular markings.

Contours of skull (Fig. 5.20)

A number of abnormalities of shape and contour of the cranial cavity of the skull occur. In hydrocephalus starting in childhood obvious enlargement of the cranial cavity may be present. Changes in the shape of the pituitary fossa may occur with pituitary tumours, or with hydrocephalus, or mass lesions above the fossa (craniopharyngioma). Basilar invagination (platybasia) may be seen in both Paget's disease and as a congenital abnormality of the foramen magnum. In this condition, associated with tonsillar ectopia, more than one-third of the odontoid peg protrudes above a line from the bulk of the hard palate to the posterior margin of the foramen magnum (Chamberlain's line) (Fig. 5.20).

Scrutiny of the paranasal sinuses and mastoid regions for abnormal opacification or erosion is of particular importance in patients with suspected intracranial abscess or nasopharyngeal carcinoma.

Indications

Unfortunately, major structural abnormalities of the cranial cavity and its contents may occur without detectable changes in the skull X-ray. The likelihood of abnormality in the skull radiograph increases with the length of time for which an abnormality is present. Thus the major indication for skull X-ray is as a screening test for benign

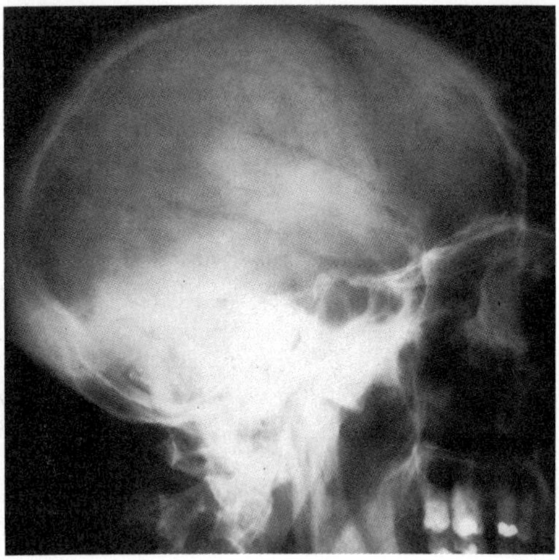

A

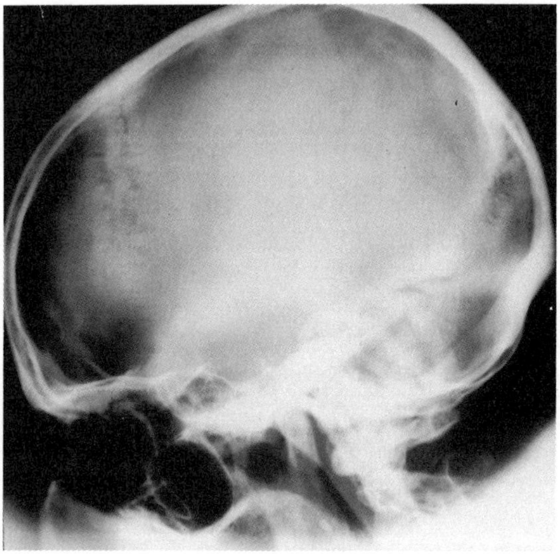

B

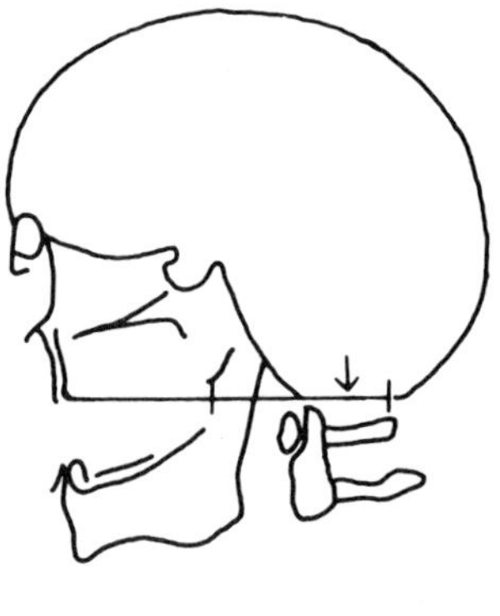

C

Fig. 5.20 Abnormal skull contours. **A** Gross enlargement of the pituitary fossa which is associated with enlarged frontal sinuses in acromegaly, **B** basilar invagination demonstrating protrusion of the odontoid above Chamberlain's line (see diagram **C**). Note also flattening of posterior clinoid processes due to long-standing hydrocephalus. The line diagram illustrates the normal position of the odontoid to the line drawn between the hard palate and occipital protuberance. (Reproduced from Sutton D (ed) 1980 *A Textbook of Radiology and Imaging*. Churchill Livingstone Edinburgh, with permission.)

pathologies which may sometimes be associated with epilepsy and headache; in such circumstances a single lateral skull film is all that is required.

There is probably no longer a place for routine skull radiography in patients where further investigation (with CT scanning, etc.) is necessary. There are, however, situations in which the skull radiograph is of specific value: these include the investigation of patients with cranial nerve palsies due to nasopharyngeal carcinoma, or to cerebellar pontine angle tumour, or tumours of the optic nerve. In such instances specially directed plain or tomographic examination of the base of the skull, internal auditory meati, and optic foramina, may be of value.

PLAIN RADIOGRAPHS OF THE SPINE

Plain radiographs of the spine are most usually biplanar (postero-anterior and lateral views). Adequate views of intervertebral foramina require oblique views.

A variety of abnormalities may be detected on radiographs of the spine (Fig 5.21).

Abnormal calcification

Abnormal calcification in and around the spine is less commonly seen than in skull radiographs. However, calcification within the spinal canal may occasionally be seen in patients with arachnoiditis, dermoid or epidermoid tumours, and meningioma.

Bony erosions, lytic lesions

Bony erosions and lytic lesions of vertebral bodies are common in myeloma and disseminated carcinoma, but occasionally sclerosis of vertebral bodies may occur with prostatic and thyroid carcinoma. Such changes will be apparent on lateral views of the spine, but close scrutiny of well-penetrated postero-anterior views is necessary to detect erosion of pedicles or transverse processes. Lytic lesions may indicate infections such as tuberculosis, pyogenic abscess, brucellosis, etc.

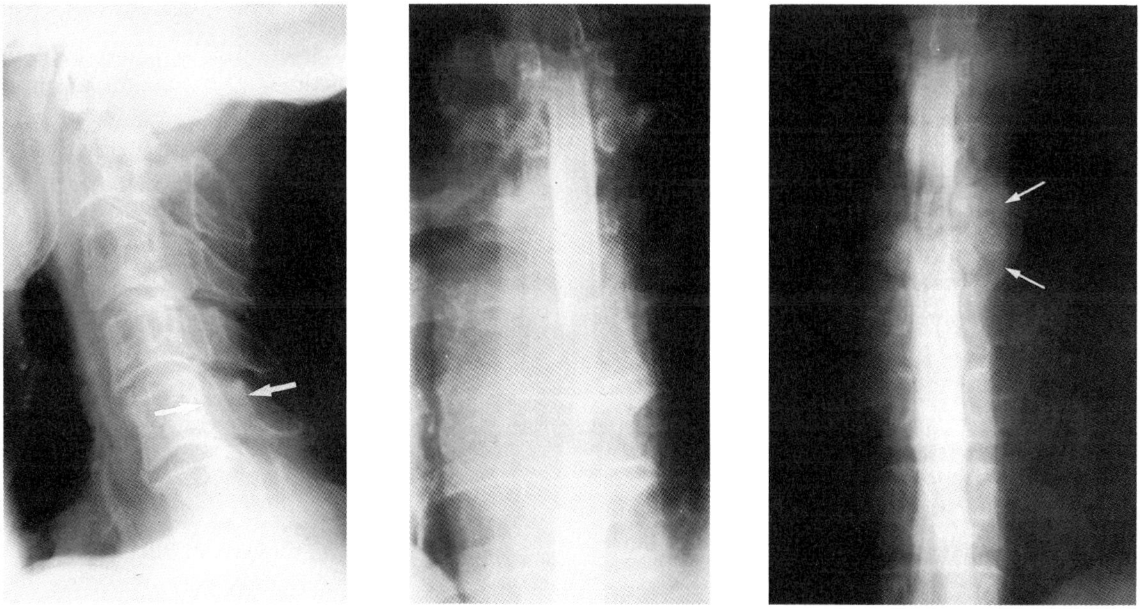

A B C

Fig. 5.21 Abnormalities on spinal X-rays. **A** Congenital canal stenosis (in an achondroplastic dwarf). Arrows delineate the A–P dimensions of the canal. **B** Myelogram showing thoracic cord compression due to extradural secondary deposit. Pedicles are seen immediately above level of block but not at level of compression. **C** Myelogram showing thoracic cord compression associated with a paraspinal mass (arrowed).

Abnormalities of bony contours

Plain films may reveal a number of congenital abnormalities of the spine, including congenital fusion of vertebrae, or the presence of neural tube defects with spina bifida. Perhaps the most important single abnormality of spinal films for the neurologist is the measurement of the antero-posterior diameter of the cervical canal in patients with myelopathy. Patients with congenital stenosis and an antero-posterior (a.p.) diameter of less than 13 mm at a C5 level are particularly prone to develop myelopathy in association with spondylotic change. Unfortunately the a.p. diameter of the canal is rarely reported outside specialist neurological and neurosurgical units. Pathological widening of the dimensions of the canal may occur with spinal tumours, and widening of intravertebral foramina in tumours of the nerve roots, e.g. neurofibromas. The detection of paraspinal shadows is of particular importance in the diagnosis of tumour and abscess.

Abnormalities of intervertebral discs

The most common abnormality is loss of intervertebral space which may indicate the presence of a prolapsed disc. Destruction of disc spaces themselves may be seen in tuberculosis of the spine, but rarely in malignant disease of the spine.

Abnormalities of spinal curvature

Kyphoscoliosis and accentuation of normal lumbar lordosis are not uncommon complications of a variety of neuromuscular disease, e.g. Friedreich's ataxia and muscular dystrophy. Instability of regions of the spine may have important consequences: thus, atlantoaxial subluxation in rheumatoid arthritis may lead to myelopathy; traumatic or rheumatoid subluxations at other levels may result in compression of the spinal cord. In such instances, adequate views with cautious flexion and extension of the spine are important.

Indications

Plain radiographs of the spine provide much more diagnostically useful information than do plain radiographs of the skull. Whereas the latter can usually be dispensed with if other investigation is available, plain films of the spine are almost always of some value, irrespective of whether myelography is being considered. It is unfortunately true that the most common deficiency in plain films of the spine is the failure to obtain radiographs of the area of the spine appropriate to the patient's problems! Thus patients are often admitted to neurological units with evidence of a spinal cord lesion, but with radiographs of the lumbar spine only!

ISOTOPE BRAIN SCANNING

Before the advent of CT scanning, isotope scanning with a technetium–99 isotope produced valuable information with a relatively non-invasive technique. The technique remains of some value for the detection of vascular lesions, particularly in centres where CT scanning is not generally available. Anterior, posterior and both lateral scans are routinely undertaken. Isotope scanning will detect a large proportion of extradural and subdural haematomas, meningiomas, cerebral abscesses and large arteriovenous malformations; it will show abnormalities in a moderate number of patients with stroke and glioma. A second scan after a few weeks' interval will often distinguish reliably between the two diagnoses. Its use, however, is limited in that little information can be gleaned about the pathology of the lesion giving rise to increased uptake of isotope.

Indications

Isotope brain scanning will seldom be necessary within neurological centres where CT head scanning is available, the latter technique providing a higher rate of detection of abnormality and possessing more pathological discrimination. However, isotope scanning may still have an occasional place: thus, some CT isodense subdural haematomas may be missed, yet detected by isotope scanning, and some cerebral infarctions may show isotope uptake when CT scans are normal.

CT SCANNING OF HEAD

Computerised tomography (CT) scanning is undoubtedly the single greatest advance in neuroradiological imaging. An X-ray tube within a tilting mobile gantry rotates through 360 degrees about the patient's head, projecting a beam through the head, on multiple occasions, at different angles to a recording instrument. Complex computing techniques then reconstruct radiodensity to provide a two-dimensional reconstruction in the form of 'slices' through the head or body. Radiodensity can be expressed in Hounsfield units appropriate to differing tissues: thus, low-density (translucent) materials include c.s.f. and fat, while grey and white matter are of differing but moderate density; the presence of oedema or infarction leads to a lower-density area. Calcification and blood are of high density on the CT scan. The plane of examination is usually axial

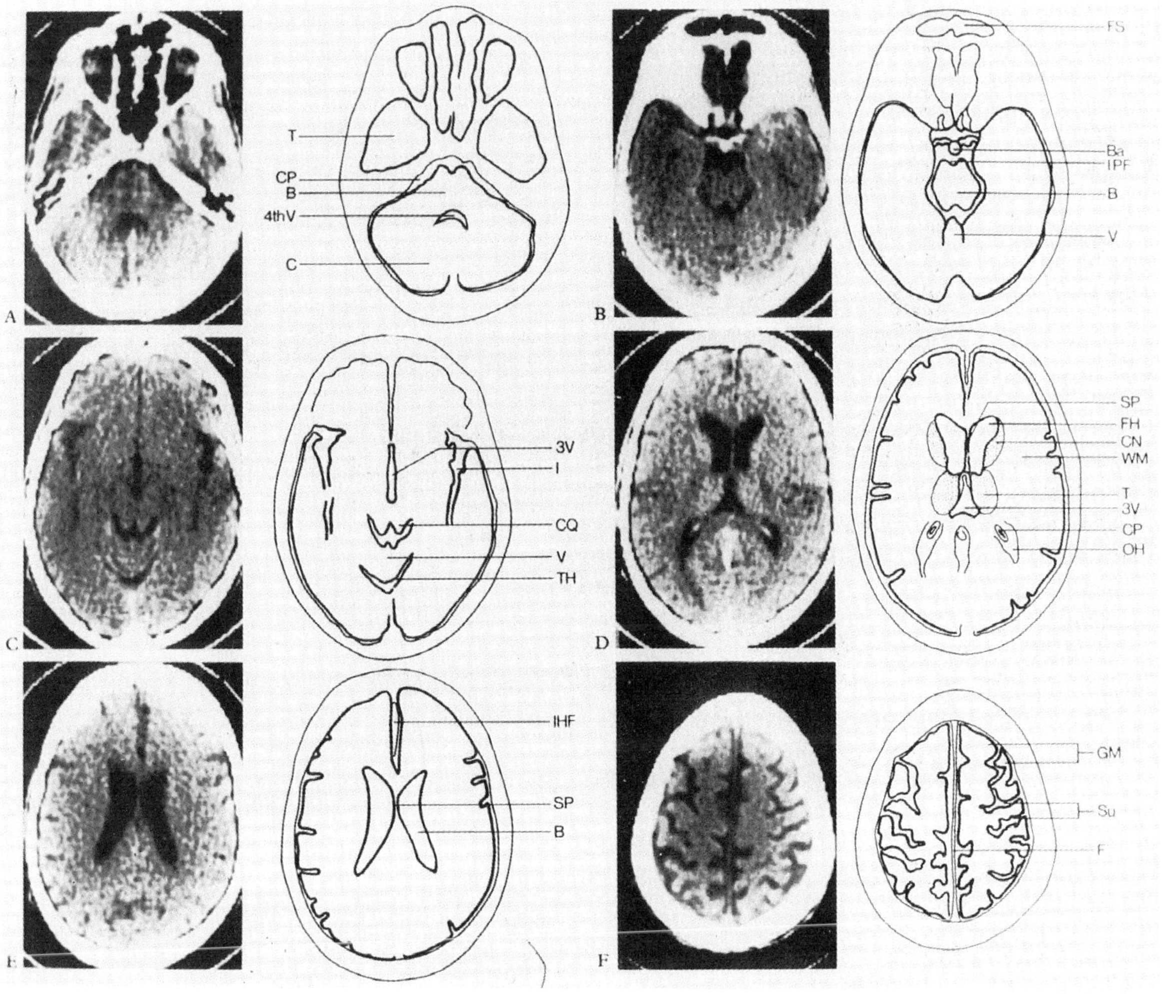

Fig. 5.22 The normal CT displaying the anatomy of the brain and ventricular system. T = temporal lobe, CP = cerebellopontine angle, B = brain stem, 4thV = 4th ventricle, C = cerebellum, FS = frontal sinus, Ba = basilar artery, IPF = interpeduncular fossa, V = vermis, 3V = 3rd ventricle, CQ = corpora quadrigemina, TH = tentorial hiatus, FH = frontal horn, SP = septum pellucidum, CN = caudate nucleus, T = thalamus, CP = choroid plexus, OH = occipital horn, WM = white matter, IHF = interhemispheric fissure, B = body of ventricle, GM = grey matter, SU = sulci, F = falx. (Reproduced from Sutton D (ed) 1980 *A textbook of Radiology and Imaging*, Churchill Livingstone, Edinburgh, with permission.)

(Fig. 5.22) but coronal scanning is possible in some individuals and sagittal reconstructions can be undertaken.

Scanning is usually undertaken before the injection of contrast medium and then after intravenous administration of iodine-containing contrast. Many vascular lesions show increased CT density often patchily following such enhancement; these include glioma, meningioma, secondary carcinoma, abscess and cerebral infarction. On occasion, water-soluble contrast may be injected intrathecally for positive contrast cisternography.

The administration of iodine-containing contrast medium during CT scanning represents the only invasive part of the investigation. A history of previous iodine sensitivity must be elicited as allergic reaction may be dangerous. In those such patients in whom contrast investigation is essential, cover with steroids should be given.

The importance of CT scanning lies in its ability to define the structure of intracranial contents (Fig. 5.22) and to make some limited differentiation between normal and pathological tissues (Fig. 5.23). Thus CT scanning is extremely sensitive in detecting displacement of intracranial contents due to mass lesions. Judgement concerning the pathology of lesions, however, remains heavily dependent on adequate clinical information concerning the patient. Some common pathologies are demonstrated in Figure 5.23. It may be impossible to differentiate between some gliomas and cerebral infarction, or between some gliomas and cerebral abscess, without adequate information about the patient. Ultimately, biopsy may be the only satisfactory method to differentiate between these.

As well as providing invaluable information about the contents of the cranial cavity, CT scanning will also define the anatomy and pathology of the orbits, extraocular muscles, sinuses and ears.

Indications

CT scanning is the investigation of choice for the localisation and characterisation of intracranial mass lesions. It is, however, less effective in the detection of vascular disease and diseases of white matter and it must always be remembered that the majority of patients with organic cerebral neurological syndromes have normal CT scans. Although CT scanning should be widely available this should not lead to abuse of this investigation. It is to be hoped that the era of 'scan-negative headache' can be avoided in the United Kingdom with the realisation that CT scanning is no substitute for clinical skills.

SPINAL CT

Spinal transverse CT has a number of potential applications, although almost all necessitate the presence of radiological contrast within the intrathecal space in order to demonstrate neural tissue:

1. It may be a useful adjunct to myelography, where this leaves questions unanswered, e.g. in the thoracic region, which is technically dificult to examine by myelography, or in spinal block, where contrast fails to pass an obstruction in adequate concentrations to allow definition by usual means.
2. It can define the bony architecture of the canal, and disc disease.
3. Following myelography, delayed CT may demonstrate contrast within a syrinx.

MAGNETIC RESONANCE IMAGING (MRI)

This revolutionary technique creates images from radiowaves absorbed and re-emitted from protons rotating about their axes in a powerful magnetic field. The intensity of the MR signal is a reflection of various tissue characteristics, including proton density, and chemical parameters known as T1 and T2 relaxation times.

The potential advantages of MRI over CT include greater differentiation between grey and white matter, lack of bone artefact and the availability of direct sagittal and coronal imaging. Furthermore, the technique appears exceptionally safe. It is already superior to CT in the demonstration of white matter disease (e.g. MS plaques) and in imaging in the posterior fossa, craniovertebral junction and cervical spine.

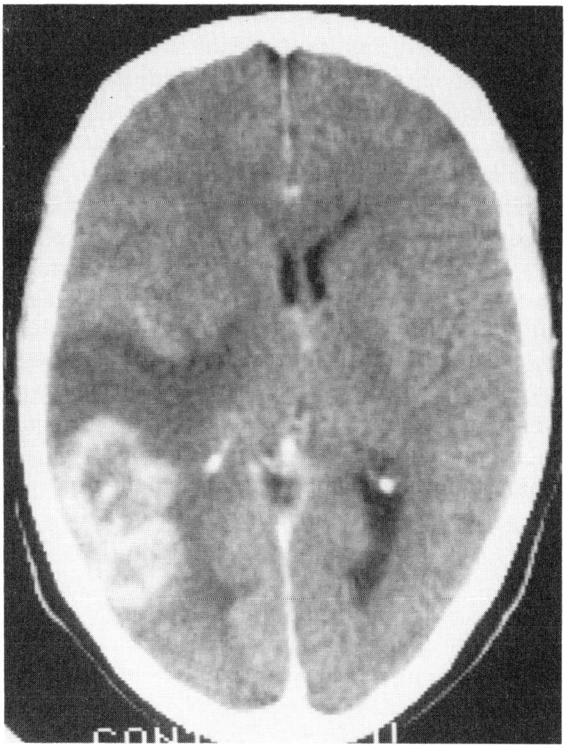

A

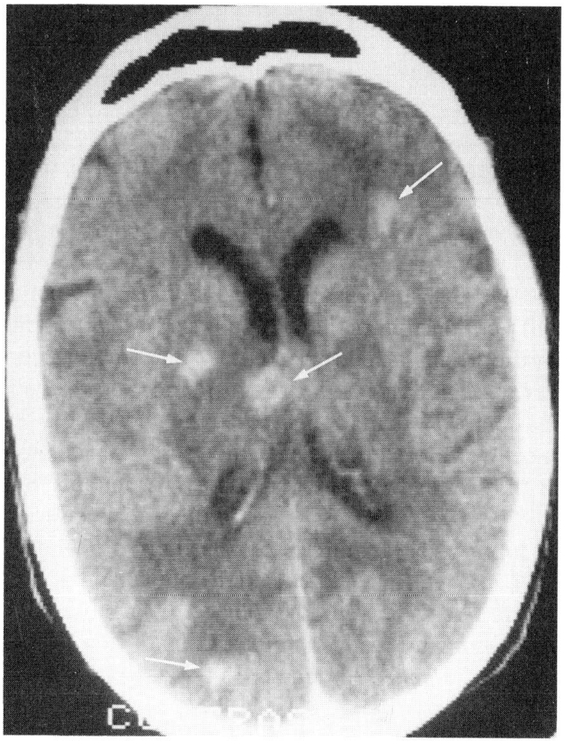

B

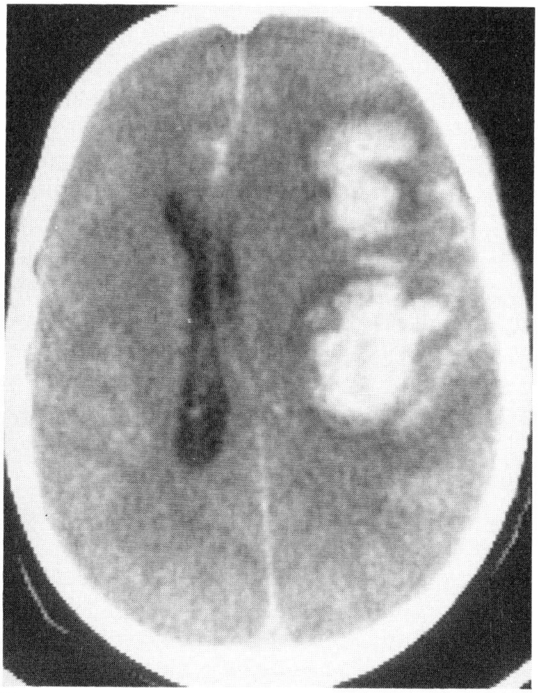

C

Fig. 5.23 Abnormal CT scans. **A** A left parieto-occipital glioma displayed after contrast enhancement. The tumour shows as high density surrounded by oedema (low density). There is a mass effect with displacement and compression of the lateral ventricles. **B** Multiple cerebral secondaries (arrowed) shown after contrast enhancement. They are surrounded by extensive low density areas (cerebral oedema). **C** Unenhanced scan showing an acute intracerebral haematoma.

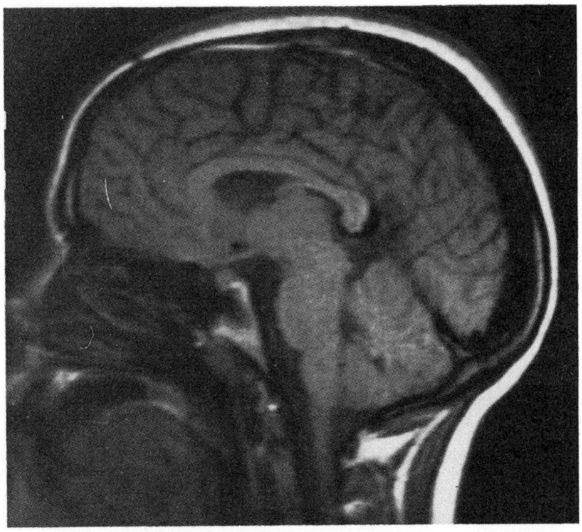

Fig. 5.24 Sagittal magnetic resonance image of the head.

At present, however, the technique is slower and more expensive than CT, but the potential of this technology also appears considerable, opening up the possibility of spectroscopic tissue analysis in vivo. An example of the quality of MR imaging is presented in Figure 5.24.

CEREBRAL ANGIOGRAPHY

Films of the cerebral vasculature may be obtained by sequential radiographs obtained following the arterial injection of radiographic contrast medium. Direct arterial puncture in the neck may be undertaken for carotid and vertebral vessels or, alternatively, and more commonly in recent years, femoral puncture with retrograde catheterisation may be undertaken. Early films reveal arterial phases followed by capillary and subsequently by venous phases. Angiography may display:

Vascular abnormalities, e.g. atheroma, aneurysm, arteriovenous malformation, arterial spasm.

Vascular displacement due to mass lesions.

Pathological circulation of tumours, infarcts and abscesses.

Angiography carries a significant mortality and morbidity: up to 5% of patients may suffer transient or permanent neurological deficit following angiography, and occasional fatal strokes can occur; patients with atherosclerosis are particularly at risk. Complications may be due to the effects of instrumentation, and chemical effects from the injection of contrast medium, platelet and fibrin emboli from the catheters or, rarely, allergic reactions to contrast media. Refinements of angiographic technique utilise computerised digital processing of images in order to obtain adequate angiographic definition following the administration of much smaller volumes of contrast medium (digital subtraction angiography). In some instances venous injection with such techniques may allow adequate definition of arterial abnormalities.

Indications

The introduction of CT scanning has enormously reduced the demand for angiography as a means of detecting mass lesions, and defining pathological circulation. It does, however, remain a necessary investigation in patients suspected of having cerebral aneurysms or arteriovenous malformations, and in patients with cerebrovascular disease in whom a surgical approach to treatment is being considered. It may be of value in detecting subdural haematomas when these are CT isodense and bilateral.

VENTRICULOGRAPHY AND CISTERNOGRAPHY

The introduction of negative (air) and positive (iodine-containing) contrast media either via the lumbar theca, or via direct ventricular injection allows the definition of the ventricular systems, basal cisterns and subarachnoid space with appropriate positioning of the patient. Whichever contrast agent is used, these investigations are unpleasant for the patient, resulting in considerable headache and vomiting. The use of excessive amounts of iodine-containing contrast media may evoke encephalopathy and seizures.

Indications

Fortunately, the requirements for ventriculography and cisternography have been greatly reduced by the introduction of CT scanning, which adequately defines the ventricular system in the vast majority of patients. However, definition of the suprasella cisterns and internal auditory meati may still require contrast cisternography and the injection of water-soluble contrast media may be helpful in the detection of communicating hydrocephalus.

MYELOGRAPHY

Radiographic contrast media may be introduced into the spinal subarachnoid space by lumbar injection utilising a routine lumbar puncture technique, or less commonly by cervical puncture under radiographic control. In the past an oily iodine-containing medium (myodil) was used: this gave rise to a discrete column of contrast media that could be screened during its passage along the spinal canal. However, it was prone to form globules, and it frequently proved difficult to demonstrate the thoracic region and obtain adequate definition of nerve roots. Over the last decade a number of water-soluble contrast media have been introduced: these give more satisfactory anatomical definition. For this reason it is important that clinicians specify the region to be examined so that radiologists can select the most appropriate mode of injection and technique of examination.

While a number of radiographs may be produced during a myelographic examination, it has to be remembered that this is a dynamic procedure and that discussion with the radiologist is an important part of reaching conclusions concerning the examination. For this reason it is always advisable to perform myelography in units where the procedure is frequently undertaken and where the radiologist is able to to discuss the results with surgical colleagues who may be involved in further management. When this rule is not followed, radiologists with little experience of the technique, acting on the advice of non-neurologists, not infrequently provide inadequate examinations which subsequently have to be repeated in a specialist centre.

Whereas use of the older oily contrast media was sometimes complicated by the development of arachnoiditis, the most recent water-soluble media seem relatively free from this side-effect. However, examination of the cervical spine and craniovertebral junction using water-soluble media may be complicated by passage of contrast into the head. On occasions encephalopathy, seizures and myoclonic jerks may result. Seizures are particularly common in patients with a previous history of epilepsy.

Indications

Myelography is currently the most generally available and satisfactory method for demonstrating structural lesions impinging on the spinal canal and proximal nerve roots. It is important in the investigation of the neurological complications of lumbar and cervical spondylosis, spinal malignant disease, intradural tumours and dysraphism. The extent to which spinal MRI may replace the more invasive technique of myelography has yet to be determined.

DIAGNOSTIC LUMBAR PUNCTURE

Local anaesthetic should be infiltrated at the site of the skin puncture: a small-bore needle can be introduced into the lumbar sac, usually through the L2/3 interspinous ligament with the patient lying in the left lateral position; in this way, samples of lumbar cerebrospinal fluid can be obtained and c.s.f. pressure measured. The landmarks for this technique are illustrated in Figure 5.25. In some instances c.s.f. may be obtained via lateral cervical puncture or cisternal puncture under X-ray control.

Headache is the most common complication of lumbar puncture. This appears to be a low pressure headache caused by continued leaking of c.s.f. through the site of the lumbar dural puncture. Characteristically, patients develop headache, nausea and faintness on standing and these symptoms resolve rapidly when the patient lies down. These symptoms usually start within 24 hours of lumbar puncture and may continue for several days, in some instances. The incidence of post-lumbar-puncture headache can probably be reduced by the use of small-bore needles. It is common practice to keep patients recumbent for

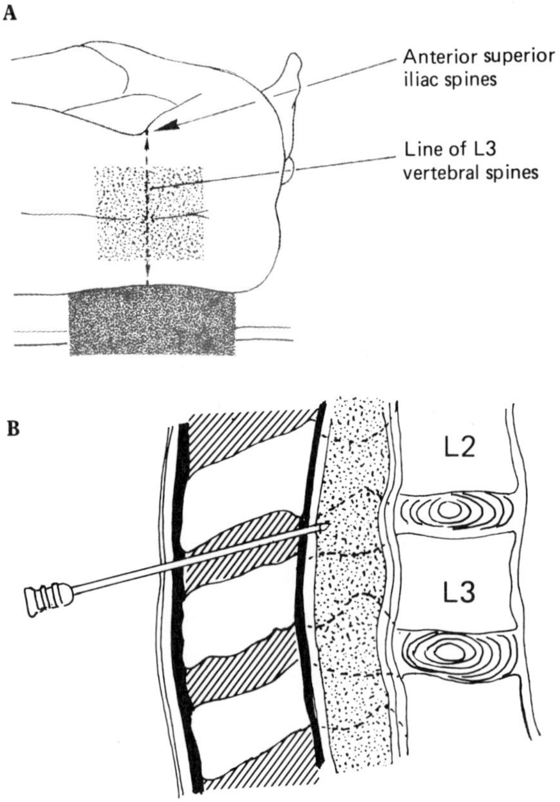

Fig. 5.25 **A** Surface landmarks **B** and technique of lumbar puncture.

24 hours after lumbar puncture in the belief that this reduces the incidence of headache. Other preventative measures include the use of blood patching into the epidural space. Once headache has developed, it can be alleviated by keeping the patient recumbent, and also by ensuring adequate hydration.

More serious complications of lumbar puncture are very rare. The most important is the precipitation of tentorial and foramen magnum coning in patients who have raised intracranial pressure. For this reason, patients in whom the presence of raised intracranial pressure is suspected should not be subjected to lumbar puncture unless the presence of hydrocephalus, or a mass lesion with displacement of the intracranial contents, has been excluded by CT scanning. It has to be emphasised that the absence of papilloedema does not indicate that lumbar puncture is a safe procedure. When papilloedema is present, lumbar puncture outside a neurosurgical centre is absolutely contraindicated. However, even in its absence, the presence of a history of raised intracranial pressure suggested by headache or impaired consciousness together with the presence of focal signs, should be sufficient in most cases to postpone lumbar puncture until adequate neuroradiological investigations have taken place.

A rarer complication of lumbar puncture is the development of epidural haematoma leading to a flaccid paraparesis or paraplegia. This complication is largely limited to patients with bleeding diatheses and lumbar puncture should be performed in such patients only after correction of any deficiencies in clotting status. Where contrast media or drugs are injected at lumbar puncture a chemically induced meningitis occasionally develops.

ABNORMALITIES OF C.S.F.

C.s.f. should be crystal clear: it may, however, appear turbid in pyogenic meningitis, or be frankly bloodstained or xanthochromic following haemorrhage. When the c.s.f. is bloodstained, it is extremely important to differentiate between blood present in the c.s.f. because of local trauma during the course of lumbar puncture and that present because of subarachnoid haemorrhage. The most important factor in differentiating these is centrifugation, which should render clear c.s.f. from a traumatic tap but, in patients with subarachnoid haemorrhage, xanthochromia will be present due to lysis of red cells in the c.s.f. This will be present from 1–2 h after subarachnoid haemorrhage for up to 1 week. Additional evidence for a traumatic tap is the maximal bloodstaining of the initial c.s.f., which is followed by subsequent clearing in successive aliquots.

In some instances it may be important to measure c.s.f. pressure. This can be done simply using a manometer but is only really necessary where it is believed that the patient may be suffering from the benign intracranial hypertension syndrome (p. 334). In the past, Queckenstedt's test has been performed routinely. This involves gentle pressure over both sides of the neck to cause an increase in venous pressure inside the head, which should then be transmitted to the lumbar sac. A negative Queckenstedt's test is indicative of a spinal block or, in some instances, of venous sinus thrombosis. There is no justification for continuing to perform this test, as lumbar puncture is not a satisfactory investigation for spinal tumours.

Full laboratory investigation of the c.s.f. will include a description and counting of any cells or organisms seen and cytocentrifugation of c.s.f. may be important in the detection of malignant cells. Estimation of c.s.f. protein and immunoglobulins, c.s.f. glucose estimation (which is of routine value in the diagnosis of inflammatory diseases of the nervous system) and adequate culturing of c.s.f., will be necessary where bacterial, viral or fungal infection are suspected. Common patterns of abnormality are described in Table 5.3.

INDICATIONS

Infection

Lumbar puncture and c.s.f. examination are essential investigations for the diagnosis of bacterial, viral and fungal infections of the meninges and c.n.s. The patient who presents with a febrile illness and meningism must have a c.s.f. examination in order to identify the causative organism and to ensure that treatment is appropriate. The only exception to the need for urgent lumbar puncture is in the presence of localised neurological signs which might suggest

Table 5.3 C.s.f. changes in disease

	Appearance	Pressure*	Cells§	Protein‡	Glucose**	Other
Meningitis						
pyogenic	turbid	+	+ to +++ (polymorphs)	++	–	organisms +ve culture
partially treated pyogenic		+	+ to ++ (lymphocytes + polymorphs)	+	normal/–	
viral		+	+ to ++ (lymphocytes + polymorphs)	+		rising antibody titres +ve cultures
tuberculous	turbid/clear	+	+ to ++ (lymphocytes + polymorphs)	++	–	AFB +ve cultures
Abscess		+	+ to ++ (polymorphs + lymphocytes)	+		CT scan +ve
Neurosyphilis			+ lymphocytes	+		↑ IgG/alb ratio oligoclonal bands+ve treponemal antigens
Multiple sclerosis			+	+		↑ IgG/alb ratio oligoclonal bands
Malignant meningitis	clear/turbid	normal/+	normal/+/++	normal/+	normal/–	abnormal cells mitoses
Demyelinating neuropathy		normal/+		+/++		

* + = >200 mm water § + = 5–100, ++ = 100–1000
‡ + = 0.4–1 g/l, ++ = >1 g/l ** – = < 2.0 mmol

abscess formation. In such instances, urgent referral to a neurosurgical/neurological centre is necessary before lumbar puncture.

Subarachnoid haemorrhage

Lumbar puncture is a valuable aid to the diagnosis of subarachnoid haemorrhage. However, its use is perhaps less essential than in the past as, in many instances, CT scanning will reveal the presence of subarachnoid blood and will also indicate the presence of any significant haematoma, which may be a relative contraindication to lumbar puncture outside a neurosurgical unit. Where the diagnosis of subarachnoid haemorrhage is unequivocal on the basis of history and signs, it is probably reasonable to obtain neurosurgical advice before lumbar puncture. It is important that either lumbar puncture or CT scanning should be performed within 24 hours of presentation, and that lumbar puncture should be performed in any patient where there is reasonable diagnostic doubt. On occasion, it may be difficult to differentiate clinically meningitis from subarachnoid haemorrhage.

C.s.f. pressure

Lumbar puncture to document raised intracranial pressure and normality of the c.s.f. is necessary for the diagnosis of benign intracranial hypertension, once space-occupying lesions have been satisfactorily excluded by neuroradiology; indeed, lumbar puncture may have a therapeutic role in this condition.

Other miscellaneous conditions

Examination of the spinal fluid can be helpful in the diagnosis of a number of conditions in which there is antibody formation within the c.n.s. Total c.s.f. protein may be considerably increased in c.n.s. infections and demyelinating neuropathies; an increased IgG/albumin ratio may be found in patients with multiple sclerosis, SSPE and neurosyphilis; oligoclonal bands may similarly be detected in these conditions; abnormal cells may be found in the c.s.f. in malignant meningitis, sarcoid and other causes of chronic meningitis.

It must be emphasised that lumbar puncture has no place in the diagnosis of cerebral or spinal tumours. Patients are still admitted to neurological/neurosurgical units in whom a diagnosis of cerebral tumour has been questioned and a lumbar puncture subsequently performed. This involves a significant risk of tentorial and foramen magnum coning if the original assumption is correct. Patients with spinal tumours require myelography rather than simple lumbar puncture.

BIOPSIES

Under certain well-defined situations, biopsy of muscle, peripheral nerve or meninges and brain may be helpful investigations.

MUSCLE BIOPSY

Muscle biopsy, obtained by either open biopsy or needle biopsy, is helpful in the diagnosis of neuromuscular disease. Conventional haematoxylin and eosin staining will provide useful morphological information and may help to differentiate primary myopathy from denervation. More sophisticated histochemical staining for NADH and ATPase will add considerable information and, in some instances, may support a specific diagnosis, e.g. absence of myophosphorylase in McArdle's disease. The presence of inflammatory infiltrate, particularly around perivascular spaces, may be diagnostic of polymyositis.

It must be emphasised that the interpretation of muscle biopsy demands a high level of skill and experience and should usually be undertaken and interpreted within specialist centres; however, this notwithstanding, it may be extremely difficult to differentiate unequivocally between primary muscle disease and denervation.

Indications

The most important single indication for muscle biopsy is the diagnosis of polymyositis and polyarteritis, because of their therapeutic implications. It is also valuable in the identification of a wide variety of uncommon primary muscle disorders characterised by specific ultrastructural or histochemical abnormalities.

NERVE BIOPSY

Biopsy of the sural nerve or terminal branches of the radial nerve may be undertaken in severe neuropathies. This may allow the differentiation between demyelinating and axonal neuropathies, and may display infiltration of peripheral nerves by abnormal substances (amyloid) or abnormal cells (lymphocytes). Loss of axons may be demonstrated in axonal neuropathies. The techniques and interpretation require that this procedure is restricted to specialist centres.

MENINGEAL/CEREBRAL BIOPSY

The main indication for cerebral biopsy is suspected tumour. Biopsy may be undertaken either via burr hole and a needle, or via open craniotomy as part of a more extensive exploratory procedure. Such procedures allow the diagnosis of the majority of cerebral tumours and, more importantly, their differentiation from abscess. More rarely, meningeal and cerebral biopsy may be helpful in the diagnosis of chronic meningitis. In the past, the diagnosis of herpes simplex encephalitis has been made by cerebral biopsy. The diagnosis of other rare conditions, e.g. cerebral angiitis and spongiform encephalopathies, may require such investigation.

OTHER MISCELLANEOUS INVESTIGATIONS

A number of other techniques are available for the investigation of cerebral function. Positron emission tomography of the brain and isotope techniques used in the estimation of cerebral blood flow and metabolism can currently be regarded only as experimental techniques and their place in the clinical management of patients has yet to be established. Spectroscopic examination of neural and muscular tissue is likely to become possible using magnetic resonance techniques.

FURTHER READING

Aminoff M J 1980 Electrodiagnosis in clinical neurology. Churchill Livingstone, Edinburgh

Fishman R A 1980 Cerebrospinal fluid in diseases of the nervous system. W B Saunders, Philadelphia

Kihoh L G, Osselton J W 1981 Clinical electroencephalography, 3rd edn. London, Butterworth.

6

Disorders of awareness and mental function

STATES OF ALTERED CONSCIOUSNESS

NORMAL CONSCIOUSNESS

Consciousness is a state characterised by awareness of self and environment, and associated with ability to respond appropriately. Two separate physiological components govern consciousness: the first is the arousal component, or wakefulness, which is behaviourally closely related to the physical manifestations of awakening from sleep, such as eyes being opened or motor activity; the second component is the content of consciousness, which governs awareness of self and environment, being the sum total of all psychological functions of sensations, emotions and thoughts. To an outsider it is the motor or verbal response of an individual which enables any assessment of the content of consciousness, or cognitive function to be made; this, of course, cannot be done without at least some degree of arousal. The sum total of cognitive functions is dependent on the activity of the cerebral cortex as a whole, and it is the cortex which can be regarded as mediating the content of consciousness or the awareness of self and environment.

Behavioural components of normal consciousness are conveniently summarised in the Glasgow Coma Scale (Table 6.1). Normal consciousness on the basis of this scale is associated with spontaneous eye opening, obedience to commands and orientation as assessed by speech. As will be seen later, this scale is not, strictly speaking, a coma scale but a consciousness scale, allowing a hierarchical grading to be made of the level of consciousness.

Table 6.1 The Glasgow Coma Scale

A *Eye opening*
1. Nil
2. Pain
3. Verbal
4. Spontaneous
B *Motor response*
1. Nil
2. Abnormal extension
3. Abnormal flexion
4. Weak flexion
5. Localising
6. Obeys commands
C *Verbal*
1. Nil
2. Incomprehensible
3. Inappropriate
4. Confused
5. Orientated fully

THE RETICULAR FORMATION

Our knowledge of the activities of the reticular formation took a major step forward with the work of Moruzzi and Magoun, who showed that electrical stimulation of the brain stem in anaesthetised cats produced changes in the EEG, similar to those observed in man on transition from a drowsy state to a state of alertness. From these and other observations it has been concluded that there is an ascending reticular system in the brain stem which can be regarded as a non-specific arousal system for the cortex.

The reticular formation anatomically is a continuous isodendritic core traversing from the medulla to the midbrain. It is continuous caudally with the reticular intermediate grey lamina of the spinal cord, and rostrally with the subthalamus, hypothalamus and thalamus. The classic view is that the anatomical basis of arousal is via projections from the reticular formation to the midline thalamic nuclei and thence to the cortex, although recent work suggests that this is an oversimplification. Neurotransmitter systems involved in the links between reticular formation and cortex are ill understood. It has been suggested that both cholinergic and monoamine systems are important in arousal.

Table 6.2 The causes of confusion and delirium (after Adams & Victor 1981)

I. *Delirium*

A No focal signs
1. Typhoid
2. Pneumonia
3. Septicemia
4. Rheumatic fever
5. Thyrotoxicosis and ACTH intoxication
6. Postoperative and post-traumatic states

B Focal or lateralising signs often present
1. Vascular neoplastic, or other diseases, particularly those involving the temporal and parietal lobes and upper part of the brain stem
2. Cerebral contusion and laceration (traumatic delirium)
3. Acute pyogenic and tuberculous meningitis
4. Subarachnoid haemorrhage
5. Encephalitis due to viral causes (e.g. herpes simplex, infectious mononucleosis)

C Miscellaneous
1. Withdrawal of alcohol (delirium tremens), barbiturates, and non-barbiturate sedative drugs, following chronic intoxication.
2. Drug intoxications: scopolamine, atropine, amphetamine, etc.
3. Postconvulsive delirium

II. *Confusion*

A No focal signs
1. Metabolic disorders; hepatic stupor, uraemia, hypoxia hypercapnia, hypoglycaemia, porphyria
2. Infective fevers
3. Congestive heart failure
4. Postoperative, post-traumatic and puerperal psychoses
5. Drug intoxication

B Focal signs often present
1. Cerebral vascular disease, tumour, abscess
2. Subdural haematoma
3. Meningitis
4. Encephalitis

III. *Decompensated dementia*, i.e. senile or other brain disease in combination with infective fevers, drug reactions, heart failure, or other medical or surgical diseases

DEFINITIONS

Confusion (clouding of consciouness)

This is the syndrome of an acute organic reaction, and the terms applied to the syndrome include the acute brain syndrome, acute organic psychosis, and the acute psycho-organic syndrome. A variety of pathological processes may induce the syndrome and these are listed in Table 6.2. It is defined as 'a disturbance of consciousness characterised by impaired capacity to think clearly, and to perceive, respond to and remember current stimuli; there is also disorientation'. Such patients have reduced awareness of self and environment, and are unable to express their thoughts clearly. Their memory is faulty and drowsiness is common with reversal of sleep rhythm. This latter component is diagnostically useful in differentiating confusion from aphasia, a restricted memory defect or an acute psychosis. As may be deduced from Table 6.2, confusion implies a generalised disturbance in cerebral function, particularly of the cortex, and is usually associated with widespread abnormalities of the electroencephalogram.

Delirium

This state is defined as one 'with grossly disturbed consciousness, associated with motor restlessness, transient hallucinations, disorientation and occasionally delusions'; it can be regarded as a state of advanced or pronounced acute confusion. Such patients may pose difficult management problems in open wards because of the intense restlessness that they often show as a pronounced feature. They are often out of touch with reality, are irritable and appear frightened with visual hallucinations. The causes of delirium are the same as those of acute confusion (Table 6.2). Most commonly delirium results from a toxic metabolic disorder and such patients usually recover within a few days. A similar syndrome is seen in patients in the recovery stage from coma after head injury and also may be a prominent feature following a subarachnoid haemorrhage. Acute schizophreniform psychosis may be differentiated from delirium by the lack of impairment of alertness. Acute mania simulates the restlessness of delirium although such patients usually have retained awareness of self and environment. Delirium implies a diffuse disorder of cerebral function and this is reflected by the EEG.

Obtundation

The obtunded patient characteristically shows a disorder of alertness associated with psychomotor retardation. This may at times be a feature of a confusional state, and the term is merely describing a clinical picture rather than a precise disorder of consciousness.

Stupor

Such patients, though not unconscious, exhibit little or no spontaneous activity. The patient appears to be asleep and yet, when vigorously stimulated, may show themselves to be alert by eye opening and eye movements. There is usually no speech and other motor activities are limited. Although stupor may result from diffuse organic cerebral dysfunction, a variety of psychiatric disorders produce an identical clinical picture. Table 6.3 lists the diagnosis in 100 patients in stupor seen in two psychiatric units in London. It is uncommon for stupor to persist for prolonged periods and 50% of those 100 patients recovered within a week.

Table 6.3 The causes of stupor in psychiatric patients

Schizophrenia	31
Depression	25
Organic	20
Neurosis	10
Unknown	14
Total	100

It may be difficult to differentiate organic stupor from that due to psychiatric illness. Those in schizophrenic stupor usually show prominent features of catatonia with negativism, echopraxia (defined as repetitive copying movements) and flexibilitas cerea. In this situation the EEG is of great value, as in organic stupor it invariably shows a diffuse abnormality, whereas in other forms of stupor it is normal. Gjessing's syndrome is a rare form of periodic stupor which may pose diagnostic difficulties as there are often minor EEG abnormalities at the time of the periods of stupor. The periodic hypersomnias are dealt with in Chapter 7.

Coma

A simple and understandable definition of coma is that of 'unarousable unresponsiveness'. This implies not only a defect in arousal, but also one in awareness of self and environment. A more practical definition may be obtained using the Glasgow Coma Scale (Table 6.1). Coma is defined as a certain pattern of behavioural responses at the lower end of the scale. In precise terms coma may be defined as the lower two responses of eye opening, the lower two verbal responses and the lower three motor responses. At best, such patients do not open their eyes to a voice or spontaneously, do not even localise a painful stimulus and utter no recognisable words. The causes of coma and the assessment of a patient in coma is dealt with below.

Vegetative state

This was the term suggested by Jennett and Plum to describe patients who recover the arousal component of consciousness but not awareness. The commonest causes are head injury, hypoxic ischaemic damage to the brain, and stroke. Such patients usually emerge from coma as evidenced by eye opening, and sleep/wake cycles may develop with periods of eye closure and spontaneous eye opening. Brain stem reflexes become brisk, and conjugate or dysconjugate roving movements of the eyes may be seen. There is, however, no evidence of response to speech or movement to command, and no evidence of cognitive activity. Flaccidity in the limbs is an early feature, although eventually there is marked increase in tone with increase in the tendon reflexes, extensor plantar responses and primitive reflexes such as a pout reflex; such patients may have an exaggerated grimace response. The whole clinical picture is a constant source of distress to relatives who find it hard to comprehend that eye opening does not indicate recovery. Persistence of this state for more than a few weeks indicates extensive cortical damage and recovery is exceptional. Patients in this condition, however, may be kept alive almost indefinitely by careful nursing. Autopsy studies show a characteristic appearance of widespread cortical damage with relative preservation of brain stem structures. A variety of other terms have been applied to this clinical picture including coma vigil, apallic syndrome, cerebral death, neocortical death and total dementia. Akinetic mutism is a behaviourally similar condition of unresponsiveness yet apparent alertness. The striking difference is the lack of any motor signs of spasticity or rigidity, despite a paucity of movement even to pain. This picture has been seen in a variety of pathological lesions, including diffuse cortical lesions, bilateral frontal lobe lesions, lesions of the deep grey matter and diencephalic lesions.

The locked-in syndrome

This term is applied to a clinical syndrome of total paralysis below the level of the third nerve nuclei. Such patients can elevate their eyelids and consistently elevate and depress their eyes, yet have lost horizontal eye movement and have no other voluntary movements. The differentiation of this condition from the vegetative state depends on the recognition of the fact that the patient is eye opening voluntarily rather than spontaneously. It is often possible to communicate with the patient by using a simple morse code as applied to eye opening. The neuropathological basis for such cases is usually infarction of the ventral pons or efferent motor tracts with preservation of the ascending reticular formation, and the third nerve nuclei. A similar clinical picture may sometimes be seen in patients with pontine tumours, pontine haemorrhage, central pontine myelinolysis, head injury or brain stem encephalitis. Patients with the condition usually die or remain tetraplegic although, with expert nursing, prolonged survival is possible; there are occasional reports of recovery.

THE PATHOPHYSIOLOGY OF COMA AND STATES OF ALTERED CONSCIOUSNESS

It cannot be overemphasised that disorders of consciousness almost invariably result from diffuse or multifocal lesions of the cerebral hemisphere; the one exception to this rule is coma itself and, as we shall see, this may result from quite discrete lesions of the brain stem.

THE ASSESSMENT OF THE UNCONSCIOUS PATIENT

History

In routine neurological practice the history is of considerable value in diagnosis. Unfortunately, it is seldom available for the unconscious patient; in these circumstances, the examination should not be delayed. Information concerning the unconscious patient may be obtained from relatives, neighbours, witnesses or even the ambulance men who brought the patient to hospital. Some of the important points to be gained from the history are:

1. Previous medical history
2. Symptoms at onset of coma
3. Circumstances of onset of coma
4. Evolution of the patient's clinical state since the onset of coma (improvement or deterioration?).

General examination

The immediate priority is the assessment of vital signs and, whatever the cause of coma, an early assessment should be made of respiratory and circulatory function. It is vital to maintain a secure airway and adequate oxygenation; similarly, blood pressure and pulse should be carefully monitored and appropriate treatment given. Once these immediate priorities have been dealt with, a more detailed general examination should be made of the patient's unclothed body. The contents of the patient's clothing should be examined, in particular looking for evidence of drugs; medic-alert bracelets, necklaces or hospital record cards may provide useful information. Evidence of external trauma to the skull or other parts of the body should be carefully sought and the neck should be examined, looking for rigidity. The remaining components of the general examination are directed at looking for two groups of clues:

1. Evidence of acute or chronic illness
2. Evidence of drug ingestion (needle marks, alcohol on breath).

The patient's temperature should be noted and, if there is any excessive coldness of the skin, a low-reading rectal thermometer should be used to exclude hypothermia.

The neurological examination

The neurological assessment of the unconscious patient will often provide clues to the cause of coma and, in particular, to the type of coma. It should be possible to differentiate coma attributable to a brain stem lesion from that caused by bilateral hemisphere dysfunction. Furthermore, the pattern of signs in these cases will differ from those in a patient in coma secondary to a unilateral hemisphere lesion with brain stem herniation. It is important to follow a systematic approach to the neurological assessment of the unconscious patient and the components of this are listed in Table 6.4.

Table 6.4 The neurological assessment of the patient in coma

General assessment
Skull
Ears
Fundi
Signs of meningism
Level of consciousness
The Glasgow coma scale:
1 Verbal responses
2 Eye opening
3 Motor responses
Brainstem function
1. Pupillary reactions
2. Spontaneous eye movements
3. Oculocephalic responses
4. Oculovestibular responses
5. Corneal responses
6. Respiratory pattern
Motor function
1. Deep tendon reflexes
2. Skeletal muscle tone

The assessment of level of consciousness

This is best assessed using the Glasgow Coma Scale (Table 6.1). In essence, the technique is to give the patient either a verbal or a painful stimulus and to observe the three possible types of response: eye opening, motor and verbal response. The maximal response must be elicited and in an unconscious patient this will require a suitably painful stimulus: supraorbital pressure with the thumb or nail bed pressure with a pen or a coin are best as they are easy to administer, very painful and do not mark the skin. It is of vital importance that the level of consciousness is recorded serially because one of the most important components of the assessment of the unconscious patient is to know whether he is improving or deteriorating.

The examination of brain stem function

The activity of a variety of brain stem structures may be assessed by the examination of evoked and spontaneous reflex activity.

The optic fundi. Although not part of the brain stem, the optic fundi are traditionally included in the cranial nerve examination and should be closely inspected in the unconscious patient. Evidence of papilloedema, hypertension, retinal ischaemia or retinal haemorrhage should be sought and, if necessary, the pupils should be dilated, although in practice this is rarely necessary.

Pupils. The pupils should be examined for size, equality and reaction to light. Before concluding that the pupillary light reflex is absent, a bright light should be used and movement of the eye assessed with a hand lens. Unilateral absence of the pupillary light reflex may result from an optic nerve lesion and this may be differentiated from the mydriasis of a third nerve palsy by the differences between consensual and direct reflex. In deep barbiturate coma the pupils may be of average size and have preserved reflexes despite absence of all other reflex activity. Bilateral small pupils may indicate pontine haemorrhage or opiate intoxication and bilateral dilated and unreactive pupils indicate upper brain stem damage. Spurious changes in the size of the pupils or the pupillary reactions may be observed in patients with iris disease, those who have received mydriatics, or pre-existing disorders such as the Adie syndrome.

Spontaneous eye movements. The assessment of spontaneous or reflex eye movements is one of the most valuable components of the examination of brain stem function and a full knowledge of the anatomical pathways subserving eye movements is necessary in order to interpret the variety of abnormalities. In the unconscious patient the spontaneous rapid eye movements of the awake individual are absent and in light coma there will often be slow conjugate or dysconjugate roving eye movements of the eyes either horizontally or vertically. Full spontaneous movements require participation of the entire conjugate gaze systems of the brain stem: the preservation of full horizontal movements indicates that the pons and midbrain are relatively intact, ruling out an infratentorial brain stem lesion as the cause of coma. In deep coma from any cause and in drug overdose coma the eyes are fixed. The resting position of the eyes should be noted: downward deviation of both eyes occurs in thalamic and subthalamic lesions but may be seen also after a seizure and in patients who have suffered extensive cerebral ischaemic damage. Upward deviation of the eyes occurs in sleep, seizures, syncope and a variety of brain stem lesions. Conjugate deviation of the eyes to one side may be indicative of either a hemisphere or brain stem disturbance and when present indicates a paralysis of gaze. A slight divergence of the eyes is not uncommon at all levels of obtundation. Certain spontaneous eye movements are of particular diagnostic value: ocular bobbing, for example, indicates an extensive lesion of the pons.

Oculocephalic response. The oculocephalic response or doll's head manoeuvre is the simplest test of reflex eye movement, but may be absent *without* brain stem damage and often requires keen observation. Another disadvantage is that the test may be difficult to perform in a patient who is intubated. In the normal conscious person when the head is rotated horizontally the eyes follow the head. In the patient with cortical depression, when the head is rotated horizontally to one side, the eyes under the influence of the labyrinths deviate briskly and conjugately to the opposite side (Fig. 6.1). Full horizontal conjugate movement on head rotation indicates normal functioning of the labyrinths, eighth nerves, conjugate lateral gaze centres, medial longitudinal fasciculi, oculomotor nerves and ocular muscles and rules out a gross lesion of the brain stem as the cause of coma.

The responses are characteristically brisk in metabolic coma and depressed in coma due to drugs. Asymmetry of the oculocephalic response is a useful sign of a brain stem lesion although this is often difficult to observe and may be seen in patients in drug-induced coma. It is possible,

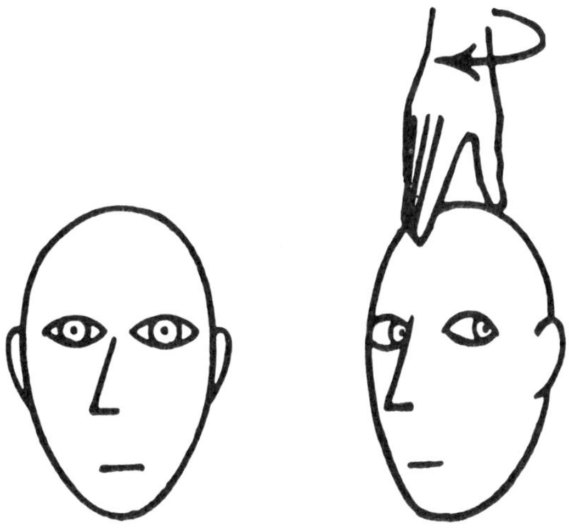

Fig. 6.1 A positive oculocephalic response

although difficult, to test vertical reflex eye movements by neck flexion and extension, but this is rarely of clinical value.

Oculovestibular response The oculovestibular response, although more time-consuming to elicit than the oculocephalic response, gives a more accurate assessment of reflex eye movements as these are usually easy to visualise. The external auditory meatus should be examined before performing the test and the best responses are obtained with ice-cold water. Although as little as 5–10 ml may produce a response, as much as 100 ml should be used before deciding whether a response is absent. Four grades of response may be recognised:

1. Nystagmus
2. Tonic deviation
3. Impaired deviation
4. No response.

In an alert normal individual, nystagmus will be seen and in an apparently unconscious patient the presence of nystagmus is diagnostic of psychogenic coma. The quick phase of the nystagmus requires cortex-brain stem connections: in coma attributable to a diffuse cortical process, the quick phase of the nystagmus is absent and the slow phase predominates, with the result that the eyes are forcibly drawn to the stimulated side (tonic deviation) (Fig. 6.2). Symmetrical tonic deviation indicates preservation of brain stem function and is characteristic of metabolic or hypoxic ischaemic coma; asymmetrical deviation is characteristic of a focal brain stem lesion, although it may be seen also in patients in drug-induced coma (Fig. 6.3). Bilaterally absent oculovestibular responses indicate either a profound brain stem disturbance, drug overdose coma, or bilateral middle-ear pathology (Fig. 6.4.). Having tested the reflex on one side one should allow a delay of 1–2 minutes before testing the opposite side. Reflex vertical eye movements may be tested using simultaneous irrigation of the external meati; warm water producing upward gaze and cold water producing downward gaze; in clinical practice, however, these are rarely used.

Corneal responses. The corneal reflexes are usually preserved, apart from those in patients in deep coma. Exaggerated responses with grimacing are characteristic of patients in the vegetative state and brisk responses in a patient in coma indicate preservation of brain-stem function. Asymmetry of the corneal responses may have localising value.

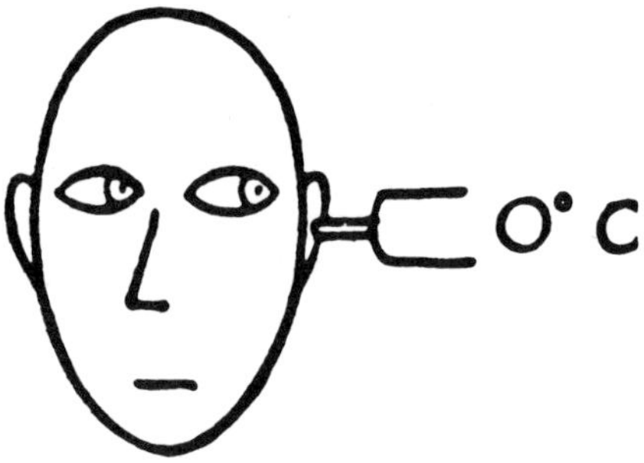

Fig. 6.2 A tonic oculovestibular response

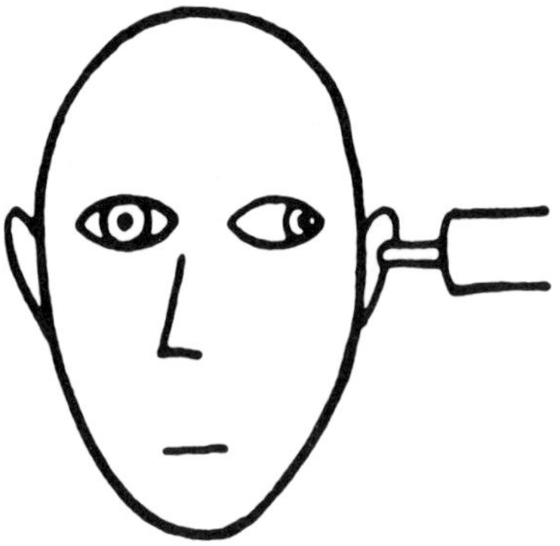

Fig. 6.3 An asymmetrical oculovestibular response

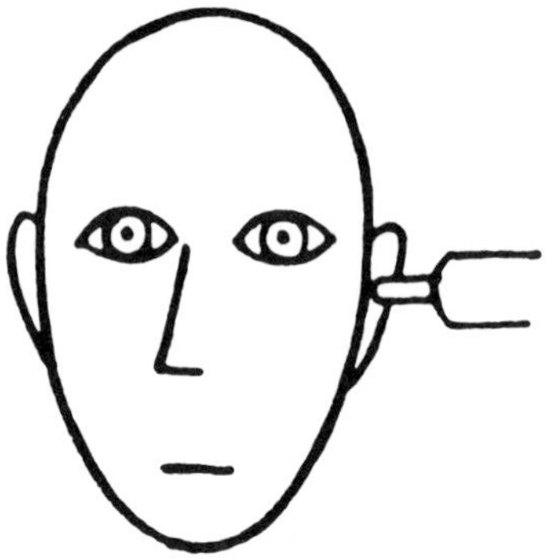

Fig. 6.4 A negative oculovestibular response

Respiratory pattern. A variety of abnormalities of respiration may be seen in coma, the best recognised of which is Cheynes–Stokes respiration.

This, contrary to common belief, usually indicates that death is not imminent. Some respiratory patterns are thought to have localising value, but these are of little use in clinical practice. Breathing which is stertorous has no special neurological significance and is due to partial respiratory obstruction.

The examination of motor function

As noted in the Glasgow Coma Scale, abnormalities of motor function are of hierarchical value, i.e. complete lack of motor response is 'worse' than an extensor motor response. In man the pathological lesions producing the so-called decerebrate and decorticate responses do not follow as precise anatomical correlates as in Sherringtonian experiments. Extensor responses, for example, may be seen in cortical, subcortical and brain stem lesions.

The major importance of the examination of motor function is in the assessment of symmetry of response. Asymmetrical responses may have considerable localising value as, with the rare exceptions of hypoglycaemia or hepatic coma, asymmetry of motor activity usually indicates focal pathology. This may be determined from the posture of the limbs, asymmetry of muscle tone, or asymmetry of responses to pain. Occasionally asymmetry of facial grimacing may be a useful localising sign.

The tendon reflexes are of limited value in the assessment of motor function as they may be present even in patients who otherwise fulfil the criteria of brain death. Brisk reflexes characteristically occur in hepatic coma and the reflexes may be selectively depressed in drug coma. The plantar responses are also of limited value in coma as they may be flexor in extensive brain stem lesions and extensor even in the absence of evidence of pyramidal tract disturbance. A unilateral extensor plantar response, however, retains its localising value. Muscle tone, like the motor responses, may be scored hierarchically in the order flexor, extensor, flaccid. Flaccid tone may be seen not only in severe brain damage but also in coma caused by drug overdose: hepatic coma characteristically is associated with increased muscle tone. Asymmetry of motor tone should be looked for not only in the limbs but also in the eyelids and is useful in localisation.

Spontaneous motor activity such as myoclonus, seizures or other involuntary movements may be of diagnostic value. Focal seizures have the same implication as focal signs and multifocal myoclonus is indicative of a diffuse cortical disturbance. Focal seizures may rarely be seen in diffuse hemisphere disturbances such as hepatic or hypoglycaemic coma.

By using the above method of assessment, it should be possible to differentiate three anatomically different forms of organic coma.

CEREBRAL HEMISPHERE COMA

To produce coma, cerebral hemisphere disturbances must be diffuse, extensive and bilateral. These may be either structural, such as diffuse anoxic damage, or metabolic, such as hepatic dysfunction or hypoglycaemia. Typically in this form of coma there is preservation of brain stem function and the patients are deeply unresponsive, yet have preserved brain stem reflexes. Tone and motor responses in the limbs are usually symmetrical and there may be flaccidity, flexor tone or extensor tone. Seizures and myoclonus may occur.

RETICULAR FORMATION COMA

Discrete brain stem lesions can readily damage the reticular formation, although damage below the level of the lower pons does not produce coma. Above this level there must be damage to both sides to produce coma, although quite a small lesion may produce this. Brain stem infarction or haemorrhage often produces coma, although it is rare with brain stem gliomas and plaques of demyelination. The important rule about brain stem coma is that any lesion which affects the reticular formation directly, inevitably will exert an effect on other brain-stem structures, as shown *at an early stage* by abnormality of the brain stem reflexes. Drug coma chiefly results from reticular formation depression, and profound metabolic or anoxic insults to the brain may also affect brain stem structures as well as the cortex; this is evidenced by disappearance of the brain stem reflexes. Large diencephalic lesions interrupting ascending efferents from the reticular formation to the cortex may occasionally be a cause of coma, although more often such lesions are associated with akinetic mutism. Bilateral thalamic damage, although rare, may produce coma and this most commonly results from vascular occlusion of perforating arteries arising from the basilar artery.

COMA RESULTING FROM A UNILATERAL HEMISPHERE OR SUPRATENTORIAL LESION

A localised unilateral supratentorial lesion will not in itself produce coma. However, a unilateral hemisphere lesion may impair consciousness by direct disruption of ascending efferents from the reticular formation to the cortex. A more common mechanism is that resulting from downward shift of the cerebral hemisphere with secondary distortion of the brain stem—the syndrome of rostrocaudal herniation or coning (Fig. 6.5). Any expanding supratentorial lesion of sufficient size to produce shift may be associated with coma, and this includes cerebral haemorrhage, cerebral infarction, tumours, subdural and extradural haemorrhage, abscesses, hydrocephalus and cerebral oedema. Coma in this situation may be recognised from the unilateral signs evident at an early stage, and the later development of brain stem signs, particularly a third nerve palsy.

PSYCHOGENIC COMA

Although this is uncommon, it may usually readily be differentiated from organic coma. Even the most florid hysteric will have difficulty in refraining from grimacing to an appropriately severe painful stimulus, and usually will try to resist when an attempt is made to open the eyes forcibly. Finally, the oculovestibular response will be diagnostic, as such patients show nystagmus. If doubt remains from the clinical examination, the electroencephalogram will be diagnostic in showing a normal pattern.

From the clinical point of view, coma can be divided into three separate groups.

AETIOLOGICAL CATEGORIES OF COMA

Drug coma

Drug coma is usually attributable to depression of reticular formation activity, although most drugs which depress cerebral function also have more widespread actions. The end result from the clinical point of view is similar in most forms of drug coma in that there is early and selective

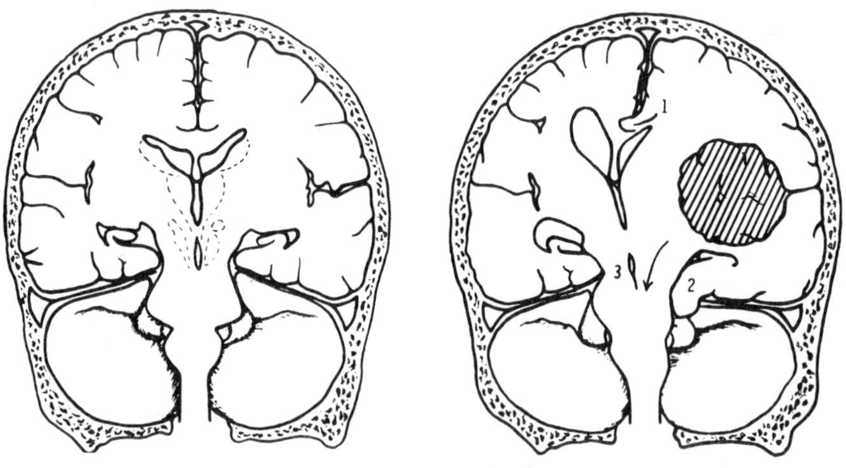

Fig. 6.5 Rostrocaudal herniation due to a mass lesion. 1—Subfalcine herniation, 2—tentorial herniation of the medial temporal lobe, 3—brain stem distortion.

depression of brain stem function, particularly of the brain stem reflexes concerning eye movement. The pupillary reflexes are often relatively spared, and this finding is so consistent that an unconscious patient with absent reflex eye movements yet preserved pupillary reflexes can be assumed to be in drug coma. In drug coma there is no direct damage to the nervous system and cerebral activity is simply depressed. The prognosis with supportive care is accordingly excellent and such patients should recover if the secondary complications of anoxia, pneumonia or cardiac arrhythmia are avoided.

Head injury

At the moment of impact there is a sharp rise in intracranial pressure and rapid movement of the brain within the skull, resulting in distortion of the cerebral hemispheres in relation to the brain stem. Disordered consciousness after head injury at least in part results from disruption of the reticular formation connections with the cerebral cortex. A rich variety of physical signs may be found in head injury coma, resulting from the variety of pathological changes such as primary brain stem damage, hemisphere contusions, secondary oedema, vasospasm and secondary haemorrhage. Penetrating head injuries are rarely associated with loss of consciousness unless there is brain stem damage, and crush injuries to the head usually produce more damage to the skull than to the brain unless the crushing impact is very severe.

Medical coma

Some of the principal medical causes of coma are listed in Table 6.5. These include a variety of different forms of coma with differing mechanisms, physical signs and outcomes. A simplification is to divide patients in medical coma into two major categories: those with and those without focal signs.

Coma with focal signs

Focal signs, such as asymmetrical motor responses or asymmetrical brain stem reflexes, are almost invariably indicative of focal pathology. From the pattern of the focal signs it should be possible to decide whether the pathology is supratentorial, with secondary brain stem herniation, or infratentorial, with distortion of the brain stem. With this information and with the information concerning evolution of the patient's symptomatology, it should be possible to reach not only an anatomical but also a pathological diagnosis. Any patient with signs indicating a progressive focal intracranial lesion producing coma should have urgent neuroradiological investigation in the form of a CT scan.

Table 6.5 Medical causes of coma

Hypoxia-ischaemia
Respiratory arrest
Cardiac arrest
Hypotension
Cerebrovascular
Occlusive
Parenchymal haemorrhage
Subarachnoid haemorrhage
Other
Hepatic
Other
Uraemic coma
Meningitis/encephalitis
Metabolic abnormalities, e.g. hypernatraemia
Endocrine abnormalities
Hypertensive encephalopathy
Diabetic coma
Hypoglycaemia
Postseizure coma

Coma without focal signs

This group may be further subdivided into patients with and without signs of meningeal irritation. Patients with signs of meningeal irritation without focal signs are likely to have had either a subarachnoid haemorrhage or to have some form of intracranial infection. A lumbar puncture in such cases is usually of diagnostic value. In the absence of signs of meningeal irritation such patients are likely to have either bilateral cortical damage producing coma or functional cortical depression from a metabolic disturbance, such as in hepatic coma. Such patients usually have evidence of brisk brain stem reflexes but are otherwise unresponsive.

BRAIN DEATH

This is a controversial subject, but is one of great practical importance. The United Kingdom Brain Death Criteria are listed in Table 6.6. These may be simplified thus:

1. Irremediable structural brain damage *of known aetiology*
2. Apnoeic coma not due to drugs, hypothermia or a metabolic disturbance
3. Absent brain stem reflexes
4. Unresponsiveness and no respiratory movements.

Because the diagnosis of brain death carries such a heavy clinical and legal responsibility, many regard additional laboratory investigations as essential. *It is generally accepted that a single series of observations should not allow a pronouncement of brain death to be made and that a second examination should be made at least 12 hours after the first.*

Table 6.6 The diagnosis of brain death (United Kingdom) criteria

Conditions under which the diagnosis of brain death should be considered:
a. The patient is deeply comatose
   i. There should be no suspicion that this state is due to depressant drugs
   ii. Primary hypothermia as a cause of coma should have been excluded
   iii. Metabolic and endocrine disturbance which can be responsible for or can contribute to coma should have been excluded
b. The patient is being maintained on a ventilator because spontaneous respiration had previously become inadequate or had ceased altogether
   i. Relaxants (neuromuscular blocking agents) and other drugs should have been excluded as a cause of respiratory inadequacy or failure
c. There should be no doubt that the patient's condition is due to irremediable structural brain damage. The diagnosis of a disorder which can lead to brain death should have been fully established

Diagnostic tests for the confirmation of brain death: All brainstem reflexes are absent:
a. The pupils are fixed in diameter and do not respond to sharp changes in the intensity of incident light
b. There is no corneal reflex
c. The vestibulo-ocular reflexes are absent
d. No motor responses within the cranial nerve distribution can be elicited by adequate stimulation of any somatic area
e There is no gag reflex or reflex response to bronchial stimulation by a suction catheter passed down the trachea
f. No respiratory movements occur when the patient is disconnected from the mechanical ventilator for long enough to ensure that the arterial carbon dioxide tension rises above the threshold for stimulation of respiration

DISORDERS OF AWARENESS AND THE CONTENT OF CONSCIOUSNESS

Disorders of awareness constitute a wide spectrum of differing clinical syndromes, some of which may result from diffuse cerebral pathology and some from localised disturbances. Confusion and delirium are states which we have considered as states of altered consciousness, but, as is discussed later, these differ only in terms of their time course from such states as dementia. The spectrum of clinical disorders considered here are those where there is an organic disturbance of cerebral function. It must be remembered, however, that a variety of psychiatric disorders may mimic closely these differing organic syndromes.

DEMENTIA

A variety of different terms are applied as equivalents of dementia and these include the chronic brain syndrome, the chronic confusional state and

Table 6.7 Causes of dementia

	Approx. incidence
Degenerative diseases (probable Alzheimer's)	40%
Multi-infarct dementia	13%
Alcoholic dementia	8%
Metabolic/toxic	5%
Hydrocephalus	4%
Tumours	3%
Huntington's disease	2%
Trauma	1%
Infections	1%
Other organic conditions	11%
Dementia associated with psychiatric disorder and pseudodementia	12%

chronic organic psychosis; such terms should *not* be used. Dementia is defined as acquired loss of cognitive skills and such a state may result from a variety of different pathological processes (Table 6.7). The clinical picture shows a considerable degree of similarity from one disease process to another in all cases resulting from diffuse or widespread involvement of the cerebral hemispheres.

Clinical features

Most forms of dementia begin insidiously with progressive impairment of memory or disorganisation of intellect. Occasionally, such states may follow acute episodes such as severe head injury or anoxia, and are then apparent when the patient recovers consciousness.

Cognitive impairment

The patient with progressive dementia often first shows failure of memory and this more often than not is noticed by relatives or workmates. As more widespread cognitive failure develops, then inability to cope at work and at home may become apparent. Change in personality may appear by this stage, with deterioration of manners, diminished awareness of the feelings of others and social blunders. Occasionally the syndrome may be disclosed by an episode of stealing or disinhibited behaviour. Although the progression is usually insidious, the illness may declare itself abruptly as a result of some dramatic instance, either at home or in a work situation. Occasionally, an intercurrent illness may precipitate confusion in what eventually proves to be a progressive dementing process.

Personality change

The general behaviour during progressive dementia may mirror the loss of intellectual ability. Loss of interest or initiative may be noted and occasionally there will be episodes of inappropriate behaviour. As the condition progresses, personal hygiene and appearance become neglected and food may be eaten sloppily in association with other uncouth habits. By contrast, some patients preserve social competence till late in the course of the disease and the diagnosis may not be apparent unless specific tests of cognitive skills are applied. Loss of insight is a hallmark of dementia, although in the very early stages in people with a high premorbid intelligence, this may be preserved, much to their distress.

Memory

The memory defect is typically global, affecting remote as well as recent events. Inability to learn new material is a most conspicuous finding, although there is rarely the sharp demarcation between remote and recent memory which characterises the pure amnestic syndrome.

Affect

The emotional reaction varies depending on the state of deterioration. At an early stage, anxiety and depression may be present, probably resulting from preserved insight into the increasing intellectual difficulties. As further deterioration occurs, a flattening of the affect becomes apparent, and this may lead to emotions taking on a child-like aspect. Emotional lability may occur with further progression, with episodes of laughing and crying for little or no cause.

Neurological signs in dementia

Diffuse impairment of cerebral function may manifest as a variety of neurological signs indicative of neuronal fall-out or disturbed neuronal function. Patients with dementia often show the presence of primitive reflexes such as a pout reflex or a grasp reflex. Profound dementia may be associated with a suckling reflex and, in cases where there is extensive interference with cortical function, there may be the development of bilateral pyramidal signs, rigidity, spasticity, increase in the tendon reflexes and extensor plantar responses.

THE DIFFERENT TYPES OF DEMENTIA

Traditionally, dementia is subdivided into presenile dementia and senile dementia, with an arbitrary cut-off point of 65 years of age. The differing syndromes which may produce either senile or presenile dementia are listed in Table 6.7, but in clinical practice the commonest cause of dementia at any age is a progressive degeneration of the brain, the so-called primary dementia. A variety of different clinical and pathological syndromes may be recognised in this group. The hallmark of all of these is that they share a hopeless prognosis and in clinical practice the main aim should be to identify and distinguish these from the secondary dementias which, in some instances, may respond to appropriate treatment.

There is some merit in differentiating different clinical syndromes in dementia according to the classification presented in Table 6.8. Cortical dementias typically are characterised by memory disorders in combination with an aphasia/agnosia/apraxia complex. The behaviour is alert and gross motor or sensory disorders do not occur. The subcortical dementias are characterised by slowness in thinking and in behaviour, forgetfulness, apathy and depression; motor disorders are present from the onset.

Arteriosclerotic dementia (multi-infarct dementia)

This is probably a much overdiagnosed syndrome and even now patients with senile dementia are often arbitrarily said to have arteriosclerotic dementia largely because of their age and known presence of vascular disease. In practice, a primary neuronal degeneration is a more common cause of senile dementia.

Table 6.8 Classification of dementias according to clinical syndromes

Cortical dementias
- Alzheimer's disease
- Pick's disease

Subcortical dementias
- Huntington's disease
- Wilson's disease
- Parkinson's disease
- Progressive supranuclear palsy
- Thalamic lesions (tumour, infarct)
- Spinocerebellar degenerations
- Toxic and metabolic encephalopathies
- Dementia syndrome of depression
- Hydrocephalus

Mixed forms
- Multi-infarct dementia
- Dementia following infection, trauma, anoxia, etc.

Arteriosclerosis is usually obvious both in the peripheral and in the retinal vessels, and hypertension is a prominent feature. There is often a previous history of minor strokes, and the onset of intellectual impairment may be abrupt and appear to follow a cerebral ischaemic episode. Typically, there is variation in the degree of cognitive impairment, although usually the course is progressive despite fluctuations.

There are often prominent signs of a disturbance of motor function with apraxia, hemiparesis or rigidity. Parkinsonian features may develop and seizures may be seen in as many as 20% of cases.

The time to death varies widely and is often a result of ischaemic heart disease or of a frank major stroke. The brain often shows areas of localised as well as generalised atrophy and on sectioning may show frank cyst formation. Typically, the atherosclerotic changes are found in other organs of the body also.

The term 'multi-infarct dementia' should probably be preferred to 'arteriosclerotic dementia', as the former indicates that the picture results not from progressive chronic ischaemia but essentially from an accumulation of multiple cerebral infarcts, both large and small. The problem of atherosclerosis and the brain and the clinical picture of so-called lacunar infarcts are discussed in Chapter 11.

Alzheimer's disease

This is the commonest of the primary presenile dementias. Typically, such cases arise sporadically although there are a very few families in which several members show the typical clinical and pathological features of Alzheimer's disease. The onset is usually between 40 and 60 years of age and women are affected more often than men, in a ratio of 2–3 : 1. The onset is insidious and the clinical features follow the course as outlined above. Occasionally signs of a focal cerebral disturbance may be obvious, and this may complicate the clinical picture. These signs are usually those of a parietal lobe disturbance with signs of dysphasia or apraxia, or occasionally signs of a non-dominant parietal lobe syndrome with constructional apraxia and topographical agnosia. In the terminal stages the patients are bedbound, mute, tetraparetic and incontinent. Fits commonly develop and death usually results from intercurrent infection.

Investigations show non-specific abnormalities: the EEG shows a diffuse abnormality and a CT scan (other than in the early stages) will demonstrate cerebral atrophy.

The disease usually runs a progressive course, with death about 2–5 years after onset, and the progression is usually inexorable. Pathologically the brain is grossly atrophic and histologically there is widespread loss of nerve cells with glial proliferation. The striking feature is the presence of so-called plaques and neurofibrillary tangles. Occasionally the cortical atrophy is more pronounced in the frontal and temporal lobes.

Many authorities believe that Alzheimer's disease and the degenerative form of senile dementia are identical in all respects other than age of onset.

Pick's disease

This is an uncommon dementing process resulting from progressive neuronal degeneration. The peak onset is between the age of 50 and 60 years and progression is somewhat slower than that of Alzheimer's disease. The condition usually manifests itself with changes indicating frontal lobe damage, with changes in personality and drive as a prominent feature. Impairment of intellect and memory tends to follow as the disease progresses. Disorders of speech with perseveration and dysphasia may become marked, although by the later stages the marked disintegration of intellect and personality results in a clinical picture similar to that seen in other progressive dementias.

The pathological features include a characteristic appearance of circumscribed shrinkage of certain lobes of the brain, most commonly frontal and temporal. The distribution of atrophy varies from case to case and the most severely affected gyri show a characteristic 'knife blade' appearance. Histological examination reveals neuronal loss accompanied by astrocytic proliferation, but in contrast to Alzheimer's disease there is a complete absence of senile plaques and neurofibrillary tangles.

It is sometimes thought that Alzheimer's disease and Pick's disease should be considered jointly, as the end result of extensive cortical atrophy is the same. However, the different histological features suggest a different causation and the differentiation of the two conditions should probably be maintained.

DIFFERENTIAL DIAGNOSIS OF DEMENTIA

Every patient with dementia should be subjected to full and comprehensive evaluation, because the label of a primary dementing illness carries a hopeless prognosis. Practices vary in relation to the age of the patient: most neurologists do not investigate in detail patients with senile dementia. Readily treatable conditions, such as pernicious anaemia or myxoedema, are probably worth excluding, even in patients in their 70s and 80s. The main aim is to exclude a remediable cause for the patient's symptoms: the value of comprehensive inpatient evaluation can be assessed from a study performed by Marsden and Harrison (Table 6.9). One hundred and six patients admitted to the National Hospital, Queen's Square, with a presumptive diagnosis of senile or presenile dementia, were studied; no fewer than 15 of the 106 patients were judged not to be demented; 8 of these had depression, 1 mania, 1 hysteria, 1 epilepsy, 2 drug toxicity and in 2 the diagnosis was uncertain. Eighty-four patients remained with evidence of intellectual impairment and *only 48* of these were shown to have cerebral atrophy of unknown cause. The importance in this study is that a number of the patients had conditions amenable to treatment.

At a very simple level a detailed history must be obtained, with particular note of symptoms suggesting raised intracranial pressure or a focal neurological disturbance. A careful neurological examination may reveal focal signs suggesting a focal disturbance and a careful evaluation of the mental state should be made looking for affective symptoms or symptoms suggesting a schizo-

Table 6.9 Final diagnosis in 84 demented patients (after Marsden & Harrison 1972)

Intracranial space-occupying mass	8
Possible normal pressure communicating hydrocephalus	5
Post-traumatic cerebral atrophy	1
Postsubarachnoid haemorrhage	1
Limbic encephalitis	1
*Dementia in alcoholics	6
**Arteriosclerotic dementia	8
Huntington's chorea	3
Creutzfeldt–Jakob disease	3
Cerebral atrophy of unknown cause	48

* Diagnosed when history of prolonged excessive consumption of alcohol was associated with one of the following: peripheral neuropathy, cerebellar ataxia affecting gait out of proportion to upper limbs, or cerebellar atrophy on AEG.

** Diagnosed when two of following were present: history of acute strokes, diastolic BP>110 mmHg, or neurological signs by way of pseudobulbar palsy or marche à petits pas.

phrenic psychosis. Psychometric testing is particularly valuable in the differentiation between organic and functional psychiatric illness (Table 6.10).

The extent of investigation of the patient depends on resources and age. In old age, even if a lesion such as a subfrontal meningioma were found, then surgical treatment would be inappropriate. Accordingly, in senile dementia routine haematological and biochemical screening investigations and a serological test for syphilis are all that is required. In presenile dementia most neurologists wish to see a CT scan and many would pursue investigation as far as a lumbar puncture if no focal intracranial pathology is shown. The EEG rarely reveals specific abnormalities, although any focal abnormalities suggest the need for further neuroradiological investigations.

Table 6.10 Psychiatric illness that may mimic dementia

Depression	Obsessive compulsive states
Hypomania	Drug addiction
Schizophrenia	Epileptic psychosis
Paranoia	Malingering
Hysteria	Compensation neurosis

Pseudodementia

A variety of conditions may mimic the organic dementias: these include the Ganser syndrome, hysterical pseudodementia, simulated dementia, depressive pseudodementia, and various forms of psychosis. To this list might be added the patients who have a degree of cognitive impairment which is not acquired and which has been present throughout their life (amentia).

Most of these syndromes are relatively uncommon, but depressive pseudodementia, as shown by the study of Marsden and Harrison, may account for as many as 10% of patients thought initially to have a progressive dementia. In most instances the clinical picture results from the psychomotor retardation which accompanies profound dementia. The importance of recognising this syndrome is obvious, as it usually responds well to either antidepressants or ECT.

MEMORY

Memory disorders are common in clinical practice and do not necessarily result from neurological lesions. Organic impairment of memory (amnesia) may result not only from diffuse cerebral problems but also from discrete lesions in particular parts of the brain.

The neurological basis of memory

In order that something may be remembered, it first has to be registered in the brain; subsequently it has to be retained, and thereafter it needs to be recollected. Conscious registration of information occurs in the cerebral cortex and this probably has a topographical representation; for example, visual information is consciously appreciated in the occipital lobe.

Retention of memory is thought initially to occur in a short-term store and thereafter in long-term stores. The long-term stores again probably have a topographical representation in that long-term visual memories are almost certainly retained in the occipital lobes, tactile memories in the parietal lobes and auditory memories in the temporal lobes.

Auditory memories in relation to language are almost certainly selectively retained in the dominant temporal lobe, while there is some evidence to suggest that memory for music is held in the non-dominant temporal lobe.

The whole neural basis for what we call short-term memory remains uncertain in man, although probably this involves a particular neural circuit including a variety of subcortical structures. These subcortical structures involve the mammillary bodies, the fornices, the hippocampus, the anterior nuclei of the thalamus and the cingulum. Although there is still debate about the precise role of these structures in memory, it is clear that localised damage to these areas is frequently associated with impaired capacity to lay down new memories. Similarly, there is also often a retrograde gap for memories laid down before the damage occurred. Remote or long-term memories, however, usually remain intact.

The current understanding is that, after cortical registration, information is transmitted to the hippocampal regions of the temporal lobe and thence to the subcortical structures of the fornices, the mamillary bodies, the anterior nuclei of the thalamus and the cingulum; some experimental evidence suggests that such short-term registration lasts for only a few minutes. Subsequently, the information appears to be channelled back to the appropriate area of cortex which then encodes long-term registration. Recollection of memory is ill understood, and the mechanism whereby long-term memory held in a particular part of the cortex may be recalled to consciousness, is uncertain. Another component of memory is immediate memory or immediate recall: that is, the ability to repeat immediately a piece of information. This almost certainly simply depends on the information being understood and appreciated in Wernicke's area, and thence being transferred immediately via the superior longitudinal fasciculus to Broca's area where it then can verbally be repeated (see section on aphasia).

Differing clinical syndromes associated with amnesia

As discussed above, a somewhat arbitrary division is made into immediate, recent and remote memory. The immediate memory span is reflected in the ability to repeat material such as brief digit sequences, within a matter of seconds; its preservation simply suggests that registration of memory is intact. Recent memory is reflected in the ability to acquire and retain new knowledge, and is assessed by noting ability to learn and retain material over short time-spans, usually for not more than a few minutes. Remote memory is reflected in the ability to recall information about long-past periods; it represents a process of retrieval of material which has been held in long-term storage.

Specific forms of memory disturbance

Amnesia in diencephalic and hippocampal lesions

Damage to the components shown in Figure 6.6 produces a specific defect in memory which most commonly is seen in Korsakoff's psychosis. Bilateral medial temporal lobe infarction or surgical trauma to the fornices may produce a similar picture. The principal defect is that there is failure of ongoing registration of current memories so that current events tend not to be available for future recall.

There is usually preservation of immediate memory and immediate recall, and a test of digit span may be normal. Recent memory, however, is defective and patients with lesions in these structures will be unable to remember events which have occurred before. In severe lesions, coherent memorising may be reduced to nil so that there is a continuing extending loss of memory for events which have occurred since the damage developed. Loss of memory for events which occur following an incident is called anterograde amnesia.

If recovery occurs, the loss of memory will be as long as the period of illness. In these cases, there may also be loss of memory for events which occurred before the development of the damage. This is called retrograde amnesia and the period may extend for days, weeks or months. Remote memory for matters beyond the period of retrograde amnesia is much better preserved and may be virtually normal.

One of the striking features of amnesias of this type can be the presence of confabulation. This

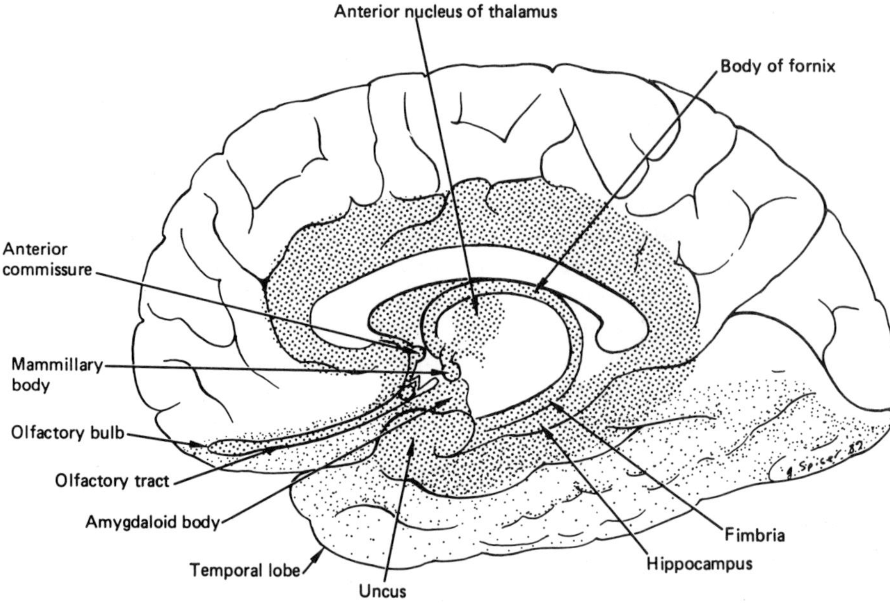

Fig. 6.6 The Papez circuit of memory in the limbic system.

most commonly results from diencephalic lesions and is not a feature of memory loss in lesions of the medial temporal lobes. Typically, the patient may give a reasonably coherent but entirely false account of recent events. Confabulation may be specifically defined as 'a falsification of memory occurring in clear consciousness in association with an organically derived amnesia'. Other cognitive functions are relatively well preserved in these patients and certainly amnestic defects are out of proportion to any other. The patients are alert and responsive and have no clouding of consciousness. Such patients are often covered by the term axial dementia.

Traumatic amnesias

Amnesia is a constant feature of a closed head injury of sufficient magnitude to impair consciousness; it is not a feature of crush injuries or penetrating head injuries as consciousness in these types of injury is usually preserved. In a head injury, the length of retrograde amnesia is usually short and the length of anterograde amnesia typically is longer than the impairment of consciousness (so-called post-traumatic amnesia) (see p. 363).

Transient global amnesia (see p. 182)

This is a condition seen in the elderly and characterised by transient global impairment of memory. It is felt in most instances to be secondary to bilateral temporal lobe ischaemia.

Memory loss in diffuse cerebral lesions

Loss of memory, as discussed previously, is a feature of dementia and often is seen in patients with diffuse cerebral lesions. It may be submerged in more widespread impairments of cognitive function, and precise analysis of the memory defects may be difficult. In acute confusional states the memory difficulties may merely be a result of the impairment of consciousness and of the defects of attention. In chronic organic reactions such as organic dementia the loss of memory often represents no more than the earliest manifestation of a general cognitive failure. Memory difficulties are often more easy to detect than other difficulties in intellectual function.

The amnestic defects of diffuse brain disease are commonly global, affecting both recent and remote events to a similar degree. When patients with dementia are tested, recent events may be the most obviously affected and remote memories may be relatively intact. However, remote memories often prove to be stereotyped and lacking in detail, and one of the hallmarks of memory loss in this situation is its variability; indeed, much of the difficulty may be due to a failure to sustain attention and concentration. However, there is some suggestion that in certain dementing processes, such as Alzheimer's disease, the amnestic component may reflect a differential involvement of areas of the brain concerned with memory. For example, in Alzheimer's disease the pathological changes may be particularly marked in the hippocampal regions. It is possible that the common memory defects of old age may similarly depend on such changes.

Psychogenic amnesia

Rarely does a week pass without a case being described in a newspaper of a person being found wandering in a dazed state claiming not to know who he or she is. Although occasionally such cases may occur as a result of organic disease, more often than not these are examples of psychogenic amnesia. Such memory loss may either be global, or restricted to certain circumscribed areas. When global, it may involve loss of long periods of past life, or loss of personal identity as described above. The diagnosis is usually clear as the loss of memory is inconsistent with the general preservation of intellect. More restricted amnesias may be found in relation to particular events at work or in marriage.

Psychogenic amnesia may be suspected when profound difficulty with recall of past events is coupled with normal ability to retain new information. Alternatively, it may be suspected when there is loss even of immediate recall. A common situation where such amnestic defects may be seen is in the field of head injuries in relation to medicolegal practice. In these instances, there may be diagnostic difficulties because of the combination of both psychogenic and organic aspects of the memory loss.

DISORDERS OF LANGUAGE

Introduction

The production of language may be subdivided into a number of separate different areas. The first requirement is to produce a sound, and this results from the passage of air over the vocal cords. Movement of the vocal cord changes the pitch of the sound and the production of such sounds is known as phonation. Certain changes in the sound may be attributable to movement of the pharynx, but the neurological basis of phonation can be regarded as being largely due to movements of structures supplied by the vagus nerve.

The next stage in the production of language is the manipulation of the sound as it passes through the upper air passages. Movement of the palate, tongue, jaw and lips may alter a sound quite considerably and the manipulation of these structures is termed articulation, leading to the production of what we know as phonemes.

The organisation of phonemes into words and the linking of words into sentences is the next stage and this requires careful programming for repeated co-ordination of the movements of the structures producing phonemes. The central mechanism controlling this programme is a function of the dominant cerebral hemisphere.

Disorders of phonation

Impairment of the production of sounds is known as dysphonia or aphonia. It may result from difficulty in respiration and a failure of the passage of air across the vocal cords. Neurologically it most commonly results from a disturbance of the nerve supply to the vocal cords, and in clinical practice this is most common in any lesion involving the recurrent laryngeal nerve. Such patients also lose the ability to cough. Local lesions of the vocal cords may produce a similar disturbance of voice: hysterical aphonia sounds identical but is differentiated by the patient's ability to cough. In pseudobulbar palsy with an upper neurone paresis of the vocal cords, there is spasticity of the cords resulting in the strangulated voice of a spastic dysphonia. A similar voice disturbance occasionally may also be simulated, although this is relatively uncommon.

Disorders of articulation

The muscles involved in the production of sound are supplied by the fifth, seventh, tenth and twelfth cranial nerves. Disorders of articulation are known as dysarthrias and are characterised by imprecision in production of the various phonemes and hence words. The neural control of these muscles involves the upper motor neurone pathway, the lower motor neurone pathway, the cerebellum and the extrapyramidal system.

Spastic dysarthria

The upper motor neurone supply to these bulbar cranial nerves is largely bilateral: consequently, a unilateral hemisphere lesion will rarely result in significant dysarthria. A so-called spastic dysarthria is usually only seen in bilateral hemisphere lesions, or in brain stem lesions damaging the corticobulbar tracts. Typically, it will be part of a pseudobulbar palsy with associated difficulty with swallowing and emotional lability. The speech sounds strained and patients usually have evidence of pyramidal signs in the limbs. Common causes are bilateral strokes, brain stem strokes, motor neurone disease or multiple sclerosis.

Flaccid dysarthria

A disorder of any part of the lower motor neurone supply to these cranial nerves may be associated with a so-called flaccid dysarthria. The cranial nerve nuclei may be damaged in poliomyelitis or in motor neurone disease; the cranial nerves themselves in a cranial polyneuropathy; the myoneural junction in myasthenia gravis, and the muscles themselves in so-called oculopharyngeal muscular dystrophy. The speech is typified by imprecision and, if the palate is involved, by a nasal quality to the speech. If facial weakness is marked, then a difficulty in producing the sound 'p' and similar sounds known as the labials will be evident.

Ataxic dysarthria

Disturbance of the supply of the cerebellar input to these cranial nerves produces so-called ataxic dysarthria or scanning dysarthria: this is most commonly seen in multiple sclerosis. The speech shows variation in rate and pitch and at times may have an explosive element. A cerebellar dysarthria is most readily recognised by the difficulty that the patient has in performing a repetitive sound such as 'p, p, p, p,'.

Akinetic/hyperkinetic dysarthria

Extrapyramidal disorders may significantly impair speech. Most common are speech defects in Parkinson's disease, where akinesia in the bulbar muscles is reflected in hypokinetic speech. In the early stages this is most evident as loss of the cadence and variation in the pitch of speech, leading to a rather monotonous voice. Extrapyramidal disorders characterised by excessive movement such as chorea may interrupt speech, and may even produce a variety of added sounds.

Disorders of the central control of speech
(language)

Historically, disturbances of language function provided the chief impetus for attempts at correlating focal psychological deficits with localised pathological changes in the brain. Unfortunately, the neural control of language is exceedingly complicated and our ability to understand this is limited.

Cerebral dominance

It is now clearly recognised that the left hemisphere in most individuals has some special function in language. The dominant hemisphere is that hemisphere which controls language, and to a certain extent cerebral dominance relates to handedness: in a right-handed individual it is virtually certain that the left hemisphere will be dominant. In a left-handed individual there is something like a 60/40 split dominant for left hemisphere versus dominant for right hemisphere. Bilateral speech representation is rare but appears to be more common in left-handed individuals.

A variety of techniques are available to determine which is the dominant hemisphere: one of the best that has been tested is the Wada technique using an intracarotid injection of sodium amytal. Cerebral dominance appears to become fixed by the age of 7–10 years: before this time there is some evidence that the opposite hemisphere may take over the control of speech if the other is damaged.

We have little actual knowledge about the underlying mechanisms for language production within the dominant hemisphere and a variety of theories exist, one of the most popular being that provided by Geschwind. In Geschwind's model, certain of the speech functions are localised in particular areas: for example, Broca's area, just anterior to the lower end of the motor cortex contains the programme to manipulate the motor cortex and thence the motor cranial nerve nuclei to produce language. Wernicke's area in the superior temporal gyrus is the auditory appreciation area where sounds are appreciated as words. More complex comprehension of words or of series of words is appreciated in regions at the posterior end of the Sylvian fissure (the region of the angular gyrus and supramarginal gyrus). In this scheme the importance of the anatomical link between Broca's and Wernicke's area (the superior longitudinal fasciculus) is obvious.

Dysphasia or aphasia may be defined as language that is not grammatical speech. That is to say, if the words are written down one after the other, they do not make correct English. Using the Geschwind model, a variety of individual speech defects may be recognised (Table 6.11).

In lesions of Broca's area the programming is impaired and the output of speech is sparse, laboured and with poor articulation. Comprehension of the spoken and written word, however, is relatively well preserved, because Wernicke's area will allow verbal comprehension and the incoming auditory signals can be recognised and conveyed elsewhere in the brain to arouse meaningful associations. In a Wernicke's aphasia, speaking is impaired because, in simple terms, Broca's area is not receiving feedback concerning its own programming. Speech may be fluent but the words may be faulty and the sequencing of the words may be incorrect.

In clinical practice, most disorders of language result from cerebral infarction and, in such cases, often there is global impairment of speech functions (so-called global aphasia). Occasionally, however, a number of isolated syndromes may be seen and these are listed in Table 6.11.

Examination of the aphasic patient

The first difficulty when faced with an aphasic patient is to recognise that he is aphasic rather than confused. Not infrequently, patients who suddenly develop a fluent dysphasia as a result of a lesion of Wernicke's area are thought to be confused. In practice, the sudden development of disorganised speech with preserved consciousness suggests a disorder of language function rather than confusion. The recognition of the speech as

Table 6.11 The differing clinical features of specific forms of aphasia. (After Benson, 1985)

Aphasia	Spontaneous speech	Fluency	Comprehension	Repetition	Naming
Broca's	Hesitant; agrammatic	Poor	Good	Poor	Poor
Pure motor	Phonetic errors	Impaired	Good	Impaired	Impaired
Global	Sterotypic utterances	Poor	Poor	Poor	Poor
Wernicke's	Paraphasic, jargon	Good	Poor	Poor	Poor
Word deaf	Normal	Good	Poor	Poor	Good
Conduction	Phonemic errors	Good	Good	Poor	Good
Transcortical sensory	Normal to semantic jargon	Good	Poor	Good	Poor
Transcortical motor	Scant, mute	Poor	Good	Good	Impaired
Isolation	Mute	Poor	Poor	Good	Poor
Anomic	Circumlocutory	Good	Good	Good	Impaired

dysphasic may result from the recognition that the patient's language is non-grammatical speech: the patient's meaning may be clear, but the sequence of words incorrect. An attempt should then be made to determine whether the production of words is fluent or non-fluent. In this instance, fluency refers not to the content of speech, but to the numbers of words or phonemes produced per unit time. Non-fluent speech suggests a Broca's aphasia, whereas fluency suggests aphasia resulting from lesions of other parts of the speech apparatus. The next stage should be to test comprehension of the spoken or written word. The patient should be asked to perform simple movements to command, such as to put his index finger on his nose, and the complexity of commands may be increased. Impairment of verbal comprehension in an aphasic patient suggests a lesion of the temporal or parietal lobes producing the speech disturbance. Next, repetition should be tested, with initially the ability to repeat single words, then phrases and finally sentences. Inability to repeat is seen in any aphasia resulting from disruption of the circuit linking Wernicke's area to Broca's area. When impairment of repetition is very prominent, this suggests a lesion of either Wernicke's area or of the superior longitudinal fasciculus. One of the most traditional facets of speech assessment is the testing of naming ability: in fact, the inability to name objects is a non-specific finding in a patient with aphasia and, although tending to confirm the diagnosis of aphasia, it has no particular localising value.

Further testing of language functions may require the testing of reading and writing and also the use of specialist tests such as the Tokan test. Disordered reading and writing is the rule in the aphasic patient. Isolated dysgraphia and dyslexia is rare.

Disorders of the development of language in children

A number of such disorders have been described and these are defined below.

Stammering or stuttering

This characteristic abnormality can be regarded as a disorder of respiratory co-ordination during speech. Its cause is uncertain but there is overwhelming evidence to suggest that emotional tension or undue concentration by parents may precipitate a stammer if a child is predisposed to this symptom.

Dyslalia

This is the term that is applied to a developmental speech disorder characterised by retardation of an acquisition of word sounds. Language is normal and with speech therapy there is improvement with time.

Developmental dyslexia and dysgraphia

These terms are applied to a group of children without gross physical defects who appear to have a specific difficulty in learning to read or write.

CLINICAL SYNDROMES ASSOCIATED WITH SPECIFIC FOCAL HEMISPHERE DYSFUNCTION

A variety of symptoms and signs may be of localising significance in patients with disturbed function of the brain. One clear example of this is the disturbance seen in the different forms of epilepsy resulting from focal discharges in different parts of the brain. It should be remembered that such focal signs and symptoms serve only to indicate the site of pathology and are of little value in suggesting the nature of the lesion.

Frontal lobe syndromes (Table 6.12)

Damage to the frontal lobes may result in significant changes in personality, most noticeable as change in temperament and disposition. Disinhibition and tactlessness may be evident, with diminished social control and lack of concern for the consequence of actions. Errors of judgement with regard to financial and personal matters may be prominent and this may be combined with marked indifference or unconcern for the feeling of others. Outbursts of irritability may occur, interspersed with periods of apathy. This may progress to profound slowing of psychomotor activity leading to stupor.

Table 6.12 Frontal lobe syndromes (after Adams & Victor, 1977)

Unilateral damage
- Contralateral hemiplegia
- Slight elevation of mood, increased talkativeness, tendency to joke, lack of tact, difficulty in adaptation, loss of initiative
- Grasp and suck reflexes
- Anosmia with involvement of orbital parts

Damage to non-dominant frontal lobe (as above)

Damage to dominant frontal lobe; additional phenomena include:
- Motor speech disorder with agraphia, with or without apraxia of the lips and tongue
- Loss of verbal associative fluency
- Sympathetic apraxia of left hand

Effects of bifrontal disease
- Bilateral hemiplegia
- Spastic bulbar (pseudobulbar) palsy
- If prefrontal, abulia or akinetic mutism, lack of ability to sustain attention and solve complex problems, rigidity of thinking, bland affect and labile mood, and varying combinations of grasping, sucking, decomposition of gait, and sphincteric incontinence

Table 6.13 Parietal lobe syndromes (after Adams & Victor, 1977)

Effects of unilateral damage of the parietal lobe
- Cortical sensory syndrome and sensory extinction (or total hemianaesthesia with large acute lesions of white matter)
- Mild hemiparesis, unilateral muscular atrophy in children
- Homonymous hemianopia (incongruent or inferior quadrantic) or visual inattention, and sometimes anosognosia, neglect of one-half of the body and of extrapersonal space (observed more frequently with right than with left parietal lesions)
- Abolition of optokinetic nystagmus to one side

Damage to dominant parietal lobe; additional phenomena include:
- Disorders of language (especially alexia)
- Gerstmann syndrome
- Tactile agnosia (bimanual astereognosis)
- Bilateral ideomotor apraxia

Effects of damage to non-dominant parietal lobe; additional phenomena include:
- Topographical memory loss
- Agnosognosia and dressing apraxia. These disorders may occur with lesions of either hemisphere but have been observed more frequently with lesions of the non-dominant one

Performance on tests of formal intelligence is often well preserved although attention span and the ability to concentrate and to carry out a series of activities may be impaired. The overall picture may at first sight resemble a dementing process, although psychometry may show little impairment. Encroachment of a frontal lesion into the motor cortex will produce contralateral weakness, most evident in the face at an early stage. A contralateral grasp reflex may be present, as may the typical pyramidal signs of increase in the tendon reflexes and an extensor plantar response. Medial frontal lesions may produce impairment of gait, and occasionally incontinence, which often occurs to the accompaniment of quite striking indifference. The involvement of Broca's area in the dominant hemisphere will produce the typical speech defect.

Parietal lobe syndromes (Table 6.13)

Parietal lobe lesions produce a variety of differing syndromes. Common to both dominant and non-dominant sides are contralateral hemisensory disturbances in the form of astereognosis and agraphaesthesia. Visual inattention on the contralateral side may be found, and loss of optokinetic nystagmus with the drum rotating to the affected lobe. Dominant parietal lobe lesions are associated with dysphasia and also with a bilateral apraxia. Non-dominant parietal lobe lesions may produce disorders of body image, such that a paralysed limb is ignored, or half of a body felt to be absent. Disordered appreciation of three-dimensional sense may show itself in the form of dressing apraxia and topographical agnosia.

Discussion of disorders of parietal lobe function involves consideration of the term agnosia: this is defined as an impaired recognition of an object which is sensorially presented while at the same time the impairment cannot be attributed to sensory defects, mental deterioration, disorders of consciousness and attention, or to a non-familiarity with the object. It implies, therefore, a disorder of perceptual recognition which takes place at a higher level than the processing of primary sensory information. Lesions producing such a restricted form of defect are rare, with the exception of visuospatial agnosia, and examples reported in the literature are open to argument. A variety of such types of agnosia are described, such as visual object agnosia, prosopagnosia, agnosia for colours, simultanagnosia and topographical agnosia. Rarer examples are auditory agnosia and finger agnosia, as part of the Gerstmann syndrome.

Many of the agnosias are said to result from parietal lobe dysfunction but some, such as auditory agnosia, are thought to result from temporal lobe dysfunction and others, such as the various types of visual agnosia, are thought to result from occipital lobe lesions.

Temporal lobe syndromes (Table 6.14)

Lesions restricted to the anterior parts of the temporal lobe may be entirely asymptomatic. Deep temporal lobe lesions may involve the optic radiation and produce a contralateral hemianopia. Non-dominant temporal lobe lesions, even if extensive, may be associated with a paucity of physical signs. On the other hand, dominant temporal lobe lesions typically will involve Wernicke's area and will produce aphasia. Bilateral temporal lobe lesions involving the hippocampus will produce impairment of memory.

Perhaps one of the best localising clues to a temporal lobe lesion is the presence of temporal lobe seizures (see Ch. 7). Personality changes may be seen in temporal lobe lesions, although these most commonly occur in association with temporal lobe epilepsy.

Occipital lobe syndromes (Table 6.15)

Lesions of the occipital lobe usually result in visual field defects. Disorders of visual recognition may result from anterior occipital lobe lesions in the absence of visual impairment: these may include prosopagnosia, which occurs most commonly in non-dominant lesions where the individual is unable to recognise faces. Bilateral occipital lobe lesions may result in total blindness with reserved pupillary reflexes. Other syndromes include Anton's syndrome, where the patient who is cortically blind denies this, and the syndrome of visual agnosia where the patient can see but cannot recognise.

Disconnection syndromes

The term 'disconnection syndrome' has been applied by a number of authors to a group of disorders resulting from disconnection of one part of the brain from another. The best-recognised of these are the syndromes resulting from hemisphere disconnection following section of the corpus callosum. Other isolated syndromes that are recognised are the syndrome of alexia without agraphia (Fig 6.7). In this particular syndrome there is damage to the left occipital lobe and the

Table 6.14 Temporal lobe syndromes (after Adams & Victor, 1977)

Unilateral damage to dominant temporal lobe	
Homonymous upper quadrantanopia	
Wernicke's aphasia	
Amusia (some types)	
Impairment in tests of verbal material presented through the auditory sense	
Dysnomia or amnesic aphasia	
Unilateral damage to non-dominant temporal lobe	
Homonymous upper quadrantanopia	
Inability to judge spatial relationships in some cases	
Impairment in tests of visually presented non-verbal material	
Effects of disease of either hemisphere	
Auditory illusions and hallucinations	
Psychotic behaviour (aggressivity)	
Effects of bilateral disease	
Korsakoff amnesic defect	
Apathy and placidity	Kluver-Bucy syndrome
Increased sexual activity	Kluver-Bucy syndrome
'Sham rage'	Kluver-Bucy syndrome

Table 6.15 Occipital lobe lesions (after Adams & Victor, 1977)

Unilateral damage
- Contralateral (congruent) homonymous hemianopia which may be central (splitting the macula) or peripheral
- Irritative lesions—elementary (unformed) hallucinations

Damage to left occipital lobe
- Right homonymous hemianopia
- If deep white matter or splenium of corpus callosum is involved, alexia and colour-naming defect
- Object agnosia

Damage to right occipital lobe
- Left homonymous hemianopia
- With more extensive lesions, visual illusions (metamorphopsias) and hallucinations; more frequent with right-sided than left-sided lesions
- Loss of topographic memory and visual orientation

Bilateral occipital damage
- Cortical blindness (pupils reactive)
- Loss of perception of colour
- Prosopagnosia, simultanagnosia
- Balint syndrome

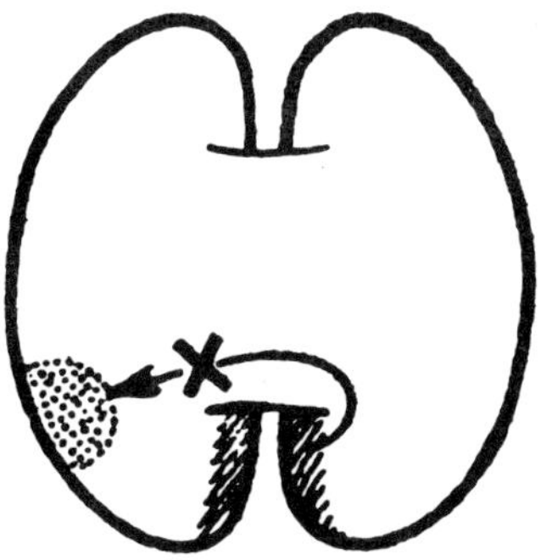

Fig. 6.7 Alexia without agraphia. Lesion of the posterior corpus callosum and dominant occipital lobe with interruption of connections between the visual cortex and the angular gyrus/Wernicke's area. Characterised by: inability to read, to name colour, to copy writing, but with normal spontaneous writing and the ability to identify colours. (Reproduced from *Neurology & Neurosurgery Illustrated* by Lindsay K W, Bone I, Callander R. Churchill Livingstone, Edinburgh, 1986, with permission.)

splenium of the corpus callosum. All visual information is thus fed into the right occipital lobe but, because the splenium is destroyed, visual information cannot be given to the left hemisphere and thus the patient cannot read.

FURTHER READING

Adams R D, Victor M 1977 Principles of Neurology. McGraw-Hill, New York

Benson D F 1985 Language and its disorders. In: Swash M, Kennard C Scientific basis of clinical neurology. Churchill Livingstone, Edinburgh, ch 19

Lishman W A 1978 Organic psychiatry. Blackwell Scientific Publications, Oxford

Marsden C D, Harrison M J G 1972 Outcome of investigation of patients with presenile dementia. British Medical Journal 2, 249–252

Plum F, Posner J B 1983 Diagnosis of stupor and coma, 3rd edn. F A Davis Company, Philadelphia

7

Paroxysmal disorders

INTRODUCTION

The diagnosis of episodes of alteration or loss of consciousness is one of the most difficult aspects of clinical neurology. Whereas in most neurological conditions the clinical history is of great importance, in the diagnosis of paroxysmal disorders we are often solely dependent on obtaining a good history, not only from the patient but also from eyewitnesses. The majority of patients complaining of episodes of disturbed consciousness will have no neurological signs and investigation may be of little help.

It must be emphasised that in some patients there may be insufficient evidence upon which to base an adequate and firm diagnosis. In such instances labels should not be attached to patients but time should be allowed to elapse, in order to gain more information. Too many patients are diagnosed as having epilepsy and started on long-term anticonvulsant therapy on insufficient evidence: once made, the diagnosis may be extremely difficult to alter.

EPILEPSY

Epilepsy was defined by Hughlins Jackson in physiological terms as a 'recurrent, disorderly discharge of nerve tissue'. The clinical manifestation of this is at least two seizures; a single isolated seizure is not epilepsy.

PHYSIOLOGY AND BIOCHEMISTRY

There is now greater insight into the phenomena which control the seizure threshold at a cellular level. Normal cells have both inhibitory and excitatory influences causing excitatory and inhibitory postsynaptic potentials (EPSPs and IPSPs). Once a critical membrane depolarisation occurs, an action potential is propagated. This leads to firing of individual neurones in a repetitive fashion, with quiescence, usually for more than 5 ms between action potentials.

Neurones in epileptogenic foci (as produced experimentally by penicillin or aluminal gel) exhibit different patterns of firing. The prime characteristic of epileptic neurones is the paroxysmal depolarisation shift which is more prolonged than the EPSP. It results in burst firing of neurones with interspike intervals of less than 5 ms instead of isolated spike firing. Bursts of action potentials from epileptic neurones terminate spontaneously and the cell then remains refractory for a prolonged period until the next burst of action potentials.

Such epileptic neurones (group I) are found at the centre of an epileptic focus and fire spontaneously: they act as an epileptic 'pacemaker'. Immediately surrounding such a population, group II neurones are found: these can fire in normal patterns and can be influenced by afferent inputs, but can be recruited to burst firing by primary neurones at the centre of a focus. It appears that burst firing by neurones at the centre of a focus may be the basis of the cortical spike. When surrounding group II neurones are recruited this may then result in a focal seizure and corresponding EEG discharge.

There is evidence that neurones can be conditioned to adopt 'epileptic' patterns of firing. A phenomenon of kindling can be demonstrated in animals, in which repeated subconvulsive electroshock results in a progressive lowering of convulsive threshold, even to the point at which spontaneous seizures begin to occur. The relevance of this experimental model to human epilepsy is uncertain, but could explain 'mirror imaging'. Here a unilateral temporal focus can give rise to contralateral spikes, which at first seem dependent on the 'leading' focus, but which may ultimately show independent activity.

The molecular basis for the paroxysmal depolarisation shift and burst firing of epileptic neurones is less certain. This may result from direct damage to membrane ionic channels themselves, or be secondary to loss of inhibitory neurotransmitter (e.g. GABA), or increased excitatory neurotransmitter (e.g. aspartate) function within a focus. There is some evidence from cortical foci in both animals and man to suggest a specific loss of gabaergic neurones within epileptic foci.

Classically, two patterns of physiological organisation of epileptic discharge have been recognised: those arising from focal cortical disturbances (as above) (Fig. 7.1A) and those characterised by immediate synchronous spike-wave discharge of both hemispheres (Fig. 7.1B); these correspond to focal and generalised seizure and epilepsies. The latter pattern (often termed centrencephalic epilepsy) has classically been thought to originate from a primary discharge in the brain stem reticular formation and to spread to the cortex via central thalamic relays. Some authorities have always been of the opinion that all seizure disorders start at a cortical level and that centrencephalic disturbances differ only in the speed at which cortical disturbance spreads centrally, evoking a secondarily generalised response.

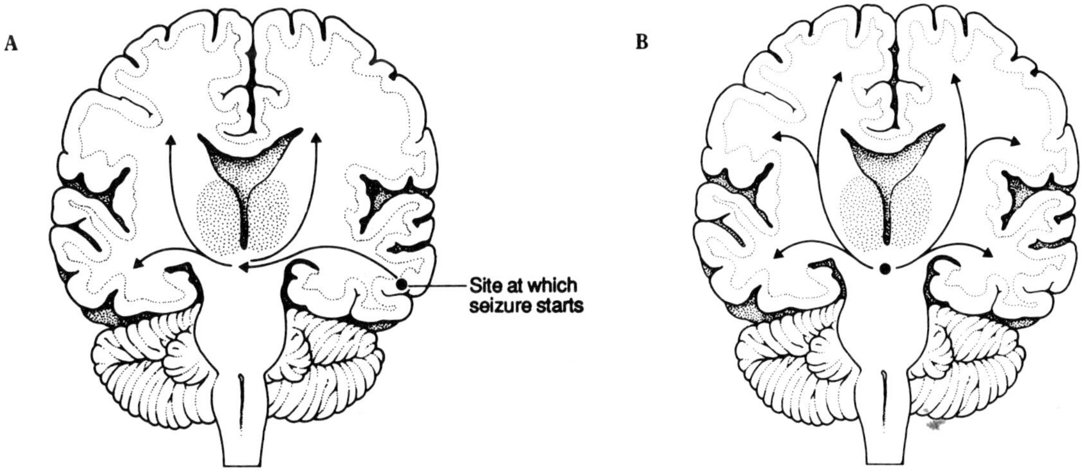

Fig. 7.1 Localisation and pathways of spread of abnormal discharge in: **A** partial seizures; **B** generalised seizures. (Reproduced from Chadwick D, Usiskin S 1986 *Living with Epilepsy*. McDonalds, London, with permission.)

EPIDEMIOLOGY OF EPILEPSY

Epilepsy is a common symptom of cerebral disorder which frequently occurs in the absence of demonstrable pathology. Incidence rates for epilepsy approximate to 20–50 per 100 000 per annum. Higher rates of 120 per 100 000 have been recorded in series which include febrile seizures and single seizures.

There is a marked variation in age-specific incidence, with the highest rates being found below the age of 10 and a rise in incidence above the age of 60.

Prevalence figures show even greater variation because of different criteria used for the assessment of activity of epilepsy in any one given year: overall figures vary between 2 and 6 per 1000 of population; again, prevalence figures are strongly influenced by age (Fig. 7.2). The differing shapes of age-related incidence and prevalence curves are dictated by the relatively good prognosis of epilepsies beginning in childhood (see below).

Total or lifetime prevalence patterns suggest that between 1 in 100 and 1 in 200 of the population will suffer from epilepsy at some time in their life, and up to 5% may suffer a single seizure.

CLASSIFICATION OF SEIZURES

No easy *clinical* definition of a seizure can be proposed because of the infinite variety of clinical manifestations. Table 7.1 summarises a 1981 international classification of seizures. The major division in this classification is between partial seizures and generalised seizures. Partial seizures begin locally at the cortex and include an aura which reflects the functional role of that part of the cortex in which the seizure discharge begins. Such seizures may also be associated with postictal focal disturbances (Todd's phenomenon). These are differentiated from generalised seizures which begin bilaterally and in which consciousness is lost suddenly and the patient therefore experiences no aura. Any partial seizure may spread to become generalised with a secondary tonic-clonic (grand mal) seizure.

The electroencephalographic (EEG) findings also help to differentiate between partial and generalised seizures. Interictal EEGs tend to show localised spikes and, on occasion, associated focal slow waves in patients with partial seizures, but synchronous high amplitude generalised spike-wave discharge in patients with generalised seizures.

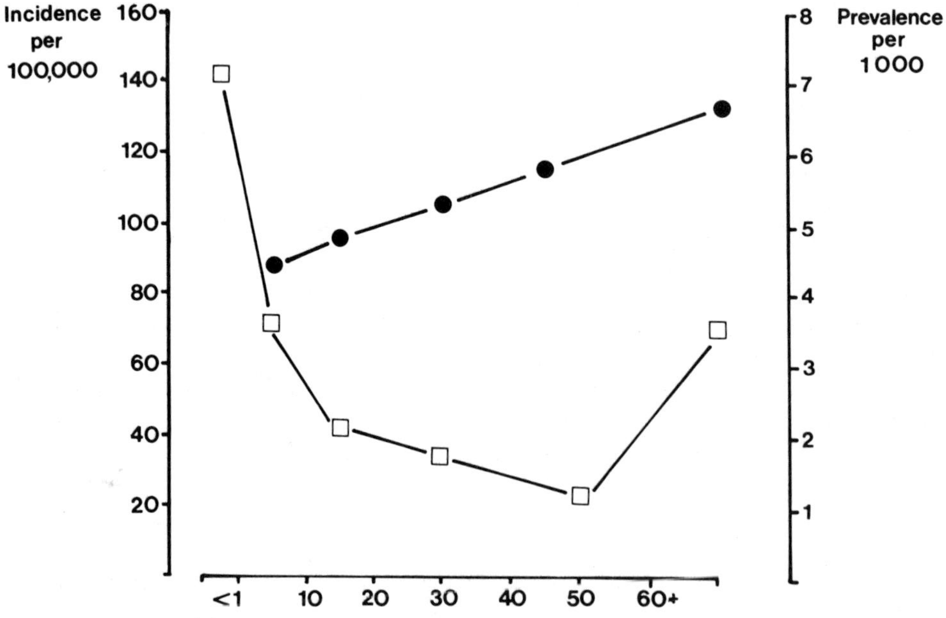

Fig. 7.2 Age (in years) specific incidence (□—□) and prevalence (•—•) rates for epilepsy (after Hauser & Kurland 1975.)

Table 7.1 Classification of seizures

Partial seizures (seizures beginning locally)
Simple (consciousness not impaired)
With motor symptoms
With somatosensory or special sensory symptoms
With autonomic symptoms
With psychic symptoms
Complex (with impairment of consciousness)
Beginning as simple partial seizures (progressing to complex seizure)
Impairment of consciousness at onset
1. Impairment of consciousness only
2. With automatism
Partial seizures becoming secondarily generalised
Generalised seizures
Absence seizures
Simple (petit mal)
Complex
Myoclonic seizures
Clonic seizures
Tonic seizures
Tonic-clonic seizures
Atonic seizures

Partial seizures

The most common sites of origin for simple partial seizures are within the frontal or temporal lobes.

Frontal lobe seizures

Frontal seizures manifest most commonly as adversive attacks. These comprise tonic or clonic deviation of the head and eyes to one side, often associated with jerking of the arm of that side or the adoption of a raised flexed posture of the arm. On occasion seizures may begin similarly in the leg. This form of frontal lobe seizure is more common than the classically described Jacksonian seizure with a recruiting march over the motor cortex. Both types of motor seizure may be followed by a Todd's hemiparesis. Involvement of the frontal speech areas may give rise to sudden speech arrest or unintelligible muttering.

Temporal lobe seizures

A greater variety of simple partial seizures are due to temporal lobe disturbance. When the uncus is involved the patient may experience abnormalities of taste or smell, usually of an unpleasant nature. Epigastric disturbances are common and pallor, flushing and changes in heart rate and other autonomic changes can accompany temporal lobe disturbances making their differentiation from syncope difficult. Furthermore, a variety of psychic phenomena may be experienced in seizures with temporal lobe origin without consciousness being impaired. Déjà vu and jamais vu are common, but patients may also perceive auditory or visual hallucinations which seem to represent some form of 'memory playback'. Commonly these experiences may be 'indescribable'.

Parietal and occipital lobe seizures

Other types of simple partial seizures are less common. Those arising from the parietal region are characterised by positive sensory disturbance and paraesthesiae. They may be difficult to differentiate from sensory ischaemic symptoms. Occipital seizures are even more uncommon and cause the patient to see balls of lights or colours, which usually are confined to the contralateral half visual field.

Complex partial seizures

Complex partial seizures, previously termed psychomotor seizures, are differentiated from simple partial seizures by the varying degrees of impairment of consciousness which they produce. This impairment of consciousness may be preceded by symptoms of a simple partial type, usually those associated with a temporal lobe origin. However, in some instances consciousness may be lost at the outset of the seizure.

Such seizures are not infrequently associated with ictal automatism, which usually is crude and stereotyped (smacking of the lips with facial movements, fidgeting and picking at the clothes). Occasionally more complex behaviour is seen which on occasions may lead to arrest for shoplifting, or indecent exposure. Complex partial seizures are frequently succeeded by postictal confusion. It is generally believed that the impaired consciousness and automatism of complex partial seizures result from a spread of ictal activity from temporal lobe cortex to the limbic system, either unilaterally or bilaterally.

Both simple and complex partial seizures may spread more generally to involve both hemispheres and result in a tonic-clonic seizure.

Generalised seizures

The tonic-clonic seizure

The most common form of generalised seizure (whether this occurs in a primary fashion or following generalisation after a partial seizure) is the *tonic-clonic* (grand mal) seizure. When this is of primary origin the patient experiences no aura but may describe a more non-specific and longer-lasting prodrome of general malaise. The patient initially cries out during a tonic phase of extension and opisthotonus associated with respiratory arrest and cyanosis; reflex emptying of bladder and bowel may occur. Next the patient enters a clonic phase of rhythmic generalised jerking lasting for a variable length of time. Less commonly only tonic or clonic phases may be seen. Deep coma follows with an ascending conscious level which often includes a postictal phase of confusion and automatic behaviour. On becoming fully conscious, usually within 15–60 minutes, the patient may experience generalised aches and pains consequent on uncoordinated muscle activity, become aware of a bitten tongue and have a generalised headache and feeling of lethargy with a desire to sleep.

Other types of generalised seizure always occur on a primary basis and are characterised by briefer attacks, which invariably begin during childhood and rarely persist into adult life.

Simple absence (petit mal)

The most classic but rare type of childhood generalised seizure is the petit mal seizure. This is characterised by sudden, usually momentary, absence during which a child loses contact with the surroundings and stops the activity he was engaged in. There may be some minor myoclonic activity around the eyelids. The attacks may occur very frequently during the course of the day and the child is often unaware of their occurrence. These seizures may declare themselves as learning difficulties at school due to the effects that frequent seizures have on ability to concentrate.

Complex absence

Complex absences are more common, and usually occur as a symptomatic epilepsy in children with pre-existing brain damage. They are more prolonged and frequently associated with myoclonic activity or atonic attacks, both of which may result in the child being thrown to the ground, frequently suffering trauma.

Myoclonic jerks

Brief myoclonic jerks occur in a number of differing epileptic syndromes (Table 7.2). They may be associated with absence (as in complex absences), or more commonly occur without impairment of consciousness. The arms tend to be most frequently involved in a sudden flexion movement.

Many seizures, when infrequent and less than fully observed, may prove difficult to classify. It is therefore inevitable that seizure classification itself is biased towards being most effective in the classification of seizures occurring frequently in patients with severe epilepsy and in whom there is a greater likelihood of observing an EEG correlate of the seizure.

Table 7.2 Myoclonus and the epileptic syndromes

Infantile and childhood epilepsies
Infantile spasms
Lennox-Gastaut syndrome
Cryptogenic myoclonic epilepsy
Adolescent epilepsies
Early morning myoclonus associated with tonic-clonic seizures (Juvenile myoclonic epilepsy)
Myoclonus plus simple absence
Progressive myoclonic epilepsies
Due to metabolic disorders
Lipidoses
Ceroid-lipofuscinosis
Lafora body disease
Sialidosis
Other often genetic syndromes
Ramsey-Hunt syndrome
Baltic myoclonus
Other multisystem disorders

Status epilepticus

Seizures are almost always self-limiting. Rarely one may follow another in close succession, resulting in status.

Convulsive status is a state of recurrent tonic-clonic seizures without recovery of consciousness between attacks; it represents a medical emergency with a high morbidity and mortality. Status occurs in approximately 3% of epileptic patients, but is most common in those patients with severe epilepsy who are non-compliant with drug therapy. It may also occur in alcohol withdrawal, as well as in acute meningitis or encephalitis or other metabolic disturbance. An initial presentation with status epilepticus is particularly common with frontal lobe lesions such as tumour and abscess.

Absence status may be seen in children who exhibit confused behaviour and an epileptic basis for this mental state may not be immediately apparent. The presence of blinking or minor myoclonic jerks may be helpful and the EEG will show continuous spike-wave activity. The condition usually responds to intravenous diazepam and is much more commonly seen in secondarily generalised epilepsies of childhood rather than true petit mal epilepsy.

Complex partial status is rarer than absence status. Patients exhibit an abnormal mental state with confusion and disorientation, which is frequently associated with automatic behaviour and with subsequent amnesia for the period of time during which these events occurred.

Epilepsia partialis continua consists of repetitive rhythmic jerking of a group of muscles in the arm, leg or face, originally described in association with epidemic encephalitis in Russia. However, the syndrome is seen most frequently in association with vascular disease and with tumours. The jerking may last for hours or days at a time and tends to be highly refractory to conventional anticonvulsant drugs, although it may be suppressed for a short time by treatment with diazepam.

EPILEPTIC SYNDROMES

Seizures may occur in response to systemic disturbance, for example hypoglycaemia. In such cases the patient cannot be said to have epilepsy or to require any investigation or treatment for epilepsy, only the correction of the underlying disorder.

Patients with epilepsy are subject to recurrent seizures unrelated to systemic disturbance. By classifying epileptic syndromes in such patients we shall more easily identify those patients who may have underlying progressive pathology and be able to offer a more satisfactory prognosis.

The main criteria used to define epileptic syndromes are:

1. Seizure types
2. Age of onset
3. EEG
4. The timing of seizures.

Inevitably there are patients whose epilepsy fails to correspond to rigid classification, but the following represents a description of the more common epileptic syndromes, their prognosis and their significance. Table 7.3 presents, in simplified form, a proposed international classification of epilepsies.

Table 7.3 Classification of the epilepsies

Generalised epilepsies
Idiopathic
Childhood absence
Benign myoclonic epilepsy of adolescence
Tonic-clonic awakening epilepsy
Symptomatic
Infantile spasm syndrome
Lennox–Gastaut syndrome
Other specific syndromes
Partial epilepsies
Idiopathic
Benign focal motor epilepsy of childhood
Benign occipital epilepsy of childhood
Symptomatic
Simple partial epilepsies
Complex partial epilepsies
Specific epileptic syndromes
Febrile convulsions
Reflex epilepsies
Stress-induced seizures
Unclassified epilepsies
Neonatal seizures
Nocturnal tonic-clonic seizures (normal EEG)

In this classification we have used 'symptomatic' to include epilepsies which are often symptomatic, but can also on occasion be apparently idiopathic.

It will be recognised that three major factors interact in an individual patient to determine the manifestation of seizure disorder. These are:

1. The genetic predisposition towards seizures
2. The age of the patient
3. Underlying cerebral pathology.

Thus similar degrees of head injury may or may not be complicated by post-traumatic epilepsy, depending on the presence or absence of a family history of epilepsy. The presence of a similar cerebral pathology may result in a symptomatic generalised epilepsy if the pathology is present from early life, or a partial epilepsy if the pathology develops in later life. These differences probably reflect maturation of the brain in the developing individual.

The generalised epilepsies

Idiopathic generalised epilepsies

These epilepsies occur in subjects without neurological disease on an apparently genetic basis. The prime EEG characteristic is the generalised spike-wave discharge (Fig. 7.3). Onset before the age of 3 years is uncommon and after the age of 25 years these epilepsies decrease progressively in incidence.

Most commonly such epilepsies present with tonic-clonic seizures beginning in childhood or adolescence. There is no aura, although myoclonus may precede seizures (see below). Seizures tend to be infrequent and to occur shortly after waking; they respond well to therapy and become less frequent or cease with maturity.

Childhood and juvenile absence (petit mal) epilepsy is a relatively rare syndrome which occurs in the absence of identified cerebral disease. There is a positive family history in up to 40% of cases: twin studies have shown a concordance rate as high as 75% and siblings of children with true petit mal have the characteristic EEG disturbance of 3 c/s spike wave in up to 80% of cases, even in the absence of clinical seizures.

Simple absences begin between the ages of 3 and 15 years. They rarely persist into adult life and only 30% of patients develop grand mal seizures during early or later life.

A prime requirement for the diagnosis of true petit mal is the observation of generalised 3 Hz

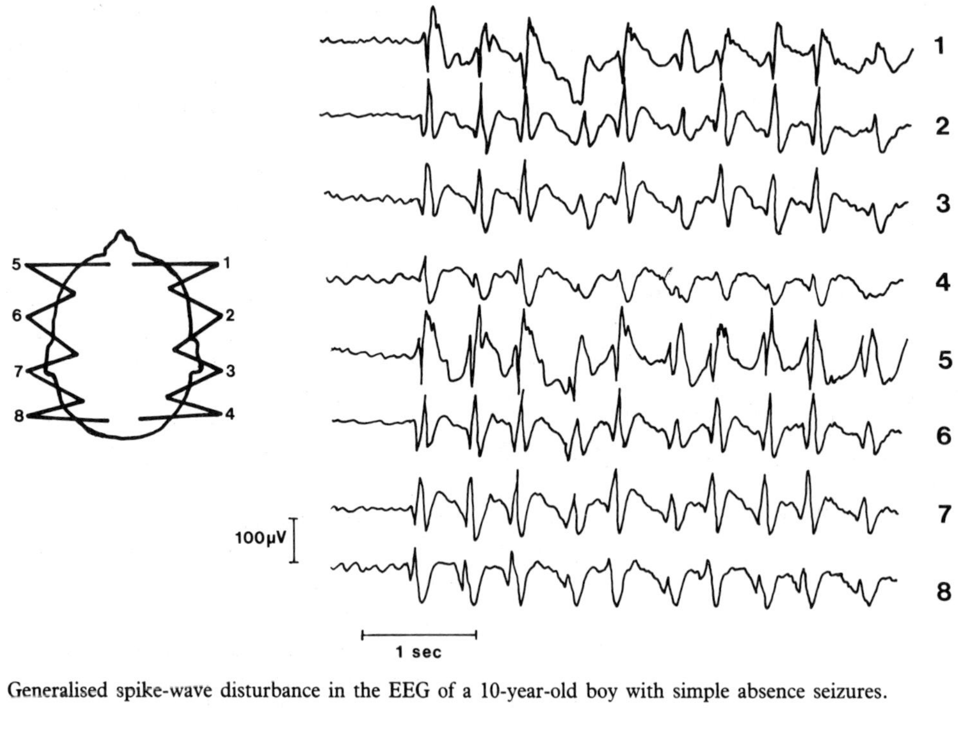

Fig. 7.3 Generalised spike-wave disturbance in the EEG of a 10-year-old boy with simple absence seizures.

spike waves on the EEG (Fig. 7.3), often provoked by hyperventilation. This is a relatively rare syndrome; it is still true that any minor seizure may be described by non-neurologists as petit mal. The diagnosis can practically be excluded if the attacks are occurring in adult life, when such minor seizures are invariably a form of complex partial seizure.

Juvenile myoclonic epilepsy is seen beginning in children and adolescents and characterised by early morning myoclonic jerks, mainly of the upper limbs, usually without absence. On occasion the jerks build up in frequency and merge into a generalised tonic-clonic seizure. The EEG shows regular 3–6 Hz spike and wave activity often associated with a myoclonic response that is particularly easily induced by photic stimuli, but which may also occur in response to other sensory stimuli, e.g. sudden noise and movement. The syndrome frequently has a familial basis, and responds well to anticonvulsant drugs with a good long-term prognosis. Valproate seems particularly effective, but withdrawal of drug treatment, even after long periods of remission, almost always results in relapse.

The symptomatic generalised epilepsies

These syndromes start in young children who frequently (but not always) have pre-existing cerebral damage or disease. They are characterised by the occurrence of more complex absence and myoclonic seizures frequently interspersed with tonic, clonic or tonic-clonic seizures.

Infantile spasm (West) syndrome represents the most severe part of the spectrum of secondary generalised epilepsy in childhood. The disorder is almost universally associated with severe pre-existing cerebral damage (prenatal or more commonly perinatal); up to 25% of cases may be caused by tuberous sclerosis.

Onset is between the ages of 4 and 7 months in half the cases and onset is rare after 1 year. The clinical hallmark of the syndrome is spasms consisting of sudden massive forward flexion of the head associated with bending of the knees and flexion and abduction of the arms (jack-knifing). This may result in brief lightning spasms or more sustained movements. Other seizure types including simple motor and tonic seizures may also occur; tonic-clonic seizures are rare.

Retardation is often obvious before the onset of the disorder, but even in previously normal infants behavioural regression is frequently seen.

The interictal EEG shows a severe disturbance devoid of normal background activity, consisting of chaotic high-amplitude and synchronous slow waves mixed with multifocal sharp waves and spikes (hypsarrhythmia).

Conventional anticonvulsant drugs have little effect on infantile spasms, but treatment with ACTH (20–60 units per day) appears to be helpful, particularly when started early in the course of the disorder. However, up to 90% of patients show severe mental retardation and death may occur.

Lennox–Gastaut syndrome usually begins before the age of 2 years and onset is uncommon after the age of 7 or 8 years. This syndrome may account for up to 10% of all epilepsies. It is twice as common as true petit mal epilepsy.

Children suffer frequent seizures of diverse symptomatology, but usually characterised by absence with brief massive bilateral myoclonus, tonic seizures or atonic drop attacks. These result in numerous falls causing multiple injuries, particularly to the head, often necessitating the wearing of a protective helmet. More conventional tonic-clonic, simple motor and complex partial seizures may occur. Absence status is much more common in this disorder than in true petit mal. The interictal EEG typically shows bilateral synchronous spike-wave complexes between 1 and 2.5 c/s (see Fig. 5.5).

The prognosis for both development and seizure control is poor in contrast to true petit mal. Retardation is present from the onset in up to half of the patients and may be severe. Where the disorder has been present for some time, retardation can be seen in up to 90% of patients. Seizures usually persist into adult life, but change in character, often with the development of complex partial seizures.

As well as these more stereotyped syndromes, which are commonly associated with underlying cerebral disease, other forms of myoclonic epilepsy are seen which appear to represent a spectrum between the above disorders. Some children are seen with 'myoclonic-astatic epilepsy' characterised by massive myoclonus or atonic seizures with interictal polyspike-wave bursts. However, the outlook appears better than for the Lennox–Gastaut syndrome, both in terms of seizure control and subsequent retardation.

There is also a group of progressive myoclonic epilepsies which present in childhood as a result of metabolic or storage diseases. These include lipidoses and mucopolysaccharidoses, as well as other progressive degenerative disorders with onset in early life. They are discussed in Chapter 15.

The partial epilepsies

These epilepsies are characterised by the occurrence of partial seizures with or without secondary tonic-clonic seizures. Where tonic-clonic seizures do occur they often do so during sleep, so much so that patients presenting with nocturnal tonic-clonic seizures should be regarded as having a partial epilepsy unless proved otherwise. This form of epilepsy may develop at any age, but it accounts for an increasing proportion of new cases with increasing age. Partial epilepsies are often symptomatic of structural brain disease.

An exception is *benign focal motor epilepsy of childhood*. In this syndrome, which is as common as petit mal epilepsy, simple motor seizures are seen, starting between the ages of 8 and 12 years in an otherwise normal individual. Seizures tend to be few in number and to remit without a risk of late epilepsy.

Tonic-clonic seizures are unusual and Rolandic spike discharges occur in the EEG. Partial seizures in childhood may also be symptomatic of structural disease, but very rarely of tumours because of the rarity of supratentorial tumours before adolescence. Similar forms of benign focal epilepsy in childhood may more rarely result in somatosensory or visual seizures.

The significance of partial epilepsy starting in adult life is the relatively high expectation of finding a tumour. Approximately 10% of patients with late-onset epilepsy (over the age of 25) have brain tumours; this incidence rises to 30% or 40% where there is a clear history of partial seizures. Complex partial seizures are by far the commonest kind of partial epilepsy beginning in adult life, but only 10–15% of such epilepsies are associated with tumours. Simple motor, somatosensory and visual partial seizures carry a higher risk of tumour association (40–60%) (Table 7.4). It must be remembered that the majority of tumours causing partial epilepsies are gliomas (particularly more benign gliomas) rather than surgically treatable meningiomas, which account for only 10% of supratentorial tumours.

Table 7.4 Types of partial seizures and tumour aetiology (after Mauguierre & Courjon 1978)

	No. patients	Identified tumour (%)
Simple partial seizures		
Motor	1211	21
Somatosensory	98	56
Other (olfactory, visual gustatory)	148	24
Complex partial seizures	228	13

Complex partial epilepsy

Complex partial epilepsy demands particular discussion because of its significance, associations and poor response to medical therapy. In this syndrome complex partial seizures occur, with or without tonic-clonic seizures, and present the most frequent management problem for the adult neurologist. Whereas associated tonic-clonic seizures are usually suppressed by anticonvulsant therapy, complex partial seizures often continue, with a tendency to show clustering. Neurological clinics are full of such patients with continued attacks in spite of large and frequently changed doses of anticonvulsants.

The aetiology of complex partial epilepsies remains obscure in the majority of patients (Table 7.5), even in the era of CT scanning. The possibility that Ammon's horn sclerosis (neuronal loss and gliosis of the medial temporal lobe) resulting from prolonged febrile convulsions is a frequent cause of complex partial epilepsy demands consideration in view of the high incidence of this abnormality in specimens obtained at temporal lobectomy. Head injury may be another important aetiological factor.

Table 7.5 Important factors in the aetiology of complex partial epilepsy

	% cases which can be attributed to cause (%)*
Complicated febrile seizures	20
Head injury	12
Cerebral palsy	9
Encephalitis	3

* Data from a community-based case-controlled study of 82 patients with complex partial epilepsy (Rocca et al 1987). 88 patients were identified and 3 were excluded because they had a tumour, 3 because of Artenovenous malformation (AVM).

Complex partial epilepsy has particular importance because of its association with psychiatric disorders. It has long been recognised that patients with epilepsy suffer from a higher than usual incidence of psychiatric disturbance. While patients with generalised forms of epilepsy have a slightly higher incidence of disorder than is usual, the highest incidence is found in patients with complex partial epilepsy and other forms of temporal lobe seizures. In spite of a prolonged debate as to whether there is a typical 'temporal lobe personality', no specific psychiatric disorder is seen and patients may have symptoms of anxiety or depression as well as personality disturbance, hysteria and schizophreniform psychosis. The incidence of such problems is illustrated in Table 7.6.

It is uncertain whether the association between complex partial epilepsy and psychiatric disturbance reflects the fact that this form of epilepsy is more chronic and refractory to treatment than other forms of epilepsy, or whether it reflects a direct association between underlying temporal lobe pathology and both epilepsy and psychiatric disorder. Whatever the reason for the association, it has profound clinical significance as this population of patients presents the greatest management problems in adult neurological clinics.

Table 7.6 Psychiatric symptoms in 666 patients with temporal lobe epilepsy (Currie et al 1971)

Anxiety	19%
Depression	11%
Aggression	7%
Obsession	6%
Florid pschiatric disturbance	
Hysteria	3%
Schizophreniform psychosis	2%
Anxiety state	0.5%
Severe depression	0.5%

Other specific epilepsies

Reflex epilepsies

It is well recognised that in rare patients particular stimuli or tasks may reflexly induce seizures: the most common phenomena to do this are photic stimuli. This is a form of generalised epilepsy, testing for which forms a standard part of routine EEG examinations. Flash stimuli may evoke spike-wave responses, sometimes accompanied by a myoclonic jerk, which may continue after the cessation of the stimulus. This phenomenon is most frequently seen in clinical practice in television epilepsy where proximity to a faulty flickering television set may provoke a seizure in a susceptible individual. Less frequently it may be seen in drivers passing along roads with regularly spaced trees, through which bright sunlight shines. Some children learn to precipitate their own seizures by blinking while looking at a light. More rarely, seizures may be evoked by sound or music or by more complex tasks such as reading or mental arithmetic.

Febrile convulsions

This syndrome must be differentiated from childhood epilepsy because of its differing prognosis and treatment. It is common, its incidence equalling that of epilepsy at all ages.

Seizures occur with temperatures higher than 38°C. The highest incidence is between 9 and 20 months and it rarely occurs before 6 months or after 5 years. Thirty to 40% of patients may have a near relative who also suffered febrile convulsions and as many as 20–25% of relatives may suffer from epilepsy. The syndrome is slightly more common in boys than girls (1.4 : 1).

Convulsions are usually of a generalised tonic-clonic variety and frequently may be the first sign of illness in a child. They may be brief, but long-lasting severe or lateralised seizures seem to carry an adverse prognosis. The convulsion usually occurs as fever reaches its peak.

In absolute terms, febrile convulsions are most commonly seen in association with upper respiratory tract infections. However, these types of infections are by far the most common in the age group prone to febrile convulsions: a higher percentage of illnesses such as pneumonia, gastroenteritis and exanthemata are complicated by febrile convulsion and the highest incidence occurs with meningitis.

The rationale of treatment can be understood only when the prognosis for this condition is considered. The risk of a recurrence of further febrile seizures is greatest, the earlier the first febrile convulsion: thus 50% of patients with the first febrile convulsion before the age of 1 year will have subsequent febrile convulsions, whereas when the first convulsion is after the age of 3 years only 10% will suffer further convulsions.

The risk of late epilepsy is controversial but may be as low as 5–10% of patients with febrile convulsions. However, a number of factors increase the risk: these include prolonged convulsions, lateralised seizures and repeated convulsions, as well as antecedent brain damage and a family history of febrile seizures.

It is likely that the pathophysiology determining the risk of both epilepsy and permanent neurological deficit following prolonged febrile convulsions is determined by the susceptibility of the immature brain to the greatly increased metabolic demands of prolonged neuronal discharge in the face of high fever. This results in neuronal loss, which may occur particularly in the hippocampal regions resulting in the characteristic changes of Ammon's horn sclerosis.

The management of febrile convulsions has three aims:

1. To terminate the seizure as rapidly as possible
2. To determine and treat the aetiology of the fever
3. To consider means of preventing further seizures in high-risk patients.

Seizures may be most readily terminated using intravenous diazepam, although in situations where this is not available rectal diazepam may be of value. Emergency transfer to hospital is indicated with any prolonged convulsion.

The possibility of meningitis needs to be considered seriously, particularly in children below the age of 18 months as they may fail to show classic signs of meningism.

Parents of children with febrile convulsions should certainly be advised to try and reduce temperatures in children at risk by tepid sponging; they may also be instructed in the use of rectal diazepam. Prophylactic phenobarbitone may reduce the recurrence of febrile convulsion, but the use of this drug has many side effects in children and parents are rarely willing to comply with the use of this drug. Valproate is as effective and may be better tolerated. Prophylactic treatment is now reserved for patients viewed as being at high risk of further prolonged convulsions. This would include patients with pre-existing brain damage, with a first febrile convulsion early in life, and possibly those in whom there is a family history of febrile convulsion.

Relative frequency of seizure types

Information on the relative frequency of seizure types is unsatisfactory as it is based largely on populations of patients with relatively severe epilepsy, which include large numbers of patients with partial epilepsies. Furthermore, the milder the epilepsy the more difficult it may be to determine on clinical and electroencephalographic grounds whether the epilepsy is of a generalised or partial type. With these restrictions in mind, most series would suggest that approximately one-

Table 7.7 Incidence of epilepsies and seizure types from a population of 1505 patients with non-febrile seizures from Aarhus, Denmark (Juul-Jensen & Foldspang 1983)

Primary tonic-clonic	25.6%
Absence	3.9%
Myoclonic	3.1%
Simple partial seizures	4.9%
Complex partial seizures	17.9%
Partial + tonic-clonic	14.4%
Alcohol-induced seizures	6.3%
Stress-induced seizures	8.0%
Drug-induced seizures	1.3%
Isolated unprovoked seizures	13.4%
Unclassified	1.2%

half of epilepsies are of a generalised type, the other one-half being partial (most commonly with a temporal lobe origin) (Table 7.7).

THE CAUSES OF SEIZURES AND EPILEPSY

Epilepsy is not a diagnosis in itself but merely a symptom of a wide variety of cerebral diseases. Generalised or partial seizures can occur in response to practically any generalised metabolic disturbance, or cerebral pathology.

The causes of seizures in response to systemic disturbance are summarised in Table 7.8. In such instances, seizures are usually associated with encephalopathic disturbance with altered consciousness and are almost invariably myoclonic or generalised tonic-clonic seizures.

More chronic problems resulting in chronic epilepsy are associated with a variety of cerebral pathologies listed in Table 7.9. It can be seen that seizures and epilepsy can be associated with virtually any cerebral pathology: however, differing pathologies and forms of epilepsy will show a marked tendency to present in differing age groups (Fig. 7.4).

In the neonate, seizures are most usually caused by birth trauma, hypoxia, hypoglycaemia or hypocalcaemia. Intracranial haemorrhage may also present with seizures.

Within the first year of life, seizures are likely to reflect severe cerebral pathology as the

Table 7.8 Systemic disturbance causing seizures

Fever	Drugs
Hypoxia	Drug withdrawal
Hypoglycaemia	Toxins
Electrolyte imbalance	
	Pyridoxine deficiency
Renal failure	Porphyria
Hepatic failure	Inborn errors of metabolism
Respiratory failure	

Table 7.9 C.N.S. disease causing seizures and epilepsy

Congenital	Birth trauma, tuberose sclerosis, arterio-venous malformation, lipid storage diseases, leucodystrophies, Down's syndrome
Infective	Meningitis, encephalitis, abscess, syphilis
Trauma	Diffuse brain injury, haematoma (extradural, subdural, intracerebral), depressed fracture
Tumour	Glioma, meningioma, secondary carcinoma, etc.
Vascular	Atheroma, arteritis, aneurysm
Degenerative	Alzheimer's, Pick's, Creutzfeld–Jakob, etc.
Miscellaneous	Demyelination

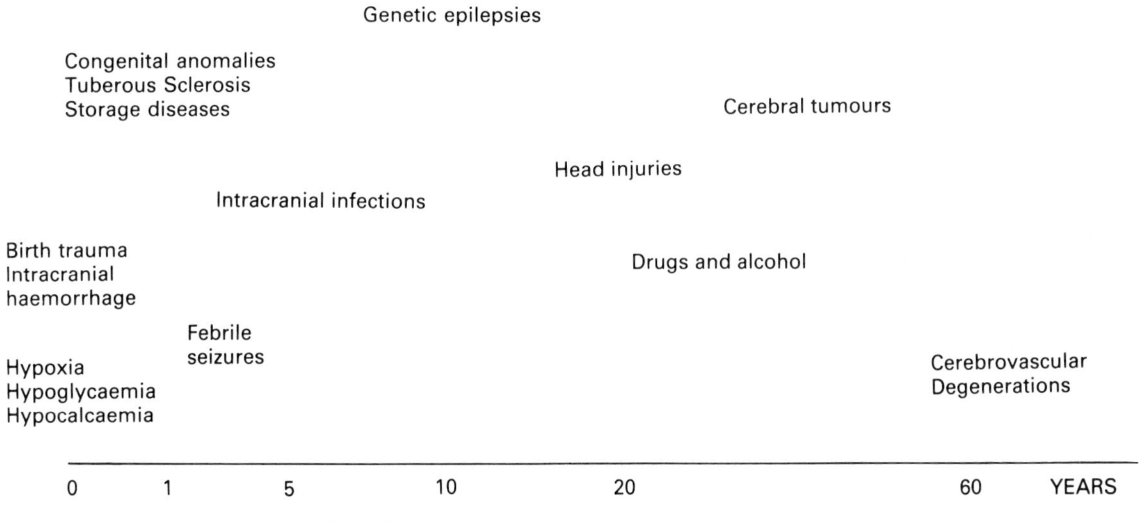

Fig. 7.4 Causes of seizures and epilepsy by age.

threshold for epilepsy in this age group appears to be relatively high: thus, seizures due to birth trauma, tuberous sclerosis, major congenital abnormalities, infective causes and the more severe storage diseases such as lipidoses and mucopolysaccharidoses may present with epilepsy at this age. Such epilepsies tend to be severe and to carry a poor prognosis.

In the toddler, idiopathic forms of petit mal and other primary epilepsies may begin, as well as more severe secondary generalised epilepsies related to pre-existing cerebral disease. Meningitis and encephalitis are also a significant cause of epilepsy in this age group.

During adolescence, primary epilepsies—particularly myoclonic epilepsies—are common, but once adulthood is attained these forms of epilepsy become rarer and partial epilepsies due to focal cerebral disease, particularly complex partial epilepsies, predominate. Over the age of 25 the onset of epilepsy is associated with an increased risk of cerebral tumour. The incidence of a tumour causing epilepsy increases with age after 25 years, but over the age of 60 years cerebrovascular disease and cerebral degenerative pathologies become an increasingly common cause of epilepsy.

FACTORS INCREASING THE SUSCEPTIBILITY TO SEIZURES

In a susceptible individual there seems little doubt that the threshold to seizures varies from day to day and even during the daily cycle. This phenomenon is often manifest by the tendency of seizures (particularly complex partial seizures) to occur in clusters over a short period with long periods of remission between. A number of factors appear to precipitate seizures.

The sleep–waking cycle

It is not uncommon for patients to have seizures only during sleep. It has been suggested that such seizures may frequently have a localised origin, which is reflected by the fact that natural sleep may well be a provocative test for focal EEG abnormalities in patients with complex partial seizures.

It is more common for idiopathic generalised seizures such as myoclonus and tonic-clonic seizures to occur within an hour or two of waking. Sleep deprivation may be important in reducing the threshold to such seizures and is a factor which should be avoided.

Alertness and the general level of interest also affect seizure threshold: the patient who is actively involved in an interesting and enjoyable pursuit is less likely to have seizures than when he is bored.

Catamenial epilepsy

It is extremely common for women with epilepsy to have seizures during the few days immediately before or immediately after the start of menstruation: this may occur in up to 60% of women with epilepsy. The reasons for this remain obscure: there is little evidence to suggest that it is due to fluid retention, but some that higher oestrogen levels may be directly associated with an increased predisposition to seizures. The effects of oral contraceptive preparations on epilepsy in these patients is, however, unpredictable—some patients apparently having more seizures, others less. Pregnancy has a similarly unpredictable effect but here, on occasions, worsening of seizure control during pregnancy may be related to falling serum drug levels in the second and third trimesters, due to increased drug metabolism.

Stress factors

Many patients with epilepsy believe that their seizures are more frequent when they are emotionally distressed or upset. This may well be true and certainly this factor may lead to disturbances in the sleep–waking cycle and drug therapy with potentially epileptogenic psychotropic drugs may complicate the underlying problems.

Drugs

Many different drugs are known to increase the susceptibility of patients to seizures (see p. 426).

Of particular importance in this respect is alcohol: alcohol withdrawal fits are a very common cause of tonic-clonic seizures without aura starting in adult life. It is of major importance to recognise this phenomenon, as alcohol-withdrawal fits do not necessitate anticonvulsant therapy, only counselling about the abuse of alcohol.

THE INVESTIGATION OF EPILEPSY

The investigation of epilepsy is undertaken to add weight to the clinical diagnosis, to aid classification of seizures and to define any underlying pathology that may require additional or alternative treatment to the patient's seizures.

It is relatively uncommon for physicians to witness seizures or to record an EEG during one. The diagnosis of epilepsy is ultimately a clinical one, therefore, based on the history obtained from the patient and his relatives. EEG recording can, however, be a useful procedure in adding weight to a clinical diagnosis, although it can never prove or disprove the clinical diagnosis of epilepsy.

Major problems arise in the interpretation of EEG recordings because mild non-specific abnormalities may occur in up to 10% of the population without a history of epilepsy, and because some patients with mild epilepsy have normal interictal records. Furthermore, in patients with complex partial seizures, medial temporal foci may be remote from conventional EEG electrode placements so that focal spike activity may not be recorded from other than sphenoidal or nasopharyngeal leads, even during a clinical seizure.

In addition to conventional EEG recording, recent technological advances have allowed the recording of EEG in combination with videotape of the behavioural responses of patients over prolonged periods, as well as less cumbersome ambulatory monitoring which can be undertaken with outpatients. With the increasing periods of EEG monitoring that these techniques allow, it is hoped that more clinically useful and relevant abnormalities will be detected. These tools may be particularly useful in differentiating true seizures from pseudoseizures (see below).

As well as helping to confirm a clinical diagnosis of epilepsy, the EEG may be of value in determining the type of epilepsy suffered by the patient. The differentiation of absence seizures associated with generalised spike waves and complex partial seizures associated with temporal lobe spikes may allow a differing therapeutic approach.

The necessity for investigation other than with an EEG in patients presenting with epilepsy will vary considerably with the age of the patient, the type of epilepsy and the presence or absence of neurological signs. It can be argued that all patients presenting with epilepsy require biochemical and haematological screening, and exhaustive neuroradiological investigation to determine a cause for their epilepsy. However, this may be economically wasteful in view of the low rate of detection of conditions demanding treatment other than by the prescription of anticonvulsant drugs. It is more important to recall that a careful history and physical examination may well reveal a cause for epilepsy, e.g. skin lesions of adenoma sebaceum in tuberous sclerosis, the findings of multiple neurofibromatosis and the characteristic facial and skeletal abnormalities that may be seen in association with a variety of storage diseases.

Biochemical and haematological screening is widely available but rarely discloses a cause for epilepsy: the exceptions to this are in neonates where hypoglycaemia and hypocalcaemia are particularly important, and in middle age where the finding of an elevated mean cell volume and abnormal liver function tests may confirm the clinical suspicion of alcohol-induced seizures. Routine serogical tests for syphilis are difficult to justify as neurosyphilis now represents an exceedingly uncommon cause of epilepsy.

Skull radiographs are routinely ordered in patients presenting with epilepsy: they may occasionally disclose evidence of raised intracranial pressure, or intracranial calcification or abnormal vascular markings from a meningioma. However, in such instances it is relatively rare for patients with such abnormalities on the skull radiographs to be free from other neurological signs or symptoms of raised intracranial pressure which should alert the clinician: it is thus debatable whether a skull radiograph is a necessary routine investigation in new cases of epilepsy.

The place of CT scanning, which in neurological centres has largely replaced radioisotope scanning in the investigation of epilepsy, remains controversial. Some have suggested that every patient with epilepsy should have a CT scan, but the costs of such a policy are difficult to justify. A number of studies of the results of CT scanning in epilepsy have been published: they indicate that CT scans are abnormal in approximately 40–50% of patients with epilepsy. However, the most common abnormalities are atrophic in nature and tumours are found in only 8–10% of patients. The percentage of patients with tumours rises to 16% in patients over the age of 20 and to 22% when only partial seizures are examined. In adult patients with late-onset epilepsy it is rare to detect tumours by CT scanning in the absence of partial seizures, focal neurological signs or a focal EEG abnormality. When all three of these features are present, CT scanning will reveal a tumour pathology in up to 70% of cases.

This provides a potent argument for restricting CT scanning in epilepsy to a selected group of patients with the onset of partial epilepsy in adult life, who also have symptoms or signs indicating progressive cerebral disease. This policy is also supported by the realisation that early and unselective CT scanning may give rise to a number of false-negative scans. Furthermore, it is salutary to recall that up to 90% of tumour epilepsies are due to gliomas or metastases, lesions which are seldom curable by a radical surgical approach. A suggested scheme for the identification of patients requiring further investigation is summarised in Figure 7.5.

THE MANAGEMENT OF THE PATIENT WITH EPILEPSY

The adequate management of the patient with epilepsy demands, first, an adequate diagnosis and

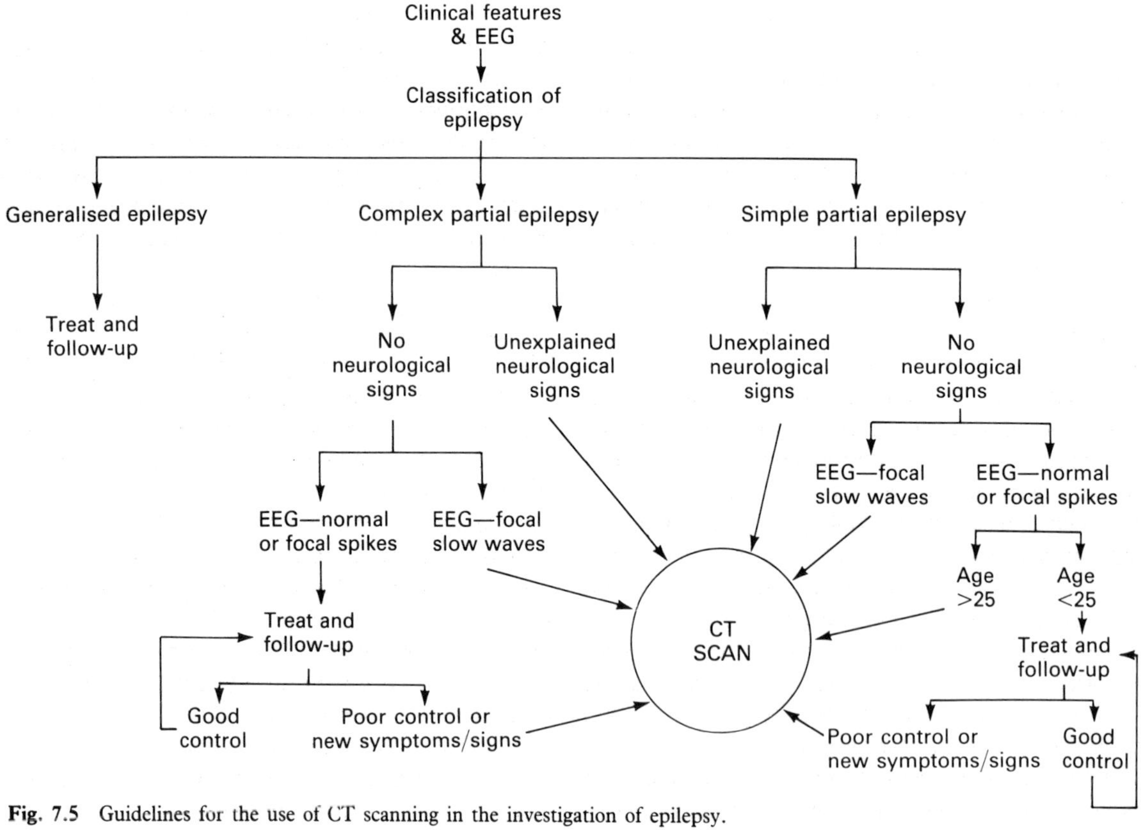

Fig. 7.5 Guidelines for the use of CT scanning in the investigation of epilepsy.

investigation of epilepsy (see above); the next step is one of counselling.

Patients and families may be taken aback by the diagnosis of epilepsy: they need to have access to satisfactory information about the subject, to avoid the commonly held myths and prejudices surrounding the condition; they need counselling on the way in which epilepsy and its treatment should or should not affect schooling, employment, leisure activities, driving, concomitant medication and pregnancy. The aim must be to encourage an informed and commonsense approach, without undue restriction of activities.

The diagnosis of epilepsy has a number of social complications: patients with a recent history of two or more seizures should not drive a motor vehicle in the United Kingdom until such time as two years have elapsed without seizures; if seizures have occurred only at night over a period of three years, then this will be treated as an exception. These facts must be explained to patients and their obligations to report the occurrence of seizures to the licensing authority emphasised; patients' motor insurance also becomes invalid. Patients presenting with a single isolated seizure should be advised to report the event to the licensing authorities, who will usually withdraw the licence for a year after such an event. The occurrence of a single seizure after the age of 5 is sufficient for a lifetime bar to holding a public service vehicle or heavy goods vehicle licence.

In a few instances the prospective risk of developing epilepsy may be such as to prevent driving: this includes patients who have cerebral tumours or metastases, or patients who have undergone craniotomy or suffered a head injury carrying a particularly high risk of epilepsy. As well as prohibiting driving, the diagnosis of epilepsy necessitates advice against working at height. Other forms of employment are more difficult to advise on: under some circumstances working close to heavy machinery may lead to problems, although usually moving parts will be adequately guarded. A full pattern of recreation and leisure pursuits should usually be possible in patients with less severe epilepsy, although such pursuits should always be undertaken in the presence of a responsible adult who is familiar with the patient's problems.

Following this the most important aspect of general management is the drug treatment of epilepsy.

Starting antiepileptic therapy

There is general agreement that a single fit does not constitute epilepsy and does not necessitate anticonvulsant treatment. Up to 40% of patients who present in adult life with an isolated seizure may suffer further attacks within the next 2–3 years. The factors which determine the risk of further seizures in such patients are poorly understood, but there is no doubt that the more time that elapses after a first seizure, the lower the risk of recurrence. It is generally accepted that at least two seizures should occur before drug treatment is started. There are, however, circumstances in which this practice may be modified (Table 7.10).

There has been an increasing practice over recent years to begin anticonvulsant treatment before the onset of seizures in patients who are at a high risk of developing epilepsy: patients with severe head injury, or patients undergoing supratentorial craniotomy. The rationale for such preventative treatment is not clear and it is impossible to know for how long such treatment should be continued. It is, therefore, more sensible to wait for the occurrence of one or more seizures following head injury or craniotomy before starting therapy.

Table 7.10 Starting antiepileptic therapy

Problem	Usual clinical practice	Factors which modify it
Prospective risk of epilepsy	No treatment	
Single isolated seizure	No treatment	Progressive cerebral disorder Clearly abnormal EEG
Two or more seizures	Monotherapy	Seizures > 1 year apart Identified precipitating factors (drugs, alcohol, photic stimuli) Patient acceptance

The aim of therapy must be to control epilepsy with the simplest possible regime. This requires institution of therapy with a single drug in modest doses, which may gradually be increased if and when further seizures occur (Fig. 7.6).

Data on the comparative efficacy of anticonvulsant drugs are extremely sparse and almost all randomised studies in adult patients fail to differentiate between the comparative efficacy of drugs tested, possibly because the numbers of patients studied are too small to achieve the necessary statistical power. It does appear that, in children, absence seizures are responsive to ethosuximide and valproate, but unresponsive to drugs effective against tonic-clonic and partial seizures, such as phenytoin and carbamazepine. ACTH seems to be of particular value in the management of the infantile spasm syndrome and valproate may have a specific role in the management of myoclonic epilepsies and other idiopathic generalised epilepsies.

In the absence of firm indications that any specific drugs are more effective than others against partial and tonic-clonic seizures, choice of drugs should probably be undertaken on the basis of their expected adverse effects (see below). The authors' preferences are summarised in Tables 7.11–7.13.

Table 7.11 Order of preference of drugs for generalised tonic-clonic seizures

	Without aura	With focal onset
1	Valproate	Carbamazepine
2	Carbamazepine	Valproate
3	Phenytoin	Phenytoin

Table 7.12 Order of preference of drugs for other generalised seizures

	Absence seizures	Myoclonic seizures	Infantile spasms
1	Valproate	Valproate	ACTH
2	Ethosuximide	Ethosuximide	Steroids
3	Clonazepam	Clonazepam	Nitrazepam
4			Clonazepam

Table 7.13 Order of preference of drugs for partial seizures

	Simple partial seizures	Complex partial seizures
1	Carbamazepine	Carbamazepine
2	Phenytoin	Phenytoin
3	Valproate	Valproate

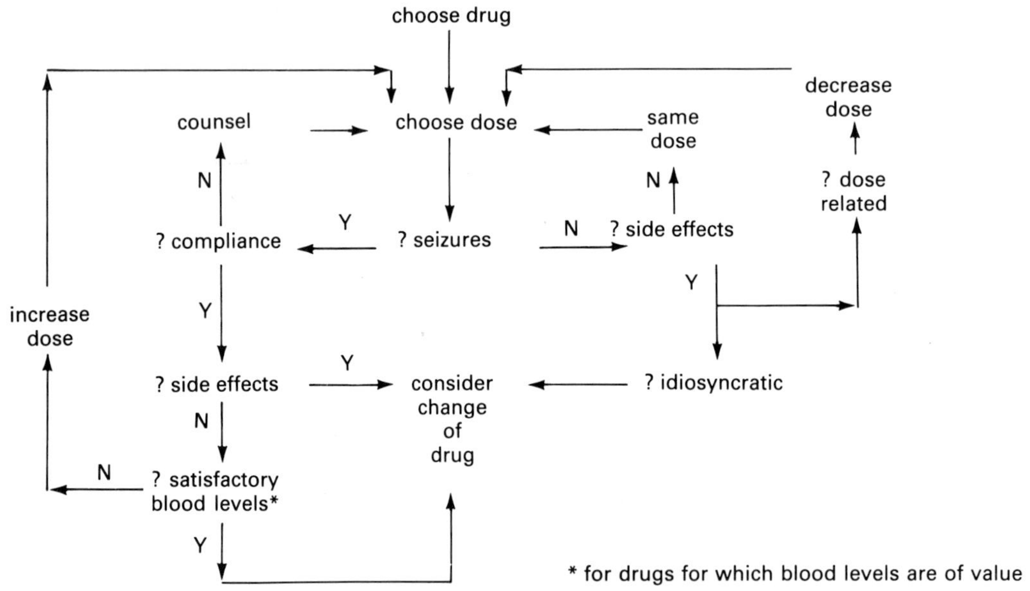

Fig. 7.6 Flow diagram of decision-taking in the use of a single antiepileptic drug.

Administering and monitoring drug therapy

Pharmacokinetics define the characteristics of drug absorption, distribution and elimination. It is most important to remember that, when measuring plasma or serum drug concentrations, one is sampling a physiological compartment far removed from the site of therapeutic drug action (Fig. 7.7). Some of the more important pharmacokinetic data on commonly used anticonvulsants are summarised in Table 7.14.

Absorption of drugs

Phenytoin and carbamazepine are relatively insoluble and are slowly and incompletely absorbed, pH may significantly influence the availability of phenytoin, which is insoluble at acid pH in the stomach and depends largely on duodenal absorption. The bioavailability of phenytoin may also be influenced by the pharmaceutical presentation of the drug: an outbreak of phenytoin intoxication occurred in Australasia because of a change in the excipient of phenytoin capsules from calcium sulphate to lactose. Phenytoin bioavailability may thus be variable and it may be important to specify a pharmaceutical preparation rather than using generics.

Particular problems occur when anticonvulsants are administered parenterally. Although such preparations of phenytoin are recommended for intramuscular administration, they are alkaline and, when buffered to physiological pH in muscle tissue, phenytoin becomes less soluble and is very slowly absorbed. Transfer from oral to intramuscular administration may lead to falling serum levels. Similar considerations apply to the intramuscular absorption of diazepam and, to a lesser degree, of phenobarbitone. Certainly, intramuscular administration of these drugs should never be used in the management of status epilepticus, although rectal administration of diazepam may be adequate under some circumstances. Intravenous administration of all anticonvulsant drugs is preferable in order to obtain a rapid onset of action,

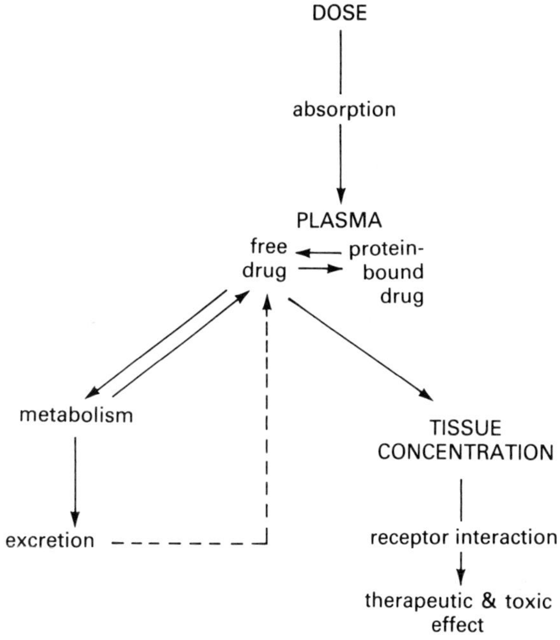

Fig. 7.7 Relationships between plasma total concentrations, free drug and therapeutic effect.

Table 7.14 Pharmacokinetics of anticonvulsants

Drug	Absorption (Time to peak serum conc. (h) after oral dose)	Protein binding (%)	Active metabolites	Metabolism (½ life (h)	doses/day)
Phenytoin	4–12	90	—	9–140	1
Phenobarbitone	1–6	45	—	50–160	2
Primidone	2–5	20	Phenobarbitone Phenylethylmalonamide	4–12	2
Carbamazepine	4–24	75	10,11-epoxide	8–30	2 or 3
Valproate	1–4	90	—	8–20	2 or 3
Ethosuximide	1–4	—	—	40–70	2 or 3

and oral administration (via a nasogastric tube) is preferable for maintaining serum levels of routinely administered anticonvulsants.

Protein binding

It is usual to measure total serum or plasma concentrations of anticonvulsants. However, phenytoin, valproate and benzodiazepines are heavily protein bound and only a small portion of the measured concentration is pharmacologically active as free drug.

Protein binding of drugs has important clinical implications in a number of situations: renal and hepatic failure, and other hypoalbuminaemic states may considerably increase the ratio of free to bound drug; bilirubin may compete for albumin-binding sites with phenytoin, while valproate is bound to albumin-free fatty-acid binding sites and interaction between drug and these endogenous substances may occur.

Protein binding of anticonvulsants may also cause drug interactions: in particular the administration of valproate may decrease the binding of phenytoin to plasma protein. Carbamazepine itself is strongly protein bound (Table 7.14), but its metabolite 10,11-epoxide is only 50% protein bound. Both are anticonvulsant, but the lesser binding of the metabolite may increase its contribution to the pharmacological activity of the drug.

Drug metabolism

Anticonvulsants are usually extensively metabolised by hepatic enzymes before excretion, and this is the rate-limiting step in the elimination of the drug. Rates of elimination vary and are usually expressed in terms of drug half-life (Table 7.14), which is important in determining:

1 The interval between doses of the drug (ideally, equal to the drug half-life)

2. The time required to reach a new steady state after alterations in drug dosage (usually five times the half-life)

3. The timing of sampling for drug-level estimation.

Phenytoin and phenobarbitone have long half-lives and can satisfactorily be given as a single daily dose without large diurnal fluctuations in drug level. Up to 14–30 days may elapse before steady-state levels are achieved following alteration in dosage although, when initiating phenytoin therapy, i.v. loading regimes will produce earlier effective steady-state concentrations. Because of the non-linear metabolism of phenytoin (see below), half-life increases with increasing serum levels and at toxic concentrations the rate of elimination and time to steady state may be unexpectedly prolonged. Rechecking serum levels after a change in dosage may therefore have to be delayed in patients taking phenytoin and phenobarbitone, but a single sample is an accurate reflection of serum levels throughout the day.

The question must be raised as to how total plasma concentrations of shorter-acting drugs are related to therapeutic effect. There is evidence that the anticonvulsant action of valproate develops slowly after a single dose of the drug and may be maintained for a prolonged period after drug withdrawal. Although valproate plasma levels vary greatly during the day, valproate is clinically effective when administered in once- or twice-daily dosage.

Within individual patients, there is a linear relationship between dose and serum level over the clinical dosage range for most anticonvulsant drugs. The important exception to this is phenytoin, which is metabolised by microsomal liver enzymes which are saturable within the therapeutic range of serum levels. Thus, with increasing doses of phenytoin, a smaller proportion of the drug is metabolised and serum levels rise quickly (Fig. 7.8). Small increments in phenytoin dosage may lead to large increases in serum level and to clinical intoxication, and it may be necessary to use increments of 50 or 25 mg per day. Unfortunately, the optimal range for the drug lies on the steep part of the curve, so that minor changes in the bioavailability of phenytoin, and drug interactions, have major clinical effects. The metabolism of ethosuximide is also non-linear in a similar fashion to that of phenytoin, but this is not of importance at therapeutic dose levels.

For all anticonvulsant drugs there is a wide interpatient variation in the relationship between dose and serum level. This is largely attributable to varying rates of drug metabolism, determined

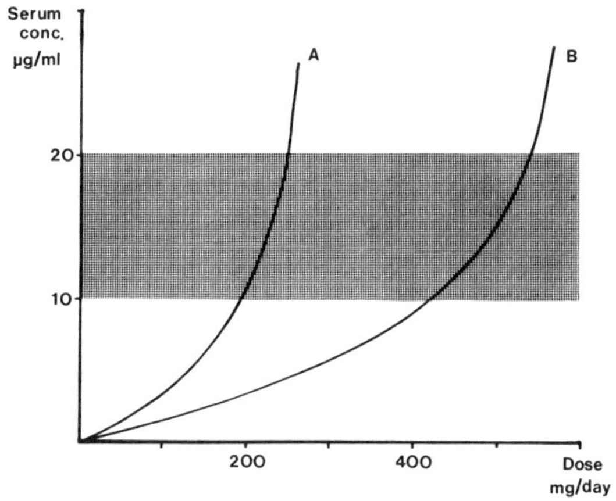

Fig. 7.8 Relationship between dose and serum concentration for phenytoin in two patients. A—with metabolism saturated at low concentration, B—with metabolism saturated at high concentration.

in turn by a number of factors, the most important of which are probably genetic, age and enzyme induction.

Phenytoin, phenobarbitone and carbamazepine are potent inducers of hepatic enzymes. Carbamazepine induces its own metabolism, so that serum levels tend to fall with time, which may account for the high incidence of adverse reactions if this drug is not introduced slowly. When multiple drug regimes are used, anticonvulsants usually interact to speed the rate of metabolism of other drugs. In particular, it may be very difficult to attain optimal serum levels of carbamazepine and of valproate in patients who are receiving other anticonvulsant drugs and larger doses of these drugs are required in patients receiving polypharmacy. This applies not only to anticonvulsants but is also responsible for increased metabolism of oestrogen preparations which leads to a higher incidence of breakthrough bleeding and to contraceptive failure in epileptic patients.

In contrast, the metabolism of phenytoin is frequently impaired by the presence of other drugs: the most clinically important of these is sulthiame, which has a potent inhibitory effect on the metabolism of phenytoin that may partly account for its clinical antiepileptic action.

Anticonvulsant drug metabolism is also important because in some cases active metabolites are produced (Table 7.14).

Pharmacodynamics of anticonvulsants

Pharmacodynamics seek to describe the interaction of drugs with tissue receptors which are responsible for drug actions. We remain comparatively ignorant of this aspect of anticonvulsant pharmacology, but must invoke it to explain phenomena such as the well-recognised tolerance to the anticonvulsant and sedative effects of benzodiazepines, which greatly limits their use. In a similar way, tolerance to the toxic effects of phenobarbitone develops with time, but is not attributable to falling serum levels.

There is increasing evidence that benzodiazepines, barbiturates, hydantoins and GABA may interact with endogenous benzodiazepine, GABA and picrotoxin receptors which are closely related to the chloride ionophor (Fig. 7.9): this may provide a common final pathway for drug action. It is known that both benzodiazepines and barbiturates facilitate the postsynaptic action of GABA and that valproate may have some anticonvulsant effect related to its ability to increase brain GABA levels. Although some anticonvulsants may

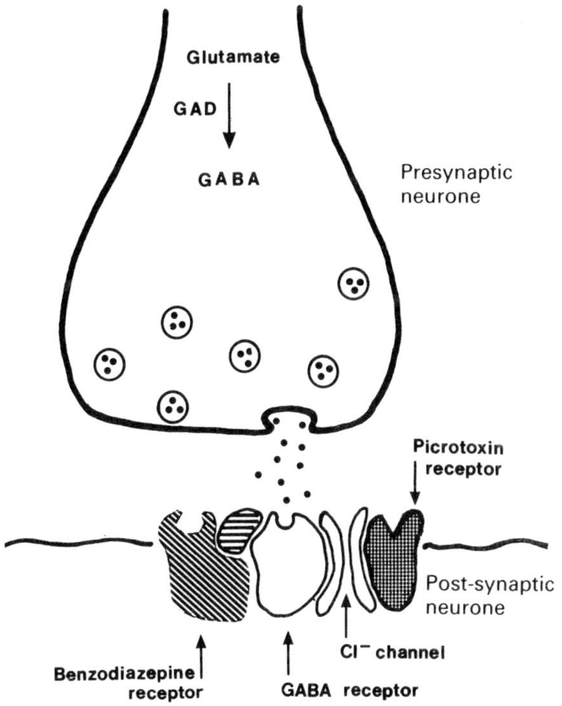

Fig. 7.9 Schematic representation of the GABA receptor, chloride-ionophor complex, benzodiazepine receptor complex.

not share this mode and site of action (e.g. ethosuximide and carbamazepine) others may well interact at the GABA receptor–chloride ionophor site in clinically important, but as yet poorly understood, ways. This increased understanding of the mode of action of anticonvulsant drugs is now leading to clinical testing of a number of new drugs with actions at the GABA receptor.

Relationship of total drug levels to therapeutic effect

Many laboratories offer a routine service for the estimation of commonly used anticonvulsant drugs. They frequently quote therapeutic ranges of serum or plasma concentration (Table 7.15) which are largely arbitrary and have, with the possible exception of phenytoin, little or no basis in controlled clinical studies. Whereas the upper limit of the therapeutic range is easily defined in terms of the appearance of toxic effects (nystagmus, dysarthria, ataxia and drowsiness in the case of phenytoin, barbiturates, carbamazepine), the serum level at which these occur can be very variable. The most consistent relationship between serum level and toxic effects is for phenytoin, but even with this drug many patients may tolerate—and indeed require—serum levels greater than 20 μg/ml for seizure control. For phenobarbitone and carbamazepine there is a wider variation in individual tolerance to serum concentration.

The lower limit to the therapeutic range is extremely difficult to define. It is evident that many patients have their epilepsy controlled by serum levels of anticonvulsants below optimal ranges and it is probably true that there are as many therapeutic ranges of anticonvulsant drugs as there are patients taking them. The major determinant of therapeutic level would appear to be the type and severity of the underlying epilepsy. Certainly, it would be absurd to suggest that a patient presenting at the age of 12 years with three or four primarily generalised tonic-clonic seizures, and who has no neurological disease, requires a serum level of anticonvulsant to control his seizures similar to that of a patient presenting at the age of 40 years with complex partial seizures due to a cerebral glioma!

An unquestioning acceptance of 'therapeutic ranges' can lead to patients who have been satisfactorily controlled on low doses and serum levels having their dose of anticonvulsant needlessly increased, thereby running an increased risk of adverse reactions and, conversely, patients who tolerate (and need) high serum levels having their dose needlessly reduced, thereby running the risk of further seizures. It is therefore of great importance to treat the patients rather than their serum levels!

Table 7.15 'Therapeutic' serum concentrations

Drug	Plasma/serum concentration (μg/ml)
Phenytoin	10–20
Phenobarbitone	15–35
Carbamazepine	4–8
Valproate	50–100
Ethosuximide	40–120

Indications for serum level monitoring

A number of factors will influence the need for anticonvulsant monitoring:

1. Use of phenytoin
2. Polypharmacy
3. In patients in whom assessment of toxicity is difficult
4. In patients with renal/hepatic disease
5. Assessing compliance
6. During controlled studies of anticonvulsants.

It is of particular importance with phenytoin because of the non-linear relationship between dose and serum level and the sensitivity that many patients show to small increments in dosage. It will rarely be necessary in patients receiving monotherapy with other drugs such as phenobarbitone, carbamazepine or valproate. In those patients who require polypharmacy, serum-level monitoring becomes essential and it may be particularly helpful in patients of low intelligence in whom the detection of toxicity presents particular problems.

Prognosis of epilepsy

There is a considerable amount of information concerning the prognosis of epilepsy. However, many problems exist in the interpretation of such data, not least the varying minimum period required as a definition of remission, and the period of follow-up: success in control of seizures is inversely proportional to both these factors. The majority of studies have been hospital based, which has an adverse effect on the outcome as patients with more severe and refractory epilepsy are more likely to be referred to specialist centres. Community-based studies are more informative. Such studies and prospective studies of newly diagnosed epilepsy suggest that long-term remissions occur in 60–70% and that the majority of patients enter remission early.

The majority of hospital-based studies are striking in that remission rates are consistent at between 20% and 30%, despite the fact that they include periods before the advent of modern anticonvulsant therapy.

A number of factors influence the prognosis for remission of seizures:

1. Age of onset
2. Classification of seizures and epilepsy
3. Duration and severity of epilepsy
4. Whether it is symptomatic or idiopathic.

The age of onset of epilepsy is perhaps one of the most important factors: there is general agreement that the onset of seizures within the first year of life (when it is usually symptomatic of cerebral pathology) carries an adverse prognosis. However, apart from this exception, childhood epilepsy is more likely to remit than adult-onset epilepsy. Both partial and generalised epilepsies have a better prognosis if they start before the age of 20.

Whatever the age of onset, the duration of epilepsy prior to treatment and remission is an important prognostic factor. Most patients who achieve remission do so early in the course of treatment; with continuing seizures and the passage of time it becomes progressively less likely that an individual patient will enter remission. Thus, there is a plateau in the number of patients in remission 15–20 years after the onset of epilepsy.

Seizure type is of major importance: remission rates range from approximately 60% for patients with only tonic-clonic seizures to between 20% and 40% in patients with complex partial seizures. The combination of complex partial seizures with secondary generalised tonic-clonic seizures seems to have a particularly adverse prognosis and in such patients it is common to find that, whereas tonic-clonic seizures come under increasingly good control with anticonvulsant therapy, partial seizures remain resistant to drug therapy. Other generalised epilepsies of childhood carry varying prognoses: between 70% and 80% of patients with simple absences (petit mal) are likely to enter remission; complex absences show a lesser remission rate (33–65%) and in patients with the West or Lennox syndromes, remission rates may be as low as 35–50%.

Epilepsy of unknown aetiology has a better prognosis than symptomatic epilepsy. In keeping with this, epilepsy complicated by an associated neuropsychiatric deficit carries an adverse prognosis.

When to stop epileptic drugs

In spite of the fact that the majority of patients with epilepsy will enter prolonged remission, few studies have been undertaken to determine the success of anticonvulsant withdrawal and the factors which identify patients likely to remain seizure free.

The factors which determine the prognosis following drug withdrawal are similar to those which determine the likelihood of remission, with the additional indication that a normal EEG immediately prior to withdrawal carries a good prognosis.

There is agreement that up to 40% of patients who become seizure free for periods of two or more years will relapse when medication is reduced or withdrawn; the risk for patients with childhood-onset epilepsy is probably about half this figure. The risks of relapse decrease rapidly with the passage of time after withdrawal and most recurrences develop either during dosage reduction or within six months of discontinuation. Patients with the onset of epilepsy during childhood, who have suffered a small number of primary generalised seizures, who have no associated neurological or psychiatric handicap and whose EEG is normal at the end of their period of drug therapy, have a high expectation of remission which will be maintained following anticonvulsant withdrawal.

Table 7.16 Stopping antiepileptic drugs

Absolute requirement	Factors in favour	Factors against
Minimum of 2 years fit-free	Childhood epilepsy	Late-onset epilepsy
Patient's informed consent	Idiopathic generalised epilepsy	Partial epilepsy
	Other idiopathic epilepsy	Symptomatic epilepsy
	Short-duration epilepsy	Long duration
	Normal EEG	Abnormal EEG
	Non-driver	Driver

Clinicians are, nevertheless, faced with the problem of advising patients who have been seizure free for long periods whether or not they should attempt anticonvulsant withdrawal (Table 7.16). Inevitably, the patient must be the final arbiter of this decision as the recurrence of seizures may jeopardise his or her work, social life and driving. In the United Kingdom, the Department of Transport suggest that patients with driving licences gained after a period during which they have been seizure free, and who wish to withdraw their anticonvulsants, should discontinue driving for at least six months. Should they experience further seizures they will be banned from driving for a further statutory period (currently 2 years). This provision will in itself often be sufficient to discourage patients with epilepsy from discontinuing their therapy.

Patients with continuing seizures

Patients with partial seizures beginning later in life and symptomatic of cerebral pathology are less likely to become seizure free. In such patients it may be important to define a 'limit' to drug therapy. If an initial drug, in doses increased to those causing dose-related adverse effects, fails to control seizures, then an alternative may be substituted, although dramatic improvement is rare. There is little evidence that adding a second drug is beneficial and this should be avoided wherever possible as polytherapy increases chronic toxic effects. In some instances, mental state and epilepsy may, in fact, improve when polytherapy is reduced. Careful review of a patient is necessary before polytherapy is ever started (Table 7.17).

Table 7.17 Management of patients with continued seizures despite adequate monotherapy

Patients with non-disabling seizures
1. Seizures infrequent
2. Only occurring during sleep or on wakening
3. Minor in their symptomatology

Changes in therapy are rarely justified

Patients with disabling seizures
Are there factors to explain poor response:
1. Known brain disease or damage
2. Partial seizures
3. Poor compliance

If not:
1. Review diagnosis—they may not have epilepsy
2. Consider further investigation—they may have unsuspected cerebral pathology, e.g. tumour
3. Is the drug used appropriate? Differentiate between absence and partial seizures

Only after this consider two drugs for a trial period; revert to monotherapy if unsuccessful

Surgical treatment of epilepsy may be considered in carefully selected patients. Anterior temporal lobectomy in patients with long-standing complex partial epilepsy, resistant to drug therapy, is sometimes successful.

Careful assessment of patients is essential to obtain satisfactory results. In particular, the clinical features of attacks need to be documented and correlated with a focal EEG abnormality, which should be mainly unilateral and ideally non-dominant. In order to localise the focus accurately, sphenoidal recordings and operative electrocorticography are frequently necessary. Assessment should also include CT scanning as the finding of hamartomas, benign tumours and other structural lesions including Ammon's horn sclerosis carry a particularly favourable prognostic significance. Detailed psychomotor assessment of memory and language functions are essential in assessing risks of surgery to the patient.

The results of anterior temporal lobectomy would suggest that, with careful selection of patients, 50–60% either become seizure free or at least have a significant reduction in seizure frequency. Psychiatric disturbance may also improve.

Focal cortical resections of epileptogenic foci in frontal, parietal and occipital areas are less frequently practised; on occasion, however, they may be of value.

Treatment of status epilepticus

Convulsive status epilepticus—the recurrence of seizures without the patient regaining normal consciousness—has a continuing mortality (10%) and morbidity (10%) and represents an acute medical emergency.

Status may occur in patients without a previous history of epilepsy, when it may be due to frontal tumour, abscess, encephalitis or drug abuse; it may also occur in patients with previously diagnosed epilepsy where non-compliance, intercurrent infection and alcohol abuse are usually implicated (see Table 7.18).

A scheme for the management of convulsive status is suggested in Figure 7.10. The first step will be an intravenous bolus of a rapid-acting agent such as diazepam or clonazepam; it is also reasonable to give intravenous phenytoin at this stage to provide a longer-lasting antiepileptic regime. Should this not abort the status, an intravenous infusion of a benzodiazepine or of chlormethiazole should be started at such a rate as to abolish seizures. One drug should be used in adequate dosage: the commonest problem in controlling status is the administration of too many different drugs in too-small doses. The patient should be placed in an ITU, where ventilation can be undertaken if respiration becomes depressed. The importance of the prevention of hypoxia, dehydration and hyperpyrexia cannot be overemphasised as all these factors have a significant effect on outcome.

From the outset, background antiepileptic medication (the patient's usual regime) should be given either intravenously or via a nasogastric tube. Adequate blood levels should be established before the acutely administered short-acting drugs are gradually tailed off.

Table 7.18 Causes of status epilepticus*

	Preceding seizure disorder	No previous seizures
Non-compliance	27	—
Alcohol	11	4
Drug overdose	0	10
Stroke	4	11
Metabolic	3	5
Hypoxia	0	4
Tumour	0	4
Trauma	1	2
Infection	0	4
Unknown	11	4

*In 98 patients. Totals are greater because more than one factor might be present in an individual patient; alcohol abuse occurred with non-compliance in 5 cases (Aminoff & Simon 1980).

COMPLICATIONS IN PATIENTS WITH EPILEPSY

Complications of epilepsy and seizures

It is widely assumed that, as a consequence of epilepsy, patients have lower than the normal IQ. There is, in fact, little objective evidence to substantiate this: the mean IQ in populations of patients with epilepsy approximate to the lower end of the normal range. A small proportion of patients with epilepsy (10–15%) may show severe mental retardation, but in the majority this results from underlying brain pathology, which is responsible for both retardation and epilepsy. In only a few instances where seizures are prolonged, associated with fever and occurring during early childhood, does retardation result from seizures themselves.

Seizures themselves rarely cause death, but epilepsy does carry an increased mortality (approximately three times greater than the expected mortality in any given year): approximately one-quarter of these excess deaths may be due to seizures themselves, particularly status epilepticus; 20% of deaths are related to suicides and approximately 10% may be accidental; 10% may result from previously unsuspected brain tumour. There remains a small number of unexplained deaths that occur each year in patients with epilepsy; it may be that these result from

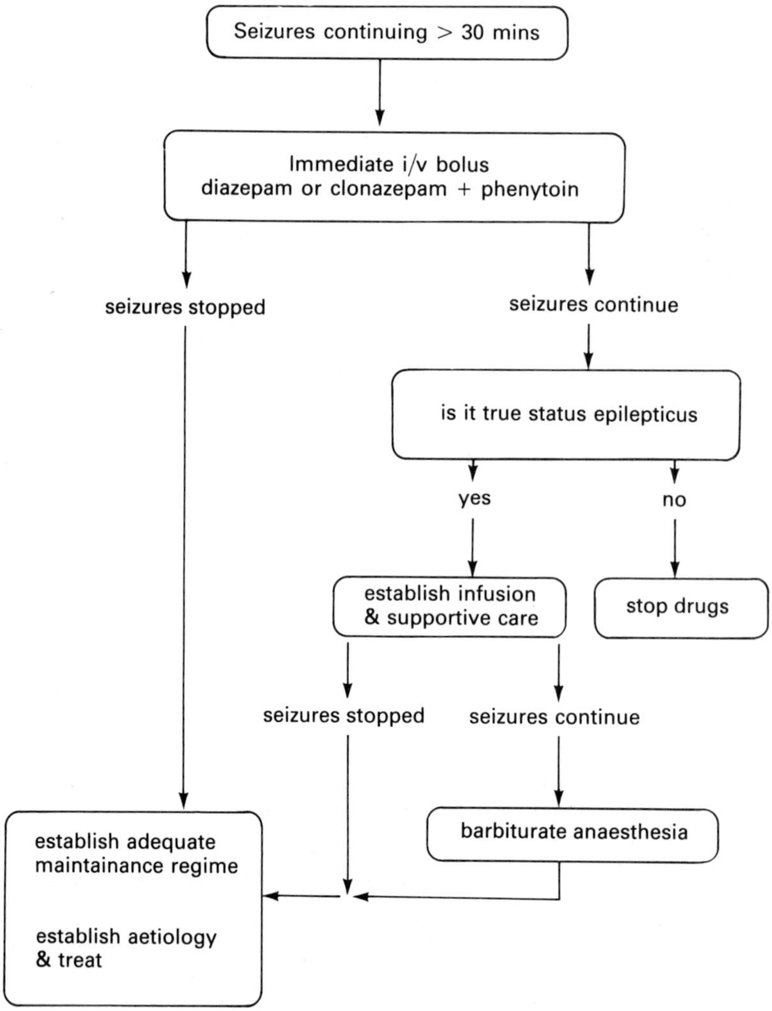

Fig. 7.10 Flow diagram of the management of status epilepticus.

inhalation or cardiac dysrhythmia occurring during a seizure.

Complications of anticonvulsant therapy

Complications of anticonvulsant therapy may be classified into three differing types:

1. Acute dose-related side effects
2. Acute idiosyncratic side effects
3. Chronic toxicity.

Acute dose-related side effects

Anticonvulsants, including phenytoin, carbamazepine, phenobarbitone, primidone and benzodiazepines, give rise to a non-specific encephalopathy associated with high blood concentrations of the drug concerned. Patients initially present with increased tiredness and show a gaze-paretic nystagmus. With increasing serum levels the patients become ataxic, dysarthric, and ultimately confused and drowsy. The syndrome is usually associated with the presence of asterixis. More rarely, patients (particularly those with pre-existing brain damage) may exhibit a variety of involuntary movement disorders including chorea and dystonia. Phenytoin is the drug most likely to be associated with the development of such reactions. On occasion, patients with high serum levels paradoxically may experience an exacerbation of their seizures. Status epilepticus may occur as a result of large overdoses taken with suicidal intent. Valproate does not appear to be associated with a typical anticonvulsant encephalopathy, but patients with high serum levels may exhibit restlessness, and irritability and, at times, a frank confusional state. The cerebellar signs and symptoms associated with other anticonvulsants do not appear to occur with this drug.

While intoxicating concentrations of anticonvulsants are inevitably associated with difficulty with concentration and memory, there is now increasing evidence that many anticonvulsant drugs, even within the therapeutic range of serum concentration, may adversely effect both behaviour in children and cognitive function. These effects seem to be greatest with phenytoin and barbiturate drugs, and are less marked with newer drugs such as carbamazepine and valproate.

Acute idiosyncratic side effects

The commonest acute idiosyncratic reaction to anticonvulsant drugs is a *maculopapular exanthematous eruption*, which usually occurs within a month of initiating treatment. Such reactions are most commonly seen with phenytoin (incidence up to 10%) and carbamazepine (incidence up to 15%). High initial serum concentrations of these anticonvulsants may increase the risk of such skin eruptions. More rarely, more severe skin eruptions may occur which include exfoliative dermatitis and the Stevens–Johnson syndrome.

Aplastic anaemia occurs very rarely with most anticonvulsant drugs, but has attracted particular attention in the case of carbamazepine. In fact, the association between carbamazepine and aplastic anaemia in patients with epilepsy remains extremely rare and most of the initial reports were related to use of the drug in elderly patients who were suffering from trigeminal neuralgia. Aplastic anaemia has also been reported with phenytoin, ethosuximide and primidone.

An *acute hepatitis* may occur with a number of anticonvulsant drugs. It is usually associated with fever, lymphadenopathy and skin eruption and has been recorded as occurring with phenytoin, trimethadione and phenobarbitone. The changes are usually reversible on withdrawal of the offending drug, but occasional fatalities do occur.

Particular concern has arisen because of reports of fatal cases of *acute liver failure* in association with valproate treatment. Some 40 or more cases have now been reported with many puzzling features. The syndrome is usually somewhat delayed and occurs most frequently after 3–6 months' treatment. It is restricted to younger patients and occurs almost exclusively in children below the age of 2. Most patients have been taking multiple anticonvulsant drugs, of which valproate is one. There has been a high incidence in patients with the Lennox–Gastaut syndrome or other neurological handicaps. Differing syndromes occur and include a syndrome of acute hepatic failure as well as, on occasions, a Reye-like syndrome. In some instances a pre-existing underlying metabolic abnormality may be responsible.

Chronic anticonvulsant toxicity

As a chronic (in many patients, lifelong) condition, epilepsy is unusual in that drug treatment may be necessary for several decades of a patient's life. Over the years, a wide range of chronic toxic effects of anticonvulsants have been recognised. Usually these effects are subtle, but on occasions they may become clinically important. It seems that the incidence of chronic toxicity is likely to increase with increasing doses of anticonvulsants and with multiple drug therapy. Indeed, because of the common practice of treating epileptic patients with multiple drugs, it is at times difficult to attribute a given symptom of toxicity to any one specific drug. The chronic toxic side effects of anticonvulsants are summarised in Table 7.19.

Nervous system. An unusual syndrome of pseudodementia, declining cognitive function and increasingly frequent seizures may be seen in younger mentally retarded patients receiving phenytoin. These patients usually have intoxicating serum concentrations of the drug.

It has long been recognised that there is a high incidence of cerebellar atrophy at postmortem in epileptic patients. Histologically this is associated with loss of Purkinje cells.

A mild, mainly sensory neuropathy, usually with loss of lower-limb reflexes, may occur in up to 10% of patients receiving phenytoin over long periods. Usually such patients are receiving other anticonvulsant drugs.

Table 7.19 Chronic toxicity of anticonvulsants

Nervous system	
	Memory and cognitive impairment
	Hyperactivity and behavioural disturbance
	Pseudodementia
	Cerebellar atrophy
	Peripheral neuropathy
Skin	
	Acne
	Hirsutism
	Alopecia
	Chloasma
Liver	
	Enzyme induction
Blood	
	Megaloblastic anaemia
	Thrombocytopenia
	Lymphoma
Immune system	
	IgA deficiency
	Drug-induced SLE
Endocrine system	
	Decreased thyroxine levels
	Increased cortisol and sex hormone metabolism
Bone	
	Osteomalacia
Connective tissue	
	Gum hypertrophy
	Coarsened facial features
	Duphytren's contracture
Pregnancy	
	Obstetric complications
	Teratogenicity
	Fetal hydantoin syndrome

A variety of behavioural changes may be seen with anticonvulsant drugs: in particular, phenobarbitone is well recognised to cause a syndrome of hyperactivity and behavioural disturbance in children.

Skin disorders. Acne and hirsutism are commonly seen following treatment with phenytoin and possibly also with barbiturates. These effects are so troublesome that it would seem unreasonable to treat young girls with phenytoin if this can be avoided in any way. Valproate may on occasion be associated with alopecia, which is usually temporary even when the drug is continued.

Hepatic metabolism. Some clinical changes in enzymes occur very commonly in anticonvulsant-treated patients. Gamma-glutamyl-transpeptidase may be increased in a high percentage of patients, but the incidence of changes in plasma alkaline phosphatase and aspartate transaminase levels are less frequently seen.

Many anticonvulsant drugs (most notably phenytoin, carbamazepine, and barbiturates) are potent liver-enzyme inducers. This increased microsomal liver enzyme activity may contribute to many other aspects of chronic anticonvulsant toxicity.

Haematological disorders. There is a well-documented trend for mean cell volume to rise following the initiation of anticonvulsant treatment, usually with phenytoin. Frank folate deficiency may develop and lead to a megaloblastic anaemia. The manner in which phenytoin leads to folate deficiency remains uncertain, but enzyme induction may be important. Sodium valproate may occasionally be associated with a thrombocytopenia, which (very rarely) may result in bleeding disorders in children.

There is an increased incidence of lymphoma in patients treated for epilepsy, which may be two to three times the expected incidence.

Endocrine system. It is well recognised that anticonvulsant-treated patients have lowered plasma thyroxine levels. This fact is not clinically significant and, like the increased excretion of steroid metabolites in epileptic patients, is probably due to hepatic enzyme induction. The latter has clinical significance in causing an increased incidence of breakthrough bleeding and contraceptive failure in anticonvulsant-treated patients taking oral contraceptive preparations. Increased metabolism of vitamin D is probably responsible for anticonvulsant-induced osteomalacia which is sometimes seen in patients with severe epilepsy.

Connective tissue changes. Gum hypertrophy may occur in up to 50% of patients treated with phenytoin and is exacerbated by poor dental hygiene. Many epileptic patients, usually those with severe epilepsy and receiving multiple drugs, develop coarsened facial features with thickening of the lips, widened nose and thickening of subcutaneous facial tissue. Many of these changes may be drug related, but a similar epileptic facies was also documented before the advent of modern anticonvulsant therapy.

Disorders of pregnancy. Studies show that epileptic women suffer a higher rate of obstetric complications including antepartum haemorrhage, premature labour and a higher rate of caesarian sections. The children of epileptic mothers tend to have lower birth weights and smaller head circumference than that expected.

Children of epileptic mothers show an increased rate of major fetal abnormality (between two and three times the expected rate). These most commonly take the form of hare lip, cleft palate abnormalities and cardiovascular anomalies, usually associated with phenytoin and older anticonvulsant drugs. A milder pattern of fetal abnormality has been associated particularly with phenytoin treatment during pregnancy: this includes facial abnormalities with hypertelorism, flattened bridge to the nose and epicanthic folds with low-set ears and wide mouth. These changes may be associated with a retarded growth and a degree of mental retardation. Recently it has been suggested that valproate is associated with an increased incidence of spina bifida abnormalities (approximately 1–2% of pregnancies, 2–3 times the expected rate).

Although the increased incidence of these complications in pregnancy is partly related to drug treatment, other factors are almost certainly involved: these include genetic associations between epilepsy and fetal abnormalities, as well as complications to the pregnancy and the child resulting from seizures during pregnancy. For this reason, while it is sensible to withdraw anticonvulsant therapy before a pregnancy in women with prolonged remissions in their epilepsy, most patients who are clearly dependent on anticonvulsant drugs to control their epilepsy should be maintained on anticonvulsant therapy during their pregnancy. It is, however, prudent to avoid using trimethadione, which has been associated with a particularly high incidence of fetal malformation. In the case of valproate, screening for spina bifida with ultrasound, amniocentesis and α-fetoprotein estimation should be undertaken at an early stage of pregnancy. A plan for the management of the pregnant epileptic patient is presented in Table 7.20.

Table 7.20 Management of the pregnant epileptic patient

Before pregnancy
1. Consider drug withdrawal where remission > 2 years
2. Reduce polypharmacy wherever possible
3. Avoid use of: trimethadione (risk of multiple congenital defects), phenytoin (cleft palate and hare-lip, cardiac anomalies)
4. If possible use carbamazepine alone (or, where necessary for idiopathic generalised epilepsies, valproate)

During pregnancy
1. Screen pregnancies on valproate for neural tube defects by 16 weeks
2. Ensure folate supplements are given
3. Monitor blood drug levels during last trimester when they may fall and increased dosage may be necessary
4. Epilepsy may become worse in approximately 25% of patients, improve in 25% and remain unchanged in the rest

After delivery
1. Check blood levels in puerperium and readjust dosage as necessary
2. Consider administration of vitamin K to child at delivery
3. Reassure about breast feeding and drugs

NON-EPILEPTIC CAUSES OF ALTERED CONSCIOUSNESS

The diagnosis of epilepsy has such profound implications for the social outlook of patients and for treatment that in every case the diagnosis must be definite. In particular, epilepsy must be differentiated from a variety of other causes of loss of consciousness. This presents problems because of the wide variety of clinical manifestations of epilepsy. The major syndromes to be differentiated from epilepsy include syncope, hypoglycaemia, transient cerebral ischaemia, transient global amnesia and a variety of psychiatric disturbances which include hyperventilation syndrome, rage outbursts and pseudoseizures.

The difficulty in correctly diagnosing epilepsy is emphasised by the significant numbers of patients with apparently resistant epilepsy, admitted for intense investigation either to neurological or to specialist epilepsy centres, and in whom a diagnosis of epilepsy is eventually refuted. Thus, if doubt remains about the diagnosis, a label of epilepsy should not be attached: the term 'known epileptic' is to be avoided at all costs. Furthermore, because of the excellent response of epileptic disorders starting in adolescence or adult life, continuation of apparent seizures in spite of adequate anticonvulsant treatment should either stimulate the search for a structural cause for the epilepsy or, perhaps more importantly, lead to a questioning of the original diagnosis (Table 7.17).

SYNCOPE AND FAINTNESS

The physiological basis of fainting is a sudden hypotension and cerebral hypoperfusion associated with vasodilatation in muscle and in central organs, which leads to a sudden fall in blood pressure.

Syncope may occur in a number of circumstances (see Table 7.21). It is associated with characteristic premonitory symptoms, which include a feeling of lightheadedness, blurred vision (becoming monochrome), vertigo, tinnitus and a feeling of detachment. The patient may feel the blood draining away from his face and may feel cold and begin to sweat. If the patient does not heed these warning symptoms and either put his head between his knees or lie down, unconsciousness may occur with the patient slumping to the ground in a flaccid state. Consciousness returns within a few seconds, but the patient is pale, sweaty and may be nauseated. Occasionally one or two convulsive jerks may occur and rarely there may be urinary incontinence. There is no postictal confusion and the patient is frequently able to proceed with his normal business within a very short period.

The major criteria for differentiating between syncope and seizure disorders are summarised in Table 7.22. Particular problems may arise in patients with temporal lobe epilepsy who may experience quite profound autonomic disturbances during their seizures, and in patients who faint but who are maintained in an upright position,

Table 7.21 Causes of syncope

Reflex syncope
- Postural
- 'Psychogenic'
- Micturition syncope
- Cough syncope
- Valsalva
- Carotid sinus sensitivity

Cardiac syncope
- Dysrhythmias (heart block, tachycardias, etc.)
- Valvular disease (particularly aortic stenosis)
- Cardiomyopathies
- Shunts

Perfusion failure
- Hypovolaemia
- Syndromes of autonomic failure

Table 7.22 Factors differentiating between syncope and seizures

	Syncope	Seizures
Posture	Upright	Any posture
Pallor and sweating	Invariable	Uncommon
Onset	Gradual	Sudden/aura
Injury	Rare	Not uncommon
Convulsive jerks	Rare	Common
Incontinence	Rare	Common
Unconsciousness	Seconds	Minutes
Recovery	Rapid	Often slow
Postictal confusion	Rare	Common
Frequency	Infrequent	May be frequent
Precipitating factors	Crowded places Lack of food Unpleasant circumstances	Rare

either by their surroundings, e.g. in a toilet, or by enthusiastic ill-informed bystanders. Under these circumstances cerebral perfusion may be diminished for a sufficient period to cause a generalised seizure secondary to anoxia.

Although syncope most commonly occurs in normal subjects as a psychogenic reflex in unpleasant or painful circumstances, or as a response to standing in hot or crowded surroundings, it may also be a symptom of pathological significance. Syncope may occur in response to pressure on the particularly sensitive carotid sinus that is sometimes seen in elderly patients with atheromatous disease of the carotid bifurcation. This form of carotid sinus syncope is said to be associated in particular with the wearing of tight collars and may be induced by changes in head posture.

Micturition syncope occurs often in elderly men who rise during the night to micturate. It is probably a mainly postural response which may, however, be exacerbated by the effect of straining leading to a rise in intrathoracic pressure and thereby reducing venous return to the heart. Attacks may be prevented by advising the patient to sit while micturating. Similarly, a rise in intrathoracic pressure associated with a prolonged paroxysmal bout of coughing may be sufficient to cause syncope in some patients.

In some circumstances syncope may occur with cardiac dysrhythmias, structural heart disease, or autonomic paresis (see p. 88). As convulsion may occur due to cerebral hypoxia consequent on cerebral dysrhythmias, seizures beginning in late adult life may require cardiological investigation. In some series up to 20% of patients referred with a primary diagnosis of epilepsy to a neurological clinic had major dysrhythmias during the course of 24 hours ambulatory monitoring of the ECG.

PSYCHIATRIC DISTURBANCES RESULTING IN ALTERED CONSCIOUSNESS

Hyperventilation syndrome

This common accompaniment of anxiety states is probably greatly underdiagnosed. The classic symptoms are of difficulty in breathing associated with paraesthesiae and occasionally frank carpopedal spasm. Less specific feelings of dizziness, blurred vision, palpitation, weakness and fatigue may also be described. The basis for these symptoms is hypocapnoea, which can be reversed by asking the patient to rebreathe into a paper bag placed over the nose and mouth.

Rage outbursts

It is widely, and probably erroneously, believed that epilepsy is associated with increased tendency to violence. In recent years this has led to a questioning of whether violent behaviour per se can occur as a direct result of epileptic cerebral dysrhythmias, and, in its most extreme form, has led to the suggestion that patients with episodic outbursts of rage (episodic dyscontrol) may be suffering from an epileptic equivalent. There is no clear EEG evidence to support this theory and the rarity with which epilepsy is associated with major crimes of violence is a strong argument against this hypothesis. Although rage outbursts have been treated with anticonvulsant drugs with occasional success, this should not be viewed as a strong argument that such outbursts have an epileptogenic basis.

Pseudoseizures

The occurrence of pseudoseizures as an hysterical conversion symptom has a well-founded history which was emphasised by Charcot's demonstrations of hysteroepilepsy. Differentiation of feigned (pseudoseizures) from genuine seizures still represents particular difficulties as, not infrequently, both genuine and pseudoseizures may occur side by side in an individual patient.

Most commonly, pseudoseizures attempt to mimic a generalised tonic-clonic seizure. Pseudoseizures differ from genuine tonic-clonic seizures in that the pattern of the attack is much more variable, tends to be much more frequent, occurring up to many times a day, and is often precipitated by emotional disturbances. They usually occur in the presence of observers; any aura tends to lack the stereotyped nature of the true epileptic aura. The convulsion itself tends to comprise more random struggling and thrashing movements than a typical tonic-clonic seizure and, although tongue biting, incontinence and injury are rare in hysterical seizures, they occur occasionally. The attacks tend to be longer lasting than genuine tonic-clonic seizures and no pupillary dilatation or extensor plantar response is seen. Pseudoseizures most commonly occur in patients with a pre-existing psychiatric history: there is a high incidence of preceding depression and suicidal attempts. On occasions, hysterical seizures may be so frequent as to mimic status epilepticus and to provoke an inappropriate therapeutic response.

A number of investigations may be helpful in differentiating pseudoseizures from true seizures. Standard EEGs may occasionally capture a pseudoseizure; 24-hour ambulatory monitoring and telemetry is more likely to be successful. While the EEG may be obscured by muscle artefact during an apparent tonic-clonic seizure, no postictal slowing is seen following a pseudoseizure. Serum prolactin levels may rise 1–2 hours after a true tonic-clonic seizure, but not after a feigned seizure.

Although all these rules should suffice to differentiate between feigned convulsive seizures and tonic-clonic seizures, particular problems still occur in the differentiation of pseudoseizures from complex partial seizures.

TRANSIENT GLOBAL AMNESIA (TGA)

This is a rare but striking syndrome occurring in middle-aged to elderly patients who develop sudden amnesia. They are obviously bewildered, typically asking questions about their circumstances: 'Where am I, what should I be doing?', over and over again. Normal memory function returns from a few minutes up to several hours later and the patient has no subsequent recall for the period of amnesia. Most patients suffer only a single attack but up to 20% of patients may have recurrent episodes.

There is considerable debate about the pathophysiology of this condition. Undoubtedly, typical TGA syndromes can occur with patients who have temporal lobe seizures, when there may be some symptomatology to suggest this, the patient complaining of olfactory hallucination or some other similar symptom; however, such patients are rare and it is much more common to assume a cerebrovascular basis for TGA. It is most likely that they occur as a result of posterior circulation ischaemia to the medial temporal lobes, but in spite of this the risk of future stroke seems low (approximately 5%).

Transient global amnesia should be differentiated from alcoholic 'blackouts' (which are periods of amnesia occurring in patients during the course of heavy bouts of drinking) and from hysterical fugue states in which both short- and long-term memory is apparently impaired, the amnesia is long lasting, the patient apparently calm and relatively unconcerned and in which the return of memory is sudden rather than gradual.

HYPOGLYCAEMIA

Hypoglycaemia and associated neuroglypenia gives rise to striking symptomatology: patients become confused as blood sugar falls and they have associated pallor, sweating and tachycardia. Subsequent coma may occur, with seizures which are usually generalised but on occasions may be focal.

Symptoms of hypoglycaemia occur most commonly in diabetics due to relative overdosage of either insulin or oral hypoglycaemics and more rarely, in patients with insulinomas. In the latter instance up to 10% may be malignant and up to 20% may have multiple endocrine adenomas. The diagnosis is particularly suggested by confusional episodes and seizures occurring during the night or early hours of the morning, or when meals are missed or delayed.

Prolonged fasting of up to 72 hours may be necessary in order to provoke attacks of hypoglycaemia, but the diagnosis of insulinoma can satisfactorily be made on finding the appropriate clinical symptoms of hypoglycaemia in association with low blood sugar which is reversible on administration of glucose.

SLEEP

NORMAL SLEEP

Sleep does not represent a uniform state and descriptions and classification of sleep have been conventionally based on EEG recordings. While the subject is awake with the eyes closed, the EEG is usually dominated by an alpha rhythm, maximal posteriorly at 8–11 cycles per second.

Stage 1 Sleep

As the patient becomes drowsy the EEG becomes of lower voltage with more mixed frequencies and shows a loss of alpha rhythm.

Stage 2 Sleep

The overall background activity remains similar to stage 1 sleep, but in addition there are bursts of higher-frequency activity (12–16 cycles per second) known as sleep spindles with, in addition, occasional higher-amplitude slow-wave complexes (K complexes).

Stages 3 and 4

During these stages there is increasing high-amplitude slow-wave activity in the frequency range of 1–3 cycles per second.

REM sleep

This stage of sleep is characterised by rapid eye movements (REM) but otherwise total muscular relaxation. The EEG becomes of much lower voltage and higher frequency and has many characteristics similar to the EEG seen in the awake subject.

The normal adult passes in sequence through stages 1, 2, 3 and 4 of non-REM (NREM) sleep and after 1 to $1\frac{1}{2}$ hours may enter the first period of REM sleep, usually preceded by a shift from the stage 4 to the stage 2 EEG pattern. Further similar, usually longer-lasting, periods of REM sleep may occur three or four times during the course of a night. In the newborn, approximately 50% of sleeping time is spent in REM sleep, but this proportion falls progressively with increasing age so that the young adult spends 20–25% of sleeping time in REM sleep, but over the age of 70 little or no REM sleep occurs.

Dreaming is closely associated with REM sleep and dreams may be recalled if the subject is either awakened, or awakes spontaneously from REM sleep.

A variety of *movements* may occur during normal sleeping. Gross body movements and changing in position may occur during any stage of sleep, but frequency is maximal during the transition between REM and NREM sleep. REM sleep is characterised by absence of major limb muscle activity, by rapid eye movements and by small-amplitude distal twitching and trembling of the limbs. As subjects enter the twilight state of drowsiness between being fully awake and fully asleep, body *jerks* may occur leading to arousal. These are often associated with a sensation of falling and involve a flexion of one or both legs and sometimes the trunk; on occasion they may occur in response to some external stimulus. These 'starts' have been referred to as *nocturnal myoclonus* and have, it has been suggested, been related to an epileptic phenomenon; this is erroneous. Other movements termed '*slow periodic movements of sleep*' are slower and characterised by repetitive flexor or extensor movements of the legs, occurring once or twice a minute.

There can be no doubt that sleeping is an important and necessary part of the sleep–waking cycle. Deprivation of sleep for periods over 60 hours lead to increasing fatigue, irritability and difficulty in concentration. Sensory hallucinations may occur and, in extreme circumstances, psychosis may be provoked. Deprivation of REM sleep tends to lead to hyperactivity and impulsiveness, whereas deprivation of NREM sleep instead leads to hyporesponsiveness and excessive sleepiness.

Recovery from prolonged sleep deprivation shows that initial sleep largely consists of stage 4 sleep to the exclusion of REM sleep; however, subsequent sleeping contains a proportionate excess of REM sleep.

Sleep requirements are markedly age dependent: the newborn child sleeps during both day and night, while the adult will usually sleep for approximately 7 hours; in old age the sleep requirement may be further reduced.

DISORDERS OF SLEEP

These are summarised in Table 7.23.

Insomnia

Subjects differ in their expectations of what is a normal amount of sleep and, indeed, some subjects appear to need only as little as 3 or 4 hours sleep a night. However, insomnia is a major source of complaint, although when it occurs it is usually a result of other disturbances rather than a disorder of sleep itself.

Secondary insomnia is most commonly seen in patients with anxiety or depression. The anxious patient complains of difficulty in getting to sleep, with frequent waking during the course of sleep.

Table 7.23 Disorders of sleep

Insomnia
Anxiety and depression
Pain syndromes (carpal tunnel syndrome, rest pain)
Sleep apnoea
Hypersomnia
Primary
Narcoleptic syndrome
Kleine–Levin syndrome
Secondary
Metabolic encephalopathy
Intracranial mass lesions
Sleep apnoea
Others
Sleep walking
Enuresis

In contrast, the depressed patient complains of early morning waking with inability to return to sleep; frequently these two problems can be combined in an individual patient. When those normal movements associated with sleep occur with increased frequency, these may also cause arousal and interruption of sleep. Similarly, the restless leg syndrome may be important in delaying the onset of sleep. A variety of pain syndromes such as the carpal tunnel syndrome, migraine, and cluster headache, may also characteristically interrupt sleep. Insomnia may also be a symptom of obstructive sleep apnoeas.

It must be remembered that many individuals tend to exaggerate the amount of time they lose from their normal sleeping.

Treatment of insomnia should always be directed at the underlying cause for the insomnia. Hypnotic agents are overprescribed and widely abused.

Syndromes of hypersomnia

Hypersomnia is an important part of the drowsiness and confusion that characterise altered states of awareness. While all cerebral mass lesions may lead to obtundation and increased daytime sleepiness, it does appear that tumours of the posterior hypothalamus and midbrain are likely to lead to hypersomnolence. Hypersomnia may also occur in trypanosomiasis and historically formed an important part of the syndrome of encephalitis lethargica.

Sleep apnoea may be complicated by daytime hypersomnia. Sleep apnoea is most commonly obstructive and frequently seen in the obese 'Pickwickian syndrome'; however, it may also occur in patients of normal stature. Subjects exhibit episodes of respiratory arrest lasting up to 1–2 minutes at a time, though usually briefer and occurring many times during sleep. These apnoeic periods may be associated with upper airways obstruction and with cessation of diaphragmatic movements and snoring. It may be that sleep loss due to subsequent arousal is sufficient to cause daytime somnolence. In severe cases tracheostomy may be necessary to reverse the hypersomnia and also to prevent the development of pulmonary and systemic hypertension. Daytime sleepiness may also be a symptom of central sleep apnoeas, though this is less common.

The *narcoleptic syndrome* probably represents the most common cause of hypersomnia: it is characterised by the association of *narcolepsy, cataplexy, sleep paralysis* and *hypnogogic hallucinations*. Symptoms do not usually start before adolescence or early adult life and narcolepsy is usually the major presenting symptom. Subjects experience an overwhelming desire to sleep during the course of the day, but such sleep rarely lasts longer than 20 minutes at a time. Most patients with such symptoms will usually admit to some form of cataplexy, a loss of postural tone caused by laughter, excitement or emotion during which the patient may fall to their knees with, however, no impairment of consciousness. Sleep paralysis consists of brief periods of inability to move (not, however, affecting respiration), either during the period of falling asleep or, perhaps more commonly, on awaking. Hypnogogic hallucinations represent particularly vivid dreamlike hallucinations, often occurring in association with narcolepsy or an episode of sleep paralysis.

The narcoleptic syndrome is never associated with structural cerebral disease and it appears to be a functional sleep disturbance with a very strong association with the HLA-DR2 group. Narcoleptic episodes bear a very close similarity electroencephalographically to periods of REM sleep and hypnogogic hallucinations may be viewed as a dreaming phenomenon. Cataplexy and sleep paralysis may have a basis in anterior horn cell inhibition that occurs during normal sleeping.

Treatment of the narcoleptic syndrome is unsatisfactory. Narcolepsy itself may be benefited by stimulant drugs such as dextro- and laevo-amphetamine and methylphenidate. Tricyclic drugs such as imipramine and chlorimipramine may be effective in suppressing cataplexy when it becomes frequent.

Hypersomnia occurs as part of the rare *Kleine–Levin syndrome*. In this condition subjects exhibit periods of several days at a time when they have prolonged sleeping with awakening for periods which are associated with increased appetite and libido. The condition is most commonly seen in young adult males and the basis is uncertain.

Miscellaneous sleep disorders

Sleep walking is a phenomenon that is largely restricted to children, occurring most usually during stage 3 or 4 sleep. Occasionally, patients may arise and walk, usually with eyes open, most commonly avoiding familiar objects in their path; they may verbalise and repeat phrases over and over or exhibit repetitive acts. They can usually be led back to bed and will return to sleep with no memory of the incident. Sleep automatism may be a closely related phenomenon occurring in adults, and occurs when half-roused subjects exhibit some brief automatic behaviour with subsequent incomplete recall for this. Parents of children can be reassured that the disorder rarely, if ever, persists into adult life.

Enuresis is a disorder of childhood and adult life is discussed in Chapter 4.

FURTHER READING

Aminoff M J , Simon R P 1980 Status epilepticus: causes, clinical features and consequences in 98 patients. American Journal of Medicine 69: 657–666

Chadwick D, Reynolds E H 1985 When do epileptic patients need treatment? Starting and stopping medication. British Medical Journal 290: 1885–1888

Currie S, Heathfield K W G, Henson R A, Scott D F 1971 Clinical course and prognosis of temporal lobe epilepsy. Brain 94: 173–190

Hauser W A, Kurland L T 1975 The epidemiology of epilepsy in Rochester, Minnesota, 1935 through 1967. Epilepsia 16: 1–66

Juul-Jensen P, Foldspang A 1983 Natural history of epileptic seizures. Epilepsia 24: 297–312

Maugierre F, Courjon J 1978 Somatosensory seizures. Brain 101: 307–332

Rocca W A, Sharbrough F W, Hauser W A, Annegers J F, Schoenberg B S 1987 Risk factors for complex partial seizures: A population-based case-control study. Annals of Neurology 21: 22–31

Schmidt D 1982 Adverse effects of antiepileptic drugs. Raven Press, New York

8

Pain and headache

INTRODUCTION

The symptom of pain is probably the main reason for the existence of medicine and doctors. All pain has two components: the direct effect of some stimulus on nerve endings and the resulting transmission of impulses to the cerebrum, and the quality of pain, which is an attitude of mind embracing the fears and interpretations of the pain by the patient. It is recognised that the appreciation of pain varies from person to person and the sensation which might be an irritation to some may to others be an unbearable pain. Thus the clinical reaction to pain will vary and an understanding of those factors which may modify these reactions is important to the physician.

ANATOMY AND PHYSIOLOGY

Many of the factors involved in the transmission of the sensation of pain from the periphery to the cerebrum have already been dealt with in the section on sensory function (Ch. 2). Only those factors which are specifically important in the transmission of the painful impulse will be described in this section.

FIRST ORDER NEURONE

The sensation of pain is not appreciated in specific sensory receptors but rather by bare nerve endings in the skin and other organs. These nerve endings are of sensory neurones of the C (0.3–1.5 μm diameter) or A (1.0–5 μm diameter) type. The cell bodies of these neurones lie in the dorsal root ganglion and the central projections of the afferent neurones enter the dorsal root of the spinal cord to gain access to the dorsal horn. Whether there are specific pain fibres, or pain is merely recognised as a pattern of impulses, is uncertain. It is suggested in the 'gate theory' that cells in the substantia gelatinosa determine whether or not there is onward conduction of the original sensory input to the cord and that such transmission is facilitated (that is the gate is opened) by activity in the small C fibres and inhibited (that is the gate is closed) by activity in the A afferents (Fig. 8.1). The sum of the effects of the various fibres then determines whether the second-order sensory

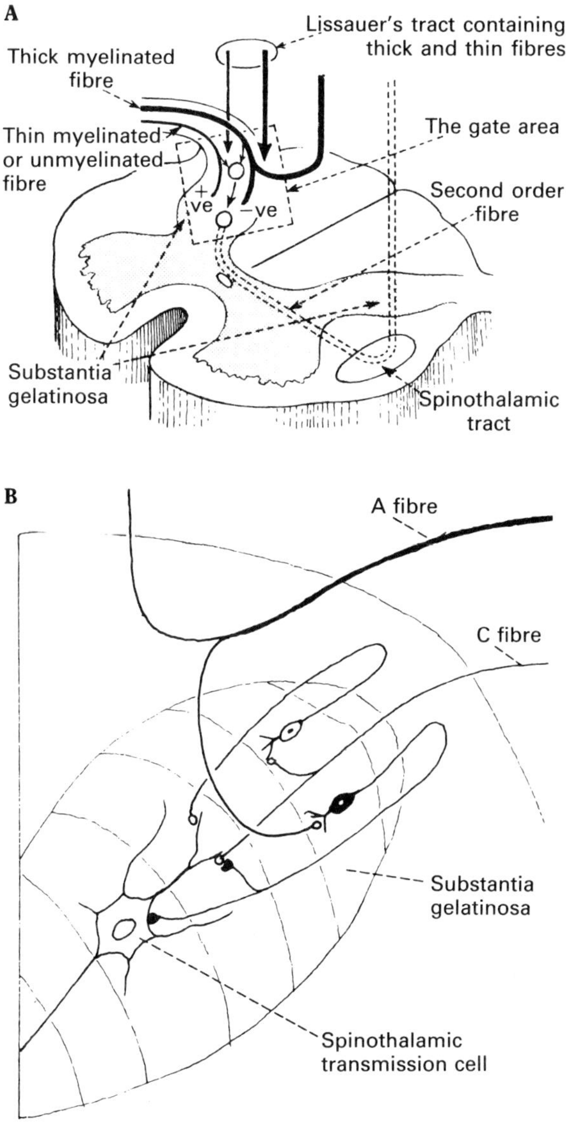

Fig. 8.1 **A** Cross-section of spinal cord showing the 'gate theory' connections of thick myelinated and thin myelinated or unmyelinated fibres. (Reproduced from Lindsay K W, Bone I, Callander R 1986 *Neurology and Neurosurgery Illustrated*, Churchill Livingstone, Edinburgh.) **B** Excitatory (clear) and inhibitory (black) neurones of the substantia gelatinosa in the gate control theory.

neurone in the substantia gelatinosa conducts the original impulse to the thalamus via the contralateral spinothalamic tract. Although the physiology suggested in the gate theory has not been confirmed, the idea of organisation at a spinal level is not novel in the animal kingdom and seems a reasonable way to explain the phenomenon of hyperpathia (excessive painful feelings) either by continuing activity of the C fibres or by a selective reduction in the firing of the A fibres. It also explains why apparently unrelated stimuli such as vibration (transmitted by A fibres) can reduce the sensation of pain and may explain the phenomenon of referred pain.

The dermatomal representation of pain is identical to that for other somatic sensations and is described on p. 27.

SECOND ORDER NEURONE

Whatever the precise organisation of fibres at the dorsal root entry zone and in the dorsal horn, the fibres subserving the sensations of pain synapse with secondary neurones in the dorsal horn and the axons of these neurones cross within a few segments of the cord in the anterior spinal commissure to lie in the contralateral anterolateral spinothalamic tract. There is layering within this tract such that the fibres ascending from the sacral segment lie most superficially and those from the more rostral levels lie more medially in the tract (Fig. 8.2). Although some of these second order sensory neurones in the spinothalamic tract may

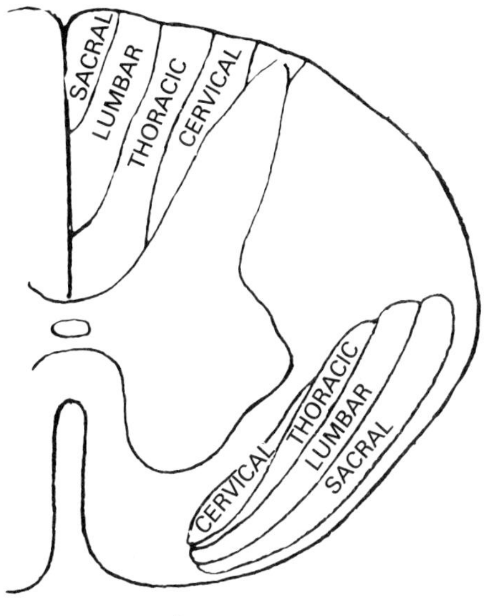

Fig. 8.2 Cross-section of the spinal cord showing layering of fibres in the anterolateral spinothalamic pathway.

relay in nuclei in the brain stem and project to the cerebellum, the great majority concerned with pain enter the nucleus ventralis posterolateralis and intralaminar nuclei of the thalamus where the second synapse occurs.

THIRD ORDER NEURONE

The appreciation of pain is almost certainly at the level of the posterior thalamus where there is the synapse between the second- and third-order sensory neurones. However, precise localisation of painful stimuli depends upon an intact cortex, which is the destination of the third-order sensory neurone travelling from the posterior thalamus to the postcentral gyrus in the parietal lobe. Thus the crude sensation of pain may be appreciated in the thalamus, but its interpretation and localisation, together with that of other relevant sensory information, occurs in the parietal lobe which is necessary for precise localisation of the site of pain.

NEUROTRANSMITTERS

The stimuli which are appreciated as pain vary from site to site. Thus in the skin any cause of trauma or destruction of tissue, be it cutting, stretching, pinching or burning, is likely to cause pain, whereas in the intestine and deeper structures, stretching is a much more effective painful stimulus. When tissues are damaged the pain is believed to be caused by the release of proteolytic enzymes which liberate kinins, irritating to the free nerve endings. More central neurotransmission of pain sensation probably involves the neurotransmitter substance 'P' which is found in high concentrations at the free nerve endings and also at the posterior horn of the spinal cord. Substance P appears to be the excitatory neurotransmitter of the pain system in the spinal cord and diencephalon; the inhibitory neurotransmitter appears to be an endogenous opiate-like compound or endorphin. The concentration of these two agents within the spinal cord and brain is known to vary in response to a variety of different stimuli and might explain why the phenomenon of pain varies so much from patient to patient and even in one individual from time to time. This variation may be explained by an alteration in the levels of different neurotransmitters.

THE CLINICAL ASSESSMENT OF PAIN

The absence of an objective physical sign of pain means that the assessment of pain is subjective and depends solely upon obtaining an adequate history from the patient. Different patients will describe pains in different ways and be troubled to a greater or lesser extent by them. The reaction to pain is undoubtedly affected by personality and the physician is entirely reliant upon the patient for accurate information about the nature and severity of the pain. Those factors which are invariably important in the history are the site and radiation of the pain, its character, severity and periodicity. In addition it is important to ascertain which factors alleviate or exacerbate the pain. This information is vital in taking a history about pain in any part of the body and may lead the physician towards an accurate diagnosis. From the patient's description it should be possible to recognise a particular variety of pain which may then help to localise the underlying pathology both in site and nature.

LOCAL PAIN

Local pain may be caused by any pathological process which irritates sensory nerve endings. Pain from the skin or a joint is usually well localised and either sharp or burning in character. Those structures which contain no pain fibres, such as bone, will not cause pain until the periosteum is involved, when pain will be well localised. Such a pain may often be associated with local signs of inflammation, including redness and swelling, local muscle spasm and disuse of the affected part.

Ischaemic pain from muscle may have more of an aching or cramping character and is usually less well localised. Pain from deeper structures in the abdomen or thorax has an aching quality and is also poorly localised by the patient, partly due to its depth from the surface and partly because of reference to the dermatomal site of the relevant roots which subserve the intrathoracic and intra-abdominal viscera. One of the usual accompaniments of pain, whether superficial or deep, is that pressure over the site of the painful tissue will cause tenderness.

NERVE PAIN

Pain arising from damage to the peripheral nervous system in general or from individual peripheral nerves may have differing characteristics; pain of diffuse peripheral neuropathy is frequently burning and tingling (paraesthesia) in nature and may be associated with hyperpathia in that areas of disturbed sensation will be hypersensitive to touch. Individual nerve pain, such as that seen with entrapment neuropathies, is also usually paraesthetic or dysaesthetic in nature and may again be associated with hyperpathia. *Causalgic pain* is the name applied to a form of peripheral nerve pain caused by partial injury to a peripheral nerve. The trauma which occasions the painful syndrome can be relatively minor and the syndrome is characterised by persistent severe pain, most usually in the digit of one of the hands, with a burning quality which may radiate beyond the territory of the injured nerve. The involved skin is exquisitely sensitive to touch and the part is usually kept protected and immobile, showing various sudomotor and vasomotor abnormalities which suggest that there may be autonomic disturbance. The skin of the affected part is moist and warm, frequently becoming shiny and smooth; occasionally scaly and discoloured. It is believed that this character of pain is due to short-circuiting of impulses or ephaptic conduction between nerve fibres in the peripheral nerve involving both efferent sympathetic and sensory somatic fibres. This mixture of autonomic and sensory nerve fibres would explain the evident autonomic abnormalities and account for the severe pain which results. Control of the pain is frequently difficult and the syndrome may be associated with other phenomena of disuse, including trophic change and Sudeck's atrophy (Fig. 8.3).

Another variety of peripheral nerve pain is seen in patients who develop a neuroma on the terminal part of a damaged nerve most often after ampu-

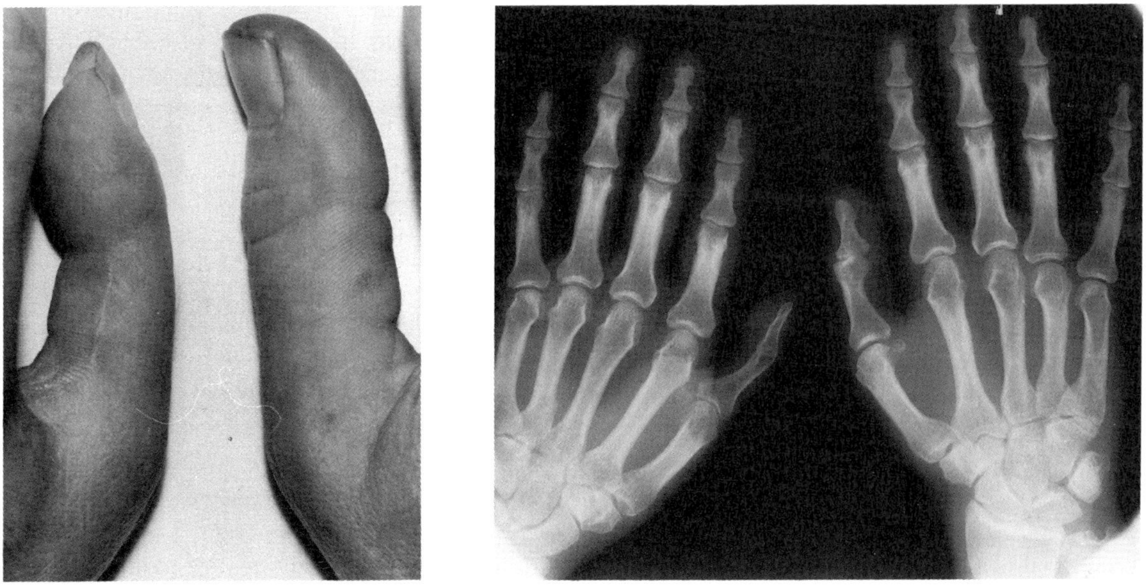

A B

Fig. 8.3 **A** Wasting and trophic change in the left thumb of a patient with causalgia. **B** Radiograph of hands of the same patient showing Sudek's atrophy with marked osteoporosis of phalanges of the left thumb.

tation, when the syndrome of *phantom pain* develops. The patient will then develop pain in the distribution of the nerve which has been sectioned and, in the case of amputation, may be associated with an abnormal sensation of the presence of the phantom limb. It can develop months or years after the original amputation. The pain is believed to have its origin in the site of the neuroma which forms at the end of the damaged nerve and it may be stimulated by tapping over the site of this traumatic neuroma. Refashioning of the stump or exploration of the site of injury to the nerve can occasionally help, although the symptom may be intractable even to nerve section or to proximal lesions within the spinal cord or thalamus.

RADICULAR PAIN

This pain, which is usually related precisely to the distribution of a single nerve root, may be due to stretching, irritation or compression of a spinal nerve root, either within the spine or at the intervertebral foramen. The pain is usually sharp and radiates from the central position near the spine out in the direction of the radicular distribution of the nerve. It is made worse by those factors which increase intraspinal pressure, such as coughing, sneezing and straining, and any manoeuvre which stretches the nerve root, such as flexing or extending the cervical spine, or bending the lumbar spine, may increase the pain. Such pain is frequently associated with paraesthesia or superficial sensory loss and there may also be reflex loss and weakness and atrophy of the involved muscles. Radicular pain involving the thoracic roots will tend to spread in girdle-like distribution around one or both sides of the thorax or abdomen.

REFERRED PAIN

Referred pain may occur either with damage to abdominal or thoracic viscera, when the pain may be related to the area of spine from which the innervation occurs, or from lesions within the spine, which can cause referred pain into the viscera which they subserve.

A further variety of referred pain will occur when abdominal viscera are irritated and the pain is referred to the dermatomal site supplied by the same roots. Perhaps the most common example of this is when irritation of the diaphragm, which is supplied by the cervical second, third and fourth nerve roots, is referred to the shoulder tip, or pain from the heart, supplied by the thoracic first to fifth nerve roots, is felt in the wall of the chest and the inner aspect of the left arm. Thus pain due to disease in the upper part of the lumbar spine may be reflected into the flank, lumbar region, groin and anterior thigh. Pain of this nature is usually deep and aching in quality and will be increased by those features which tend to affect spinal pain.

TRACT PAIN

Disease processes which involve the spinal tract subserving painful sensations may cause symptoms referable to the whole of the limb or limbs below the site of involvement. The nature of spinal tract pain is frequently dysaesthetic in character and may be intermittent and searing in nature. A typical example of this form of pain is seen in multiple sclerosis when sharp, shock-like sensations of pain may occur, which are believed to be due to the phenomenon of ephaptic transmission across the site of a demyelinated plaque. The patient may then appreciate searing pain occurring in a leg or arm and a leg below the site of involvement.

One particular form of painful syndrome due to irritation of spinal tracts occurs in Lhermitte's phenomenon in which flexion of the cervical spine, which may be the site of a plaque of demyelination or occasionally of a cervical tumour or spondylosis, results in dysaesthesiae passing down the spine and into the lower limbs.

THALAMIC PAIN

A lesion, frequently ischaemic or haemorrhagic in nature, which damages the posterior lateral part of the thalamus is at first characterised by hemianaesthesia. In time some aspects of sensory function return and pain develops in a hemisensory distribution involving the arm and leg and less frequently the face. The symptom may occasionally arise spontaneously, but usually follows an evident hemianaesthesia and is believed to be attributable to irritation at the level of the thalamus. The characteristics of the pain are its relentless dysaesthetic nature and it frequently poses a considerable clinical problem which may respond to therapy with carbamazepine, but which can become intractable.

CORTICAL PAIN

Pain arising from lesions within the cerebral cortex or hemispheric white matter structures may resemble thalamic pain in nature but frequently is less well localised, variable in its site and of a deep burning nature. It is also difficult to control and may be described by the patient in various bizarre ways.

PAIN WITHOUT ANATOMICAL CAUSE

The most common forms of persisting pain without evident anatomical cause are pain in the cervical or more commonly the lumbar spine. It is reasonable to begin each assessment of a patient by assuming that there is an underlying cause for the pain in the cervical or low spinal regions, but after careful examination there will remain a group of patients in whom no pathological basis can be found for the back pain. On occasions the pain may be related to abnormalities of posture either of the cervical or lumbar spine, but such pain may be a major symptom in patients with hysteria, malingering, anxiety, depression and hypochondriasis. The most difficult problem arises when patients have had a minor injury or illness to account for the initial pain, but whose pain then persists beyond that for which the physician can find a reasonable organic explanation. This problem is most apparent in those patients seeking compensation for industrial or accidental injury, although it is also common in the depressed and anxious patient. In such patients there is a reasonable indication to prescribe a trial of antidepressant drugs which will alleviate most causes of depression and in many instances also have an effect in reducing the chronic pain.

It is apparent from the descriptions above that the localisation and nature of the pain will frequently give information as to the type of cause. The terms hyperaesthesia and hyperalgesia are frequently used to describe a lowering of the normal threshold to tactile and painful stimuli. Hyperpathia is occasionally used in the same context, though it ought really to be reserved for those situations in which the reaction to normal pain or touch is excessive. The phenomena of hyperpathia and hyperalgesia tend to occur with lesions peripheral in the nervous system and is probably due to the continuous stimulation of second order neurones and thereby of the thalamus.

Assessment of the symptom of pain in any individual patient must take into account the fact that, unlike most sensory stimuli, persistent pain does not tend to become less significant but rather adopts a greater degree of importance to the patient. This affective factor in painful stimuli results in psychological state being of enormous importance in conditions of chronic pain.

The persistence of pain in any individual will increase irritability, disturb sleep and result in profound depression and anxiety as to the nature of the symptom. Although it is well recognised that the effect of pain may to some extent be ameliorated by the personality of the individual and by factors of race and culture, there is no doubt that chronic pain is one of the most disabling of all symptoms and physicians must be willing to use several different therapies in an attempt to control and reduce persisting pain.

PAINFUL SYNDROMES

HEADACHE AND FACIAL PAIN

Headache is perhaps the most common and most worrying of all painful symptoms to the patient. Despite this, it is usually poorly described by the patient and not well localised. It should be remembered that isolated headache is not usually indicative of any serious or significant intracranial pathology but that most headaches represent reactions to anxiety, tension and depression.

Headache never originates from the brain itself, which is devoid of the relevant sensory endings, but is due to other factors such as distension or stretching of intracranial vessels, pressure or inflammation of the meninges or of certain intracranial sensory nerves, spasm in muscles in the head and neck, irritations of the linings of sinuses, ear or orbit, or lesions of the bone of the cranium. Wolf suggests that headache or facial pain (and the two are not always seen as distinct by patients) is usually due to one of the following mechanisms:

1. Alterations in intracranial pressure or meningeal irritation
2. Distension, traction or dilatation of the intracranial or extra-cranial arteries
3. Traction or displacement of large intracranial veins or their dural envelopes
4. Compression, traction or inflammation of the sensory cranial and spinal nerves
5. Voluntary or involuntary spasm or inflammation of cranial or cervical muscles.

Altered intracranial pressure or meningeal irritation

Raised intracranial pressure

The most important worry in the mind of the patient developing headache is that it might indicate the presence of cerebral tumour and, consequently, the most important headache which the physician must be able to identify is that due to raised intracranial pressure from tumour, haematoma, abscess, cerebral oedema or hydrocephalus. The pain of raised intracranial pressure is frequently poorly localised and only occasionally relates to the site or side of the cerebral tumour. Classically, with raised intracranial pressure there is a tentorial or foraminal pressure cone and the meninges in the occipital region are therefore stretched, resulting in a typically occipital headache. As intracranial pressure is most elevated when the patient is lying flat, the pain tends to begin during the night and frequently wakens the patient from sleep early in the morning. It will tend to lessen during the day when the patient assumes the upright posture and, like most organic pains, will respond to some extent to the use of analgesics.

The headache will typically be made worse by those manoeuvres which increase intracranial pressure such as bending, coughing, stooping or straining. There may be associated features related to the high pressure, including vomiting, the symptom of dizziness or lightheadedness due to pressure at the level of the brain stem, visual disturbances due most commonly to sixth nerve problems resulting in blurred vision and double vision and, very occasionally, episodes of blindness, termed visual obscurations, occurring due to sudden increases in intracranial pressure. These, together with the headache, are the non-specific symptoms of raised intracranial pressure. Obviously, with a structural lesion within the cranium, focal symptoms may also occur related to the particular site of the lesion: these focal symptoms may be either positive or negative depending on the irritative or destructive nature of the lesion. Positive symptoms such as focal seizures will indicate irritation of the contralateral hemisphere; negative symptoms such as loss of vision, speech, sensation or motor power will identify destructive lesions in appropriate areas.

On examination, the cardinal finding in raised intracranial pressure is the presence of papilloedema. It should be remembered that papilloedema due to raised pressure does not cause disturbances of visual acuity and it should also be remembered that the absence of papilloedema is no guarantee of the absence of raised intracranial pressure. Other findings may include the presence of a sixth nerve palsy resulting in failure of abduction of the eye or of a partial third nerve palsy with a dilated and unreactive pupil. Other cranial nerve signs may exist which can reflect the localisation of the tumour, or be non-specific or false lateralising signs due to pressure upon structures within the cranium. The presence of neck stiffness, due to a foraminal pressure cone, is a common finding in raised intracranial pressure, and deep tendon reflexes will usually be brisk, possibly asymmetrically, where they will serve as lateralising signs which may also identify the site of the lesion causing the raised pressure.

In general, description of symptoms of raised intracranial pressure is more important than the signs of raised pressure. Whilst it is unusual to see patients with raised intracranial pressure in the absence of localising signs, patients may have raised intracranial pressure without papilloedema or false localising signs. Where the history strongly suggests raised intracranial pressure patients must be regarded as having this condition until it is excluded by investigation. The investigation of patients with raised intracranial pressure is now ideally by computerised axial tomography and will be dealt with in greater detail in Chapter 13.

Low pressure headache

This headache is believed to be due to a negative intracranial pressure when in the upright position which exerts traction on dural attachments and dural sinuses because of caudal displacement of the brain. It is most commonly seen following lumbar puncture, where it is believed to be attributable to a persistent leakage of c.s.f. into the lumbar tissues along the needle tract. It may occasionally follow spontaneous rupture of the spinal arachnoid or be due to the development of fistulae from the arachnoid into the tissues allowing leakage of cerebrospinal fluid. Characteristically it is alleviated by lying down and made worse by standing. It can be controlled by advising the patient to remain recumbent, although in those cases due to spontaneous fistulae there may occasionally be the need for surgical correction.

Such low pressure headaches have also been recorded in patients who have undergone ventriculoatrial or ventriculoperitoneal shunting where the problem is usually corrected by the insertion of a higher pressure system. The syndrome of post-alcohol or hangover headache may also be due to a lowering of intracranial pressure due to dehydration and should respond to rehydration. The syndrome of post-lumbar puncture headache is more complex than simple lowered intracranial pressure and occasionally patients are seen who have significant neck stiffness and paraspinal spasm together with the headache following lumbar puncture. A repeat lumbar puncture in these patients may reveal low pressure but can also show a pleocytosis and there is obviously the possibility of a mild meningeal irritation without there being a true meningitis.

Meningism

Meningism is the syndrome of irritation of the meninges most commonly seen as the result of meningitis or subarachnoid haemorrhage. Occasionally there may be a chemical irritation of the meninges in patients who have epidermoid or dermoid cysts, or in whom drugs or contrast media have been injected intrathecally.

Meningitis. Acute viral or bacterial meningitis causes a headache which is diffuse although predominantly localised to the occiput. It is usually associated with photophobia, pyrexia and general malaise and may be associated with signs of systemic infection and exanthemata.

Examination will usually reveal a patient who is febrile with a tachycardia and who may show evidence of redness of the optic disc or frank papilloedema due to the development of hydrocephalus, the presence of significant cerebral oedema or a high c.s.f. protein. Neck stiffness and a positive Kernig's test will be present. (Kernig's test, which consists of the attempted extension of the knee joint when the hip joint has been flexed, is of some use in differentiating the presence of neck stiffness due to raised intracranial pressure from that due to meningitis. If Kernig's test is positive, i.e. the knee cannot be extended fully when the hip is flexed to 90 degrees due to pain and tension in the hamstrings, then this indicates the presence of irritation of the lumbar roots which, together with neck stiffness, indicates the presence of meningitis. If Kernig's test is negative, i.e. the leg can be extended fully when the hip is flexed to 90 degrees, then the neck stiffness is more likely to be due to raised intracranial pressure and a tonsillar pressure cone.) There may be also be focal neurological signs which will suggest the possibility of collection of pus, a focal encephalitis, a thrombotic infarction due to arteritis or venous sinus thrombosis or developing hydrocephalus.

More chronic meningitis may be seen with some bacterial infections such as tuberculosis, with fungal infections and also with neoplastic infiltration of the meninges. In these situations there may be less evidence of systemic illness and headache may be more focal and more insidious in onset. The most significant features of meningeal irritation are those of neck stiffness together with irritation of the lumbar roots as revealed by Kernig's sign.

Subarachnoid haemorrhage. This is probably the most dramatic of all headaches and results from rupture of a berry aneurysm or arteriovenous malformation, or after head injury. Meningeal irritation can also be due to blood released into the subarachnoid space following a parenchymal haemorrhage, but in this case focal features usually dominate the clinical picture and the patient will often suffer loss of consciousness. In a typical subarachnoid haemorrhage there is acute onset of severe headache which is occasionally likened to a blow to the head. There may be loss of consciousness but, if the patient is able to give a description of the onset, its abruptness and rapid evolution to become a diffuse head pain with pain in the neck which occasionally radiates down the back, usually makes the diagnosis apparent. Vomiting is common.

Clinical findings in subarachnoid haemorrhage are neck stiffness together with a positive Kernig's sign. Examination with an ophthalmoscope may reveal evidence of subhyaloid haemorrhages in the area around the optic disc. If focal signs are also present then they may give a clue as to the site of the ruptured aneurysm or of the presence of a haematoma. The clinical syndromes of patients with subarachnoid haemorrhage and the management of these patients is dealt with in Chapter 11.

Distension, traction or dilatation of the intracranial or extracranial arteries

Migraine

Migraine is an overdiagnosed cause of headache which has become socially more acceptable than tension headache. Migraine syndromes are estimated to occur in between 5% and 10% of the population and a classification of the different types of migraine is given in Table 8.1.

Table 8.1 Classification of migraine

Common migraine
Classic migraine
Complicated migraine
Ophthalmoplegic
Hemiplegic
Basilar
Symptomatic
AVM
Aneurysm
Meningioma
Periodic migrainous neuralgia

Common migraine. The term 'common migraine' has been applied to periodic headaches which may be unilateral in site and associated with nausea and photophobia, but which have few of the other characteristic features of migraine. There can be little doubt that some of these headaches have a vascular basis similar to that of classic migraine but others may be varieties of tension headache or related to depression. They rarely require treatment with more than symptomatic therapy and frequently respond best to common analgesic preparations.

Classic migraine. Classic migraine is a frequently familial syndrome in which the patient suffers periodic, unilateral headaches which may begin in childhood or early adult life and tend to reduce in frequency, usually ceasing at about the time of the menopause. Patients who later develop classic migraine frequently have a history in childhood of biliousness or acute attacks of abdominal pain with nausea and vomiting. The typical attack of classic migraine develops with an aura consisting of disturbances of vision, photopsia, teichopsia, scotoma or hemianopia and occasional disturbances of sensation, motor function or aphasia. This aura is followed by a hemicranial headache, nausea and vomiting associated with photophobia. The syndrome will commonly last for between 6 and 48 hours and rarely occurs at intervals of more than 7 days. It most characteristically occurs when the patient is resting and has occasionally been referred to as the 'weekend headache'. There is a family history in some 60–80% of cases and the condition is more common in women than men. In general, migraine is more likely to occur in women at times of menstruation, although there is an interesting and variable relationship with the menstrual cycle and with hormonal changes. Some women will develop migraine only during pregnancy whereas others become free from attacks during a pregnancy; similarly, there are undoubtedly patients whose migraine presents for the first time when they take the contraceptive pill and others in whom such treatment results in cessation of attacks. In addition to classic migraine, there are two other forms of migraine which are of clinical significance:

Complicated migraine. Complicated migraine describes the situation in which focal neurological disturbances, other than visual, either herald the attack, coexist with the attack, or follow an attack of migraine headache. Occasionally episodes of focal neurological disturbance may occur without headache—the syndrome of migraine sine headache in which the differential diagnosis from transient ischaemic attacks may be difficult. These focal attacks occurring in the context of migraine imply a degree of cerebral ischaemia which may occasionally be severe enough to result in permanent loss of function. Thus, a hemianopia is a not uncommon prodrome to a migraine attack, and a permanent hemianopia can occur as a result of cerebral infarction during a migraine episode (Fig. 8.4).

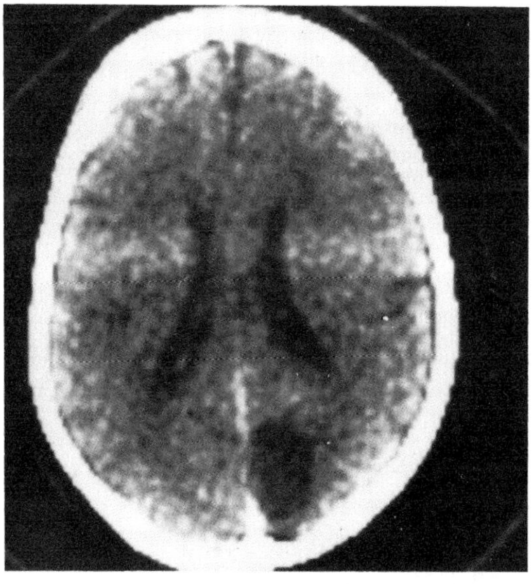

Fig. 8.4 CT scan showing occipital infarction in a patient with a migrainous stroke.

The forms of complicated migraine which are recognised include: *ophthalmoplegic migraine*, which is most common in children and which results in the symptom of diplopia, ptosis and an evident external ophthalmoplegia; *hemiplegic migraine*, a rare familial condition in which transient hemiparesis may occur; *basilar migraine*, in which bilateral visual symptoms, unsteadiness, ataxia, dysarthria and vertigo may be recorded together with sensory and motor disturbance of both upper or both lower limbs. Rarely, loss of consciousness may occur with this form of migraine which is most common in young women.

Symptomatic migraine. Migraine may also be symptomatic of underlying cerebral pathology, most commonly berry aneurysm or arteriovenous malformations. The factors which make the physician suspect the presence of some structural abnormality to account for migraine are identical attacks occurring in the same patient with a headache always on the same side and the complicated symptoms always contralateral to the headache. Other factors are the finding of bruit over cervical or cranial vessels and evidence of persisting neurological deficit. Migraine occurring in a patient with focal epilepsy may indicate a significant underlying cause. It should be emphasised that symptomatic migraine is rare and routine investigations of patients with uncomplicated migraine are rarely justified.

Aetiology. There will frequently be a family history of migraine or of 'bilious attacks' in other family members, though no recognisable pattern of inheritance has been identified. Occasionally the occurrence of intermittent abdominal pain in childhood is thought to represent abdominal migraine. The cause of migraine remains unknown although the classic attack appears to be biphasic with an initial phase of relative ischaemia to the cerebrum followed by a phase of presumed vasodilatation and consequent pain. This phenomenon may be a response to a vasogenic amine, probably serotonin. It has been shown that some patients with migraine excrete increased amounts of metabolites of serotonin (5-hydroxyindoleacetic acid) during an attack and there is a corresponding reduction in the level of platelet serotonin. This, taken together with the fact that reserpine (which depletes platelet serotonin) can provoke migraine and that antiserotonin agents can apparently reduce the occurrence of migraine seems to suggest some sort of relationship between monoamines and migraine.

It has recently been suggested that substance 'P' (already mentioned in terms of a pain neurotransmitter) is present in high concentrations close to cerebral blood vessels during migraine attacks and, as it has a vasogenic effect, it may also be involved in the mechanism of the unilateral headache. The problem with these theories has always been why only some vessels appear to respond in this way, resulting in the focal symptoms and unilateral headache, but not others. A recent suggestion that migraine may be a cerebral rather than a vascular disturbance, with a central cause for pain due possibly to serotonin acting upon pain pathways, would go some way towards explaining the peculiar unilateral character of the headache. It is recognised that migraine may be precipitated in some patients by external factors such as coffee or chocolate or particular episodes of mental or physical stress. It seems likely that the way in which these exogenous agents affect the development of migraine is probably through the activity of various neurotransmitters and the fact that many of the foods which have been identified to cause episodes of migraine contain agents which affect biogenic amines would be in keeping with this theory.

Investigation. The diagnosis of migraine is usually made historically and investigation is not normally indicated. Those features which make the physician consider further investigation, including CT scan and even angiography, would be the presence of complicated migraine which persistently involved the same area of brain, especially if associated with focal seizures or subarachnoid haemorrhage.

Therapy. In the majority of patients with migraine, the frequency of attacks is such that an adequate explanation of the nature of the headache together with the provision of symptomatic treatment is all that is required. Only occasionally is it necessary to use interval therapy in an attempt to prevent the occurrence of migraine attacks, though this is reasonable in patients with frequent attacks or in those with prolonged or severe complicated migraine. In the main, therapy for migraine can be divided usefully into three categories (Table 8.2). Firstly, in those patients in whom some external factors can be identified to cause the syndrome, the relevant factor should be removed: this is obvious in patients who get attacks related to taking coffee or to eating certain identifiable items, but may be less obvious when related to drug therapy such as antihypertensive treatment. In patients whose attacks are related to taking a contraceptive pill a particular problem ensues: there seems no doubt that in women who develop complicated migraine with evidence of cerebral ischaemia while taking the contraceptive pill there is an absolute contraindication to the continuation of therapy; the risk of cerebral infarction seems sufficient to advise the withdrawal of treatment although there is little actual evidence that patients with complicated migraine are in fact more likely to have cerebrovascular accidents. Patients who develop common migraine or classic migraine without significant neurological defects while taking a contraceptive pill may be regarded as having a relative contraindication to using this agent but many prefer to continue taking the pill and use symptomatic treatment for the migraine.

The second line of treatment in migraine is the use of symptomatic therapy for the attack. Most episodes are helped significantly by common analgesic preparations occasionally taken in associ-

Table 8.2 The treatment of migraine

Avoidance of precipitants
Chocolate
Alcohol
Cheese
Oranges, etc.
Symptomatic therapy
Analgesics
Analgesics + metaclopramide
Prochlorperazine
Ergotamine
Oxygen
Interval therapy
Antiserotonin agents
Beta blockers
Tricyclics
Progesterones

ation with an agent to reduce nausea and improve gastric emptying. The most common combination therapies would be the use of aspirin or paracetamol together with metoclopramide. More complex combinations of therapy are available but appear to give little significant benefit. The use of ergotamine and its derivatives in the symptomatic treatment of migraine is questionable. This agent, which causes significant vasospasm, certainly gives relief from headache in many patients with classic migraine; the risks of peripheral, cerebral or cardiac ischaemia arising as a result of the use of these agents must, however, be remembered and some patients complain of increased nausea. The major concern is the use of these agents in patients with complicated migraine in whom there is evidence for a presumed cerebral ischaemic episode during the attack. Most neurologists would now regard such complicated migraine as being a contraindication to the use of vasospastic agents such as ergotamine. Patients who use ergotamine chronically may find that the headache returns as the drug wears off and this postergotamine headache should be recognised and is best managed by withdrawal of the drug.

The third form of therapy is confined to those patients who have either frequent attacks or attacks which are associated with disabling complications. In this group of patients consideration needs to be given to the use of interval therapy with agents that are designed to prevent the development of migraine. The most effective of these agents to date appears to be methysergide, an antiserotonin agent which has significant benefits in preventing the development of migraine. The drawback to methysergide is that a certain proportion of patients will develop retroperitoneal fibrosis and, although this is rare (except in prolonged usage of the drug) and can usually be identified early by the finding of a high ESR, it is a factor which causes most physicians to be very guarded in its use. It may be avoided by restricting its use to periods of 4–6 months. Pizotifen is a less effective serotonin antagonist which appears relatively free from side effects and which gives benefit as an interval therapy to many patients with frequent episodes of migraine. Alternative interval therapies consist of the use of beta-blocking agents such as propranolol, although paradoxically this can occasionally cause episodes of migraine in susceptible individuals; occasional patients will respond reasonably to the use of tricyclic agents. Many different agents have been used as interval treatment in migraine but few have stood the test of time and most have little rationale (Table 8.2).

Periodic migrainous neuralgia (cluster headaches). This form of headache, which is also termed Horton's histamine cephalgia, is a syndrome which occurs chiefly in young men and is typically a unilateral periorbital pain developing in the early hours of the morning and waking the patient from sleep. The pain is felt in and around the eye and often radiates into the temple and forehead on the same side. The patient will usually describe epiphora, redness of the eye, ptosis, nasal stuffiness, rhinorrhoea and possibly meiosis during the attack. Episodes last for hours at a time and tend to occur daily for a matter of weeks or months. There is then usually a spontaneous resolution of the symptom which may recur a year or more later.

Although occasionally this form of headache has a focal cause, no abnormal pathology is detected in the majority of patients and the syndrome responds well to the use of an antiserotonin agent such as methysergide or pizotifen, or to the use of nocturnal ergotamine, frequently in suppository form, in the days following an initial attack.

Temporal arteritis

This syndrome occurs in patients over the age of 50 years and is due to a subacute, granulomatous, inflammatory infiltration of lymphocytes and other mononuclear cells and giant cells in the walls of the external carotid arteries. The most severely affected parts of the artery may become thrombosed and even cause ischaemic necrosis of the tissues supplied. The condition is peculiar in being confined to the extracerebral arteries, although involvement of the vessels outside the cerebrum itself may occasionally give rise to ischaemic damage to the tissues of the brain and eye. It most usually presents as a severe, and frequently very well localised, headache usually described as head pain or tenderness over the scalp and related to the distribution of one of the extracranial vessels. The most common site for such headache is in one or other temporal region, although occasionally the pain may be felt over the occiput. The patient will often appear generally ill and will frequently describe pain on brushing or combing the hair, bathing or washing the affected area of scalp and while chewing or talking. The temporal or occipital arteries may be palpated and are frequently exquisitely tender and may be non-pulsatile.

The diagnosis is supported by the finding of a high ESR, an investigation which is mandatory in patients over 60 presenting with headache. Temporal arteritis may be confirmed by biopsy of the affected vessel, although, as the condition is patchy, a negative biopsy does not exclude the diagnosis. In some instances there may be the association of systemic symptoms including fever, anorexia, weight loss, malaise and anaemia. Occlusion of the branches of an affected artery may result in ischaemic damage to the skin, leading to necrosis, or more importantly affect the ophthalmic artery, causing blindness. Occasionally the arteries which supply the cranial nerves may be involved leading to cranial nerve paresis, most commonly ophthalmoplegia. Cerebrovascular accidents may occur due to occlusion of an internal carotid or vertebral artery, although such complications are rare. Occasionally the syndrome may overlap with a more generalised inflammatory arteritis, as in polyarteritis, or with more systemic illness, such as polymyalgia rheumatica. Early diagnosis is vital and rapid treatment with steroids is obligatory to prevent the dangerous complications. Patients respond dramatically to treatment with steroids and their progress can be monitored by symptomatic improvement and by measuring the ESR. It is frequently possible to reduce the steroids to an alternate-day regime within a matter of weeks and ultimately to wean patients from the drug. Monitoring the ESR and clinical condition enables the physician to determine when it is possible to begin to withdraw the drug. Some patients will relapse as the prednisone is withdrawn and will then require restitution of the therapy.

Cough or exertional headache

Occasionally patients will complain of transient severe headache when coughing, sneezing, stooping or straining at stool. The pain is usually occipitofrontal in nature, lasts for a few seconds and is described as bursting in nature. Its cause is uncertain but it is rarely associated with significant intracranial disease, although it is reasonable to undertake a lateral skull radiograph in patients with this symptom. The syndrome appears to be self-limiting, which is fortunate in view of its lack of response to therapy.

Headaches related to sexual activity

Men may occasionally complain of headaches at the time of sexual activity, which may either occur with sexual excitement (in which case they are believed to be of a tension nature), or at the time of orgasm (when they are more explosive in nature and may raise the question of subarachnoid haemorrhage). Investigations of such patients seldom reveal any evidence of significant intracranial pathology and there is frequently a reasonable response to prophylactic treatment with a beta blocker.

Traction and displacement of large veins or dural envelopes

Extradural haematoma

The syndrome of extradural haematoma commonly occurs in a young child or adult complicating a skull fracture. There is pain at the site of the injury which increases gradually over the succeeding hours as consciousness deteriorates. This condition, which represents a surgical emergency, is described more fully in the section on vascular disease.

Subdural haematoma

Acute and subacute subdural haematoma tend to present with localised headache and most typically follow trauma. Altered consciousness and focal neurological signs dominate the clinical picture.

Chronic subdural haematoma in the elderly may of course present with confusion, drowsiness and stupor, with or without significant headache. This syndrome is described in Chapter 11.

Venous-sinus thrombosis

In states of dehydration, pyrexia, malaise and local intracranial sepsis, the occurrence of a localised severe headache together with focal disabilities or seizures raises the possibility of cortical venous-sinus thrombosis. The site of the pain is usually relatively well localised and the associated clinical features should give a clue to the diagnosis. Occasionally this form of disturbance may occur in young women taking the contraceptive pill or during pregnancy. It is dealt with fully in the section on cerebrovascular disease.

Pain syndromes related to specific cranial nerves

Trigeminal neuralgia (Tic douloureux)

This classic painful syndrome affects predominantly the elderly in the population and is rare under the age of 50 years. It is frequently overdiagnosed and many patients with atypical facial pain (p. 203) are initially considered, incorrectly, to have trigeminal neuralgia. Patients under the age of 50 years with trigeminal neuralgia must be considered as having symptomatic pain due to trauma, vascular, neoplastic or demyelinating conditions. The incidence of the disease is approximately 15 per 100 000 per year and it is almost one and a half times as common in women as in men.

The pain is lancinating in nature, unilateral in site, and arises in the maxillary or mandibular division of the trigeminal nerve. Its severity is such as to make the patient grimace and the acute pain may occur either spontaneously or in response to external stimuli, including talking, chewing, cold and touch. The patient may frequently be able to identify a trigger point within the distribution of either the second or third sensory division of the trigeminal nerve and touching or pressing upon this point may cause the pain. It can be sufficiently severe to stop the patient bathing, talking and feeding. The pain is rare in the ophthalmic division of the nerve and its presence in this area should raise the suspicion that the pain is symptomatic of some other disease.

Aetiology of the pain is unknown and several different pathologies may play a part. It is recognised to occur with increased incidence in multiple sclerosis where, presumably, plaques in the brain stem are responsible for the pain. Its usual occurrence in patients over the age of 50 suggests a vascular or degenerative cause and it has recently been suggested that irritation of the trigeminal nerve by a kinked blood vessel may be responsible for the intermittency and frequency.

The differential diagnosis of idiopathic trigeminal neuralgia from the symptomatic forms of facial neuralgia is not difficult in the typical form. Conditions which should be considered to cause symptomatic trigeminal neuralgia include injuries to the cranial nerves and skull fractures which most commonly affect the most superficial nerves in the supratrochlear, supraorbital and infraorbital regions; these conditions are usually associated with a sensory loss in the distribution of the nerve involved. Tumours in the sinuses and metastatic disease of the bone may also involve divisions of the trigeminal nerve which cause continuous pain and a progressive sensory loss: they are also more likely to involve other cranial nerves. Inflammatory causes such as herpes simplex and infections of the middle ear with inflammation of the petrous apex can also cause irritation of the trigeminal nerve and consequent pain. Other conditions which should be considered include pressure on the trigeminal nerve from intracranial neoplasms such as meningiomas, acoustic neuromas, trigeminal neuromas, cholesteatomas and chordomas. Very occasionally, trigeminal neuralgia may occur in association with sensory loss in the distribution of the trigeminal nerve, when the condition of sensory neuropathy should be considered.

In general, the pain of trigeminal neuralgia will respond well to therapy with carbamazepine so dramatically that such treatment acts almost as a diagnostic test. However, if patients are unable to tolerate carbamazepine or if the pain is refractory to this therapy, the possibility of radio frequency lesions of the Gasserian ganglion, which run the risk of leaving an area of numbness or even anaesthesia dolorosa on the face, or of formal posterior fossa craniotomy with exploration of the trigeminal nerve root and removal of any aberrant vessel from it, needs to be considered. The technique of nerve section which was formerly practised is now not recommended and was also associated with a significant residue of anaesthesia dolorosa.

Glossopharyngeal neuralgia

A rare syndrome identical in character to trigeminal neuralgia can occur in the back of the throat and tonsillar fossa spreading into the throat or into the ear. This is termed glossopharyngeal neuralgia and is, again, of uncertain aetiology, although the suggestion has also been made that it may be due to a kinked blood vessel impinging upon the glossopharyngeal nerve. This syndrome also tends to respond well to carbamazepine but, if it is refractory to such therapy, then section of the root of the glossopharyngeal nerve or posterior fossa exploration of the nerve and freeing the nerve from aberrant blood vessels may be considered.

Painful ophthalmoplegia

The most common form of pain in the eye together with abnormal movement of the eye is due to local orbital causes such as *orbital myositis* or *orbital infections*. Pain in and around the eye may also occur with periodic *migrainous neuralgia* as described above and can also indicate disease or disturbance of the cranial nerves within the cavernous sinus due to *cavernous sinus thrombosis*, *intracavernous aneurysm of the carotid artery* or a *caroticocavernous fistula*. The gross oedema and venous engorgement with evidence of infection is indicative of the first of these causes, pain in the distribution of the first branch of the trigeminal nerve is typical of the second and the third can be recognised by pulsatile proptosis and a bruit over the orbit.

The development of a third nerve palsy together with pain in and behind the eye, should always raise the possibility of a *posterior communicating artery aneurysm* and it may also be seen, although rarely, in the condition of *ophthalmoplegic migraine*, which is most common in the young. In addition, the presence of pain in an eye, together with proptosis or disturbance of eye movement, raises the possibility of Grave's disease or of the Tolosa–Hunt syndrome of *orbital apicitis*: this latter syndrome is a granulomatous condition which causes pain and ophthalmoplegia and is due to a lesion at the apex of the orbit. Any *tumour* growing in the orbit is liable to produce disturbance of eye movement together with pain in the eye. The *paratrigeminal syndrome of Raeder* in which there is a Horner's syndrome of ptosis and meiosis together with pain in the eye is believed to be of vascular origin. The causes of painful ophthalmoplegia are detailed in Table 8.3.

Table 8.3 Painful ophthalmoplegia

Intraorbital
Dysthyroid eye disease
Orbital myositis
Orbital infection
Tumours
Secondary tumours
Pseudotumour
Orbital apex
Tolosa–Hunt syndrome
Retro-orbital
Cavernous sinus thrombosis
Aneurysm of internal carotid
Caroticocavernous fistula
Posterior communicating artery aneurysm
Raeder's syndrome

Shingles

Involvement of the Gasserian ganglion with herpes zoster virus results in a vesicular eruption over the distribution of branches of the trigeminal nerve. It usually involves the ophthalmic division of the nerve and more rarely the mandibular or maxillary branches. It is usually unilateral and of most immediate importance because it may result in scarring of the cornea. Involvement of the dorsal root ganglia of the upper cervical roots can result in a similar rash over the occipital region, together with pain in the back of the head and cervical areas. Involvement of the geniculate ganglion may result in blisters over the external auditory meatus and a facial nerve palsy in the *Ramsay Hunt syndrome*. This form of herpes zoster infection can occasionally extend to involve the brain stem and may result in more marked symptoms related to the disturbance of other cranial nerve functions. The most troublesome effect of shingles affecting the cranial nerves is the persistence of pain after the acute infection has settled; presenting as postherpetic neuralgic. This intractable and lancinating pain in the distribution of the nerve involved is usually refractory to treatment and may cause patients to become depressed and even suicidal.

Nasopharyngeal tumours

Direct extension of tumours in the nasopharynx into the base of the skull, orbit or ear may result in involvement of cranial nerves and commonly causes severe local pain. The pain may radiate into the distribution of the nerve involved, most commonly the trigeminal nerve.

Malignant meningitis

Secondary tumours commonly from the bronchus or breast may cause deposits in the meninges, particularly around the base of the skull. In this situation there is localised pain which may become more widespread and again may involve individual sensory cranial nerves resulting in typical pain syndromes. It is frequently associated with cranial nerve lesions resulting in ophthalmoplegia, facial palsy and hearing loss.

Voluntary or involuntary spasm of cranial and cervical muscles

Cervical spondylosis (p. 225)

Chronic headache is not infrequently attributed to nipping of cervical nerve roots due to arthritis of the cervical spine. In practice, it is more likely that spasm of paraspinal muscles in the high cervical region causes pain as a result of cervical spondylosis and this pain is related to the occiput and gives rise to long-standing headache. Occasionally more specific pains can arise when the C2 nerve root is specifically involved in spinal disease but this is relatively uncommon.

Tension headache

Perhaps the most common of all headache causing referral to neurological clinics is tension headache. It may occur in patients who suffer from significant tension or depression and is typically diffuse, ill-defined, of long standing and often difficult for the patient to describe.

The symptoms which are used to describe such headache include those of band-like pain persisting day after day and unrelieved by simple analgesics. The history is characteristically long, the patient has frequently undergone numerous investigations and the problem is usually refractory to therapy. The pain tends to be continuous night and day and may be associated with a significant sleep disturbance in the form of early morning waking. This form of headache is more common in women than in men, is most commonly seen in middle life and frequently coincides with periods of anxiety or depression, although these may be denied by the patient.

There are no signs of raised intracranial pressure nor evidence of focal neurological problems and the periodicity of migraine, the specificity of other organic headaches and the associated symptoms of significant neurological disease are absent. Although such headaches are frequently refractory to therapy, the use of anxiolytics or antidepressants is sometimes helpful in their management.

Post-traumatic headache (p. 366)

The precise cause of post-traumatic headache is uncertain, although there are reasons for believing that local tissue damage may result in irritation or scarring of meninges, muscles or the skull itself to result in the persisting symptoms. Typically the headache will persist from a few months to 2–3 years after the head injury but there can be no doubt that other features, such as the mental state of the patient, the circumstances of the injury and the possibility of litigation, may play a part in the persistence of such headaches. There are frequently associated features such as lightheadedness, dizziness and memory disturbance and once again an organic pathology is usually absent.

Other causes of headache and facial pain

As headache is one of the most common of all presenting symptoms it is inevitable that it can occasionally occur as the result of more systemic illness. Perhaps as many as 50% of patients with hypertension have a complaint of headache and many other patients with respiratory, renal or hepatic failure will also mention headache among their complaints. Thus a full general examination is necessary in the assessment of headache. The identification of the many different forms of headache frequently causes problems and is detailed in Table 8.4.

The facial pain of *sinusitis* is usually not difficult to diagnose. It occurs in the context of upper respiratory tract infections, frequently results in the patient being febrile and able to localise the pain very accurately to the area of one of the sinuses and is made worse by bending or by pressure or tapping over the infected sinus. Although many facial pains, and indeed some headaches, are attributed to sinusitis this condition is in fact extremely rare and is only commonly seen in the presence of lesions within the sinus such as mucoceles or tumours.

The possibility of *dental pain* needs to be borne in mind with many of the facial pain syndromes. Usually the occurrence of pain with eating or chewing, relationship to items which are extremely hot or extremely cold and localisation of the pain enables a diagnosis to be made. Nonetheless, many patients with trigeminal neuralgia and some with atypical facial pain or other facial pain syndromes will present to the neurologist only after undergoing numerous dental extractions.

Pain in the *temperomandibular joint* (Costen's syndrome) may occur in patients with malocclusion or in those with generalised joint disease. It has been occasionally suggested that malocclusion of the dentures can give rise to migraine-like syndromes but the evidence for this is lacking.

Table 8.4 Classification of headache

	Type, site and character	Associated features	Treatment
Migraine	Frontotemporal, uni- or bilateral, throbbing	Nausea and vomiting, visual symptoms	Analgesics, ergotamine, antiserotonin agents, propranolol
Periodic migrainous neuralgia	Orbitotemporal, unilateral, intense and episodic	Lacrimation, blocked nostril, rhinorrhea, injected conjunctiva	Prophylactic ergotamine, antiserotonin agents, steroids, lithium
Tension headache	Generalised, continuous pressure	Depression, worry, anxiety, fatigue and fear of brain tumour	Reassurance, anxiolytics and antidepressants
Meningeal irritation	Generalised, occipital or frontal, intense and persistent	Neck stiffness, Kernig and Brudzinski signs	Antibiotics, antifungal, anticancer, or surgery as indicated
Raised intracranial pressure	Unilateral or generalised, frequently occipital, variable intensity, frequently worse in the morning	Papilloedema, vomiting, impaired mentation, seizures, focal signs	Corticosteroids, mannitol, treatment of underlying cause
Low pressure headache	Temporal, unilateral or bilateral, intermittent then continuous	Recent lumbar puncture or dehydration	Analgesics and rehydration
Temporal arteritis	Unilateral, temporal headache, occasionally occipital, continuous	Loss of vision, polymyalgia rheumatica, fever, weight loss, increased ESR	Cortico steroids

Atypical facial pain is a chronic continuous aching pain usually seen in late middle life, frequently bilateral, relentless and unresponsive to drug therapy. This is commonly a reflection of an affective disorder within the patient but which frequently results in them becoming edenturelate before referral to the appropriate clinic. The many varieties of facial pain frequently cause difficulty in differential diagnosis and their characteristics are considered in Table 8.5.

PAIN IN THE BACK

A significant proportion of people presenting with the symptom of pain in the cervical, dorsal or lumbosacral regions will not be found to have underlying evidence of organic disease. This situation is most commonly seen in patients who have suffered back injury where litigation is involved or blame is implied. In such patients the pain is frequently ill-defined in nature and extensive. It may be associated with exquisite tenderness of the skin over the area of the pain and marked limitation of movement of the spine which is apparent in formal examination but not apparent in the gait and posture of the patient when not being examined. Such problems are difficult to manage, and patients will frequently be submitted to a variety of investigations and some even to operation. The only consistent feature is the refractory nature of the pain to medical therapies and most success is likely to be achieved with the use of a tricyclic agent.

Table 8.5 Classification of facial pain

Type	Site and character	Associated features	Treatment
Trigeminal neuralgia	2nd and 3rd divisions of trigeminal nerve, paroxysms of stabbing pain, trigger points	Women more than men, over 50 years, idiopathic, MS in young, vascular anomaly, tumour of V cranial nerve	Carbamazepine, phenytoin, radiofrequency lesion of Gasserian ganglion. Posterior fossa decompressive surgery
Atypical facial pain	Unilateral or bilateral, continuous, intolerable pain	Depressive and anxiety states, dental therapy	Antidepressant and anxiolytic medication
Postherpetic neuralgia	Unilateral, ophthalmic divison, aching, burning pain with lancinating episodes	Herpes zoster	Carbamazepine, tricyclics, opiates
Sinusitis	Acute localised pain over sinus made worse by local pressure	Fever and malaise	Antibiotics, surgical drainage
Costen's syndrome	Unilateral, behind or in front of ear, severe aching pain increased by chewing	Loss of teeth, rheumatoid arthritis	Correction of bite, surgery
Tolosa–Hunt syndrome	Unilateral and retro-orbital. Sharp, aching pain	Ophthalmoplegia and sensory loss over forehead, lesions of cavernous sinus or superior orbital fissure	Corticosteroids, analgesics
Raeder's paratrigeminal syndrome	Unilateral, frontotemporal and maxillary. Intense, sharp or aching pain	Ptosis, meiosis, preserved sweating, tumours, granulomatous lesions, injuries to parasellar region	As appropriate for underlying cause, corticosteroids
Carotidynia	Unilateral, face, ear, jaws and teeth, extending to upper neck. Constant, dull ache	Rarely with cranial arteritis, carotid tumour and migraine	Ergotamine, anti-serotonin agents
Migrainous neuralgia	Orbitofrontal, acute, nocturnal pain	Epiphora, injection of conjunctiva, nasal stuffiness, rhinorrhoea	Ergotamine or serotonin antagonists before anticipated attack

The commonest cause of organic backache is musculoskeletal pain associated with spondylosis or arthritis in the spine with consequent muscle spasm. Such pain is constant and aching in nature and relatively localised usually to the lumbar region. It may be associated with local paravertebral spasm and induced by exercise or movement of the affected part. Spinal deformities and spinal injuries make the development of such syndromes more likely.

Most neurological back pain is caused by disease within the spinal canal, vertebrae or pressure upon a spinal nerve root. Diseases affecting the bones themselves will be associated with paravertebral spasm and occasionally with local deformity at the site of the lesion. Pressure on the bones involved will usually cause pain and movement of the spine will result in an increase in symptoms. Lesions in the spinal canal are usually associated with some radicular and some myelopathic features and, like those of pressure upon a spinal nerve root, will tend to be increased by those factors which increase intraspinal pressure such as coughing and sneezing. There will be a characteristic radiation of the pain along the distribution of the nerve root involved and this pain, which is sharp and lancinating in nature, will be increased by coughing, sneezing and straining.

When examining a patient with the symptom of backache it is important to observe the resting position of the spine with the normal cervical and lumbar lordosis and mild dorsal kyphosis. The presence of scoliosis either at rest or on movement implies an underlying abnormality and tenderness or deformity of the spine is an important sign.

Neck pain

Cervical spondylosis is by far the commonest cause of pain in the neck and is a common finding radiologically in patients over the age of 50. Patients who are involved in heavy manual labour, who have suffered accidents, or who have congenital abnormalities of the spine are more prone to the development of spondylosis and the consequent pain. This is often localised to the neck, although it occasionally radiates into the occipital region and may spread into the arms in radicular fashion.

Whiplash injury is the term given to patients who sustain cervical injury occurring during road traffic accidents (p. 372). It is common with head-on crashes or when one vehicle is struck by another vehicle from behind. The patient suffers a hyperflexion-hyperextension injury to the neck as the body moves forwards followed by the head and is then restrained by the seatbelt. This form of injury may occasionally cause dislocation of the cervical spine or an acute disc prolapse and even in the most severe cases a haematoma within the cervical cord. It is more common, however, for there to be no objective neurological evidence of damage but for the patient to suffer presumed soft tissue trauma to the ligaments and muscles of the cervical spine. Radicular pain may be present in the upper limbs and there has been some histopathological evidence to suggest that tiny petechiae may arise in the dorsal root ganglion. In the majority of cases, however, there is no evidence for structural abnormality and the persistence of problems after this sort of injury is in part related to the recognised problems of litigation and in part due to the chronic persistence of pain following soft tissue injury. Patients occasionally also complain of dizziness, which may be due to abnormalities in cervical reflex pathways to the brain stem.

An *acutely prolapsed cervical disc* is a relatively uncommon cause of cervical pain, but usually follows an injury and will result in pain in the neck together with acute radicular pain which is unilateral and extends into an arm following the distribution of the dermatome. It is frequently associated with the loss of reflex or reduction in power and wasting of the relevant muscles.

Other causes of cervical pain include *intrathecal tumours*, which may be extramedullary, commonly causing radicular pain, or intramedullary, frequently causing a more generalised and less well localised aching burning sensation. Such lesions are also associated with myelopathic disturbances below the level of the lesion. Other structural abnormalities such as syringomyelia or haematomyelia should be relatively easy to diagnose in view of the associated symptoms and signs of a central cord lesion.

Sometimes an acute cervical spine lesion such as a *transverse myelitis* or a plaque of *multiple sclerosis* may begin with severe localised cervical pain, due presumably to irritation of the meninges in this region. The signs of cervical cord and root damage together with the examination of such patients is documented in the section on spinal cord disease.

Pain in the thoracic spine

Pain in the thoracic spine is less common than that in the cervical or lumbosacral regions. When present, it should always raise the possibility of an *intra-abdominal* or *intrathoracic tumour* or of a *secondary deposit within the vertebral body*. Extradural lesions in the dorsal spine such as *dorsal discs, extradural haematomas* or secondary deposits may occur and will then tend to cause radicular symptoms such as girdle pain. Such pain may be occasionally misdiagnosed due to lesions within the thorax or abdomen itself and examples abound of patients who have girdle pain in the thoracic region but who are thought to have pleurisy, and those with girdle pain in the lumbar region who are mistakenly diagnosed as having renal colic.

Intradural lesions in the dorsal spine such as *neurofibromas* and *meningiomas* may also cause pain, the former more commonly in men and the latter in women. These tumours are likely to present with radicular symptoms and also with an evolving paraparesis.

Pain in the dorsal spine and radicular distribution may occur with *shingles* of the dorsal root ganglia in this region and will usually declare itself with a rash within a few days. The characteristic of neurological lesions in the dorsal spine is that they present with local pain, radicular pain and an evolving paraparesis which makes radiology and myelography obligatory.

Pain in the lumbosacral spine

Low back pain is a common cause of prolonged disability, particularly among patients involved in heavy manual industries. Most patients do not have a significant neurological lesion and many do not have an organic cause at all. The presence of pain in the low back without radiation into the legs, although occasionally seen in *tumours of the conus medullaris*, is usually not neurological in origin and is due to musculoskeletal problems.

Symptoms which indicate a potentially neurogenic pain include radiation of pain into the legs in either sciatic or femoral nerve distribution, disturbances of bladder or bowel function, or the development of a motor or sensory disturbance in the lower limbs. Together with this is a history of increase in pain by those manoeuvres which increase intraspinal pressure such as coughing, sneezing and straining. Lesions occurring below the first lumbar vertebra will tend to involve the cauda equina and result, apart from pain, in a typical flaccid paresis of both lower limbs together with bladder and bowel disturbance. Those at the lower portion of the dorsal spine may involve the conus medullaris and result in a mixture of upper and lower motor neurone signs together with sensory symptoms.

One relatively recently recognised syndrome of low back pain with radiation into the legs is the syndrome of intermittent claudication of the cauda equina in which, due either to congenital narrowing of the spine or to localised lesions in the spine, there is a relative ischaemia to the lumbar region which becomes more evident when the patient stands, walks or lies with the back extended. Positions of flexion, such as sitting or bending forwards, give relative relief from symptoms and the possibility of laminectomy to reduce intraspinal stenosis should be considered.

PAIN IN THE ARM

The symptoms of pain in a limb may be local or referred. Local causes, such as bone and joint disease, ischaemic and rheumatological problems, should be excluded by examination and investigation. The possibility of referred pain from intrathoracic organs must also be considered. There are three causes of neurological pain in the arm.

Spinal cord or root pain

Damage to the cervical roots or cervical spinal cord may cause pain radiating into the arm.

Radicular pain tends to be sharp and constant and spreads in the distribution of the individual root involved into the arm and is made worse by neck movement, coughing, sneezing and straining. It is well localised and is more common in the fifth, sixth and seventh cervical segments. It may occur with an acute cervical disc prolapse, cervical spine tumour or secondary tumour in the vertebra. It is also seen in patients who have suffered from shingles affecting the roots of the upper limb.

Spinal cord pain such as that due to an intramedullary lesion like a syrinx, or an ependymoma or haematoma, is usually more constant in nature and more burning in character. Neurofibromas and meningiomas may also occur at this site and can, similarly, cause both localised spinal pain and radiation of a radicular nature into the limbs.

Plexus pain

Lesions of the brachial plexus which are painful may be postinfective, as in the syndrome of brachial plexitis, or *neuralgic amyotrophy* when most commonly the fifth and sixth cervical roots are involved, causing exquisite pain for several days followed by wasting of the relevant muscles. Neuralgic amyotrophy is a proximal demyelinating condition which most commonly follows an upper respiratory tract infection or inoculation. It is believed to be due to an autoimmune process causing demyelination of cervical roots within the brachial plexus resulting in initial pain and later wasting. Alternatively, structural damage related to a cervical rib or, in the lower roots of the plexus, involvement of the plexus in a Pancoast tumour from the apex of the lung, may also occur. The latter condition tends to involve the first thoracic root and will therefore also be associated with a Horner's syndrome and loss of sweating in the hand.

Nerve pain

The most common causes of pain in the peripheral nerves of the upper limb are due to entrapment neuropathies. The radial nerve may be trapped in the radial groove of the humerus and, although this lesion is usually painless, it can cause pain in the back of the hand. The ulnar nerve may be damaged at the elbow in the olecranon groove which results in pain and numbness in the little and ring finger and weakness of the majority of muscles in the hand. The median nerve is most commonly compressed in the carpal tunnel at the wrist, which problem may occur in relation to myxoedema, pregnancy, acromegaly, rheumatoid arthritis or old fractures of the wrist. It tends to occur in the dominant hand and causes dysaesthesiae most prevalent at night in the thumb, index and middle fingers of the hand.

The anterior interosseous nerve may be trapped in the interosseous membrane or at the head of the pronator teres and typically causes pain on pronation and supination of the forearm with weakness of the long flexors of the hand.

These mononeuropathies occur due to local pressure, but they can also be the result of more generalised conditions such as arteritis or diabetes, causing nerve infarcts. There are also certain familial conditions, such as tomaculous neuropathy, in which patients are particularly prone to pressure palsies. Some more peripheral lesions involving digital nerves in the hand may result in the development of causalgia, which has been described earlier.

Other neurogenic pain

Other causes of neurogenic pain in the arm include spasticity, when the cramp in the muscle may result in a significant degree of pain. In addition polymyositis, an inflammatory myopathy, is frequently associated with pain in the muscles particularly on palpation and exercise.

PAIN IN THE LEG

Although it is always necessary to exclude from consideration those local painful syndromes of bone, joint and blood vessels in the lower limbs, it should be remembered that exercise-induced pain is not always diagnostic of ischaemic disease of the legs but, as mentioned above, can occasionally be due to ischaemia arising in the cauda equina and may be seen in patients with spasticity in the lower limbs or with polymyositis or metabolic myopathies.

Spinal cord or root pain

Prolapsed intervertebral disc is the most common cause of radicular pain in the lower limbs. The most common discs to prolapse are those between the lumbar fourth and fifth and the lumbar fifth and first sacral vertebrae resulting in the syndrome of sciatica. Pain will characteristically radiate down the posterior aspect of the leg into the ankle or foot. It is made worse by those factors which increase intracranial intraspinal pressure such as coughing or sneezing and may also cause limitation of flexion of the lumbar spine, loss of the normal lumbar lordosis and limitation of straight leg raising to less than the normal 90 degrees. There will usually be an associated loss of reflexes in the appropriate segment of the lower limb and there may be sensory loss and wasting and weakness of muscles. More rarely, the roots of the femoral nerve are involved in a prolapsed intervertebral disc, causing pain radiating to the front of the thigh and associated with loss of the knee jerk and wasting of the quadriceps. Femoral nerve involvement may also occur in the presence of diabetes mellitus when the lesion is believed to be attributable to infarction of the nerve. This condition of diabetic amyotrophy is usually associated with an initial severe pain in the region of the quadriceps followed by weakness of the muscle.

Intraspinal tumours will cause a less well localised pain which may radiate into the lower limbs or into the perineum and is frequently associated with loss of sensation, wasting and weakness of muscles and with reflex loss. Ischaemia within the lumbosacral spine may cause pain on exercise, together with symptoms of weakness and sensory disturbance. Occasionally, bladder and bowel disturbances may occur on exercise or when assuming the erect posture. Other intraspinal causes of pain radiating into the leg include arachnoiditis in the lumbar spine and occasional sharp lancinating pains in the legs are found in the condition of tabes dorsalis.

Plexus pain

The most common causes of pain in the lumbosacral plexus are the presence of *infiltration of tumours* from the pelvis. The most important part of examination is rectal or pelvic examination and other methods of examining the pelvis such as ultrasound or body scanning are obligatory in such cases. The pain in this situation is usually intractable, unilateral, gnawing and related to signs of lower motor neurone damage with areflexia and flaccidity and disturbances of bladder and bowel function with a flaccid bladder and patulous anus. Pain in the anterior aspect of the thigh together with weakness of the quadriceps may occur in the syndrome of *diabetic amyotrophy*. Whilst this may occur in the context of a patient recognised to be diabetic, it can also be the presenting feature of the disease particularly in the elderly and is believed to be due to ischaemic lesions occurring in the plexus or femoral nerve. *Neuralgic amyotrophy*, though less common than in the brachial plexus, may also affect the lumbar plexus presenting with acute pain and progressive muscle weakness.

Peripheral nerve pain

Pain in the lower limb due to peripheral nerve damage is less common than that in the upper limb but similar causes of mononeuropathy need to be considered. Entrapment of the lateral cutaneous nerve of the thigh at the inguinal ligament results in the syndrome of meralgia paraesthetica with pins and needles over the outer aspect of the thigh. Digital pain in the foot may be caused by the presence of a neuroma on one of the digital nerves, as in Morton's metatarsalgia, and generalised peripheral neuropathies characteristically of axonal type can cause dysaesthetic pain in both lower limbs and in the hands. Such conditions are seen in diabetic neuropathy, some paraneoplastic neuropathies and other more diffuse causes of generalised peripheral neuropathy.

Other neurogenic pain

Intermittent claudication of the cauda equina has already been mentioned and, although this syndrome may present with pain in the back, it will also tend to cause pain in the lower limb which will increase with extension of the spine and with exertion. In addition, cramp in the lower limb will tend to result from any condition causing spasticity and the metabolic and inflammatory myopathies may again cause pain in the lower limbs, particularly on exercise or palpation.

Pain of uncertain nature

There are two syndromes which occur in the lower limbs and which are of uncertain and possibly multiple aetiology. The first of these is the *restless legs syndrome*, or Ekbom's syndrome, and is a usually benign syndrome which may frequently be most prominent at night and can cause sleep disturbance. It may occasionally indicate the presence of a subclinical peripheral neuropathy or even myelopathy, but most commonly no significant cause can be found and the symptoms will respond to low doses of phenothiazines or occasionally tricyclic agents.

The second syndrome of painful feet and moving toes is also of uncertain aetiology but may be particularly distressing, especially when resting. It is difficult to control and is of uncertain cause.

PAIN IN AN ARM AND LEG

The occurrence of pain in a hemidistribution is uncommon but occurs in patients who suffered thalamic infarcts or haemorrhage where the contralateral side may be rendered both anaesthetic and dysaesthetic. This particular type of hyperpathic pain is termed the thalamic syndrome and is frequently intractable to therapy although carbamazepine, phenytoin and tricyclic medication can be used. In patients with multiple sclerosis, lesions in the spinothalamic tract may occasionally be associated with painful tonic spasms on the contralateral side of the body, which symptoms usually respond to treatment with carbamazepine.

MANAGEMENT OF PAINFUL SYNDROMES

The management of the patient with chronic pain syndromes is complex and outside the scope of this chapter. In essence three major principles of management should be considered.

DIAGNOSIS

Although it is recognised that the cause of chronic pain may not always be identifiable, it is imperative that the physician make an attempt to understand any underlying organic basis. Not only is this important in devising the most appropriate therapy, but it may indicate a cause which requires surgery and enable a prognosis to be given to the patient. It is frequently of help in being able to provide a patient with an explanation for the nature of their chronic pain and it is a common finding for patients in whom there is no evident cause of pain to declare that they wish there had been some sort of disease process discovered.

The investigations to be undertaken will include biochemical, haematological, radiological and even electrophysiological studies to trace the nerve pathways and to assess the damage.

THERAPY

Where possible, specific therapy should be applied to treat the cause of the painful syndrome. If this is not practicable, then the use of adequate analgesic agents should be considered up to and including the opiates. If these agents are ineffective, or if it is more appropriate to consider ablative surgery to either peripheral nerve, cord or thalamus, then these procedures should be undertaken.

The recent development of pain clinics has given rise to a considerable number of alternative therapies, including transcutaneous electrical stimulation and the use of local anaesthetic injections. The tendency for the patient with chronic pain to turn to alternative medicine such as acupuncture, chiropraxy and faith healing is of course well recognised.

SUPPORT SERVICES

When pain is constant and cannot adequately be relieved by the physician it is important that adequate support be given, whether this be at a practical level, with therapeutic agents, or by paramedical intervention. Many patients who have intractable pain syndromes can be helped by adequate supportive care and advice from trained professionals and in many respects it is this aspect which has been most successfully fulfilled by the hospice movement.

FURTHER READING

Lance J W 1982 Mechanism and management of headache, 4th edn. Butterworths, London

Lipton S 1977 Persistent pain—modern methods of treatment, vol 1. Academic Press, London

Wall P D 1970 The sensory and motor role of impulses travelling in the dorsal columns towards cerebral cortex. Brain 93: 505–524

Wolff H G 1963 Headache and facial pain, 2nd edn. Oxford University Press, Oxford

9

Disorders of the spinal cord and cauda equina

ANATOMY

The adult spinal cord is oval in shape and approximately 1 cm in diameter. It extends from the foramen magnum, where it is continuous with the medulla, to the upper border of the second lumbar vertebra below which descend the lumbosacral roots which make up the cauda equina (Fig. 9.1).

The spinal cord is surrounded by meninges, the outermost layer of which, the dura, extends to the sacrum. The cord is supported by ligaments within the intraspinal canal (Fig. 9.2). The anatomy of the motor sensory and autonomic pathways is covered in Chapters 1, 2 and 3

BLOOD SUPPLY

A diagrammatic representation of this is depicted in Figure 9.3. The upper thoracic cord is a watershed zone between supply from the anterior spinal artery and supply from the intercostal arteries, the largest of which enters in the low thoracic or upper lumbar region (the artery of Adamkiewicz). At L2 the vessels entering through the intervertebral foramen join to form the lowermost portion of the anterior spinal artery which runs along the filum terminale.

The direction of blood flow in the anterior spinal artery varies depending on the level. In the cervical and upper dorsal cord the flow is rostrocaudal whereas below this the flow is upwards.

The spinal veins exit from the substance of the cord and terminate in a plexus in the pia mater. In the cervical and upper dorsal cord, channels pass upwards into the corresponding veins of the medulla. Segmental veins pass outwards along the nerve roots to join the vertebral venous plexus which is continuous throughout the level of the spinal cord and joined rostrally to the intracranial venous sinuses. Venous drainage through the intervertebral foramina is relatively unimportant.

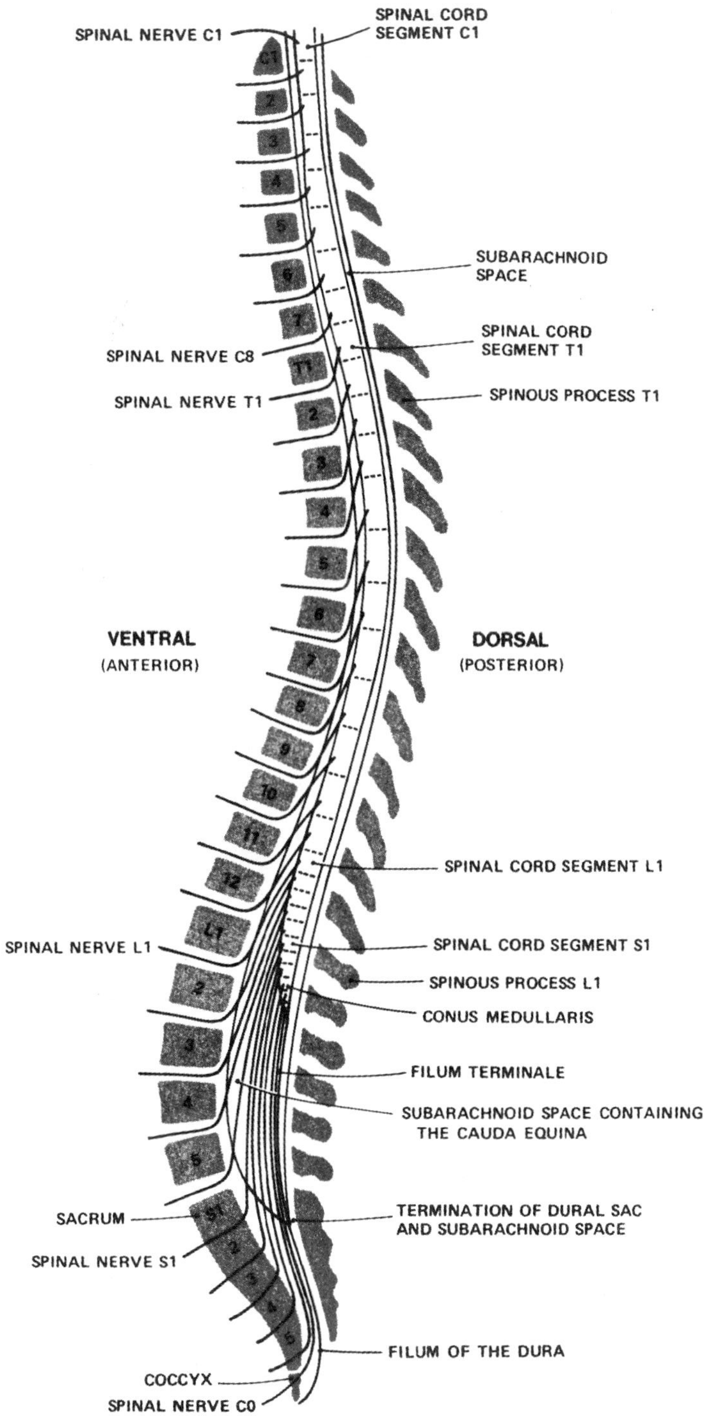

Fig. 9.1 General anatomy of the spinal cord and its segments in relation to the vertebral bodies.

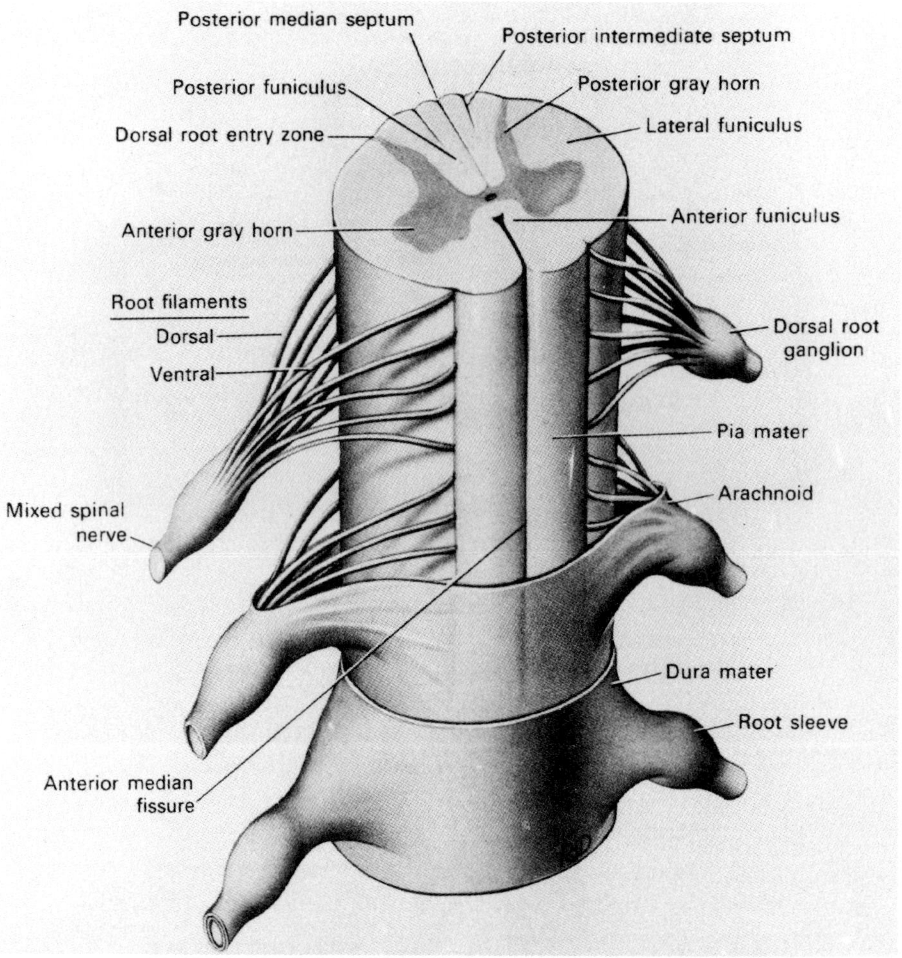

Fig. 9.2 General anatomy of the spinal cord and meninges (Reproduced from Carpenter M B, Sutin J 1983 *Human Neuroanatomy*, 8th edn. Williams and Wilkins, Baltimore, with permission).

CLINICAL FEATURES OF SPINAL CORD DISTURBANCES

Damage to the spinal cord may produce deficits due to involvement of the descending motor pathway, the ascending sensory pathways, the pathways concerned with autonomic function and the nerve roots. Complete transection of the cord at a single level will produce paralysis of all motor function below that level (paraplegia or tetraplegia), complete anaesthesia below that level, loss of bowel and bladder function, impairment of sweating and vasomotor control and, due to damage to the anterior horn cells, segmental lower motor neurone motor dysfunction. If the dorsal root is damaged there will be segmental sensory loss at the affected level.

EVOLVING PARAPARESIS

Spinal cord compression is among the most urgent of neurological emergencies and it is of considerable practical importance to recognise the clinical features of this syndrome. Without appropriate treatment patients with progressive spinal cord compression may be rendered permanently paraplegic whereas, in many instances with appropriate treatment, this may be prevented.

A

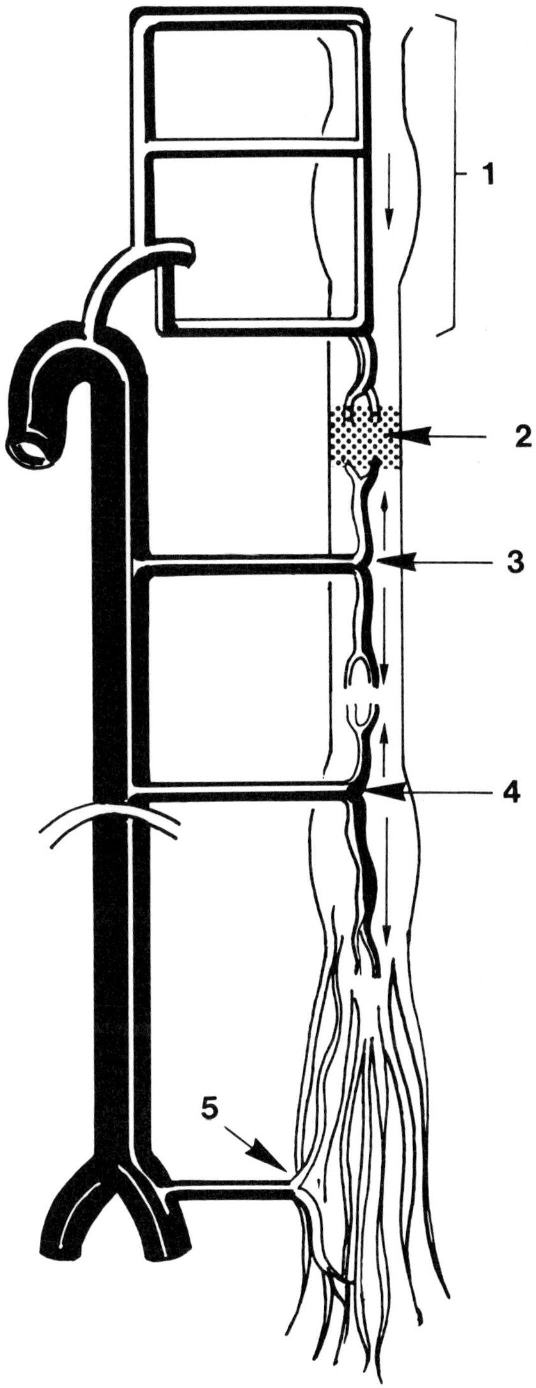

B

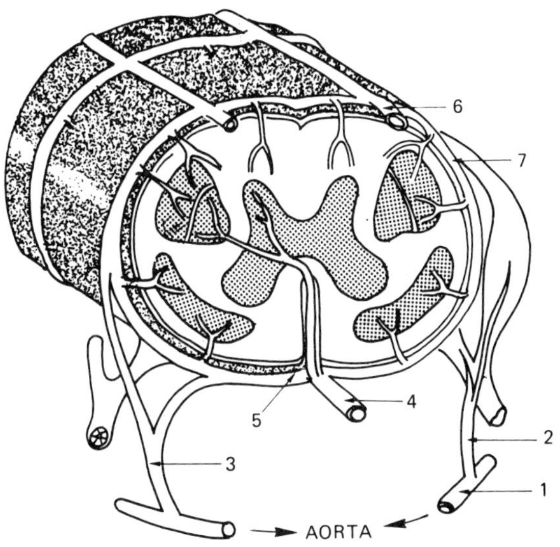

Fig. 9.3 Arterial supply of the spinal cord. **A** 1—Cervical and upper thoracic cord supplied by branches of the vertebral ascending cervical and superior intercostal arteries, 2—watershed zone at level of fourth thoracic segment, 3—mid-thoracic cord supplied from a single intercostal artery 4—thoracolumbar region supplied by a large vessel near the diaphragm, 5—cauda equina supplied from lower lumbar, ileolumbar and lateral sacral arteries. **B** 1—Intercostal artery, 2—posterior branch supplying nerve roots only (the usual pattern), 3—posterior branch supplying cord (e.g. arteria magna), 4—anterior spinal artery, 5—anterior sulcal artery supplying one-half of cord, 6—posterior spinal artery, 7—circumflex vessel supplying surface of cord. (Reproduced from Henson R A, Parsons M 1967 Ischaemic lesions of the spinal cord: An illustrated review. *Quarterly Journal of Medicine* 142: 205–221, with permission.)

Compression of the spinal cord may produce any combination of the signs and symptoms referred to above with, in many instances, the additional symptom of local pain.

Symptoms

Local

Back pain may be present in a spinal cord lesion when due to compression from a tumour, disc or abscess. Referred pain due to root irritation may occur in the thoracic region (girdle pain), cervical region (brachialgia), or lumbar region (sciatica). Typically the pain is brought on by movement or a Valsalva manoeuvre, or may occur at rest, the latter being suggestive of a tumour. Tingling down the spine or into the arms and legs on flexing the next (Lhermitte's sign) indicates cervical cord pathology and may occur not only in spinal cord compression but also in multiple sclerosis.

Weakness of the legs may be a symptom of damage to the cord *at any level* or damage to the cauda equina and this differentiation should be obvious from the signs. Sensory disturbances due to spinal cord compression typically begin in the feet and ascend.

Signs

The most obvious signs are usually those of weakness in the legs. When the cord itself is damaged there will typically be signs of an upper motor neurone disturbance with increased tone, increased reflexes and extensor plantar responses. Damage to the cauda equina produces lower motor neurone signs with depression of the tendon reflexes. Damage at the level of the conus may produce a combination of upper and lower motor neurone signs. If there are signs to indicate a cord disturbance it is important to remember that the damage has occurred *above* the level of the second lumbar vertebra.

Root signs may be of value in determining the level of the spinal cord pathology. Loss of upper limb reflexes or inversion of the biceps reflex are important signs of cervical cord dysfunction. Segmental loss of motor function in the thoracic region is rarely detected because of the overlap of the intercostal muscles although damage at the level of the tenth thoracic segment of the spinal cord may produce a Beevor's sign, i.e. the navel moves upwards when the patient attempts to sit up.

The level of the sensory loss may be helpful in indicating the site of damage but it is important to remember that the sensory level may be many segments *below* the actual area of damage in incomplete lesions. As compression becomes more severe, sensory levels tend to ascend progressively to approach their true anatomical level. Occasionally a segmental sensory loss may be helpful in estimating the spinal level, as may a level for loss of sweating.

The functional level of the spinal cord does not correspond to the bony level of the vertebra (Fig. 9.1), e.g. damage at the level of the fourth thoracic vertebra produces signs at a functional level of T6.

CLINICAL SYNDROMES (Fig. 9.4)

Partial lesions

Partial lesions of the cord may produce differing clinical syndromes depending on the tracts involved. Intrinsic spinal cord lesions, often termed intramedullary, tend to produce a different pattern from extrinsic or extramedullary spinal cord lesions. Intrinsic disorders of the spinal cord often produce precipitancy or urgency of micturition as an early symptom. Extrinsic lesions compressing the spinal cord more commonly produce motor signs and sensory symptoms as early symptoms. Root pain and local back pain are more common with extramedullary lesions.

Anterior cord syndromes

Damage predominantly to the anterior parts of the spinal cord will be associated with motor weakness and loss of spinothalamic sensation.

Posterior cord syndromes

Damage to the posterior parts of the cord produce proprioceptive impairment and such patients often have a Lhermitte's sign. As well as symptoms of

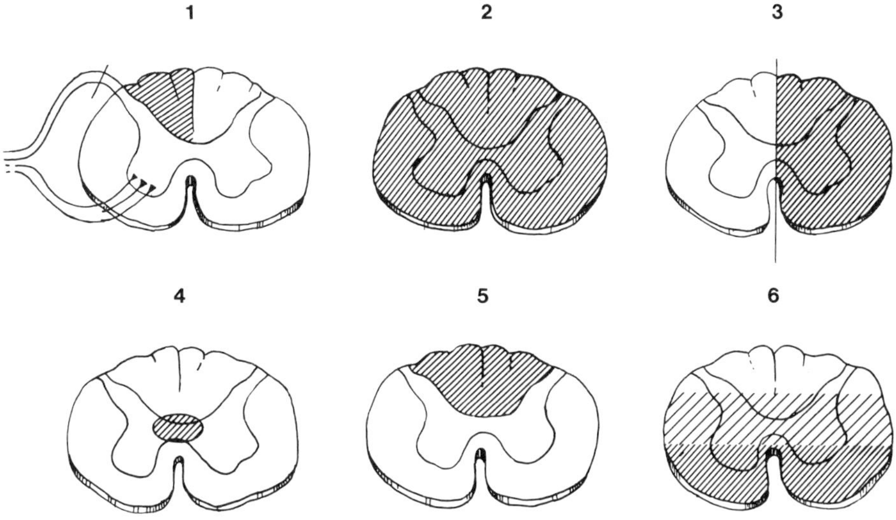

Fig. 9.4 Some characteristic spinal cord syndromes. 1—Tabetic syndrome, 2—complete transection, 3—hemisection of the cords, 4—syringomyelic syndrome, 5—posterior cord syndromes, 6—anterior spinal artery syndrome. (After Adams R D, Victor M 1981 *Principles of Neurology*. McGraw-Hill, New York, with permission.)

unsteadiness due to proprioceptive loss, there are often positive symptoms such as feelings that the legs are swollen or encased in tight bands.

Foramen magnum compression

Compression of the posterior part of the spinal cord at the craniovertebral junction may produce a very characteristic pattern of sensory loss in a 'round the clock pattern', proprioceptive symptoms appearing first in one leg then the ipsilateral arm, then the contralateral arm and finally the contralateral leg.

Hemisection of the spinal cord

The Brown-Séquard syndrome is the syndrome of hemisection of the spinal cord. It is rarely seen in its pure form and most commonly results not from spinal cord compression but from multiple sclerosis. The features are:

1. Ipsilateral paralysis of the upper motor neurone type below the level of the lesion with lower motor neurone signs at the level of the lesion.
2. Ipsilateral loss of tactile sensation, joint position sense, two point discrimination and vibration sense below the level of the lesion.
3. Contralateral loss of pain and temperature sensation below the level of the lesion. Spinothalamic fibres cross to the opposite side within a few segments of entering the cord and thus it is usual to find that the level of the contralateral spinothalamic sensory loss is a few segments below the level of the causative lesion.

There may be some ipsilateral impairment of pain and temperature sense at the level of the lesion because of interruption of the fibres at the dorsal root entry zone.

Central cord damage

A central cord syndrome occurs when the damage is predominantly in the central portions of the spinal cord. This most typically results from syringomyelia, but intrinsic tumours and trauma may produce a similar pattern of signs. The damage typically first occurs to the crossing spinothalamic fibres producing an expanding suspended loss of pain and temperature sense; this may be associated with pain. Damage to the reflex arc at the level of the expanding central cord lesion produces loss of the tendon reflexes at the affected segment and in most instances there is compression of the descending motor pathways producing upper motor neurone signs in the legs.

Conus damage

Damage at the level of the conus produces a mixed pattern of upper and lower motor neurone signs. Typical causes are an ependymoma or a glioma, though occasionally developmental anomalies of the lower spine such as dysraphism associated with a lipoma at the lower end of the cord may produce a similar picture. Characteristically, the patient complains of pain and lower sacral segment sensory loss is present. The tendon reflexes in the legs are diminished or absent yet the plantar responses are extensor. Sphincter problems and, in the male, impotence are common.

Cauda equina compression

Cauda equina compression results most commonly from either a tumour or from a central disc prolapse. Both local and root pain are usually a prominent feature. Damage to the roots usually is associated with lower motor neurone paralysis of the affected segments with muscle weakness, wasting and loss of tendon reflexes. The pattern of sensory loss depends on the roots involved: compression of the lower sacral roots leads to a characteristic saddle-shaped area of anaesthesia extending over the perineum, buttocks and backs of thighs; disturbance of bladder, bowel and sexual function is a common and early symptom.

Any of these syndromes of incomplete spinal cord damage may progress to paraplegia and appropriate investigation and treatment may be required to prevent this.

Complete transection

Complete transection most commonly results from trauma (p. 368). This results in total loss of function below the level of the damage and spinal shock.

INVESTIGATIONS

Depending on the speed of onset of symptoms, it is important to await the return of routine investigations as these may give important clues as to the diagnosis; for example, a high ESR might indicate a malignancy or myeloma, a raised MCV might indicate pernicious anaemia or an abnormal chest X-ray might indicate a bronchogenic carcinoma suggesting the diagnosis of a spinal metastasis.

All such patients should have plain radiographs of the appropriate area of the spine. In a patient with a paraparesis, but no definite level, both cervical and thoracic spine radiographs should be obtained. Even if these are normal, patients with suspected spinal cord compression should undergo more definitive investigations: these most commonly will include a myelogram. A lumbar puncture alone should not be performed in a patient suspected of having spinal cord compression. The major reason for this is that the patient's neurological deficit may become worse due to a change in the intraspinal pressure with coning.

AETIOLOGY

Table 9.1 lists the many and varied causes of spinal cord dysfunction. Many of these are covered in other chapters and here we shall concentrate on developmental disorders, spinal tumours, disc disease and vascular disease affecting the spinal cord.

DEVELOPMENTAL DISORDERS (Table 9.2)

SPINAL DYSRAPHISM (Spina bifida)

Closure of the neural groove occurs within a few weeks of fertilisation and failure of neural groove closure is the cause of neural tube defects, the most common of which is spinal dysraphism. A wide variety of differing conditions occur, the most common of which is a defect in the lumbosacral region (Fig. 9.5).

In severe forms, a sac protrudes through the bony defect and is apparent as an obvious mass in the midline. The sac may contain meninges and cerebrospinal fluid (a meningocele) or, in addition, neural tissue (meningomyelocele). Occasionally the cutaneous covering is incomplete and there is discharge of the cerebrospinal fluid. In less severe cases there is no protrusion, but a defect in the

Table 9.1 Causes of spinal cord dysfunction

Developmental disorders
e.g. Chiari malformation
Diastematomyelia
Trauma
Mechanical
Physical—radiation myelopathy
Spondylosis and disc disease
Tumours
Primary
Secondary
Infections
Viral myelitis
Bacterial—epidural abscess
Syphilis
TB
Demyelination
Multiple sclerosis
Transverse myelitis
Metabolic
e.g. Hepatic myelopathy
Paraneoplastic
Subacute necrotising myelopathy
Degenerative
Familial–Hereditary spastic paraplegia
Motor neurone disease
Deficiency disorders
Pernicious anaemia
Vascular diseases
Cord infarction
Haematomyelia

Table 9.2 Developmental disorders of the spinal cord

Neural crest malformation
Arnold–Chiari malformation
Syringomyelia
Hydromyelia
Spinal dysraphism
Spinal cord agenesis
Bifid cord
Myelodysplasia
Diastematomyelia
Cysts
Dural/arachnoid cysts
Lipomas
Dermoids
Enterogenous cysts
Vascular
Vascular malformations
Bony disorders
Achondroplasia
Klippel–Feil anomaly
Congenital spinal stenosis

lamina may be palpable as a depression. Occasionally there is only a bony defect which is visible radiographically (spina bifida occulta). In the lumbar region this is a frequent incidental radiological finding and in the absence of any obvious clinical abnormality of the lumbar spine it is most unlikely that such an incidental finding will be associated with any symptoms (Fig. 9.6).

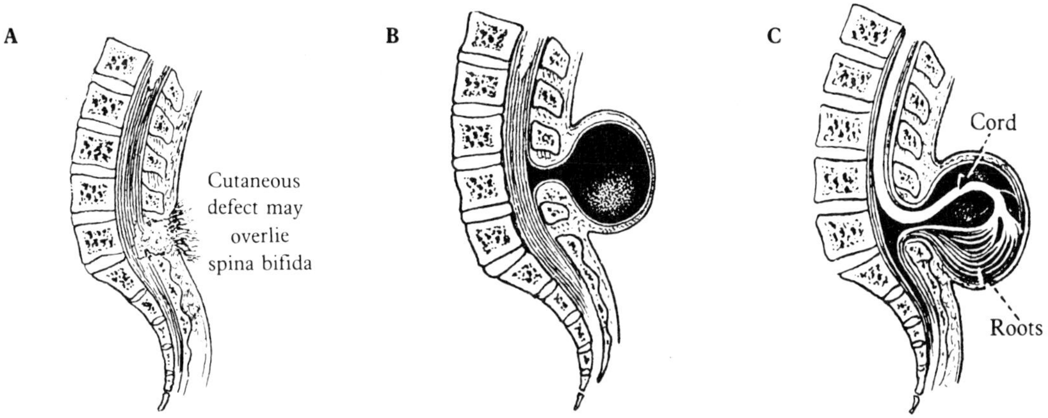

Fig. 9.5 Types of spina bifida—**A** in association with cutaneous defect; **B** meningocele; **C** meningomyelocele. (Reproduced from Lindsay K W, Bone I, Callander R 1986 *Neurology and Neurosurgery Illustrated*. Churchill Livingstone, Edinburgh, with permission.)

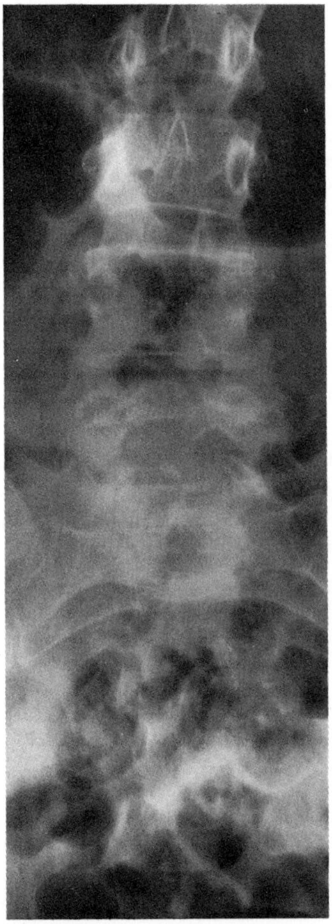

Fig. 9.6 Radiograph of lumbar spine showing spina bifida occulta.

In patients with spina bifida which shows itself with a palpable bony defect or a tuft of hair over the defect (spinal bifida operta) there may be a variety of intraspinal lesions including intrathecal dermoids, fibrous bands, lipomas or ectopic nerve roots. Spina bifida is frequently associated with other congenital abnormalities, particularly hydrocephalus. Severe degrees of spina bifida may be incompatible with survival, the victim being stillborn or surviving only a short time.

Symptoms

The neurological deficit in spina bifida may vary considerably. At one end of the spectrum there is the patient with asymptomatic spina bifida occulta and at the other end the patient with a gross deformity and a meningomyocele resulting in total paraplegia and sphincter paralysis. In most instances of those with a neurological deficit, this is stable, present from the time of birth and does not progress. The deficit may take the form of incontinence of urine, weakness of one or other leg, often with maldevelopment of the leg, or simply a degree of slowness in learning to walk.

In some instances patients with a minor degree of neurological deficit since the time of birth may show progression in later life. This may occur at any stage and may in unusual cases be delayed until middle or later life. Later deterioration in spina bifida is usually due to the effect of growth causing tension upon the lower cord or to the development of a lipoma, dermoid or constricting band compressing the cauda equina. The symptoms are those of a cauda equina disturbance but pain is not usually a feature. Bowel and bladder symptoms commonly occur and impotence may be present in the male. Trophic changes in the skin may become evident.

A diagnosis of spina bifida in obvious cases with a palpable deficit is easy. The bony abnormalities may usually readily be seen on routine radiographs of the lumbosacral region and normal radiographs exclude the diagnosis. In patients with deteriorating symptoms, myelography is needed to delineate the intraspinal anomaly.

The prognosis in spina bifida is directly related to the degree of the deficit. Children with severe defects will die without treatment and many may be saved but left totally paraplegic, and in some instances retarded as a result of associated hydrocephalus. Table 9.3 lists some of the indications for surgical treatment.

Table 9.3 Indications for surgery in spina bifida

Early
No neurological deficit
Open deficit
Mild/moderate deficit
Myeloschisis
Myelodysplasia
Late
Late deterioration of neurological deficit
Intraspinal lipoma or other pathology

MYELODYSPLASIA

This is a variety of spinal dysraphism which is present from the time of birth and is a form of maldevelopment of the spinal cord alone. The commonest anatomical abnormality of the cord is diastematomyelia (a bifid state of the lower cord). In some instances the two separate parts of the spinal cord are contained within a single dural tube, but in others each of the two cords has its own dural sheath and these are separated by a bony or fibrous septum. Such abnormalities most commonly occur in the lumbosacral region but may be present at any level of the spinal cord.

Clinically, myelodysplasia presents as a non-progressive spinal cord disturbance and it is often associated with deformities of the feet such as pes cavus or syndactyly. Radiological spina bifida is a common accompaniment.

SYRINGOMYELIA AND THE ARNOLD CHIARI MALFORMATION

Syringomyelia is a chronic disease characterised by the pressence of long cavities within the spinal cord; in many instances such cavities are related to the central canal of the spinal cord. Recent work has shown that in many cases there is an associated abnormality at the craniovertebral junction such as the Arnold–Chiari malformation. Table 9.4 lists the differing types of syringomyelia.

Table 9.4 Varieties of syringomyelia

Communicating syringomyelia
With Chiari malformation
With acquired abnormalities at foramen magnum
Syringomyelia after spinal trauma
Syringomyelia after arachnoiditis
Syringomyelia in association with spinal tumours
Idiopathic syringomyelia

In the normal development of the ventricular system the cerebrospinal fluid drains through foramina in the roof of the fourth ventricle (the foramina of Luschka and Magendie). Total failure of development of these foramina results in the Dandy Walker syndrome and partial failure in one of the various types of Chiari anomalies (Fig. 9.7) of which there are three types:

Type I	Descent of cerebellar tonsils into spinal canal
Type II	Descent of part of cerebellum and fourth ventricle into spinal canal
Type III	Descent of brain stem into spinal canal.

Figure 9.8 gives a diagrammatic representation of one theory of the pathogenesis of communicating syringomyelia.

Pathology

Syringomyelic cavities in the cord most frequently are found in the cervical and upper thoracic

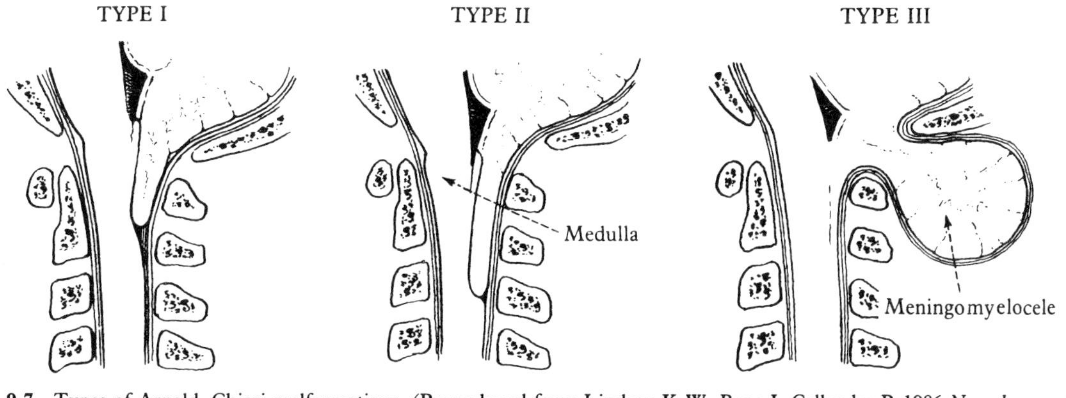

Fig. 9.7 Types of Arnold–Chiari malformations. (Reproduced from Lindsay K W, Bone I, Callander R 1986 *Neurology and Neurosurgery Illustrated*. Churchill Livingstone, Edinburgh, with permission.)

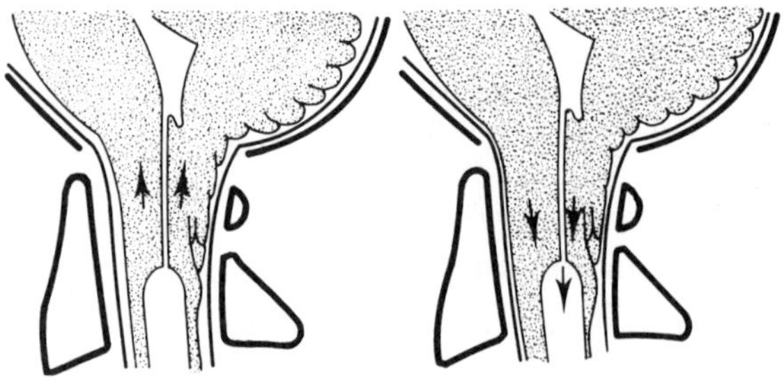

Fig. 9.8 The pathogenesis of syringomyelia. Schematic illustration of the potential ball and socket valve mechanisms thought to be present in syringomyelia associated with tonsillar ectopia. (Reproduced from Williams B 1970 Current concepts of syringomyelia. British Journal of Hospital Medicine 4: 331, with permission.)

regions. Extension into the medulla (syringobulbia) or thoracolumbar region may occur. The affected portion of the spinal cord is swollen and there may be enlargement of the bony canal. The cavity of the cord is lined by gliosis and contains clear or yellow fluid. Expansion of the cavity and resulting gliosis leads to compression of the antèrior horn cells and the major ascending and descending fibre pathways. Occasionally there may be haemorrhage into a syringomyelic cavity, constituting one of the rarer forms of haematomyelia.

Symptoms

Symptoms may begin between the ages of 10 and 60 and most commonly occur in the third and fourth decades, with males being affected more than females.

Sensory symptoms and signs are prominent due to damage to the crossing spinothalamic fibres resulting in typical cases with half cape dissociated sensory loss. Pain may be a prominent feature and, because of the sensory loss, trophic changes may occur, most commonly in the fingers. The commonest motor symptoms are weakness and wasting, which are most apparent in the hands, and tendon reflexes in the arms are typically absent. This more commonly begins on one side and spreads to the other. As the cavity extends, wasting and weakness spread to involve proximal muscles and if the cavity extends into the medulla there will be wasting and weakness of the tongue and soft palate and other muscles supplied by the vagus nerve. In those cases with an anomaly at the craniovertebral junction nystagmus is a common finding due to distortion of the vestibular nuclei in the floor of the fourth ventricle.

The enlarging cavity may compress the descending motor tracts, producing upper motor neurone signs in the legs, and loss of the descending sympathetic fibres produces a Horner's syndrome or lack of sweating over the affected limb. The sphincters are rarely involved until late.

Skin and skeletal changes

Trophic changes in the affected limbs take the form of painless burns and trophic ulcers and one fifth of patients show evidence of Charcot's joints (Fig. 9.9). Scoliosis is not infrequent and in severe cases the deformity is marked.

Diagnosis

In most instances the diagnosis is straightforward as the combination of wasting and trophic lesions in the hands with extensive sensory loss and upper

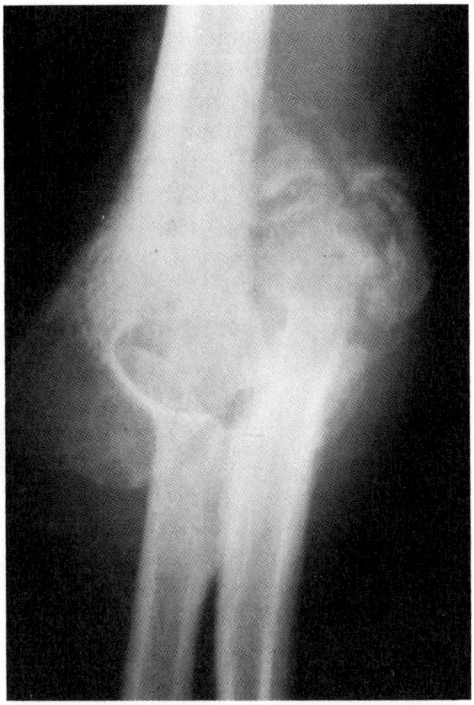

Fig. 9.9 Radiograph of an elbow joint showing disorganisation due to loss of pain sensitivity (Charcot's joint).

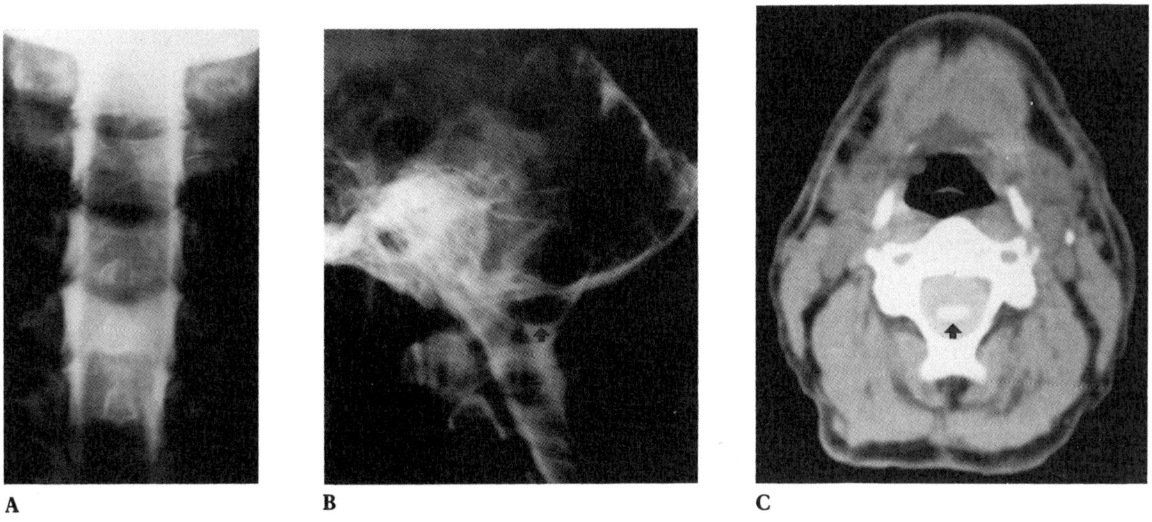

Fig. 9.10 Contrast radiography in syringomyelia. A Radiograph in AP plain showing intrinsic swelling of the cervical cord; B lateral radiograph showing protrusion of cerebellar tonsils through the foramen magnum (arrowed); C delayed contrast CT scan 12 hours later showing collection of contrast within the cavity within the spinal cord at a high cervical level.

motor neurone signs in the legs is highly distinctive. Intramedullary tumours of the spinal cord may produce a similar pattern of physical signs but these usually progress more rapidly. Cervical spondylosis may produce the combination of lower motor neurone signs in the arms and upper motor neurone signs in the legs but the sensory loss is rarely extensive. Motor neurone disease may simulate the motor but not the sensory signs.

Investigations

Plain radiographs of the cervical spine may show congenital anomalies and in chronic cases the anteroposterior diameter of the spinal canal is enlarged. Myelography will usually confirm that the spinal cord itself is enlarged but supine examination is necessary to demonstrate the region of the foramen magnum and show the Chiari malformation. Radiographically this appears as descent of the tonsils below the level of the foramen magnum. Other more sophisticated techniques using the spinal CT scan may demonstrate passage of a radio opaque medium from the subarachnoid space into the central cavity (Fig. 9.10). Because patients with Chiari malformations and syringomyelia may have hydrocephalus, it is usual to perform a CT scan of the head as an initial investigation before performing myelography. The technique of magnetic resonance imaging in the future will almost certainly be the investigation of choice as this produces detailed pictures with clear delineation of the anatomical structures (Fig. 9.11).

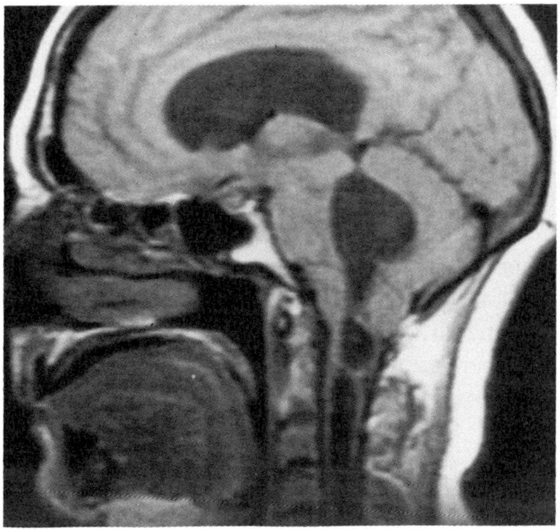

Fig. 9.11 Magnetic resonance image in syringomyelia.

Prognosis

Prognosis in variable and in a number of instances progression is so slow that treatment is neither required nor justified; other patients, however, may deteriorate quite rapidly and without appropriate treatment will become severely disabled.

Treatment

A variety of surgical procedures have now been developed to deal with syringomyelia. In those patients with a demonstrable Chiari malformation, decompressive surgery at the level of the foramen magnum will often halt progression of the condition and occasionally will lead to some improvement. Alternative treatments are some form of surgical drainage to the cyst itself.

The Chiari malformation without syringomyelia

Occasionally patients are seen with a Chiari malformation who do not have the signs or symptoms of syringomyelia. It is thought that in these cases the syringomyelia has not developed because the central canal of the cord has closed. Neurological deficits occur in later life due to compression of the spinal cord at the level of the foramen magnum by the tonsils themselves. This produces a clinical picture similar to that of a spinal tumour occurring at the level of the foramen magnum, with progressive motor and sensory deficit affecting all four limbs. Surgical decompression of the foramen magnum may lead to resolution of the symptoms.

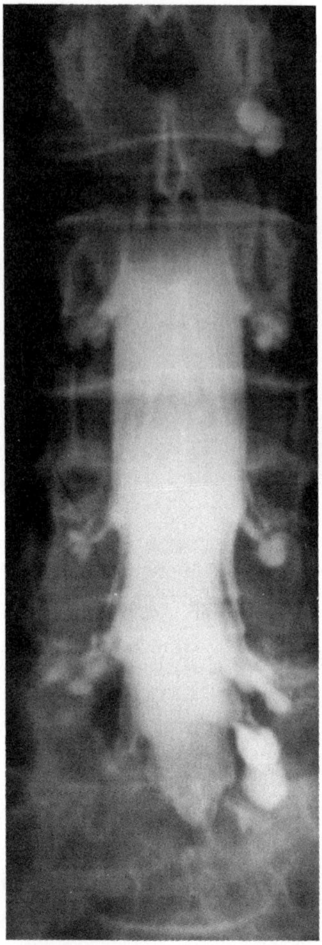

Fig. 9.12 Myelogram showing Tarlov's cysts.

OTHER DEVELOPMENTAL DISORDERS

A variety of other intraspinal developmental anomalies are occasionally encountered, including dural cysts, arachnoid cysts, lipomas and dermoids. Although these may in some instances be associated with radiological spina bifida, occasionally they occur in isolation and present with signs and symptoms of spinal cord decompression. At myelography it is not infrequent to find a number of such developmental arachnoid cysts which, in most instances, do not produce clinical abnormalities: these are so-called Tarlov cysts (Fig. 9.12).

ARTERIOVENOUS MALFORMATIONS

One developmental anomaly that may present in later life and which merits special consideration is that of a vascular malformation of the spinal cord. This is occasionally encountered in association with spina bifida but is more often present in isolation. In some cases there is an angioma in the skin over the area involved. These most commonly occur in the thoracolumbar regions and appear to increase in size gradually with the passage of time. They may present with signs and symptoms of progressive spinal cord dysfunction, although occasionally they may present acutely as a result of haemorrhage into the subarachnoid space or into the cord itself. The development of progressive cord symptoms in malformations may be due either to direct compression of the cord by the malformation, or to ischaemic myelomalacia. They produce a very characteristic picture on a myelogram, and in some instances surgical removal of the malformation is possible.

ACHONDROPLASIA

This dominantly inherited syndrome of dwarfism is associated with a failure of metaphyseal development resulting in impaired growth of cartilagenous bones. Not only are the long bones short, resulting in dwarfism, but the laminae of the spine are smaller than normal resulting in spinal stenosis. When the normal process of spondylosis develops, spinal cord compression results. A very high percentage of patients with achondroplasia who survive long enough become paraplegic. Treatment is very difficult.

Table 9.5 Types of spinal tumour

Intramedullary tumours
Primary
Gliomas
Ependymomas
Medulloblastomas
Lipomas
Angiomas
Haemangioblastomas
Secondary
Lung
Breast
Gastrointestinal tract
Melanoma
Lymphoma
Myeloma
Extramedullary (Extradural–Intradural)
Primary
Neurofibroma
Meningioma
Ependymoma
Secondary
Lung
Breast
Gastrointestinal tract
Melanoma
Lymphoma
Myeloma

TUMOURS

Primary tumours developing in and around the spinal cord are relatively uncommon, but the spread of malignant tumours to the vertebrae is not infrequent and these may present with signs and symptoms of spinal cord compression before the primary tumour has become manifest.

Tumours affecting the spinal cord are traditionally divided into intramedullary, intradural and extramedullary and extradural (Table 9.5, Fig. 9.13).

INTRAMEDULLARY TUMOURS

The commonest of these are ependymomas and gliomas, although very occasionally metastatic spread

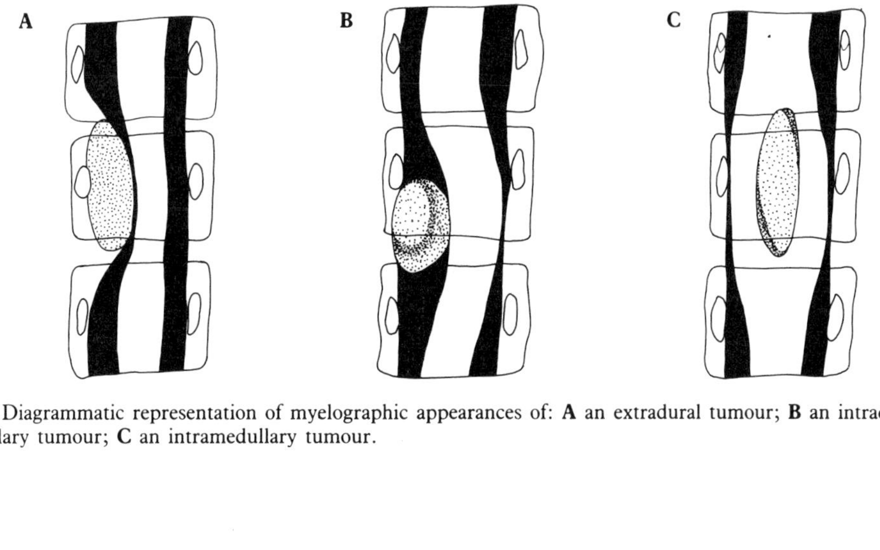

Fig. 9.13 Diagrammatic representation of myelographic appearances of: **A** an extradural tumour; **B** an intradural extramedullary tumour; **C** an intramedullary tumour.

may lead to the development of an intramedullary secondary. Other rare intramedullary tumours are lipomas and haemangioblastomas. Tumours may develop at any level in the spinal cord and ependymomas are sometimes seen at the level of the conus producing symptoms of conus or cauda equina compression.

The symptoms are those of spinal cord compression at the appropriate level and there is usually inexorable progression. Intramedullary tumours produce a characteristic myelographic appearance (Fig. 9.13C), but surgical removal is often difficult without considerable damage to the spinal cord. Radiotherapy is usually given postoperatively in patients who have a glioma or an ependymoma.

INTRADURAL AND EXTRAMEDULLARY (Fig. 9.13B)

The two common benign tumours of the spinal cord, the neurofibroma and meningioma, are seen in this site, as may be the occasional metastasis. These benign tumours characteristically progress slowly and are associated not only with signs of spinal cord compression, but also with radicular or girdle pain or local back pain. Meningiomas most typically occur in the dorsal region in middle-aged and elderly women whereas neurofibromas may occur at any level and may be multiple in patients with neurofibromatosis. Surgical removal of neurofibromas and meningiomas is usually complete, so that a cure may be anticipated.

EXTRADURAL (Fig. 9.13A)

The commonest extradural tumour is a metastasis. The tumour may originate in the bones of the vertebra and expand to compress the spinal cord or may develop from a blood-borne metastasis in the venous plexus in the extradural space. Tumours that show a predilection for bone commonly produce spinal cord compression and these include carcinoma of the prostate and lung; however, any malignant tumour may metastasise to produce this effect. The differential diagnosis of metastatic spread to the spinal column includes the solid malignancies, multiple myeloma, leukaemia and the lymphomas. Where the vertebral body is involved, symptoms may develop rapidly at the time of vertebral collapse, with an acute paraplegia developing within hours. More commonly the signs develop over a matter of weeks and local pain is often a prominent feature.

The diagnosis is usually obvious in patients who have a known malignancy; occasionally, however, the development of a spinal metastasis may be the first sign of an underlying malignancy. The radiological appearance of the changes in such cases may give a clue to the diagnosis, but in some instances the only way of making the diagnosis is by surgical biopsy.

In patients with secondary carcinoma involving the spine, survival is uncommon beyond 12 months; the aggressiveness of the treatment should thus be determined by the general health and outlook for the patient. The treatment of choice for most patients is radiotherapy: this may improve cord function and usually will alleviate pain. For patients where the pathology is uncertain, then surgical decompression may be considered. High-dose steroids occasionally produce temporary improvement and should be considered in all cases.

DISC DISEASE AND SPONDYLOSIS

Without question disc prolapse and the effects of spondylosis at various levels in the spine are the commonest cause of spinal symptoms. Acute disc prolapse commonly occurs under the age of 40 as the ageing processes in the spine are associated with reduced spinal mobility and a number of other changes which reduce the risk of disc prolapse.

ACUTE INTERVERTEBRAL DISC PROLAPSE

Acute intervertebral disc prolapse most commonly occurs under the age of 40 and symptoms are often precipitated by trauma. The commonest site for prolapse is in the lumbar region between the fifth lumbar vertebra and the first sacral vertebra.

The disc may prolapse directly backwards to compress the cauda equina or more commonly protrude laterally to compress the exiting lumbar root. Symptoms often develop following sudden lifting and consist of local back pain with radiating pain in the segment of the compressed root. Central disc prolapse may be associated with less pain, but with symptoms of compression of the cauda equina such as weakness of the legs, sensory disturbance or sphincter involvement.

The pain of lumbar disc prolapse is characteristically made worse by movement or by adoption of the erect posture. Pain of a similar type, which is more evident when the patient is resting, should suggest that the diagnosis is that of a tumour.

The signs of an acute lumbar disc prolapse are those of immobility of the lumbar spine, impairment of straight-leg raising on the appropriate side and motor and sensory signs due to damage to the affected root. In most instances these signs will be simply those of loss of the ankle jerk or some loss of sensation in the S1 segment over the lateral aspect of the foot.

A lateral disc protrusion is best treated conservatively with bed rest and immobilisation and the indications for further investigation by myelography with a view to surgery are persistence of pain despite rest, the development of neurological deficit such as foot drop, or intractable pain. Acute disc prolapse uncommonly occurs in the thoracic region, although when it does it may compress the spinal cord producing the clinical picture of spinal cord compression. Surgical removal of the disc is usually required but this is technically difficult with a significant morbidity.

Acute cervical disc prolapse may occur either spontaneously or as a result of trauma. It is associated with acute neck pain and if the protrusion is lateral with symptoms of root compression at the affected level. This most commonly is at the C5/6 or C6/7 levels with pain radiating into the appropriate dermatomes. Movement of the neck characteristically increases the pain and there is loss of the appropriate reflexes and occasionally sensory loss and muscle weakness. The treatment of acute lateral cervical disc prolapse is immobilisation by a collar and if necessary bed rest. If symptoms do not settle rapidly then myelography should be undertaken with a view to surgical removal of the disc. Posterior cervical disc protrusions often occur in the absence of pain and present with signs and symptoms of cervical cord compression, which are indistinguishable from those of a tumour in the cervical region. Such cases warrant early myelography with a view to surgical removal.

AGEING IN THE SPINE (Spondylosis)

A number of characteristic aging changes occur in the spine, most commonly in the cervical and lumbar spine areas. They are part of the normal aging process and are almost universal over the age of 60. The changes are more common in men, particularly in those who have worked in 'heavy' occupations such as mining and heavy industry. The changes of the intervertebral disc include disc degeneration with the development of anterior and posterior osteophytes from the margins of the body of the vertebra. Similar changes occur at the apophyseal joints and these restrict mobility at the affected level. In the cervical region the most commonly affected levels are C5/6 and C6/7 (Fig. 9.14) and the lumbar region L4/5 and L5/S1. Similar changes may occur at other levels in the spine, including the dorsal spine, but these are less common.

SPONDYLOSIS AND CHRONIC DISC DISEASE

Cervical spondylosis is characterised by osteophyte formation, disc degeneration and radiological narrowing of the disc spaces. There is often deformation of the ligamentum flavum and the combination of this deformation and the osteophytic protrusion into the spinal canal may produce spinal cord compression. There is evidence to suggest that the constitutional diameter of the spinal cord is important in the predisposition to spinal cord compression, as those with a constitutionally narrow canal are more likely to develop signs of spinal cord compression. There is some evidence to suggest that the osteophytes occurring

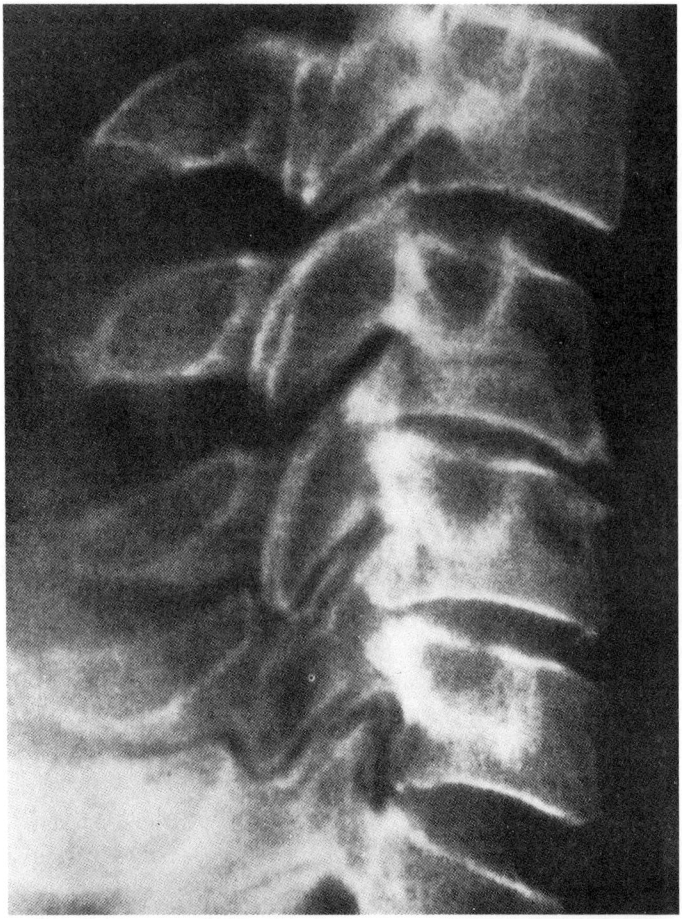

Fig. 9.14 Radiograph showing changes of cervical spondylosis with posterior osteophyte formation and loss of disc spaces.

at the level of the intervertebral foramina may compress the radicular arteries and that ischaemia is an important factor in the pathogenesis of a cervical myelopathy. What is apparent, however, is that gross cervical spondylosis may be visualised radiologically in some individuals who have no symptoms of either root or spinal cord compression and who are virtually pain free. There remains a degree of uncertainty as to why some individuals with cervical spondylosis develop symptoms and some with equally severe spondylosis remain asymptomatic.

The characteristic neurological complications of cervical spondylosis are those of a combination of motor and sensory root signs in the arms and upper motor neurone signs in the legs. Table 9.6 lists some of the common syndromes. The signs may evolve with a varying degree of rapidity and occasionally are precipitated by trauma with a rapid progression thereafter.

The indications for investigation and treatment in cervical spondylosis are progressive neurological deficits. Straight radiographs may show the affected level and the width of the cervical canal may be measured. The specific investigation of choice is myelography. A number of surgical procedures are available including cervical laminectomy to decompress the posterior aspect of the cord, or some form of anterior spinal fusion associated with removal of the degenerate disc and the osteophytes via an anterior approach.

Lumbar spondylosis

Chronic disc disease and spondylosis in the lumbar region are a common cause of symptoms

Table 9.6 Cervical spondylosis—clinical syndromes

Site of damage	Clinical features	Differential diagnosis
Motor roots	Muscle wasting and weakness of the upper limbs	Motor neurone disease, syphilitic amyotrophy
Sensory roots	Variable sensory loss in the upper limbs. Occasionally dissociated sensory loss	Syringomyelia
Mixed motor and sensory roots	Muscle wasting and weakness in the upper limbs with sensory loss	Syringomyelia
Spinal cord	Spastic paraparesis with ascending sensory level from the feet upwards. Occasionally Brown–Séquard syndrome	Any cervical cord pathology such as multiple sclerosis, spinal cord tumours, etc.
Motor and sensory roots and the spinal cord (the most common clinical picture)	Signs of root damage with muscle weakness and loss of upper limb tendon reflexes with spastic paraparesis and sensory loss in the legs. Bladder and bowel disturbances tend to develop late	Spinal tumours, multiple sclerosis

of backache and leg pain. Progressive neurological deficits due to compression of the cauda equina are relatively uncommon and merit further investigation by myelography. Occasionally gross spondylosis in the lumbar region produces encroachment upon the spinal canal and signs of cauda equina compression or the symptoms of cauda equina ischaemia (see below).

Most common of all are the complaints of back pain, with or without leg pain, in the absence of neurological abnormalities. In some instances it is impossible to be sure whether or not the symptoms are genuine and treatment of these patients is very unsatisfactory. Conservative measures including bed rest, plaster jackets and spinal epidural injections have been tried and it is often this sort of patient who ends up visiting an osteopath and having manipulation and other forms of fringe medical treatments.

OTHER FORMS OF SPONDYLOSIS

Rheumatoid arthritis and other forms of arthropathies may affect the vertebrae of the spinal cord, producing symptoms which may mimic spondylosis. Rheumatoid spondylosis typically affects the cervical spine and one common result is atlantoaxial subluxation leading to spinal cord compression. A flexion extension radiograph of the cervical spine should be taken in all patients with rheumatoid arthritis before they are anaesthetised to detect this complication; anaesthetists should receive appropriate warnings (Fig. 9.15).

VASCULAR MYELOPATHIES

The blood supply of the spinal cord has been described in an earlier section of this chapter and reference to effects on the vasculature of the spinal cord has been made in the trauma chapter and in the section dealing with spondylosis.

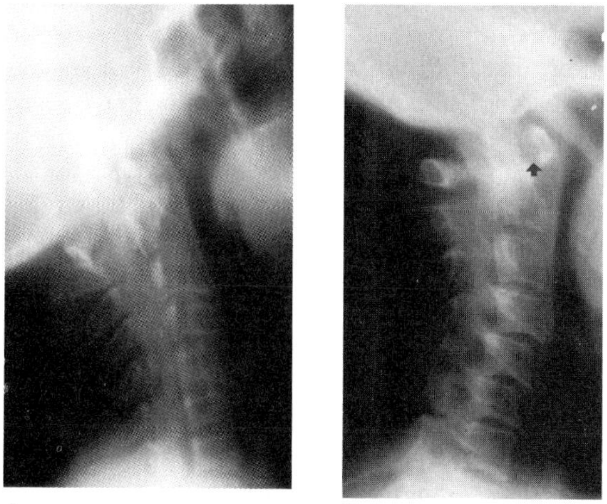

A B

Fig. 9.15 Radiographs of the cervical spine showing atlantoaxial subluxation in rheumatoid arthritis. **A** Views in extension; **B** views in flexion with arrows showing opening of space between odontoid peg and the atlas. Subluxation is also evidence at lower cervical levels.

INFARCTION OF THE SPINAL CORD OR CAUDA EQUINA

Acute infarction of the spinal cord as a result of vascular occlusion is relatively uncommon. *Anterior spinal artery occlusion* in the dorsal region may occur as a complication of dissecting aneurysm of the aorta or of surgical treatment of aortic aneurysms and spinal cord infarction occurring as a result has a bad prognosis. In patients with atheromatous vascular disease spontaneous anterior spinal artery occlusion may occur with symptoms of local pain in the back followed by the development of a rapid flaccid paralysis of the lower limbs, sphincter paralysis, and a sensory level at or about the umbilicus. There is usually some preservation of light touch and of joint position sense.

In recent years increasing attention has been paid to a variety of clinical syndromes thought to result from restricted zones of infarction in the spinal cord. These cases may result from occlusion of one posterior spinal artery or one or more feeding radicular arteries. In such cases the motor and sensory deficit is restricted to one or other limbs. Occasional examples of transient ischaemia to the spinal cord have been described.

There is now good pathological evidence to suggest that repeated episodes of such ischaemia or infarction may give rise to a gradually progressive paralysis of the legs in a stepwise direction. This is called atherosclerotic myelopathy and clinically it may mimic spinal cord compression and other inflammatory or demyelinating disorders.

Embolism to the arteries supplying the spinal cord occasionally occurs from fragments of atheromatous material in the aorta and a similar clinical picture may occur in bacterial endocarditis or as a result of air or fat embolism. One recognised example of this is decompression sickness.

INTERMITTENT CLAUDICATION OF THE CORD OR CAUDA EQUINA

In 1906 it was first suggested by Déjérine that transient weakness or numbness of one or both lower limbs occurring during exercise might be due to ischaemia of the cord or cauda equina. It is now well recognised that such a syndrome exists and the symptoms are typically those of pain, a sensory disturbance, and occasionally weakness induced by walking or even simply by standing. Exercising such affected individuals may lead to the demonstration of abnormal signs which disappear with rest.

Constitutional narrowing of the spinal canal in the lumbar region and extensive lumbar spondylosis narrowing the canal are the common two causes of this syndrome; disc disease at higher levels narrowing the canal may produce an identical picture. The precise explanation as to why exercise should produce ischaemia of the spinal cord or cauda equina is uncertain.

Appropriate radiography in such cases will usually demonstrate the spinal canal narrowing and many such patients may be cured by decompression of the spinal canal by laminectomy.

SPINAL HAEMORRHAGE

Haemorrhages, either within the cord or over the surface of the cord, are uncommon, although occasionally these may be precipitated by trauma (see p. 369).

Spontaneous haemorrhage within the spinal cord produces the syndrome of haematomyelia: this may occur spontaneously, in the haemorrhagic diatheses, in association with spinal arteriovenous malformations, or as a complication of syringomyelia. It typically presents with acute local pain in association with signs and symptoms of an expanding intramedullary lesion.

Epidural haemorrhage may occur spontaneously or in association with the haemorrhagic diatheses: it presents with local pain followed by symptoms or signs of spinal cord compression.

Spinal subarachnoid haemorrhage most commonly occurs as a result of a bleed from an arteriovenous malformation of the spinal cord. It presents with acute back pain, with radiation of the pain into the legs and ultimately the symptoms of a subarachnoid haemorrhage with headache, photophobia and vomiting. A spinal subarachnoid haemorrhage may be associated with symptoms of spinal cord dysfunction but more commonly is not.

VENOUS THROMBOSIS OF THE SPINAL CORD

Venous thrombosis affecting the vertebral venous plexus is a rare event. It may occur as a complication of epidural spinal abscess and it is thought to be one of the factors producing neurological deficit in those patients who suffer complications after injudicious intraspinal injections.

SPINAL ARACHNOIDITIS

This is a rare condition which may develop spontaneously, but most commonly is seen after some process damaging the spinal meninges. It may follow meningitis, most commonly due to TB, may be seen as a complication of intraspinal surgery, or may follow the introduction of radiographic agent into the subarachoid space at myelography.

The clinical features are usually those of a slowly progressive spinal cord syndrome with pain as a prominent feature. Typically there is extensive involvement of many segments of the spinal cord producing a combination of upper and lower motor neurone signs. There is no effective treatment.

Arachnoiditis at the level of the foramen magnum is one of the causes of a syringomyelic syndrome.

MANAGEMENT

The principles of management of spinal cord disorders are:

1. Diagnosis and treatment of the underlying cause where possible
2. Management of the paraplegia or tetraplegia either until it recovers, or in the long term.

MANAGEMENT OF PARAPLEGIA

BLADDER DISTURBANCES (see p. 93)

In the patient with a neurogenic bladder disturbance, the first priority is to maintain adequate drainage either to prevent distension of the bladder or to prevent incontinence with subsequent risk of skin excoriation. This usually will require an indwelling catheter until such time as the bladder recovers or in the long term. In the patient with permanent paraplegia and bladder problems there is some debate as to whether it is better to use a continuous indwelling catheter or to use intermittent catheterisation. In young women who are paraplegic, occasionally it is worth considering constructing an ileal conduit in order to preserve sexual function. The alternative is to teach the husband how to catheterise his wife so that he may remove the catheter at the time of sexual intercourse. For men there are many satisfactory incontinence apparatuses, such as sheaths, but there are no such equivalents for women. The atonic bladder associated with cauda equina lesions can usually be evacuated by manual compression and such patients do not require long-term catheterisation.

BOWEL

Bowel problems occur in a similar manner to that of bladder problems in patients with spinal cord damage. The commonest is constipation. In complete transverse cord lesions it may be possible to achieve reflex defaecation with stimulation to the sacral cutaneous area. In most patients with cauda equina lesions, satisfactory control of the bowels is best achieved by means of twice-weekly enemas, suppositories, or by manual evacuation of the faeces.

SKIN

In paraplegia the skin is extremely liable to injuries resulting in bed sores and the commonest cause of these is pressure due to lack of movement and anaesthesia. Most commonly such sores develop over the bony prominences of the heels, the ischeal tuborosities, the sacrum and the greater trochanters. Other factors which may be important are vasomotor paralysis, skin excoriation from incontinence and shock or anaemia.

The paraplegic skin requires extreme care: extremes of temperature should be avoided and patients should be nursed on smooth surfaces; the skin should be thoroughly cleaned and dried daily and the patient should be turned at least every 2 hours. Occasionally, where turning is not possible because of the need to immobilise limbs or of other medical problems such as respiratory insufficiency then patients need be nursed on special beds, such as the ripple bed or the clinitron bed.

SPASTICITY

In patients with transverse cord lesions, spasticity is an inevitable development once the stage of spinal shock passes. The limbs may develop spasms in either flexion or extension and these may occur spontaneously or may be precipitated by any sensory stimulus to the limbs. Physiotherapy in the form of passive movements may help, but in patients with profound spasticity it may be necessary to use intrathecal injections of phenol when there is no hope of recovery. Lesser degrees of spasticity may respond to the use of spasmolytics such as diazepam, baclofen or dantrolene. In patients with profound spasticity, contractures may develop and these make the nursing of such patients exceedingly difficult. Occasionally surgical treatment of the contractures is necessary.

PAIN

Pain is a common symptom in patients with spinal cord or cauda equina damage. The pain may be local in origin, due to root damage, or due to damage to the spinal sensory tracts. Pain is also often a feature of spasticity and that of the paraspinal muscles may produce local back pain. The treatment of the pain depends on the specific cause.

REHABILITATION

The rehabilitation of the paraplegic or tetraplegic patient involves more than simply physiotherapy to enable the patient to make the most of his or her deficit: the patient must be helped to adjust to a new mode of life and occupational therapy is important. Work at Stoke Mandeville has emphasised the importance of sporting activities. Family adjustments will need to be made and advice given about sexual activity. Detailed discussion of these aspects of the management of the paraplegic patient is beyond the scope of this section.

FURTHER READING

Barnett H G M, Foster J B, Hudgson P 1973 Syringomyelia. W B Saunders Co. Ltd, London

Guttman L 1978 Spinal cord injuries. Blackwell, Oxford

Hensen R A, Parsons M 1967 Ischaemic lesions of the spinal cord. Quarterly Journal of Medicine 26: 205–222

Hughes J T 1978 Pathology of the spinal cord, 2nd edn. W B Saunders Co. Ltd, Philadelphia

Wilkinson M 1971 Cervical spondylosis, 2nd edn. W B Saunders Co. Ltd, Philadelphia

10

Diseases of the peripheral nerves and muscle

DISEASES OF THE PERIPHERAL NERVES

INTRODUCTION

The peripheral nervous system comprises those parts of the nervous system lying outside the spinal cord and brain stem. The spinal and cranial nerve roots lie within the spinal canal or cranial cavity, and consist of a dorsal afferent root which comprises the central process of the dorsal root ganglion cell and the ventral efferent roots which are composed of the axons from the anterior and lateral horn cells and which terminate on muscle fibres, or in the ganglia of the autonomic nervous system. The dorsal root enters the cord at the dorsal root entry zone and the axons within it extend into the posterior columns or spinothalamic tracts as described in Chapter 2. The longer axon of the bipolar dorsal root ganglion cell acts as the sensory nerve fibre and terminates either as branching endings or as specialised corpuscular endings in the skin, joints and other tissues of the limbs.

The peripheral nerves are covered by supporting sheaths of perineurium and epineurium and they are richly supplied with anastomosing nutrient arteriolar branches which run throughout their course. Within the spinal canal, however, the dorsal and ventral roots lie within the arachnoid mata and are bathed by cerebrospinal fluid (Fig. 10.1).

Damage to the peripheral nerve may occur at any point from the origin of the spinal roots to the sensory or motor endings of the nerves. It is the site of such damage which determines the type of symptoms involved, and the distribution of the symptoms gives the clinician clues as to the nature of the underlying disease process. Disease processes will vary in the form of damage which they cause to the peripheral nerve. Some processes particularly those involving the vessels and compression, cause damage to all the elements within the nerve, whereas others may selectively involve either the motor or sensory elements and either the axons themselves or the myelin which surrounds those axons (Fig. 10.2). It is the determination of the site and type of the damage which allows some definition to be made of the nature of the underlying process. It should be recognised that peripheral nerve disease remains a condition in which accurate diagnosis is frequently not possible and, in approximately 40% of patients presenting to neurological departments, particularly with chronic progressing neuropathies, no cause can be determined. It is possible that, with the advances that are being made in understanding the biochemistry, physiology and function of nerves, this proportion of undiagnosable neuropathies will be reduced, but at present a significant proportion defeat even the most exhaustive of investigations.

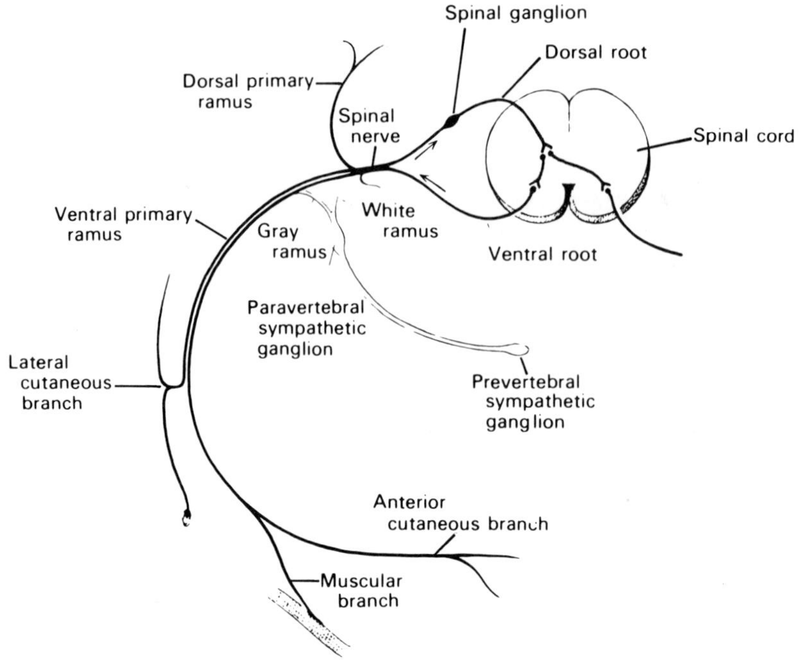

Fig. 10.1 Relationships of nerve roots and the spinal cord.

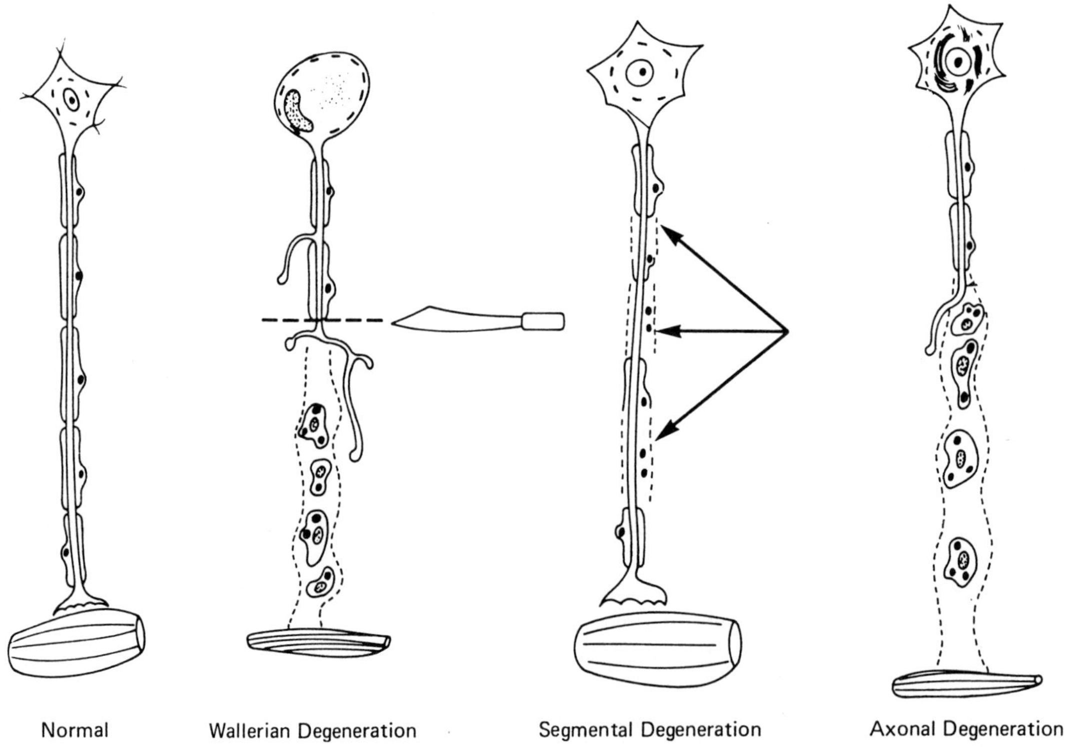

Fig. 10.2 The pathology of peripheral nerves showing Wallerian degeneration, demyelination, and axonal degeneration.

SYMPTOMS AND SIGNS OF PERIPHERAL NERVE DISEASE

Disease of the peripheral nerves is one of the conditions in which the history is of vital importance in attempting to determine the site of damage to the nervous system. There are a series of cardinal symptoms which should raise suspicion of disease affecting the peripheral nerve.

Motor symptoms and signs (see Ch. 1)

Weakness is the commonest motor symptom in peripheral nerve disease and, as it implies damage to the lower motor neurone, will usually be associated with the findings of wasting, flaccidity and absent tendon reflexes in the muscles concerned. Unfortunately, it is not possible from this weakness to determine whether the damage is due to disease affecting the axon or the myelin sheath, but the distribution of the weakness is of considerable importance in identifying the type of nerve involved. Thus, weakness which begins symmetrically and peripherally, usually in the lower limbs, implies a diffuse and generalised peripheral neuropathy, whereas that confined to the distribution of a single peripheral nerve, or motor root, implies damage to that nerve or to the root concerned. It thus becomes important that the clinician can identify which muscles are supplied by a particular nerve or by an individual motor nerve root. In general, the finding of muscle wasting is indicative of long-standing disuse or denervation and will not therefore be a feature of the acute neuropathies, but will be more marked and evident in those which are chronic in nature. Prolonged denervation of peripheral muscles will be liable to result in the development of contractures, which causes increasing problems for patients.

Although, as mentioned above, tendon reflexes tend to be absent in peripheral neuropathies, there is one class of small fibre peripheral neuropathy which is predominantly sensory in nature and which may not involve the tendon reflexes. Occasionally, muscles which are involved with damage to the lower motor neurone may show the phenomenon of myokymia, in which the muscle can be seen to be rippling, and may occasionally cause the condition of cramping. Fasciculation implies a proximal motor root or anterior horn cell disturbance.

Sensory symptoms and signs (see Ch. 2)

Sensory symptoms in the peripheral neuropathies may be divided into those which are positive, due to irritation or abnormal conduction within the nerve, and those which are negative, due to loss of function. Positive sensory symptoms include paraesthesiae and dysaesthesiae, or the feeling of intense coldness and heat. Such sensations are particularly unpleasant and may be described as aching, burning or pin-pricking; very occasionally they may be more acute and resemble the lightning pains of tabes dorsalis. Such symptoms are frequently increased by tactile stimulation and are often associated with the phenomenon of hyperaesthesiae with an exaggerated response to any sensory stimulus. Such conditions make the patient hold the hands or feet in unusual positions and may, particularly when autonomic fibres are involved, result in an abnormal shiny appearance of the skin. The cause of such abnormal painful neuropathies is not fully understood, although it seems to be a prominent feature of those sensory neuropathies which involve the unmyelinated and small myelinated nerve fibres. The most common negative sensory symptom is loss of feeling or numbness and, again, the distribution of this particular sensation is of importance in identifying the type of nerve involved. The most common finding is loss of sensation ascending from the toes to the upper calves and then beginning to involve the fingers. This results in the classic 'glove and stocking' distribution of sensory loss which is characteristic of a peripheral neuropathy.

A less common but very striking negative feature of peripheral nerve damage is related to loss of proprioceptive sensation, in which there is sensory ataxia, clumsiness of the hands and unsteadiness when walking. This can be demonstrated by the patient holding the hands outstretched with the fingers apart and eyes closed, when the phenomenon of pseudoathetosis may be seen, or by the patient standing with feet together and eyes closed when Romberg's sign of induced unsteadiness may be revealed. Occasionally, the proprioceptive loss is sufficiently severe to manifest as a tremor of the outstretched hands and the patient may complain of clumsiness in performing fine movements.

Autonomic symptoms

In certain polyneuropathies the features of anhydrosis and orthostatic hypotension are prominent and indicate an underlying disturbance of autonomic nervous function. They are most frequently seen in diabetic polyneuropathies although they also occur in amyloid and some other small fibre peripheral neuropathies. They are occasionally associated with congenital neuropathies and may be the sole manifestation of the pure autonomic polyneuropathy or Riley–Day syndrome. Bladder and bowel symptoms may be indicative of autonomic disturbance and in men impotence is a common symptom, although one which is frequently not mentioned by the patient. In general, sympathetic nervous system disturbances are more evident and more common than parasympathetic.

Trophic changes and deformity

When a polyneuropathy has been present for a considerable time, there may be evidence of trophic changes which can involve both motor and sensory phenomena. Deformity of the feet, most commonly pes cavus (Fig. 10.3), is seen in a considerable number of patients with congenital neuropathies, and spinal curvature may also be found. Less commonly, similar disturbances in the upper limb may result in claw hand, due to paralysis of the intrinsic muscles (Fig. 10.4A). In general, atrophy and wasting of muscles together with contractures are the cardinal features of longstanding peripheral neuropathic disturbance.

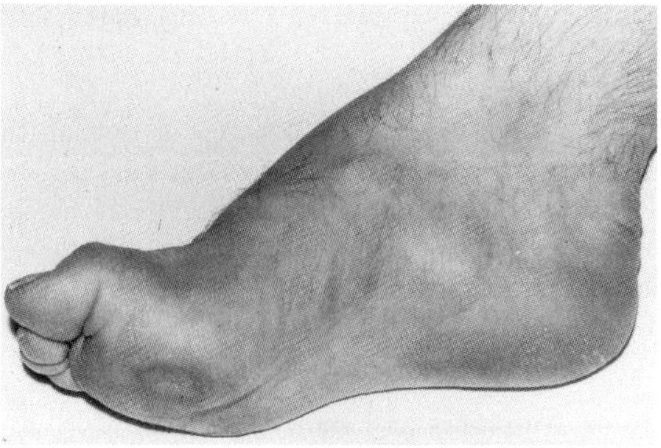

Fig. 10.3 Pes cavus.

Analgesia of the feet or hands renders them liable to pressure sores and burns which are painless and which are frequently secondarily infected. It is, therefore, important to examine the soles of the feet and the pulps of the fingers for evidence of such chronic and unhealing ulcers (Fig. 10.4B

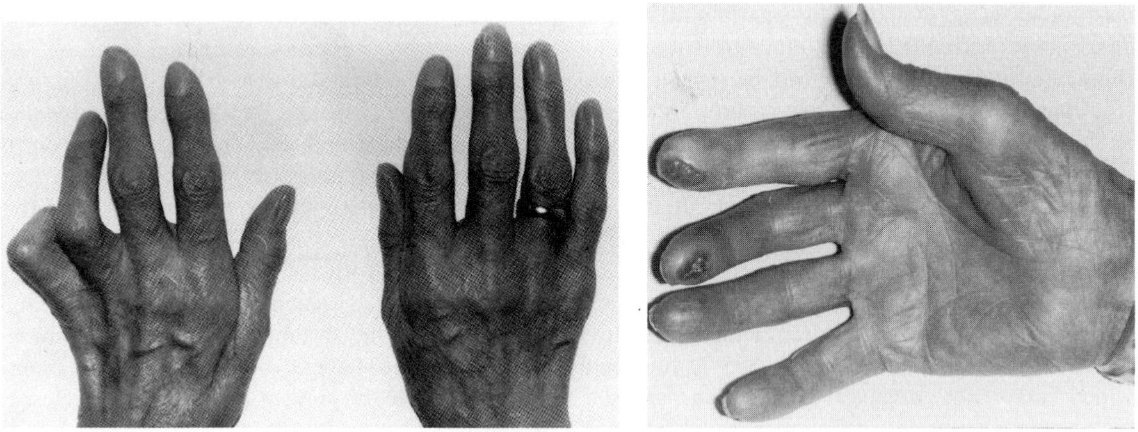

A B

Fig. 10.4 **A** Intrinsic muscle wasting of one hand with clawing of the ulnar two fingers in a patient with an ulnar nerve lesion. **B** Wasting of the thenar eminence and trophic ulcers of the index and middle fingers in a patient with a severe carpal tunnel syndrome.

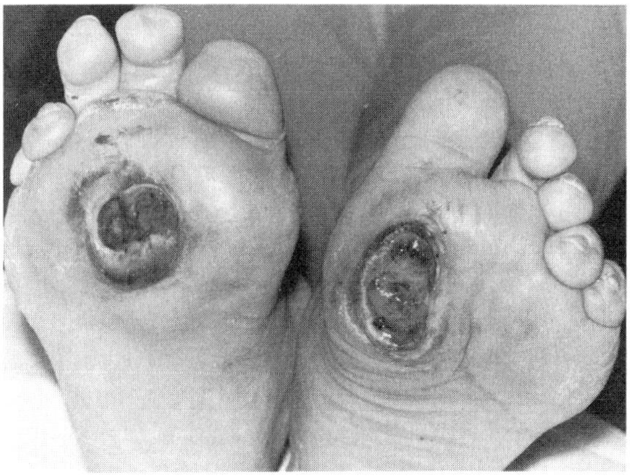

Fig. 10.5 Painless ulcers on the soles of the feet of a patient with sensory neuropathy.

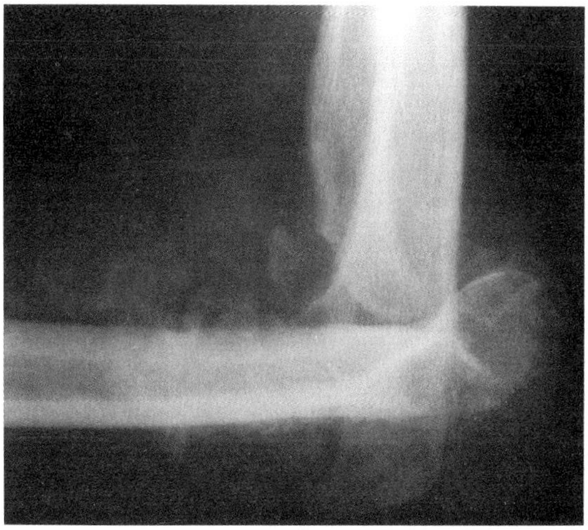

Fig. 10.6 Radiograph of a disorganised elbow joint (Charcot's joints).

and 10.5). Very occasionally analgesia and loss of proprioception in the joints will result in the development of Charcot arthropathy, which is most commonly seen in tabes dorsalis and syringomyelia, but which may also be a feature of diabetes mellitus (Fig. 10.6).

INVESTIGATION OF PERIPHERAL NERVE DISEASE

Investigation of a patient presenting with disease of the peripheral nerve depends to a considerable extent upon the clinician's ability to identify which of the syndromes of the neuropathies fit best with the clinical picture. In this respect, aspects of history are important in determining initially whether the neuropathy is diffuse, or whether it involves one or more individual peripheral nerves. It is also important to identify those neuropathies which are predominantly sensory from those which are predominantly motor; in addition, any recent exposure to infections, drugs,

Table 10.1 Clinical classification of peripheral neuropathies

Inherited neuropathies
Mixed sensory motor neuropathies
1. Idiopathic
2. Metabolic
Sensory neuropathies
Acute acquired neuropathies
Guillain–Barré syndrome
Porphyria
Toxic
Diphtheritic
Subacute acquired neuropathies
Deficiency states
Heavy metals
Drug intoxication
Uraemic
Diabetic
Arteritic
Chronic acquired neuropathies
Carcinoma
Paraproteinaemia
Uraemic
Beri-Beri
Diabetic
Hypothyroid
Connective tissue
Amyloid
Leprosy
Relapsing neuropathies
Idiopathic
Porphyria
Mononeuropathies
Pressure
Trauma
Idiopathic
Serum/postvaccinal
Herpes zoster
Neoplastic
Leprosy
Radiation
Diphtheritic
Mononeuritis multiplex
Arteritis
Diabetes

toxins, or liability to dietary deficiencies is important in the history. From the history and examination it should be possible to identify which syndrome of peripheral neuropathy (as shown in Table 10.1) fits most closely with the symptoms and signs exhibited by the patient.

Nerve conduction and electromyography (p. 106)

In general, the investigations which may be undertaken can be divided into those which will give information about the presence and nature of the neuropathy and those which may explain its underlying cause. Of the former, the most important by far are nerve conduction studies and electromyography (EMG). The former will indicate whether there is a demyelinating or an axonal process: demyelinating neuropathies tend to cause marked slowing of trunk speeds and axonal neuropathies show less evident slowing but considerable reduction in nerve action potentials. Their most common causes are listed in Table 10.2. In neuropathies with a significant sensory component it will be impossible to obtain sensory nerve action potentials. The EMG may give further information about the underlying nature of the problem, in that denervation is more commonly seen in neuropathies which are axonal in nature and EMG evidence of reinnervation would suggest a more chronic pattern to the disease. Denervation potentials in muscle will not be seen during the first few weeks of an acute neuropathy.

Table 10.2 Causes of axonal and demyelinating neuropathies

Axonal
Deficiency states
Alcohol
Toxins and most drugs
Uraemia
Collagen-vascular disorders
Carcinoma
Porphyria
Amyloid
Demyelinating
Guillain–Barré
Chronic demyelinating neuropathies
Some diabetic neuropathies
Hereditary motor and sensory neuropathies
Diphtheria
Leucodystrophies

Haematological

For detection of the underlying abnormality responsible for a neuropathy, investigations should include haematological studies assessing the level of haemoglobin, the morphology of the red cells and the MCV, together with an assessment of the ESR to indicate whether or not an inflammatory neuropathy might be present. Examination of the white cells is particularly important in patients who might suffer from infective conditions, such as infective mononucleosis, and to exclude the possibility of leukaemia (Table 10.3).

Biochemical

Biochemically there are numerous investigations which can be considered, including assessment of urine for sugar, porphyrins and heavy metals, and in the blood the level of sugar, alcohol, vitamin B_{12}, the presence of organic solvents or heavy metals, the gamma GT and liver function studies, the level of urea, the lipoproteins, phytanic acid, aryl sulphatase A and other more specific investigations, indicated in Table 10.4.

Cerebrospinal fluid examination should be undertaken as a routine in the investigation of peripheral neuropathy a high level of c.s.f. protein often indicating a demyelinating or neoplastic cause for the neuropathy and the dis-

Table 10.3 Haematological investigations in neuropathies

1. ESR	
Elevated	Arteritis
	Collective tissue diseases
	Neoplasia
	Paraproteinaemia
2. Red cells	
Megaloblastic	Vitamin B_{12} deficiency
	Folic acid deficiency
Macrocytic	Alcohol
Acanthocytes	Abetalipoproteinaemia
Rouleau	Paraproteinaemia
3. White blood cells	
Mononuclear	Infective mononucleosis
Leukaemic/lymphomatous	Leukaemia/lymphoma
4. Marrow	
Stippled red cell precursors	Lead
Fat-laden macrophages	Tangier disease

Table 10.4 Biochemical changes in the neuropathies

Increased γ-GT and liver enzymes	Alcohol Hepatitis
Elevated phytanic acid	Refsum's disease
Reduced high-density lipoproteins	Bassen–Kornzweig
Reduced aryl sulphatase A	Metachromatic leukodystrophy
Toluene	Solvents
Increased urinary porphobilinogen and δ-aminolaevulinic acid	Acute intermittent porphyria
Urinary heavy metals increased	Heavy metals
Reduced α-galactoside in fibroblasts	Anderson–Fabry disease

sociation between cells and protein being particularly important in the Guillain-Barré syndrome.

Nerve biopsy

The use of biopsy of the sural nerve or distal branch of the radial nerve is of increasing importance in the diagnosis of peripheral nerve lesions. Histological and histochemical examination of these nerves, biopsied under local anaesthesia, will usually confirm whether the abnormality is demyelinating or axonal and may show infiltration of the nerve with inflammatory or neoplastic cells or the deposition of abnormal proteins and lipids. The technique of electron microscopy may well reveal further abnormalities in the peripheral nerve and can, again, be of help in diagnosis (Table 10.5) (Figs 10.7, 10.8).

Table 10.5 Histological change in peripheral nerves

Demyelination Generalised Segmental Perinodal
Axonal degeneration
Vasculitis
Infiltrations Cellular (lymphoma, carcinoma) Paraproteinaemias Amyloid

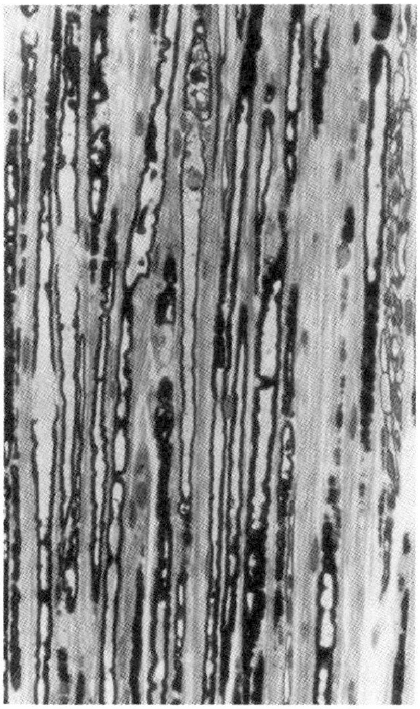

A

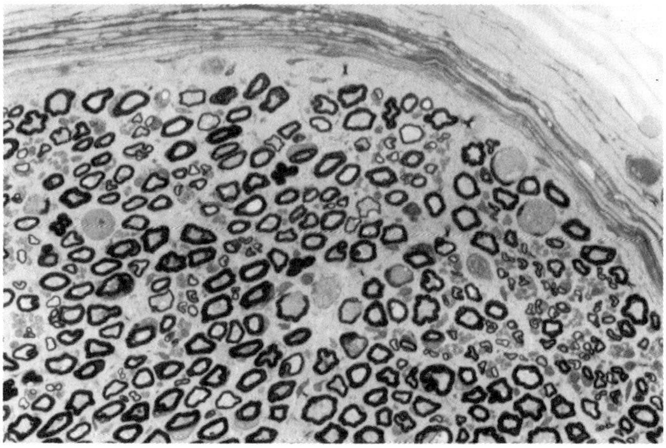

B

Fig. 10.7 **A** The histology of a demyelinating neuropathy (longitudinal section) showing the presence of myelin ovoids. **B** Cross-section of the same.

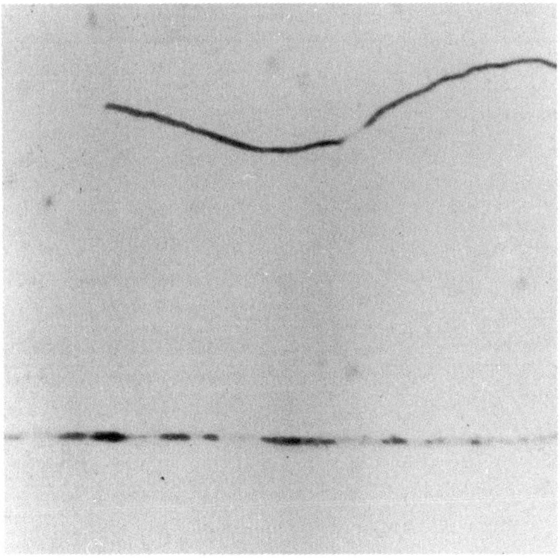

Fig. 10.8 Teased fibre of a peripheral nerve showing segmental demyelination.

Table 10.6 Genetically determined neuropathies

Inherited polyneuropathies of sensory type
Dominant mutilating sensory neuropathy in adults
Recessive mutilating sensory neuropathy in children
Congenital insensitivity to pain
Other inherited sensory neuropathies with spinocerebellar degenerations
Inherited polyneuropathies of mixed sensorimotor autonomic type
Idiopathic group
Dominant perineal muscular atrophy
Dominant hypertrophic polyneuropathy
Roussy–Lévy polyneuropathy
Polyneuropathy with optic atrophy, spastic paraplegia, spinocerebellar degeneration, mental retardation, dementia
Inherited polyneuropathies with a recognised metabolic disorder
Refsum's disease
Metachromatic leukodystrophy
Globoid-body leukodystrophy
Adrenoleukodystrophy
Amyloid polyneuropathy
Porphyric polyneuropathy
Anderson Fabry disease
Abetalipoproteinaemia and Tangier disease

CLINICAL SYNDROMES

It should be possible from the history and examination to place the patient's symptoms within one of seven defined categories of peripheral neuropathy (Table 10.1).

Inherited neuropathies

Characteristically, patients with genetically determined peripheral neuropathies will give a history of a chronic disorder frequently beginning in childhood. They may have been less able to perform sporting activities than their peers at school and may also give a history of other similar problems affecting members of the family. There will often be abnormalities in the form of pes cavus and the neuropathies tend to be progressive and symmetrical.

A satisfactory classification is not available at present, but the most clinically useful classification is that proposed by Adams and Victor, who divided these neuropathies into those which are truly idiopathic and without a known biochemical abnormality and those which are associated with a biochemical, metabolic abnormality which is known to be genetically controlled (Table 10.6). Here we shall deal only with those syndromes more commonly seen in adults.

Idiopathic inherited polyneuropathies of mixed sensorimotor type

Peroneal muscular atrophy (Charcot–Marie–Tooth disease, hereditary sensorimotor neuropathy type I). This autosomal dominant neuropathy, which tends to begin in the second decade, is occasionally associated with myelopathies and may overlap with Friedreich's ataxia. It causes a chronic degeneration of the peripheral nerve, which first affects the feet, later involving the hands. The initial symptoms are of loss of sensation in the feet accompanied by weakness and wasting of the peripheral muscles of the legs leading to foot drop and difficulty in walking. The patients commonly have pes cavus and the legs are said to have the appearance of an inverted champagne bottle (Fig. 10.9). Later, the hands become numb, the muscles of the hands and forearm may waste and there may be clawing of the hands with the development of peripheral contractures and ultimately trophic changes in the feet and hands.

Initial symptoms include complaints of difficulty of walking due both to peripheral weakness

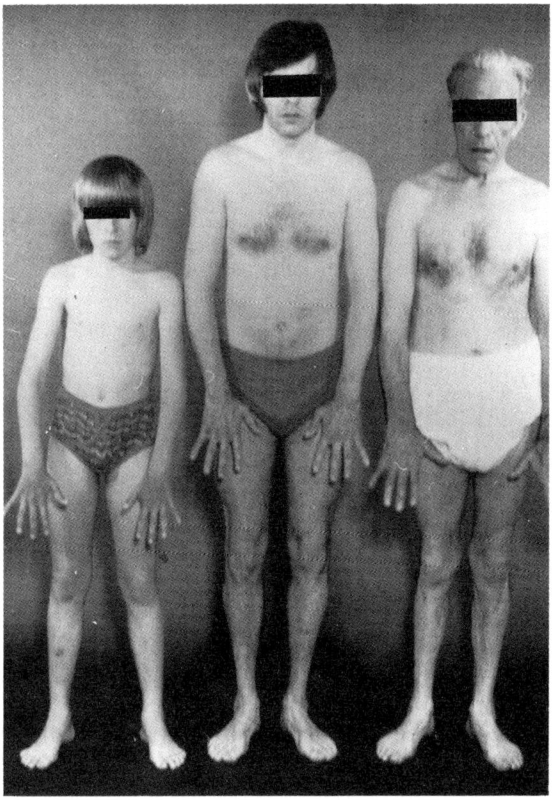

Fig. 10.9 Hereditary sensory motor neuropathy in three generations of the same family demonstrating the evolution of 'inverted champagne bottle' legs. (Reproduced from Blackwood W et al 1983 (*Slide Atlas of Neurology*. Gower Medical Publishing, London, with permission.)

and to the development of a sensory ataxia. The peripheral nerves are not tender and are not palpably enlarged, autonomic disturbances are uncommon in this condition, but occasionally there may be optic atrophy and the pupils may be unreactive. Nerve conduction studies and histological examination suggest that the clinical syndrome may be associated with either demyelinating or axonal neuropathy.

Therapy is confined to stabilising the ankles by arthrodeses and the use of leg braces. Rarely are patients likely to become severely disabled, and upper limb weakness is not often a cause of considerable disability. The differential diagnosis must always lie between demyelinating and axonal peripheral neuropathies and anterior horn cell disease as in spinal muscular atrophy. Nerve conduction and EMG examination will usually provide evidence as to the nature of the disorder.

Progressive hypertrophic neuropathy (Déjérine-Sottas disease, hereditary sensory motor neuropathy type II). This autosomal recessive neuropathy usually begins earlier than Charcot–Marie–Tooth disease and is also slowly progressive. The clinical features are similar to those of Charcot–Marie–Tooth disease, but the peripheral nerves are evidently and palpably enlarged. The progression is faster than in Charcot–Marie–Tooth disease and the patients are often wheelchair bound at an early age. There may be difficulty in diagnosing the condition differentially from other hypertrophic neuropathies such as amyloidosis and Refsum's disease, but investigations will reveal slowing of nerve conduction, indicating a demyelinating neuropathy, and biopsy will show the classic onion bulb appearance of demyelination and remyclination. The c.s.f. protein may frequently be increased as the roots are also involved and occasionally the spinal roots may be so enlarged as to compromise the spinal cord.

Hereditary areflexic ataxia (Roussy–Lévy syndrome). This is a predominantly sensory ataxia in which the patients have pes cavus and areflexia. It shows an early onset and has a relatively benign course. The presence of a kyphoscoliosis may cause the condition to be mistaken for Friedreich's ataxia, but there is no true cerebellar ataxia in this condition.

Inherited polyneuropathies with recognised metabolic causes

Refsum's disease. Refsum's disease is an autosomal recessive condition beginning in late childhood or early adolescence. The peripheral neuropathy is associated with retinitis pigmentosa, cerebellar ataxia and the pathognomonic finding of a high blood phytanic acid level. Many patients also show a cardiomyopathy and neurogenic deafness with pupillary abnormalities and cataract; ichthyosis of the skin is also common. The neuropathy is hypertrophic, the peripheral nerves are often palpable and it is possible that a diet low in phytol-containing compounds may be of benefit to the patients.

Abeta lipoproteinaemia (Bassen–Kornzweig syndrome, acanthocytosis). This condition is a rare autosomal recessive disease which causes a progressive peripheral neuropathy of mixed type and is associated with a reduction in beta-lipoproteins, with retinal degeneration and acanthocytosis in peripheral blood. The condition usually presents in infancy with the problem of steatorrhoea and areflexia; and the peripheral neuropathy and ataxia develop later. There are suggestions that treatment with vitamin E may help in this condition.

Tangier disease (an alpha-lipoproteinaemia). This is a rare autosomal recessive condition in which the combination of yellow tonsils and a sensorimotor neuropathy with areflexia is seen. There are reduced levels of high density lipoproteins in the blood and examination of the marrow reveals fat-laden macrophages. There is no therapy for this progressive condition.

Anderson–Fabry's disease (p. 385). In this sex-linked recessive disease, which is also known as angiokeratoma corporis diffusum, there is a primary deficiency in the enzyme alpha-galactosidase, which results in a build-up of ceramide trihexoside in endothelial and smooth muscle cells of the blood vessels. It may present with pain in the muscles in late childhood or early adolescence and there is loss of the small-fibre axons in the peripheral nerves.

Metachromatic leukodystrophy (p. 385). In this autosomal recessive condition there is congenital absence of the enzyme aryl sulphatase A, resulting in sulphatide accumulation throughout the central and peripheral nervous systems. The cerebral effects are often the most obvious, but in addition there is hyporeflexia, muscular atrophy and diminished nerve conduction velocities. The presentation is usually in early childhood, where the weakness, hypotonia and areflexia may cause confusion with Werdnig–Hoffmann disease. Measurement of aryl sulphatase A in the peripheral blood or the finding of metachromatically staining granules in the cytoplasm of Schwann cells on nerve biopsy will confirm the diagnosis.

Familial dysautonomia (Riley–Day disease). This recessively inherited disorder affects Jewish children. There is failure to thrive, fever and pneumonia together with hyporeflexia and loss of pain and temperature sensation. Motor fibres in the peripheral nerves are less evidently involved but nerve conduction studies will reveal reduced conduction velocity in peripheral nerves. The autonomic disturbances and repeated infections often overshadow other aspects of the illness.

Familial amyloid polyneuropathy. This is an autosomal dominant condition, which was first and most prominently recognised in the Portuguese. It causes a chronic sensorimotor peripheral neuropathy which tends to begin in the 3rd or 4th decade and frequently involves the autonomic system in a manner similar to that seen in primary amyloidosis.

Inherited sensory neuropathies

A group of inherited neuropathies present predominantly with the symptom of pain in the feet and the hands and may then progress to cause numbness, ulceration and chronic osteomyelitis. Different patterns of this condition have been recorded, one being an autosomal dominant trait, another autosomal recessive; the third possibly related condition is that of congenital insensitivity to pain.

Acute peripheral neuropathies

These are neuropathies which evolve over hours or days and may be postinfective, metabolic or toxic.

Guillain–Barré Syndrome (postinfective) polyneuropathy)

This is undoubtedly the most common form of acute peripheral neuropathy, occurring with an incidence of 1–2 per 100 000 a year. It is typically a postviral phenomenon and may be seen in patients with infective mononucleosis and cytomegalovirus infections. It may rarely be seen in patients who are convalescing postoperatively and is also related occasionally to lymphomas and to inoculation. The classic picture is of a symmetrical weakness beginning in the feet and associated with minimal sensory change. It evolves over days or weeks but occasionally may progress rapidly over hours. The weakness follows an ascending pattern and can cause a respiratory paralysis. Not uncommonly there is pain and paraesthesiae in the feet, and back pain with radicular radiation may be prominent. Objective sensory findings are, however, usually minimal. There is invariably areflexia, but the most obvious finding is of a flaccid weakness which may be more marked in the proximal than in the peripheral muscles. The disease usually evolves too rapidly for there to be significant wasting of muscles and occasionally cranial nerves are involved, although this tends to be late and is relatively uncommon. There are rare forms of the condition which predominantly affect the cranial nerves together with peripheral areflexia: a well-recognised pattern of cranial nerve involvement, ophthalmoplegia, ataxia and areflexia is the Miller–Fisher syndrome. Myelopathies may occur together with the Guillain–Barré syndrome, and urinary disturbance, although rare, is recognised.

Investigations reveal slowing of conduction in peripheral nerves and particularly, delay in F-wave latencies, indicating a proximal site of the neuropathy. The disease may be more correctly called an ascending radiculopathy. It is unusual early in the disease to find evidence of true denervation in the muscles, but some cases with early denervation have an axonal form of disease and the prognosis for recovery is poor. Examination of the c.s.f. will reveal no increase in cell count but a considerably raised protein level often above 1 gram per litre. It must be remembered that if c.s.f. examination is performed early in the course of the illness there may be no increase in protein at this stage.

The cause of the condition is almost certainly an immune-mediated demyelination of the peripheral nerve and root. There is a direct comparison with the animal model of experimental allergic neuropathy, in which a demyelinating proximal peripheral neuropathy may be caused by immunisation with peripheral nerve tissue. It appears that the specific antigen is a peptide of the basic protein of peripheral nerve myelin.

When the disease is suspected it is important that the patient is admitted to hospital and, where necessary, to an intensive therapy unit. This is necessary because there may be rapid extension of the disease to involve the respiratory muscles and respiratory support may become essential with early tracheotomy. Major therapy is directed towards nursing support of the patient. In those patients with autonomic disturbances, particularly cardiac dysrhythmias and changes in blood pressure, circulatory support may be necessary.

The place of steroids in management of the disease is uncertain: several controlled trials of steroids have failed to prove benefit for this form of therapy, but there is now a suggestion that plasmaphaeresis in the first three weeks of the disease may help to hasten recovery. There are, however, still considerable doubts about the benefit of this therapy and most physicians would not employ it in patients with mild forms of the disease. Those who have a more severe disease may be considered suitable for such aggressive therapy which appears to reduce time on a ventilator and admission time significantly. Approximately 25% of the patients will have a residual disability, but most will recover completely from this condition, although the recovery time can often be measured in months. An important aspect of management relates to the care of paralysed limbs to protect the skin and avoid the development of contractures.

Porphyria

Acute intermittent porphyria may be associated with an acute peripheral neuropathy, usually in conjunction with abdominal pain, psychiatric disturbances, confusion and, occasionally, convulsions. The condition is inherited as an autosomal dominant trait and is associated with the increased production and excretion of porphobilinogen and δ-aminolevulinic acid. The polyneuropathy occurring in this condition is usually symmetrical and predominantly motor, although in rare cases sensory and autonomic involvement may occur. It is unusual in that the weakness may frequently be proximal and a bibrachial distribution of the weakness is quite classic.

The neuropathy has a variable course and may regress completely within a few weeks. It can occasionally progress to cause death and autonomic disturbances very occasionally may result in tachyarrhythmias. Pathological investigation reveals a mixed axonal and demyelinating neuropathy. Patients may be helped by the use of beta-blockers and glucose therapy and usually need supportive therapy, occasionally including respiratory support. Once the diagnosis of acute intermittent porphyria has been confirmed by measurement of porphobilinogen and δ-aminolevulinic acid in the urine, the most important aspects of management are to avoid precipitating factors such as barbiturates, sulphonamides, phenytoin, oestrogens, griseofulvin and succinimide.

Toxic

Most toxins will tend to cause relatively chronic peripheral neuropathies, but thallium may produce a peripheral neuropathy which can rapidly be progressive and may mimic the Guillain–Barré syndrome (p. 439).

Diphtheria

Although rare in Western practice, the demyelinating effects of diphtheria toxin are well recognised and diphtheritic neuropathy is an acute though usually focal neuropathy with a significant relationship to the site of growth of the diphtheria organisms. The typical involvement of the fauces in children was a cause of flaccid bulbar palsy and death.

Subacute peripheral neuropathies

The majority of subacute neuropathies, i.e. those developing over a period of weeks to months, are due to deficiency states, toxins, metabolic disturbance or inflammatory conditions. In general, the symptoms begin with dysaesthetic pain, paraesthesiae or numbness in the feet gradually spreading upwards to the knees and then involving the fingers and hands. The picture is of the typical glove-and-stocking distribution of sensory symptoms, which are later accompanied by weakness and wasting of the peripheral muscles. The clinical findings of sensory loss or alteration in sensation, wasting of muscles and areflexia indicate the presence of a peripheral neuropathy and the underlying pathology must then be identified by relevant investigations including electrophysiological studies and biochemical tests. Occasionally, certain features in the clinical assessment will help to pin-point the underlying cause.

Alcoholic neuropathy (p. 436)

The neuropathy in alcoholics is believed to be nutritional rather than due to a direct toxic effect of alcohol. The syndrome is similar to neuropathic beri-beri and due to a B vitamin deficiency, predominantly of thiamine. Pain and paraesthesiae are common initial symptoms and are later accompanied by weakness and the signs of wasting and areflexia. In rare cases there may be involvement of the autonomic nervous system with excessive sweating or dryness of the limbs, postural hypotension and tachyarrhythmias. Nerve conduction studies will reveal an axonal neuropathy and the findings of other stigmata of alcoholic disease including a raised MCV and abnormal liver function tests including elevated gamma GT, indicate the likely diagnosis. Therapy consists of ensuring a diet adequate in B vitamins, sometimes with added thiamine supplements, and in reducing the intake of alcohol. Recovery is slow and in the most severe cases may be only partial.

Arsenic (p. 438)

In chronic poisoning the neuropathy which occurs with arsenic tends to evolve over weeks, but in patients surviving an episode of acute poisoning there may be a more rapid development of a diffuse peripheral neuropathy, possibly associated with gastrointestinal symptoms, seizures, mental changes and coma. There is classically a brownish skin pigmentation, hyperkeratosis and the development of white lines on the nails (Mees' lines). Arsenical poisoning is diagnosed by increased levels of arsenic in hair and urine and there may be increased levels of c.s.f. protein. There is little evidence that chelating agents (e.g. British anti-Lewisite) affect the peripheral neuropathy, which recovers slowly if the toxic substance is withdrawn.

Lead (p. 438)

Lead neuropathy is rare and tends to affect motor function in the upper limbs, most commonly presenting with wrist drop. It is associated with anaemia, stippling of the red cell precursors in the marrow, a lead line on the gingival margins and the excretion of lead and copper porphyrins in the urine. Blood levels of lead are increased and treatment is by the use of chelating agents.

Industrial solvents (p. 438)

Although there are occasional examples of acute poisoning with solvents in industrial processes and accidents the most common agent involved in causing solvent neuropathy is *n*-hexane, which is used in contact cement or glues and which is responsible for the neuropathy of glue-sniffers. The neuropathy is due to axonal damage with a classic histological appearance of perinodal swelling and demyelination. Withdrawing the agent allows recovery of the neuropathy, although again in severe cases recovery may be slow and incomplete.

Drugs (p. 431)

Many different drugs may cause a neuropathy and, in the case of some agents such as the anticancer drugs, the neuropathy may be an acceptable part of treatment, but in others such as the antibiotics, antianginal agents and some antihypertensives, such a side-effect is unacceptable. The majority of drug-induced neuropathies are axonal in nature though some, notably perhexilene and amiodarone, can cause a demyelinating neuropathy. The commonly recognised drug-induced neuropathies are listed in Table 17.3, and the management in all cases is the withdrawal of the offending agent which results in a resolution of the neuropathy. In some cases, as with isoniazid neuropathy, it is possible to provide specific treatment as isoniazide causes a neuropathy by interfering with the phosphorylation of pyridoxine, and the administration of pyridoxine to the patient prevents the development of this complication.

Diabetes mellitus (p. 461)

Almost 50% of the patients with diabetes mellitus have electrophysiological evidence of a demyelinating neuropathy, but less than 20% will be symptomatic. Several different forms of neuropathy are recognised to occur in diabetes mellitus:

Autonomic neuropathy
Diffuse sensory peripheral neuropathy
Sensorimotor peripheral neuropathy
Mononeuritis multiplex
Entrapment neuropathies
Femoral neuropathy (diabetic amyotrophy)
Intercostal neuralgia.

The above are discussed in Chapter 18. It should be remembered that more than one form of neuropathy may coexist in a single patient. The pathology of the diabetic neuropathy is believed to be due to disease of the vasa nervorum resulting in ischaemia to the nerve, which pathologically shows both loss of axons and secondary demyelination; it is possible that a metabolic factor is also involved. C.s.f. protein is usually raised in this condition due to involvement of the spinal roots in the ischaemic process. Therapy is directed at optimal control of the blood sugar and the provision of B vitamin supplements. Specific symptomatic treatment for the pain may be necessary with agents such as carbamazepine and in some instances consideration should be given to the possibility of changing from an oral hypoglycaemic agent to insulin, which may improve diabetic control.

Arteritis (p. 467)

Several diseases which are associated with an arteritis also cause a peripheral neuropathy. In many instances the neuropathy is a form of mononeuritis multiplex, but more generalised subacute motor and sensory neuropathy may occur. The diseases involved are listed in Table 10.8 and the diagnosis is often made by specific blood tests and the finding of a high ESR and is confirmed by nerve biopsy. Treatment usually involves steroids, or occasionally cytotoxic agents such as azathioprine.

Chronic peripheral neuropathy

Chronic neuropathies arise over months or years and cause the development of symptoms and signs similar to those in a more acute neuropathy. The varying pathologies which may be involved are listed in Table 10.6. The nature of the neuropathy is shown by electrophysiological studies and the precise diagnosis necessitates a search for the possible underlying causes.

Carcinomatous neuropathy (p. 465)

Approximately 5% of patients with carcinoma will develop a form of neuropathy and almost one-half of these are suffering from carcinoma of the lung. The neuropathy is commonly mixed sensorimotor in type and seldom purely sensory. It is usually painful, tends to progress over months and may be severely disabling, with marked weakness and sensory ataxia. It may occasionally occur with other forms of paraneoplastic disease such as the Eaton–Lambert syndrome, involving disturbances of neuromuscular conduction, cerebellar ataxia, limbic encephalitis or multifocal leucoencephalopathy. The prognosis is poor and treatment is directed toward removing the underlying cause, providing symptomatic therapy for the pain and occasionally using steroids. The pathology is variable, usually involving an axonal loss and occasionally associated with segmental demyelination. There may also be degeneration within the dorsal root ganglia and dorsal columns. The c.s.f. often shows an increased level of protein.

Paraproteinaemias and dysproteinaemias (p. 456)

A variety of conditions in which there are abnormal proteins present in the blood may be associated with the development of a chronic neuropathy. The most common of these is multiple myeloma, in which 15% of patients will show a significant symptomatic peripheral neuropathy. There is some evidence that the neuropathy may be due to infiltration of protein into the axons of the damaged nerves, and recovery from the neuropathy has been reported with adequate treatment of the underlying paraproteinaemias. Neuropathy may also be seen in macroglobulinaemia and in cryoglobulinaemia, in which conditions it is probably ischaemic in nature.

Benign monoclonal gammopathy may also be associated with a peripheral neuropathy, most commonly in the elderly population. It is most commonly associated with an IgM monoclonal gammopathy and the protein may have antimyelin activity. The neuropathy may occasionally be hypertrophic. Ataxia telangiectasia, which is characterised by a specific decrease in IgA, is associated with evident hyporeflexia and a slowly evolving peripheral neuropathy.

Uraemic polyneuropathy (p. 463)

Patients with chronic renal failure have a high incidence of peripheral neuropathic abnormalities. As many as 70% of patients undergoing regular dialysis will show evidence of a neuropathy, which is usually painless although it may occasionally give rise to the 'restless leg syndrome' of distressing dysaesthesiae in the legs at night-time. The neuropathy appears to be related to the renal failure itself rather than to the underlying cause and, with long-term haemodialysis, transplantation or peritoneal dialysis, there is evidence that the symptoms may stabilise and occasionally improve. Pathological investigation shows axonal degeneration with secondary demyelination. Although the cause of the neuropathy is unknown it is believed to be due to the accumulation of toxic substances of molecular weight 300–2000 (the middle molecules). These are not removed by dialysis, but are cleared by the transplanted kidney, thus accounting for the improvement seen after transplantation.

Chronic idiopathic neuropathy

A significant proportion of patients presenting with chronic mixed sensorimotor neuropathy of either axonal or demyelinating type will not be found to have any evident underlying cause. These patients are said to have 'idiopathic neuropathy', which obviously reflects an inability to identify the cause of a particular neuropathy in their case. Some such patients will eventually be shown to have a neoplastic cause for their neuropathy and a significant proportion are shown to have abnormalities of protein metabolism. None the less, a proportion of patients (varying from 25% to 50%) with such chronic peripheral neuropathy will have no apparent cause for the symptoms. In such cases the only management is symptomatic in an attempt to reduce the distress and discomfort of the patients.

Mononeuropathies and mononeuritis multiplex

The presence of motor, reflex and sensory changes confined to the territory of a single nerve or several individual nerves identifies the syndrome of mononeuropathy or mononeuritis multiplex respectively. The diseases may involve individual roots or plexuses. They may be due to local trauma, entrapment or involvement of a single nerve in an ischaemic process due to arteritis, diabetes, or atherosclerosis, or to an episode of postinfective demyelination. There are some families in which damage to peripheral nerve myelin is relatively common and this may present with repeated episodes of mononeuropathy or plexopathy. The common forms of mononeuropathy are listed in Table 10.7 and the causes of mononeuritis multiplex in Table 10.8.

The diagnosis is undertaken in two parts. Initially the site of the lesion is identified by clinical examination and nerve conduction studies, or by EMG identification of the distribution of muscles showing total or partial denervation; secondly the underlying source of the lesion must be identified. This may be apparent, as in those cases due to local trauma, or less apparent when the lesion is due to an arteritis, diabetes or a postinfective demyelinating condition. The sites at which nerve entrapment commonly occurs are relatively few and this will in turn suggest the local pathology in that case. It should be remembered that, in the presence of a mild or subclinical neuropathy, entrapment neuropathies are more commonly seen and therefore an underlying cause should be sought, even in patients with evident entrapment syndromes. In those conditions in which multiple neuropathies are seen it is even more important to seek underlying disease processes which render the nerve liable to such damage.

Table 10.7 Common entrapment and pressure mononeuropathies

Nerve	Site of entrapment/pressure
Suprascapular	Spinoglenoid notch
Radial	Humeral groove
Median	Carpal tunnel
Ulnar	
Elbow	Cubital tunnel
Hand	Palmar fascia/pisiform bone
Anterior interosseous	Between heads of pronator muscle
Lateral cutaneous of thigh	Inguinal ligament
Obturator	Obturator canal
Lateral popliteal	Head of fibula
Posterior tibial	Tarsal tunnel, medial malleolus, flexor retinaculum

Table 10.8 Causes of mononeuritis multiplex

Collagen vascular disorders
Polyarteritis nodosa
Rheumatoid disease
Systemic lupus erythematosus
Wegener's granulomatosis
Diabetes mellitus
Sarcoidosis
Carcinoma
Paraproteinaemias (+ cryoglobulinaemia)
Leprosy
Intravenous drug abuse

Brachial plexus lesions

Lesions of the *whole plexus* are most often seen as the result of road traffic accidents and the identification of the site of the trauma, in terms of the roots involved and whether the damage is pre- or postganglionic, is important in management. Lesions which are postganglionic will result in loss of the weal and flare reaction in the area of anaesthetic skin, which indicates trauma to the brachial plexus itself. Although it is reasonable to wait for a period of months to enable observation of any spontaneous recovery indicating neurapraxia or axonotmesis, a persistence of the problems indicates the need for exploration in case neuronotmesis has occurred and the nerve can be surgically repaired. Apart from neurophysiological studies, myelography may be indicated in this situation to identify whether or not there has been avulsion of the nerve root within the spinal canal, with a resulting meningocele, which indicates the hopelessness of a surgical approach. If the lesion is preganglionic, that is proximal to the dorsal root ganglion, the weal and flare reaction will be retained in the anaesthetic skin; such lesions have a poor prognosis and are not amenable to surgery.

Lesions of the *upper brachial plexus* may occur in road traffic accidents but are also seen following forceful separation of the head and shoulder during difficult delivery, when they result in the classic *Erb's palsy* with weakness of deltoid, biceps, supraspinatus, infraspinatus and rhomboids. The arm is internally rotated and extended at the elbow but hand function is unaffected.

Lower brachial plexus palsy, or *Klumpke's paralysis*, is usually due to traction of the abducted arm, either peroperatively or as the result of local trauma, or occasionally with infiltration or compression by tumours in the apex of the lung (Pancoast's syndrome). In this instance, weakness is confined to the small muscles of the hand, giving rise to a characteristic claw-hand deformity. There may be an associated Horner's syndrome. A group of conditions referred to as the thoracic outlet syndrome frequently cause pain, dysaesthesiae and paraesthesiae in the upper limbs and occasional weakness. One of these syndromes has a neurological basis when there is damage to the lower cord of the brachial plexus due to the presence of a cervical rib or band. This may be suspected clinically and diagnosed either radiologically or electrophysiologically.

Dislocation of the head of the humerus, cervical ribs and local compression during anaesthesia may result in damage to the cords of the brachial plexus which can be identified: *lateral cord damage* results in weakness of flexion and pronation of the forearm; *medial cord damage* causes weakness of the small muscles of the hand; *posterior cord lesion* results in weakness of deltoid, triceps and the extensors of the wrists and fingers.

Neuralgic amyotrophy or brachial neuritis is the term given to a postinfective or postvaccinal demyelinating lesion of the brachial plexus, which usually begins with exquisite pain at the shoulder and neck followed within a few days by the development of muscular weakness and subsequent wasting. The lesion is usually unilateral and tends to be confined to the muscles of the shoulder. Sometimes an area of sensory disturbance in the distribution of the circumflex nerve is evident, but reflexes are usually maintained. In general the pain lasts for only a matter of days and recovery of power occurs within a 6–12 week period. Sometimes the weakness persists for longer and, occasionally, pain may be a prominent feature for several weeks. The condition is sometimes complicated by the development of a pericapsulitis which tends to cause continuing pain and lack of evident recovery.

Particular clinical problems arise with lesions of the brachial plexus in patients who have undergone *radiotherapy* following mastectomy. The difficult differential diagnosis in such patients is between a radiation-induced neuropathy and one due to carcinomatous infiltration. In general, the latter pathology tends to cause more pain and usually involves the lower roots of the plexus. However, it may be clinically impossible to separate the two potential causes, although the use of CT scanning through the brachial plexus may give some evidence of the development of neoplasia.

In some families there is an *autosomal dominant* tendency to *brachial plexus neuropathy* with repeated episodes of weakness of one or other shoulder muscles. Some of these patients will have evidence of neuropathies occurring in other nerves and may on biopsy show evidence of segmental demyelination and remyelination to which appearance the term tomaculous neuropathy has been applied.

Brachial mononeuropathies

The *long thoracic nerve of Bell* which supplies serratus anterior may be injured by carrying heavy weights on the shoulder or, occasionally, in a form of neuralgic amyotrophy. It results in the phenomenon of winging of the scapula and requires no treatment.

The *suprascapular nerve* which supplies supra- and infraspinatus is commonly involved in brachial neuritis and may occasionally be damaged with trauma to the shoulder. It may occasionally be compressed where the nerve crosses the spinoglenoid notch and may require decompression.

The *axillary nerve* may be damaged in dislocation of the shoulder joint and fractures of the neck of the humerus. It supplies the teres minor and deltoid and results in failure of abduction of the shoulder.

The *radial nerve* may be compressed in the axilla with a crutch palsy but is more frequently damaged in the radial groove of the humerus. Such pressure palsies may occur during sleep, where the arm is rested against the arm of a chair, and may also be damaged in fractures of the humerus. Damage results in weakness of the extensors of the wrists and fingers and there may be weakness of triceps. The most impressive finding is therefore of a wrist drop.

The *median nerve* is most commonly damaged in the carpal tunnel where it is liable to repeated trauma, infiltration of the transverse carpal ligament with amyloid or thickening of connective tissue as in rheumatoid arthritis, acromegaly and hypothyroidism. Carpal tunnel syndrome is most commonly seen in the dominant hand and results in dysaesthesiae most often at night over the thumb and lateral two and a half fingers of the hands on the palmar surface. There is also loss of power in the median nerve innervated muscles of the thenar eminence, namely the abductor pollicis brevis and opponens pollicis. The diagnosis can be confirmed by neurophysiological tests, showing increased latency at the wrist, and although symptomatic relief may be given by the provision of a cock-up splint to the wrist to wear at night, by the use of diuretics or by local steroid injections, decompression of the carpal tunnel is the most definitive therapy.

The *ulnar nerve* is most commonly damaged in the olecranon groove at the elbow, either by repeated trauma or by fracture or dislocation of the elbow joint. It may be seen some considerable time after damage to the elbow, when it is referred to as a tardy ulnar neuropathy. It results in loss of sensation over the medial aspect of the little finger and half of the ring finger on the palmar surface. It is associated with weakness of the majority of small muscles of the hand and may result in a claw hand deformity. Treatment may involve transposition of the nerve from the olecranon groove more anteriorly on the medial aspect of the elbow.

The ulnar nerve may also be damaged in the palm where the deep palmar branch of the nerve is liable to suffer damage after prolonged pressure on the ulnar part of the palm. This results in weakness of the small hand muscles but no sensory loss and the site of a lesion should be localised by nerve conduction studies.

The *posterior interosseous nerve* which is a branch of the radial nerve passing between the two planes of the supinator may be trapped at this site or damaged in supracondylar fractures of the humerus. Damage to this nerve results in weakness of the extensors of the wrist, thumb and fingers but can be differentiated from radial nerve palsies by sparing the triceps muscle.

The *anterior interosseous nerve* (a branch of the median nerve) may be compressed between the two heads of pronator teres or at the interosseous membrane where it may cause weakness of flexor digitorum profundus resulting in inability to flex the index and middle fingers.

Although each of these upper limb neuropathies may occur due to trauma or local entrapment, they may also occur with other underlying conditions which damage the peripheral nerve. Thus, the alcoholic with a subclinical neuropathy is prone to a median or ulnar neuropathy, as is the diabetic. It is, therefore, not sufficient merely to identify the site and local cause of the neuropathy but to investigate the possibility of an underlying cause for its occurrence.

Lumbosacral plexus

In the presence of lumbosacral plexus disease it is always important to exclude the possibility of intraspinal lesions by myelography, thus excluding disease of the cauda equina. It should be noted that unilateral diseases of the lumbosacral plexus are much more common than a purely unilateral lesion caused by intrathecal disease.

Unlike the brachial plexus, the lumbar plexus is rarely involved in traumatic lesions unless there is considerable disruption of the lower spine, the pelvis and abdomen. However, lesions to the pelvic plexus do occur with operations on abdominal and pelvic organs, and postoperative weakness and pain in the lower limbs should also raise the possibility of damage to the plexus. The lumbar plexus may also be compressed by an aortic aneurysm, or infiltrated by tumours involving the pelvic organs or bowel. Such diseases commonly cause lumbar plexopathies that are identified chiefly by the intractable and persistent nature of their pain. Neuralgic amyotrophy of the lumbosacral plexus is much less common than in the brachial plexus, but may occur, as may lesions to roots of the plexus, due to more diffuse diseases such as diabetes and arteritis.

Mononeuropathies of the leg

Involvement of the *lateral cutaneous nerve of the thigh* at the level of the inguinal ligament results in paraesthesiae in the outer aspect of the thigh, which syndrome is termed meralgia paraesthetica. This condition is most commonly seen in people who are obese, but may also occur during pregnancy and with diabetes mellitus. It usually requires no treatment but may be helped by a local block or occasionally by decompression.

The *obturator nerve* of the mother may be damaged during delivery. It causes pain radiating into the knee and weakness of adduction and external rotation of the thigh.

The *femoral nerve* is the common site of neuropathy in diabetes mellitus, where it tends to present with severe pain in the thigh followed by weakness of the quadriceps. It may also be injured by bleeding into the iliac muscle in patients treated with anticoagulants, and in haemophiliacs, where a palpable mass in the iliac fossa will suggest the diagnosis.

The *sciatic nerve* may be injured by fractures of the pelvis or by dislocation of the head of the femur and by inaccurate intramuscular injections. Damage to this nerve results in weakness of the hamstrings and all muscle below the knee with considerable numbness in the lower limb. Lesions of the sciatic nerve must be differentiated from L5 radiculopathies by clinical assessment and EMG.

The *common peroneal nerve* may be damaged at the head of the fibula, resulting in numbness over the dorsum of the foot and a foot drop. This may be caused by local pressure behind the knee, as by sitting cross-legged, or by wearing a plaster cast.

The *tibial nerve* may rarely be damaged at the back of the knee but is sometimes compressed in the tarsal tunnel behind the medial aspect of the calcaneum. Here it may be compressed by thickening of the tendon sheaths or by osteoarthritis, and results in a tingling pain and burning over the sole of the foot, which develops after standing or walking for a long time. Usually there is no motor deficit and relief may be obtained by severing the flexor retinaculum.

Mononeuritis multiplex

When more than one peripheral nerve is involved in an individual patient, consideration should be given to the possibility of mononeuritis multiplex due to an underlying systemic abnormality. Some patients who present with multiple pressure palsies of median, ulnar and lateral popliteal nerves will be found to have systemic disturbances, such as diabetes mellitus, alcoholism, or other diffuse abnormalities which render the nerves more liable to pressure. The classical syndrome of mononeuritis multiplex, however, with frequently acute and often painful neuropathies developing at different sites, is most commonly due to vascular damage to the nerves occurring in the context of arteritis, diabetes mellitus or paraproteinaemias and investigations to identify such pathology should be undertaken (Table 10.8).

DISTURBANCES OF NEUROMUSCULAR FUNCTION

A group of diseases interfere with normal neuromuscular transmission at the motor end plate and have in common the cardinal symptom of fatiguing muscle weakness.

CLINICAL SYNDROMES OF NEUROMUSCULAR DISEASE

Myasthenia gravis

This disease, with a prevalence of approximately 5 per 100 000, has a bimodal spread of incidence, being most common in the third decade of life where women are affected twice as frequently as men, and a second peak in the seventh decade where the sex incidence is approximately equal.

Myasthenia gravis is now established to be due to an immunological mechanism in which circulating antibodies bind adjacent to the receptor sites at the neuromuscular junction and prevent the normal action of acetylcholine in opening the calcium entry channels in the muscle fibre. Evidence of this belief was first provided in the early 1970s when repeated immunisation of rabbits with acetylcholine receptor protein was found to cause a fatiguing muscle weakness which had the neurophysiological features of myasthenia gravis. Later studies using radioactive labelled alpha-bungarotoxin showed that acetylcholine receptor antibodies could be demonstrated in the majority of patients with myasthenia gravis.

There is still a question as to why certain patients form these antibodies and the relationship of the condition to thymic tumours and hyperplasia has long been recognised but is not fully understood.

Clinical features

The cardinal feature of myasthenia gravis is a fatiguable weakness of muscles, which may be generalised or confined to a specific group of muscles. The insidious onset of weakness developing after prolonged exercise frequently leads to a mistaken initial diagnosis of psychological disturbance and many patients are referred to psychiatrists before the true nature of the illness is determined. There is usually involvement of the muscles of the eyes, resulting in ptosis which develops during the day and occasionally the onset of diplopia in the evenings. Weakness of the facial muscles and of those in the pharynx and tongue result in the development of a flaccid dysarthria and difficulty in chewing and swallowing food. Limb involvement tends to occur later in the disease and results in fatigue on exertion, which may be difficult to identify and gives the mistaken impression of lassitude, tiredness and an inability to sustain voluntary effort.

In younger patients the eyes are commonly affected and in some patients the disease may be confined to the eye muscles (ocular myasthenia). In older patients the development of a bulbar palsy, with a typical posture of the hand being used to keep the jaw closed and the development of a flaccid dysarthria and dysphagia, should always raise suspicion of this disease.

The diagnosis clinically depends upon the demonstration of a fatiguable weakness in levator palpebrae, the tongue or pharyngeal muscles or the limb muscles. The reflexes are normal. The use of the anticholinesterase edrophonium bromide, as in the Tensilon test, with rapid resolution of symptoms confirms the diagnosis.

The course of the illness is variable. Some patients may develop no more than a mild ptosis which persists for years, whereas others progress rapidly from first symptoms to a condition which may be misdiagnosed as a bulbar palsy of vascular aetiology or due to motor neurone disease. Symptoms may become more pronounced at times of emotional or physical stress; initial symptoms may occur during pregnancy or in association with an operation where the injudicious use of curare-like agents may be associated with prolonged recovery time. The various clinical stages of the disease have been classified by Osserman (Table 10.9) and the use of the staging in assessing patients helps to give an idea of prognosis and indicate the need for various types of therapy.

Investigations

These include the use of tetanic train stimulation which reveals progressive reduction in the size of the motor action potential, or of single-fibre studies in which increased jitter and blocking confirm the diagnosis. In more than 70% of patients with generalised myasthenia, but a

Table 10.9 Classification of myasthenia gravis

1. Ocular myasthenia
2. a. Mild generalised myasthenia with slow progression
   Drug-responsive
   b. Moderate generalised myasthenia
   Severe skeletal and bulbar involvement
   Drug response poor
3. Acute fulminating myasthenia
   Rapid progression of symptoms
   High incidence of thymoma
4. Late severe myasthenia

smaller proportion of patients with ocular myasthenia, acetylcholine receptor antibodies may be detected in the blood and help to confirm the diagnosis.

A significant proportion of patients with myasthenia gravis (10%) are shown to have thymic tumours and this particular association is most common in older men who should therefore undergo routine chest radiography and CT scan of the thorax. It has been suggested that the HLA phenotype of B8 and DR3 is related to the development of disease in young women and that DR2 is more commonly found in older men. Many patients will show an association with familial incidence of other autoimmune disease, and 5% of patients with myasthenia gravis can be shown to have a history of thyrotoxicosis.

Management

The therapy of this condition is initially symptomatic, with the use of agents such as pyridostigmine; occasional benefit may be obtained from the use of ephedrine. When using an anticholinesterase agent such as pyridostigmine it is frequently of use to add atropine or probanthine to the regime to block the unwanted autonomic effects (colic and diarrhoea) of the anticholinesterase. In general, patients will respond to pyridostigmine in a dose of between 30 and 60 mg four-hourly together with atropine 0.6 mg twice or thrice daily to reduce the muscarinic effects.

There is now good evidence that the use of steroids reduces the effect of the disease and, in patients with purely ocular myasthenia, it may prove to be the most effective form of therapy. Alternative treatments with cytotoxic agents such as azathioprine are also beneficial to patients and, in the acute disease, plasmaphaeresis may give significant benefit. Plasmaphaeresis does not appear to have a part to play as regular therapy in the disease, because repeated treatments are necessary. There is increasing evidence that thymectomy is the treatment of choice, particularly in generalised myasthenia, although patients may take months or even years to show significant benefit from this procedure. It is always indicated in patients with thymoma and probably is beneficial for all patients with myasthenia.

One particular important consideration is the possible occurrence of neonatal myasthenia in a baby born to a myasthenic mother: for this reason sample of cord blood should be taken at the time of delivery for assessment of acetylcholine receptor antibodies and the infant must be carefully monitored to detect any problems with respiratory function.

Prognosis

The greatest risks to the patient with myasthenia gravis relate predominantly to bulbar and respiratory insufficiency and some patients during acute exacerbations of the disease will require respiratory support with intermittent positive pressure ventilation. When patients are receiving treatment and appear to deteriorate there arises the question as to whether the deterioration is attributable to a cholinergic crisis following excessive treatment, or a myasthenic crisis because of ineffective therapy. Although, in theory, the use of edrophonium bromide at this time can help to determine which of the two conditions is present, in practice it is safer to admit the patient to an intensive care unit, to discontinue all therapy and to observe his condition over a few days. Occasionally the withdrawal of therapy (although often necessitating ventilatory support) will give the patient the chance to recover from an acute exacerbation. Particular care needs to be taken during any anaesthetic procedure in patients with myasthenia gravis, but the avoidance of neuromuscular-blocking drugs is usually adequate to ensure patient's safety at this time.

The demonstration of acetylcholine-receptor antibodies in the serum of patients with myasthenia gravis indicates that most of these patients have an illness which is an organ-specific autoimmune antibody-mediated disease. There remains, however, the possibility that some patients with myasthenia gravis do not have an immunological form of the disease and this is certainly true of patients with congenital myasthenia. The relationship, in the majority of cases, to an immunological disorder and an abnormality of thymic function raises the possibility that thymic cells with nicotinic acetylcholine receptors might be involved in the genesis of the original antibody followed by overproduction of the antibody, which then affects the skeletal muscle receptors.

Congenital myasthenia

Some patients with myasthenia presenting in the neonate have a disease which persists throughout life and occasionally these cases are familial. Such patients may respond to anticholinesterase preparations, but rarely to thymectomy or the use of steroids. The precise cause of myasthenia in this situation is not known.

Myasthenic syndrome of Eaton–Lambert

The development of a fatiguing muscle weakness associated with oat cell carcinoma of the lung was first described by Eaton–Lambert in 1957. The muscles of the pelvic and shoulder girdles are most affected and involvement of those muscles innervated by the cranial nerves is uncommon. The syndrome is also associated with dryness of the mouth and impotence in the male. Paradoxically, patients with this condition may show some initial improvement on exercise and tendon reflexes are diminished or abolished rather than normal, as in myasthenia gravis. The onset of this condition is subacute but the progression is relentless. The response to anticholinesterase agents is poor and electrophysiological studies with tetanic train stimuli show facilitation in the size of the muscle action potential rather than the decremental response seen in myasthenia gravis.

The diagnosis requires the search for and treatment of occult malignancy. The only therapy which appears to be at all beneficial is the use of guanethidine hydrochloride or 3, 4-aminopyridine. Unfortunately, both of these agents have significant side effects in causing blood dyscrasias. It has recently been suggested that some patients with this condition may indeed have an antibody to the end plates and there has been some suggestion that the use of plasmaphaeresis may give benefit to the patients.

Drug-induced myasthenic weakness

There are occasional reports of myasthenia-like syndromes developing with certain antibiotics such as neomycin, lanomycin, streptomycin, polymyxin B and some tetracyclines. These conditions are almost certainly due to an interference with calcium ion fluxes in response to nerve stimuli at the terminals. A more classic myasthenic syndrome is produced by the administration of D-penicillamine, in which a typical myasthenia gravis may develop and antiacetylcholine-receptor antibodies are found in the serum (p. 433).

MUSCLE DISEASE

INTRODUCTION

Diseases of muscle usually result in the development of weakness which is most apparent in the largest muscle groups. For this reason the diagnosis of muscle disease must be considered in patients developing weakness in the proximal muscles of the limbs or the shoulder or hip girdles. The initial symptoms of weakness are difficulty climbing stairs, rising from a chair, or reaching to place things on a high shelf. The weakness in pelvic muscles frequently results in the development of a waddling gait with a profound lumbar lordosis and the appearance of a pot belly. Although pain and cramps may appear in the muscles there is, by definition, a complete absence of sensory signs; reflexes are usually reduced and may be absent.

INVESTIGATIONS OF MUSCLE DISEASE

The investigation of patients with muscle disease as part of a more systemic illness will necessarily involve numerous other tests, possibly relating to imaging techniques and to biochemical and haematological studies. In general, however, in those diseases confined to muscle there are three forms of investigation which are particularly important.

Laboratory investigations

In the inflammatory muscle diseases the finding of a high ESR can be important in indicating the nature of the diagnosis and in most diseases with destruction of muscle there is an increased serum creatine kinase activity and on occasion the presence of myoglobin may be detected in the blood. Certain specific tests, such as the ischaemic lactate test, may be indicated in McArdle's disease and in patients with profound muscle lysis the presence of myoglobinuria may be detected.

Electromyography

Electromyography of muscle is the single most helpful investigation in identifying those conditions caused by primary muscle disease, where myopathic potentials of small size are seen together with occasional fibrillations (which helps to differentiate these conditions from neurogenic muscle disease in which large polyphasic units may be found together with fibrillation potentials—p. 109). In some instances myotonic activity may suggest the underlying disease and newer techniques of macro-EMG recording may provide more information as to the nature of the underlying problem.

Muscle biopsy

The definitive test for muscle disease is to examine histologically, histochemically and by electron microscopy a piece of tissue excised from a diseased muscle. The various techniques used will help to distinguish between neurogenic and myopathic disease and, in the case of myopathic disease, should indicate whether that is inflammatory, dystrophic or due to some metabolic abnormality. As biochemical techniques improve, tissues from muscle biopsy may be examined biochemically as well as by histochemical means, and further information on the activity of individual enzymes may be obtained.

Magnetic resonance spectroscopy

The relatively new technique of MR spectroscopy of muscle provides further information about biochemical function within muscle tissue and, although available in few centres at present, is potentially a most useful tool in the investigation of the metabolic myopathies.

CLINICAL SYNDROMES OF MUSCLE DISEASE

Inflammatory diseases of muscle

Polymyositis

The condition may vary considerably in its clinical manifestations from a relatively benign proximal weakness seen in menopausal females to an acute fulminant variety resulting in death within weeks The condition also has a juvenile form occurring in the early part of the second decade, but is most frequently seen in adults in the fifth and sixth decades. It is more common in women than men and may occasionally be preceded by a febrile illness or mild infection. Typically, patients become aware of weakness of the pelvic and thigh muscles, often with a chronic aching pain and tenderness in those muscles. They develop difficulty in rising from a sitting or squatting position and have problems in lifting objects on to a high shelf, or in brushing their hair. The onset is usually insidious and the course progressive, usually with a symmetrical weakness of proximal limb and trunk muscles.

The facial, pharyngeal and laryngeal muscles are involved in approximately 10% of patients, but ocular muscles are almost never involved. Many patients will have minor ECG changes and some patients may have significant arrhythmias. In rare cases with more severe forms of the disease there may be overt muscle swelling, the finding of myotonia and discrete tenderness of the muscles.

Investigations will frequently reveal an elevated ESR and almost invariably a high level of creatine kinase activity. Myoglobinuria and myoglobinaemia may be found in those patients with more fulminating muscle disease. The EMG will reveal a typical myopathic pattern with many brief action potentials of low voltage and numerous fibrillation potentials with occasional pseudomyotonic potentials. Muscle biopsy will usually demonstrate inflammatory infiltration in the muscle but, as the disease is patchy, unfortunately the biopsy may occasionally be normal (Fig. 10.10).

The treatment of the disease is with prednisone and occasionally with the use of cytotoxic agents. Both azathioprine and cyclophosphamide have been used, partly for their steroid-sparing effect and partly because they appear to give a better long-term result than prednisone. Most patients (80%) will improve with the use of steroid or cytotoxic therapy and the activity of the disease is usually limited to a 2–3 year period. However, patients may be left with significant muscle weakness which may persist indefinitely and some patients with more fulminant forms of the disease may die within months, usually from cardiac or pulmonary complications. Occasional patients will show a relapse in the condition some years after initial response to therapy.

Dermatomyositis

In this condition, which may appear identical to polymyositis, there is in addition a localised or diffuse erythematous maculopapular eruption with occasionally an exfoliative dermatitis. There is a characteristic heliotrope (purple) appearance to skin over the lower eyelids, cheeks and forehead and there may be periorbital oedema. The skin lesions are most commonly seen on the extensor surface of joints and in mild cases may be overlooked. Patients with dermatomyositis more commonly have evidence of other connective tissue disease than those with pure polymyositis and almost 30% of patients will show evidence of Raynaud's phenomenon. In rare cases the condition may be associated with a form of scleroderma, and oesophageal weakness is relatively common.

Connective tissue disease with polymyositis and dermatomyositis

Patients with rheumatoid arthritis, scleroderma, lupus erythematosis and Sjögren's syndrome may also develop a form of polymyositis which may be complicated by an associated arthritis.

Polymyositis with carcinoma

The condition of polymyositis or dermatomyositis may be associated in 10–20% of adults with an occult neoplasm. The frequency of neoplasia with polymyositis appears to increase with age and is slightly more common in men than in women.

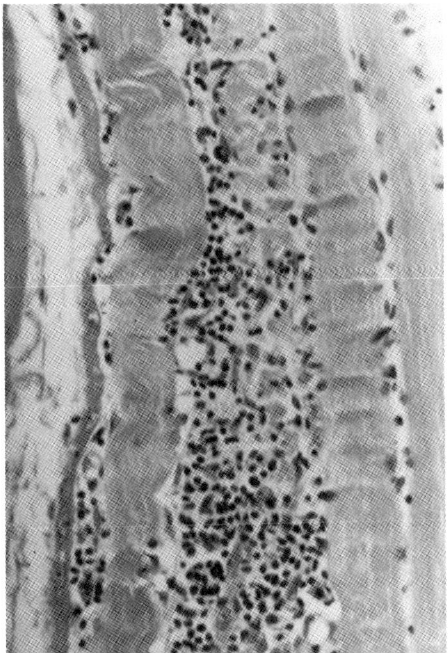

A

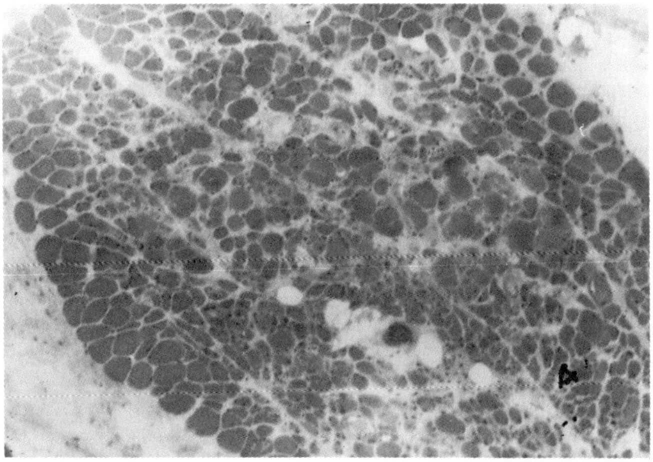

B

Fig. 10.10 Histology of muscle from a pateint with polymyositis. **A** longitudinal section **B** transverse section

The most common tumour to be associated with this condition is a bronchogenic neoplasm. The polymyositis or dermatomyositis may antedate the development of the malignancy by one or two years.

Infective myopathies

Infective myopathies are an extremely uncommon form of muscle disease, but trichinosis may present with ocular muscle weakness, pharyngeal weakness and weakness of the tongue. The muscles involved are swollen and tender and there is marked facial oedema. As the infective agents become encysted the symptoms regress and the patient recovers. Many patients will show no symptoms of this form of infection but, rarely, profound infection with cardiac involvement will cause death. Toxoplasmosis may occasionally result in the development of pseudocysts in skeletal muscle causing focal inflammation, but muscle symptoms are uncommon.

Viral infections frequently cause an acute myalgia during the course of the illness but rarely show significant muscle symptoms or signs. Infections with Coxsackie B virus in Bornholm disease involve considerable muscle pain but little evidence of muscle pathology. Some patients with persistent aches and pains after virus infections and who are diagnosed as having epidemic myalgia, can be regarded as having a chronic form of virus infection of muscle, although the proof of virus infection in this disease is lacking.

Although sarcoidosis is not usually included as an infective condition, patients may develop a syndrome similar to idiopathic polymyositis in which non-caseating granulomatous lesions are found in the muscles. This so-called sarcoid myopathy is uncommon and tends to respond reasonably to treatment with steroids.

The muscular dystrophies

This group of progressive hereditary degenerative diseases of skeletal muscle result in severe degeneration of the muscle fibres, with intact spinal motor neurones, nerves and nerve endings. The characteristic features are a symmetrical distribution of muscle weakness with atrophy, but with intact sensation, preservation of cutaneous reflexes and the occurrence of familial incidence of the disease. Only the more common and those likely to be seen in adults by neurologists are discussed here.

Duchenne hypertrophic X-linked muscular dystrophy

The prevalence of this condition is approximately 3 per 100 000; it occurs exclusively in males and may be associated with hypertrophy of muscles. The onset is in early childhood and, although classically there is an X-linked family history, more than one-third of the patients will show no significant family history and are believed to represent mutations. The disease frequently presents before the male child begins to walk and is usually diagnosed between the third and fifth year of life. The child either fails to achieve his normal motor milestones or achieves them and then fails to progress. Increasing difficulty in arising from a prone posture, the development of a waddling gait and the associated hypertrophy of muscles make the diagnosis likely. The proximal muscles of the lower limb are the earliest and most severely affected and the calves and forearm muscles may become grossly enlarged. Even these enlarged muscles however can be shown to be weak and they are usually hypotonic.

The children show an extremely lordotic posture, have a waddling gait and tend to show the classic sign of climbing up their legs as they arise from a sitting position (Gower's sign). As the disease progresses, the weakness and atrophy spread to involve muscles of the upper limb girdle where the neck flexors, brachioradialis and wrist extensors are also involved. The muscles of the eyes, face and bulbar muscles are usually spared. Contractures may develop and the feet assume an equinovarus position. Ultimately, the child is unable to walk and becomes wheelchair bound. The development of scoliosis results in considerable difficulty with respiration. Although tendon reflexes are initially present, they are lost as muscles waste, and the ECG may show abnormalities. Death usually occurs in the second decade of life and is often due to pulmonary infection or cardiac decompensation.

The disease is diagnosed by the classic clinical appearance and the finding of increased creative kinase (CK) activity in the serum. EMGs show a typical myopathic appearance and muscle biopsy reveals degeneration and regeneration of muscle fibres. There is some evidence that the female carriers of the disease may have increased CK activity in the serum. In addition to genetic counselling, the use of amniocentesis to detect potential involvement of the fetus may be of use. Gene probes are now being used to identify the linkage of the gene for muscular dystrophy and this may in time result in more accurate prediction of the disease and thereby avoidance of it.

Becker-type muscular dystrophy

This is also an X-linked disorder affecting approximately 4 per 100 000 male births. The onset is later than in Duchenne dystrophy, tending to begin at the end of the first decade; the course is more benign, the patient not becoming wheelchair-bound until the third decade and frequently surviving into the fifth decade. Increased CK activity and the findings on EMG help in the differential diagnosis from forms of hereditary spinal muscular atrophy and the female carrier may, again, show slightly increased CK activity.

Facioscapulohumeral dystrophy

This condition, which tends to follow an autosomal dominant form of inheritance, is much more slowly progressive than Duchenne or Becker dystrophy and tends to involve predominantly the musculature of the face and shoulders. It is less common than Duchenne dystrophy and the age of onset is usually in the second decade. The first symptoms are of difficulty in raising the arms above the head, together with winging of the scapulae and weakness and atrophy of muscles in the shoulder girdles and in the face. The condition may frequently show periods of arrest and rarely causes involvement of cardiac muscles. The CK activity is only slightly increased and the EMG is myopathic. The course may be very benign and rarely tends to cause significant disability to the patient.

Limb girdle dystrophy

There are many patients who show weakness of pelvic and shoulder girdle muscles but who do not fit into the categories of dystrophy described above. Some patients have myopathic disease of the muscles but others show a form of spinal muscular atrophy with a pattern of distribution remarkably similar to that of the true limb girdle dystrophies. The disease may present in late childhood or early adult life and the later the onset the more likely the course is to be benign. CK activity may be mildly increased, and the EMG in the dystrophic cases is myopathic. In the future it is inevitable that more specific syndromes will be identified from this group of diseases and thus the true limb girdle dystrophies will become a relatively smaller part of the overall problem of muscle disease.

Progressive external ophthalmoplegia

There is a form of progressive ophthalmoparesis with ptosis developing in childhood or early adult life which is autosomal dominant. Differential diagnosis is occasionally difficult from cases of the Kearns–Sayre syndrome or 'ophthalmoplegia plus', but in these conditions, which are believed to be forms of mitochondrial cytopathy, the association of other neurological abnormalities and the finding of a high c.s.f. protein tend to make the diagnosis apparent. The true progressive external ophthalmoplegia tends to progress to complete ophthalmoparesis but not to involve other muscles.

Oculopharyngeal dystrophy

This autosomal dominant condition usually becomes evident in the fifth decade of life and causes progressive ptosis together with a flaccid difficulty in swallowing and flaccid dysarthria.

Dystrophia myotonica

This autosomal dominant disease is probably the most common of all of the dystrophies and results in classic marked wasting of the sternocleidomastoid, causing the so-called swan-necked appearance, together with myopathic weakness of the facial muscles and a progressive and predomi-

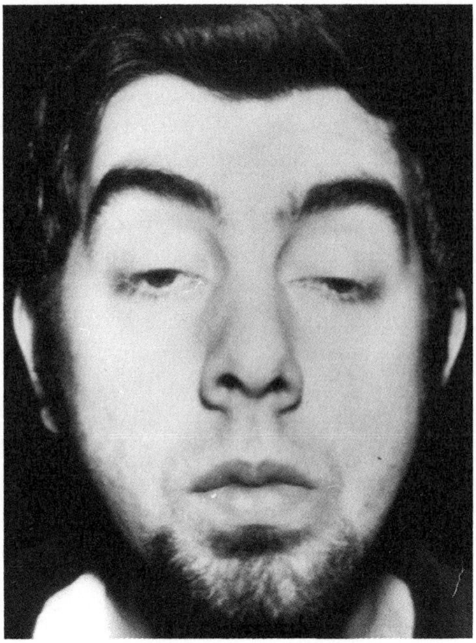

Fig. 10.11 Myopathic facies typical of dystrophia myotonica. (Reproduced from Blackwood W et al 1983 *Slide Atlas of Neurology*. Gower Medical Publishing, London, with permission.)

nantly distal myopathic weakness (Fig. 10.11). The cardinal feature of the disease is the presence of myotonia, i.e. the inability to relax a contracted muscle, and the association with frontal baldness, early cataract, diabetes mellitus, cardiac conduction abnormalities and degrees of mental retardation make the diagnosis evident.

There is usually increased CK activity in the blood and classic myotonic potentials are revealed on EMG studies. Nerve conduction studies may also show the presence of a neuropathy and, although the myotonia may be helped by the use of phenytoin, there is no treatment for the more disabling myopathy.

Congenital myotonic dystrophy

Infants with profound hypotonia and facial diplegia at birth may have a form of congenital myotonic dystrophy in which the myotonia does not become apparent for a 2–3 year period. Many children will not survive to develop this aspect of the disease and it is noted that in this congenital form of the illness the affected parent is almost always the mother. This raises the possibility of a cytoplasmic agent involved in the development of the condition and it may be that it is, in fact, one form of mitochondrial cytopathy.

In the majority of cases described in this section there is no specific therapy available for the underlying dystrophy. Medical treatment is therefore confined to symptomatic help to the patient and supportive treatment to the patient and the family. Physiotherapy has an important part to play and the provision of aids and resources to enable the disabled child or adult to adapt to the disability forms an important part of management.

Metabolic myopathies

It is inevitable that, as more is understood about the biochemistry of the muscle cell, an increasing number of diseases which were originally classified as being due to dystrophy or of unknown aetiology are recognised as being due to metabolic abnormalities (Table 10.10).

Glycogen storage myopathies

A group of diseases due to disturbance of the glycogen pathways result in classic muscle weakness with pain, and biochemical investigations identify several sites within the pathway at which problems can arise (Table 10.10).

Table 10.10 Metabolic myopathies

Defects of glycogen metabolism
Acid α-glucosidase deficiency
Amylo-1,6-glucosidase deficiency
Branching enzyme deficiency
Phosphorylase deficiency
Phosphorylase kinase deficiency
Phosphofructokinase deficiency
Phosphoglycerate kinase deficiency
Phosphoglycerate mutase deficiency
Lactate dehydrogenase deficiency
Defects of mitochondrial metabolism
Complex I–V deficiencies (individual and combined)
Defects of fatty acid oxidation
Carnitine palmitoyltransferase deficiency
Short chain acyl-CoA dehydrogenase deficiency
Median chain acyl-CoA dehydrogenase deficiency
Long chain acyl-CoA dehydrogenase deficiency
Electron-transfer flavoprotein dehydrogenase deficiency
Defects of calcium metabolism
Luft's disease and malignant hyperthermia

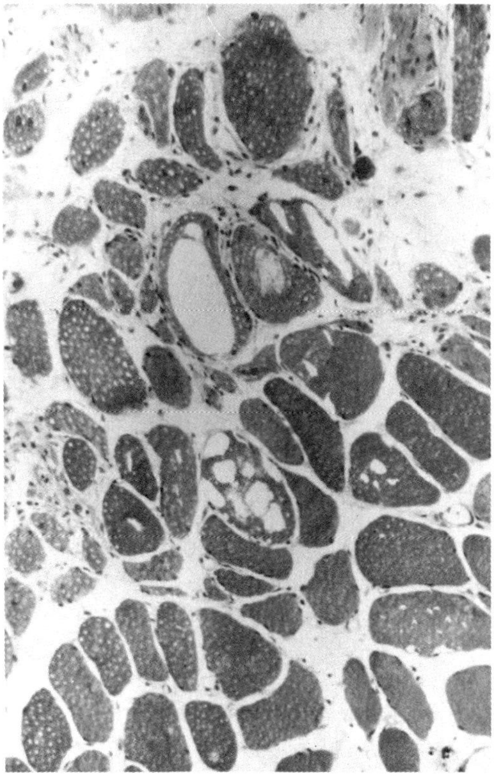

Fig. 10.12 Photomicrograph showing vacuolation in muscle fibres as seen in glycogen storage disorders.

Acid maltase deficiency. A deficiency of the enzyme alpha-1–4-glucosidase may present in three different clinical forms. The most severe develops in the first months of life and causes dyspnoea and cyanosis with hypotonia. The tongue is frequently enlarged, hepatomegaly though present is not marked and the heart may be relatively normal in size. The clinical picture must then be differentiated diagnosed from infantile spinal muscular atrophy. The disease is rapidly progressive and ends in death within a few months.

In the childhood form of the disease the onset is in the second year of life with delay in reaching motor milestones. Cardiomyopathy may be present, hepatomegaly is unremarkable and death occurs within two years.

In the adult form of the disease there is an initially mild proximal myopathy, which is slowly progressive over years and may result in death due to respiratory muscle paralysis. There is no cardiomegaly or hepatomegaly but the CK activity is found to be increased and the EMG is myopathic, with occasional myotonic discharges.

The diagnosis at all ages is confirmed by muscle biopsy, in which there is vacuolation of the sarcoplasm of muscle cells and special stains may reveal stored glycogen. Electron microscopy shows that the glycogen particles lie within lysosomal vesicles and the changes are most pronounced in type I fibres. It is believed that the difference in severity between the infantile and adult forms of the disease may depend upon the relative level of the enzyme present.

Myophosphorylase deficiency (McArdle's disease). This condition, which may present in childhood or early adulthood, causes weakness and stiffness with cramps on using muscles. It may frequently present at times of unusual exertion, when severe spasms may develop in the muscle, which may undergo myolysis, causing pain and resulting in myoglobinuria. The defect in myophosphorylase results in the inability of the muscle to convert glycogen to glucose-6-phosphate and the diagnosis may be confirmed by failure to find increased blood lactate in the cubital vein after a 3-minute period of ischaemic exercise to the forearm muscles. Histochemical stains of biopsied muscle show an absence of phosphorylase activity, which confirms the diagnosis. There is some evidence that fructose taken orally before exercise may be helpful in some cases, but in the majority of cases it is necessary to limit the amount of exercise undertaken.

Carnitine deficiency

Carnitine is necessary in muscle to allow the intramitochondrial oxidation of long-chain fatty acids. A deficiency of carnitine results in progressive muscle weakness which begins in early adult life and affects predominantly the trunk and proximal muscles. Muscle enzyme activities are found to be increased in the serum and muscle biopsy reveals excessive fat in the muscle and a reduction of muscle carnitine. There is some evidence that a high carbohydrate and low-fat diet, together with carnitine replacement, may help to reduce the effect of the syndrome.

Carnitine palmityl transferase deficiency. A deficiency of the enzyme which, with carnitine, is responsible for the influx of lipids into the mitochondria may cause an acute weakness after an infection or, more commonly, a chronic weakness of muscles. It is diagnosed on muscle biopsy which reveals the presence of excessive fat inside the muscle fibres.

Endocrine myopathies

Thyroid

Thyrotoxic myopathy. This condition in association with chronic thyrotoxicosis may cause progressive weakness and atrophy of muscles. It is associated (unusually for a myopathic disturbance) with brisk reflexes and the finding of brisk reflexes and myopathy therefore should always raise the possibility of thyrotoxicosis.

Hypothyroid myopathy. Very occasionally in hypothyroidism there will occur a form of stiffness and slowness of contraction of the muscles with percussion myoedema, which has been described as the Hoffman syndrome. There may be clinical evidence of myotonia, although none is detected on EMG, and muscle biopsy is relatively normal.

Thyrotoxic periodic paralysis. In Oriental races the occurrence of a typical periodic paralysis associated with thyrotoxicosis is well recognised. The level of potassium appears to be low during an attack and the infusion of potassium chloride may abort an episode.

Adrenal

Corticosteroid proximal myopathy. The chronic use of corticosteroid drugs may result in a situation similar to that seen in Cushing's syndrome, in which there is weakness of proximal and limb girdle muscles. An EMG will show a myopathic pattern and biopsies show variation in fibre size with atrophy. Withdrawal of steroids in such patients will result in a recovery from the weakness.

Primary aldosteronism. Patients with primary aldosteronism will develop hypokalaemia, which may present as a myopathy (p. 458).

The mitochondrial cytopathies

A group of diseases caused by abnormalities of mitochondrial enzymes are being increasingly recognised and may present at different stages in life. They may cause hypotonia in infants, muscle pain and cramps in older children and adolescents and a progressive muscle weakness in the older population. The different presentations probably result from varying severity of the defects of different enzymes and there is frequently an association with other forms of neurological disease or systemic illness.

Some forms are well recognised, such as that described by Kearns and Sayre as 'ophthalmoplegia plus', in which there is an evolving ophthalmoparesis together with ataxia, high c.s.f. protein and variable involvement of intellect, peripheral muscle and cardiac involvement. These illnesses, which were originally called mitochondrial myopathies, are now more correctly termed mitochondrial cytopathies because the involvement of mitochondria is not confined to those in the muscle cells.

Congenital myopathies

A group of conditions presenting in infancy with hypotonia and failure to thrive are diagnosed on muscle biopsy. They are described in Table 10.11 and they cause a degree of muscle weakness which is relatively non-progressive.

Spinal muscular atrophies

Although such conditions are not strictly due to disease of muscle, they are included in this section because of frequent difficulty in diagnosing them differentially from true diseases of muscle. There are essentially three different forms of spinal muscular atrophy.

Infantile-onset SMA

This condition, which is also called *Werdnig–Hoffmann disease*, begins in infancy and has a poor prognosis. The weakness develops within the first year of life and the majority of patients die within the first decade. It appears to be transmitted as an autosomal recessive condition in which there is

Table 10.11 Congenital myopathies

Diagnosis	Clinical features	Inheritance	Biopsy
Central core myopathy	Delayed motor milestones, may present from birth to middle age	Autosomal dominant	Amorphous change in myofibrils
Nemaline myopathy	Hypotonia in infancy with generally poor prognosis	Autosomal dominant and recessive	Bacilli-like rods beneath the sarcolemma
Myotubular myopathy	Hypothonia and weakness in childhood	X-linked recessive, auto dom and recessive	Central nucleation of muscle fibres
Fibre-type disproportion	Hypotonia in infancy, variable prognosis	Autosomal recessive	Small type I fibres

degeneration of the lower motor neurone; death results from respiratory complications.

Juvenile form

This condition, which is termed *Kugelberg–Welander disease*, has an onset in childhood and may initially cause difficulty because it resembles Duchenne dystrophy. The EMG is diagnostic of a neurogenic atrophy, however, and it is again due to degeneration of the anterior horn cells.

Adult form

Various forms of spinal muscular atrophy may occur in adult life. They frequently result in the slow and insidious wasting of one or more groups of muscles and loss of reflexes. The weakness may be confined to one limb or may show a pattern which resembles that of the limb girdle dystrophies. The diagnosis is made by electrophysiological studies, which show neurogenic atrophy that can be confirmed by muscle biopsy. Nerve conduction is normal or only minimally slowed. In patients in whom the condition is focal it may be necessary to undertake myelography to exclude the possibility of an intraspinal lesion.

The limb girdle syndrome

A group of patients will present with weakness of the limb girdles with or without facial weakness, the overall appearance resembling facioscapulohumeral or scapuloperoneal diseases. The question always arises in this condition as to whether the problem is a form of spinal muscular atrophy or dystrophy. It may frequently be difficult, both clinically and after investigation with electrophysiology and histopathology, to identify the precise cause of the problem, though those clinical features which would indicate a neurogenic basis for the problem are asymmetry, depressed reflexes and evidence of focal muscle atrophy.

Periodic muscle paralysis

A group of conditions occur in which muscle weakness is intermittent and variable.

Familial or hypokalaemic periodic paralysis

The onset of this disease is in late childhood or early adolescence. Symptoms frequently begin during the night after a day of unusually strenuous exercise. They may be precipitated by a meal rich in carbohydrates and the patient usually awakens with mild weakness of the limbs, which progresses to become severe. Limbs are affected more severely than trunk muscles and reflexes are abolished. Attacks of paralysis tend to occur less frequently with advancing age and ultimately the disease arrests. There may, however, be a residual myopathic weakness following the attacks of episodic paralysis. Most patients are found to have low levels of serum potassium during an attack and it is this which may be generated by the muscle exercise and high carbohydrate load. Attacks may be aborted by the infusion of potassium chloride and avoided by the use of low carbohydrate and high potassium diets.

Thyrotoxicosis with periodic paralysis

In Oriental races periodic paralysis may occur in association with thyrotoxicosis and the attacks resemble those of familial periodic paralysis.

Hyperkalaemic periodic paralysis

There is a further familial form of episodic paralysis in which the serum level of potassium is elevated during the attack. This form again tends to begin in early childhood and follows exercise; it starts within minutes of the exercise, however, and is not related to high carbohydrate meals.

Normokalaemic periodic paralysis

In this condition there is no change in the level of serum potassium during the episode of paralysis.

Hypokalaemic weakness in primary aldosteronism

The occurrence of intermittent weakness should always make one suspect primary aldosteronism which may cause hypokalaemia and result in the development of intermittent paralysis.

Drug-induced periodic paralysis

The potassium-losing diuretics may result in a condition of hypokalaemia and intermittent paralysis which is indistinguishable from the forms seen in primary aldosteronism.

Myotonic syndromes

Dystrophia myotonica

This dominantly inherited muscular dystrophy is discussed in the section on dystrophy.

Thomsen's disease (myotonia congenita)

This is a genetically inherited muscle disease of which two forms are recognised. That originally described by Thomsen is an autosomal dominant condition with myotonia beginning in early infancy, the symptoms being exacerbated by exposure to cold. Muscle hypertrophy is mild or absent and there are no episodes of paralysis.

In the second type of myotonia congenita, the inheritance is an autosomal recessive with more males being affected than females. In this condition the myotonia begins later in childhood and may not occur until adult life. It tends to be more severe, invariably associated with hypertrophy and there may be associated mild distal weakness. The condition may worsen until the end of the third decade of life and there can be increased serum CK activity. There may appear to be similarities between this condition and myotonic dystrophy, but the findings of testicular atrophy, cardiac abnormality, frontal baldness and cataracts are absent in myotonic congenita.

The cardinal features of these conditions are that the muscles are liable to tonic spasm after voluntary contractions, a phenomenon most pronounced after a period of inactivity. Repeated contractions result in a lessening of the symptom and the spasm is usually painless. In most instances myotonia may be induced by tapping the muscle belly with a percussion hammer, and myotonia, unlike myoedema, will persist for several seconds. Diagnosis may be difficult to confirm electrophysiologically although the presence of percussion myotonia is usually sufficient to establish the diagnosis.

The cause of the condition is not entirely understood, although it is assumed that there is some abnormality in the sarcolemma of the muscle fibres. EMG shows that muscle tension in contracting fibres is slow to diminish and activity continues after the volley of nerve impulses that initiated the contraction has ceased.

Therapy is with quinine sulphate or procainamide, and phenytoin may occasionally be of use.

MANAGEMENT

In most conditions involving both the peripheral nerve and muscle in which specific and treatable causes can be identified the relevant therapies should be instituted. There are, however, many similarities in terms of the disabilities sustained by patients with peripheral neuropathic and anterior horn cell, or muscle disease for whom there is no treatment available for the underlying condition. It is then appropriate that general therapy be considered in the form of splinting and calipers to aid mobility and prevent contractures, physiotherapy to maintain muscle bulk and strength and to overcome disturbances in posture, and orthopaedic procedures to lengthen tendons, fuse joints and avoid the development of progressing deformity. In patients with sensory neuropathy it is particularly important to protect the areas of skin which are most liable to pressure injury and therefore to the formation of sores.

Genetic counselling

In many of the primary diseases of muscle and nerve which are recognised to be inherited, the possibility of genetic counselling to advice on the risks for further offspring is important and the advent of techniques such as amniocentesis may allow the diagnosis of an affected child in utero.

FURTHER READING

Adams R D, Victor M 1977 Principles of neurology. McGraw-Hill, New York

Dyck P J et al (eds) 1984 Peripheral neuropathy, 2nd edn. W B Saunders, Philadelphia

Walton J N (ed) 1988 Disorders of voluntary muscle, 5th edn. Churchill Livingstone, Edinburgh

11

Disorders of the cerebral circulation

INTRODUCTION

Stroke remains one of the top four causes of death in the civilised world and an understanding of the cerebral circulation and its disorders is of considerable importance to the practising physician. Stroke prevention has produced a very significant reduction in the occurrence of stroke in the United States and the United Kingdom: the death rate from stroke has now decreased by at least 40% in the last 10–15 years. Although experimental work has increased our understanding of the control of cerebral blood flow, epidemiological and clinical studies have contributed most to this decreased incidence.

THE CEREBRAL ARTERIAL CIRCULATION

The blood supply of the brain is derived from the two internal carotid arteries and the two vertebral arteries, which originate from the aortic arch (Fig. 11.1) and which unite anteriorly to form the basilar artery. The circle of Willis, which is situated at the base of the brain, is formed by anastomoses between the internal carotid arteries, the basilar artery and their branches (Fig. 11.2). The basilar artery divides into the two posterior cerebral arteries and these are joined to the two internal carotid arteries by the posterior communicating arteries. Each internal carotid artery gives off an anterior cerebral artery and these are linked by a single anterior communicating artery, thus completing the circle.

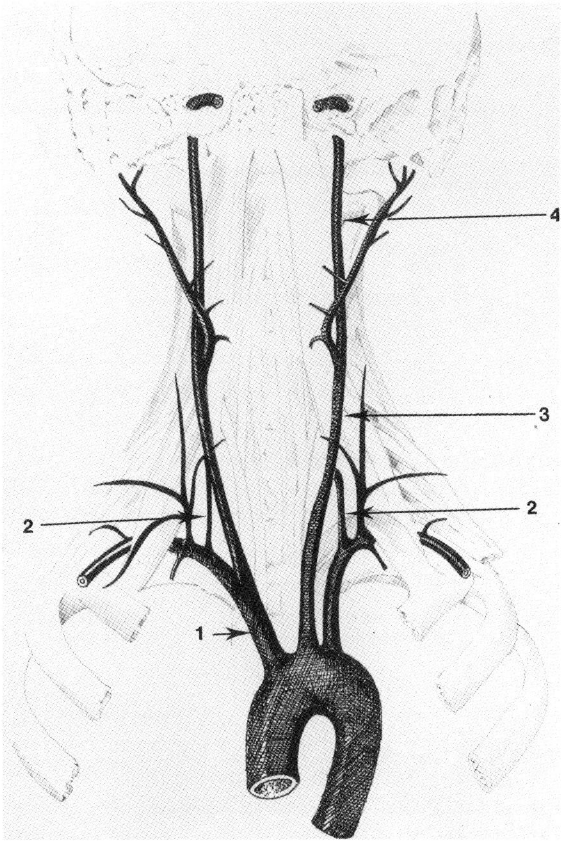

Fig. 11.1 Origins of the great vessels from the arch of the aorta. 1—Innominate artery, 2—vertebral artery, 3—common carotid artery, 4—internal carotid artery.

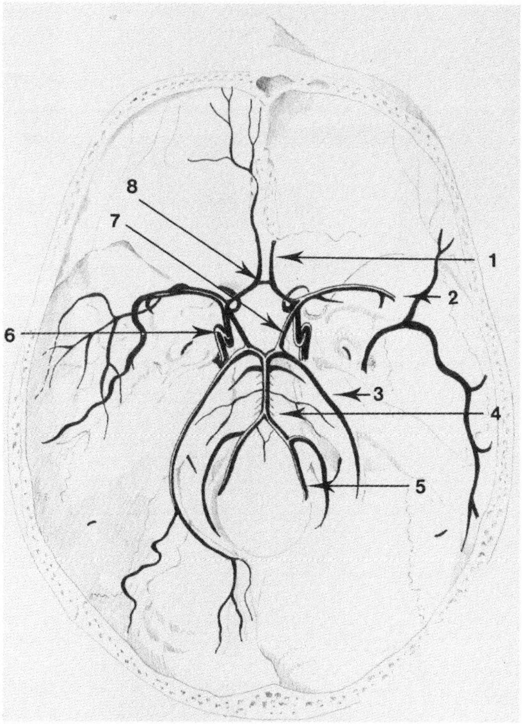

Fig. 11.2 The circle of Willis. 1—Anterior cerebral artery, 2—middle cerebral artery, 3—posterior cerebral artery, 4—basilar artery, 5—vertebral artery, 6—internal carotid artery, 7—posterior communicating artery, 8—anterior communicating artery.

It is important to remember that there is a considerable amount of variation, not only in the origins of the carotid and vertebral arteries, but also in the constituent arteries making up the circle of Willis. Fifty per cent of normal individuals have a significant anomaly of the circle of Willis and 1–5% of normal subjects have an anomaly of one of the origins of the main extracranial vessels from the aorta. The commonest anomalies at the circle of Willis are hypoplasia of either one of the posterior communicating arteries or of the anterior communicating artery. The distribution of the main areas of supply of the anterior, middle and posterior cerebral arteries is shown in Figure 11.3. The branches of the basilar artery show considerable anatomical variation but conform to a general scheme (Fig. 11.4).

COLLATERAL CIRCULATION

The blood supply of the brain has a considerable collateral circulation which provides a secondary defence mechanism against failure of the primary vessels. There is marked anatomical variation in the capability of these vessels to transport blood and often the collateral circulation becomes evident only when the intracranial arterial supply of the brain is impaired. Some of the most important collaterals exist between branches of the external carotid and branches of the internal carotid. One of the most frequently observed of these is via the ophthalmic artery linking with branches of the external carotid artery supplying the orbit (Fig. 11.5). This collateral circulation is usually most evident in cases of internal carotid artery occlusion. The importance of these

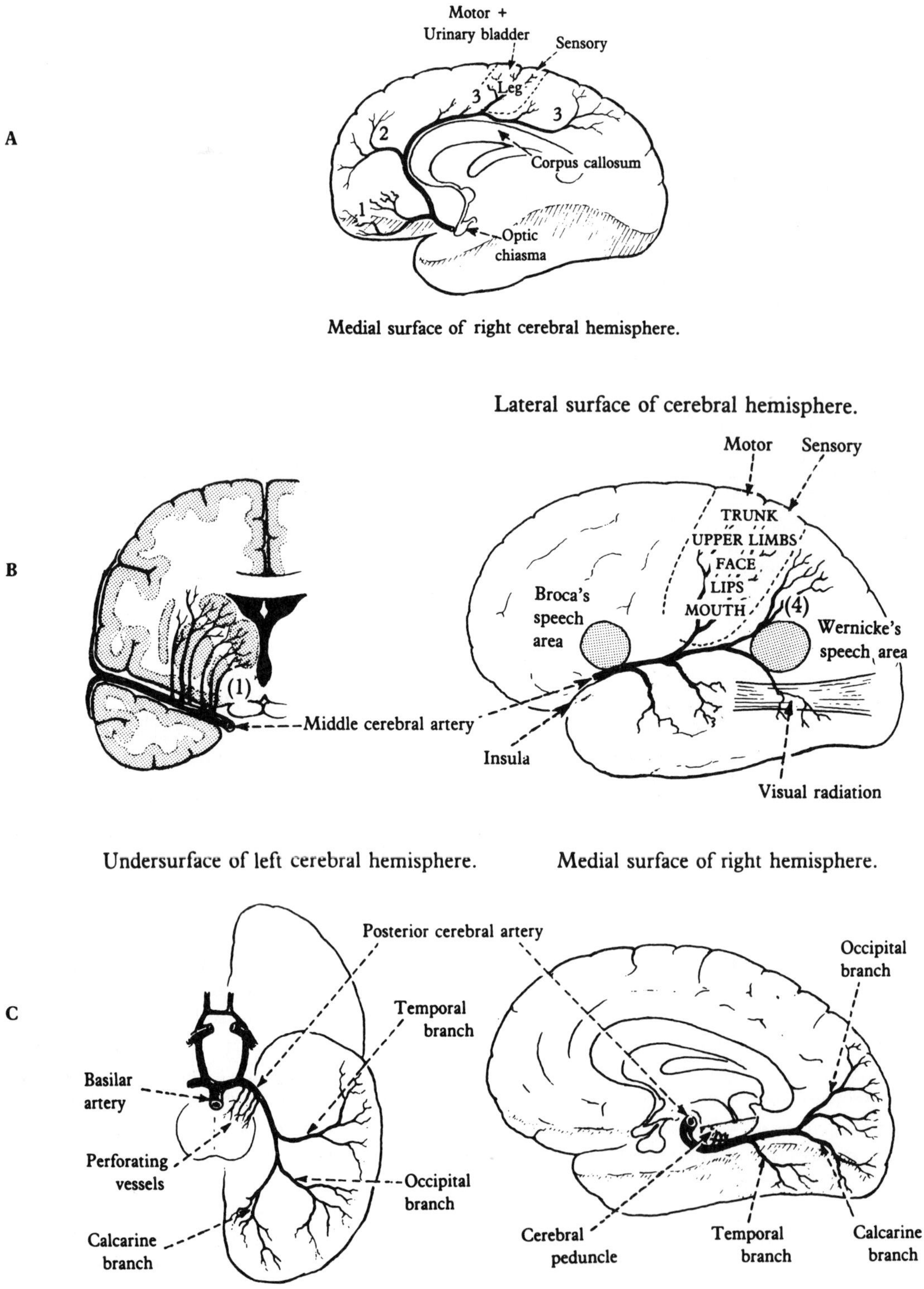

Fig. 11.3 The main areas of supply of: **A** the anterior cerebral artery, **B** the middle cerebral artery, **C** the posterior cerebral artery. (Reproduced from Lindsay K W, Bone I, Callander R 1986 *Neurology and Neurosurgery*, Churchill Livingstone, Edinburgh, with permission.)

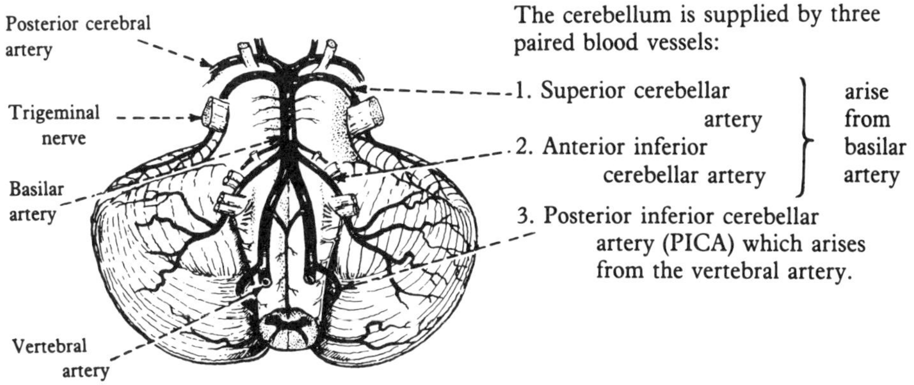

Fig. 11.4 The branches and areas of supply of the basilar artery. (Reproduced from Lindsay K W, Bone I, Callander R 1986 *Neurology and Neurosurgery*, Churchill Livingstone, Edinburgh, with permission.)

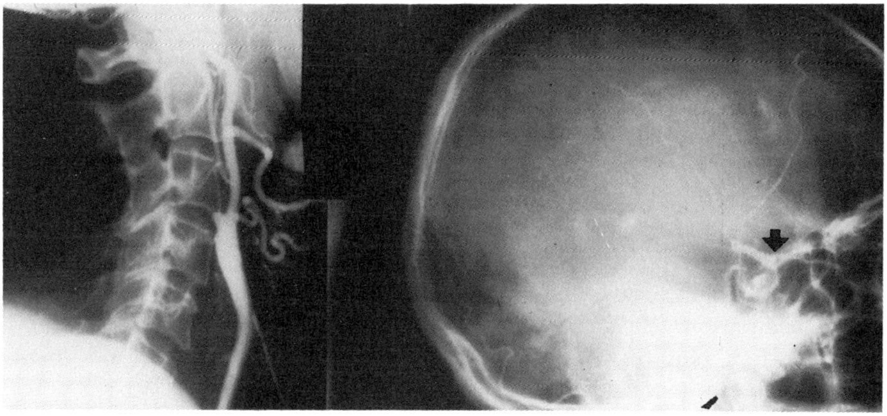

Fig. 11.5 Carotid angiogram demonstrating a complete internal carotid occlusion with filling of the internal carotid in the head via collateral circulation through the orbit (arrowed).

collaterals in attempting to maintain intracranial flow is obvious and, indeed, it was a better understanding of the development of these collaterals which led to the development of the artificial creation of such anastomoses in the technique of extracranial–intracranial anastamosis of the superficial temporal to the middle cerebral artery (see below).

THE CEREBRAL VENOUS SYSTEM

The general pattern of venous drainage from the brain is of two discrete but intercommunicating systems. The superficial set of veins drain directly into adjacent dural venous sinuses and the second system, the deep venous system, forms a single unit receiving branches from the entire brain. Both venous systems ultimately pass dorsally and join to exit as the internal jugular vein. It should be remembered, however, that the internal jugular vein is not the only source of venous drainage from the intracranial cavity (Fig. 11.6).

PHYSIOLOGY OF THE CEREBRAL CIRCULATION

The last 10 years has seen considerable research into the physiology of the circulation of the brain

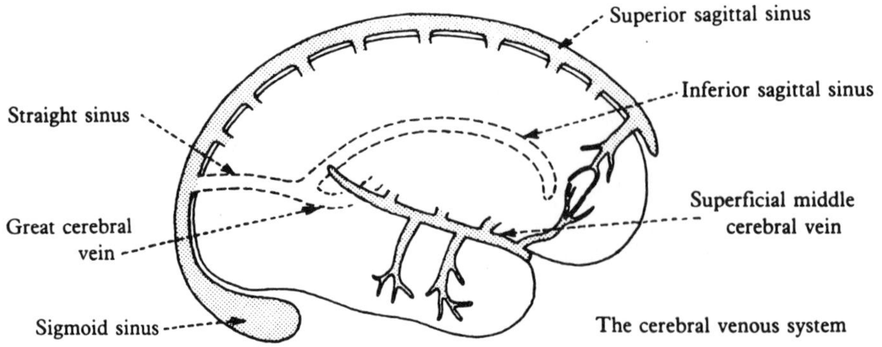

Fig. 11.6 The main cerebral veins. (Reproduced from Lindsay K W, Bone I, Callander R 1986 *Neurology and Neurosurgery*, Churchill Livingstone, Edinburgh, with permission.)

and, in particular, into the study of cerebral blood flow. Although this work unfortunately has had little clinical relevance, it has increased our understanding of the factors affecting blood flow to the brain. Most of the blood to the cerebral hemispheres is supplied by the internal carotid artery and its branches. The areas of cortex at the intersections of the differing branches, anterior, middle and posterior cerebral arteries, are called the watershed zones because hypoperfusion in the territory of one of these arteries will show itself clinically and pathologically in that area.

Normal brain function requires a continuous supply of nutrients from the bloodstream, the most important being glucose and oxygen. Although the brain constitutes only 2–3% of total body weight, 20–25% of all oxygen consumed by the human under resting conditions is utilised by this organ. Normally over 90% of cerebral energy is derived from degradation of glucose to lactate and pyruvate. There are virtually no tissue stores of oxygen and glucose in the brain and when the blood supply to the brain fails, the brain ceases to function. The brain responds to oxygen lack by mobilising its meagre energy resources and by lowering requirements through diminution of cortical electrical activity, but these mechanisms are only briefly effective.

Rates of cerebral blood flow have now been obtained for different parts of the brain under both physiological and pathological conditions; the normal being 54 ml 100 g^{-1} min^{-1}. Under normal circumstances, cerebral blood flow and intracranial arterial pressure is zealously maintained by a number of homeostatic mechanisms which begin to fail only when the arterial blood pressure falls below a level of 60–70 mm of mercury. This homeostatic mechanism depends very much on cerebral vascular resistance and there is an intrinsic nervous supply to the arterioles of the brain, the control of which has been studied in great depth. The newer techniques of nuclear magnetic resonance and positron emission tomography are allowing more detailed study of cerebral metabolism in health and disease; it is hoped that these will cast further light on the effects of impairment of the circulation to the brain.

DEFINITIONS

The term cerebrovascular disease is applied to any abnormality of the brain resulting from a pathological process implicating blood vessels. The commonest two pathological mechanisms are those of occlusion of a vessel or rupture with haemorrhage. Without question, the commonest process is that resulting in vessel occlusion and the various pathological causes of this and the other syndromes of cerebrovascular disease are considered in a later section.

The common mode of expression of cerebrovascular disease is in the form of *stroke*, defined as a sudden non-convulsive focal neurological deficit. In its most obvious form there is sudden hemiplegia, which may be associated with coma.

Table 11.1 Stroke: definitions and severity

Transient cerebral ischaemic attack	A transient focal neurological deficit of presumed vascular origin lasting for less than 24 hours (sometimes called insipient stroke or intermittent insufficiency)
Completed stroke	Focal neurological deficit of presumed vascular origin with symptoms lasting for more than 24 hours
Minor stroke	Stroke lasting for less than 7 days
Major stroke	Stroke lasting for more than 7 days
Progressing stroke (advancing stroke, slow stroke, stroke in evolution)	A focal neurological deficit of presumed vascular origin which progresses over a matter of hours or occasionally days

A number of terms, including apoplexy, stroke or cerebrovascular accident, have been used. In its mildest form the deficit may simply take the form of a trivial transient neurological deficit with complete recovery and there are all gradations of severity between these two extremes (Table 11.1). The hallmark of a vascular disorder is the abruptness of its origin, whatever the length of persistence of the deficit, the time course of evolution varying from seconds to minutes. It cannot be emphasised too often that, clinically, it may be impossible to differentiate the underlying pathological basis of an acute stroke, i.e. an acute cerebral haemorrhage from a cerebral infarct, and furthermore, even pathologically, it is often difficult to differentiate a thrombotic infarct from an embolic infarct.

EPIDEMIOLOGY

A considerable amount of information has been accumulated concerning the epidemiology of cerebrovascular disease but, as much of this is based on clinical assessment, the reliability of data from many studies is uncertain. Overall, approximately 500 000 new strokes occur annually within the United States and, in Great Britain, approximately two strokes occur each year for every 1000 of the population. Table 11.2 lists age-specific prevalence rates for cerebrovascular disease derived from a variety of sources and Table 11.3 lists mortality data.

Table 11.3 Percentage dead among cerebrovascular disease patients discharged from England and Wales hospitals during 1955, 1960, 1966, by age and sex

Year and sex	All ages	Age in years 15–44	45–64	65+
1966 Men	45.1	21.9	34.3	52.6
Women	49.6	18.7	34.8	55.9
1960 Men	45.0	24.2	32.8	54.6
Women	50.5	26.8	39.6	56.4
1955 Men	48.8	17.0	39.0	57.9
Women	53.4	35.7	42.4	59.5

Much of the epidemiological information concerning stroke has come from the Framingham study. These data show that the incidence of strokes generally, and atherosclerothrombotic brain infarctions specifically, increases with age in both sexes but more precipitously in women than in men. Only under the age of 55 years is the male preponderance characteristic of atherosclerotic disease apparent.

Table 11.2 Incidence and prevalence of cerebrovascular disease estimated for a population similar to the Tyneside conurbation (data taken from multiple sources)

Age group	Standard million population	Estimated incidence per 1000	Expected new cases per year	Estimated prevalence per 1000	Expected total cases in community
0–34	582 083	0.00	0	0	0
35–44	113 561	0.25	28	0	0
45–54	114 206	1.00	114	20	2 284
55–64	91 464	3.50	320	35	3 101
65–74	61 155	9.00	550	60	3 669
75 plus	37 531	30.00	1126	95	3 565
Total	1 000 000		2138		12 619

MORTALITY

In the United States, stroke accounts for approximately one-tenth of the total mortality. This may be an underestimate because death certification, by stating only the underlying cause of death, often fails to note the contribution of a previous stroke. Stroke fatalities rank third among all causes of death in most affluent countries, exceeded only by heart disease and cancer.

RISK FACTORS

It hardly needs emphasising that major reductions in disability and in death from stroke will come largely from prevention rather than from more effective medical or surgical treatment. Indeed, there is evidence (in the United States at least) that stroke is decreasing in frequency. This decrease is greatest in primary intracerebral haemorrhage and almost certainly this has resulted from the increasingly effective treatment of hypertension.

There is general agreement that both hypertension and cardiac abnormalities are powerful contributors to stroke incidence. Unfortunately, at present the cause of atherosclerosis remains uncertain and, hence, despite a wealth of information concerning the associated features of atherosclerosis, myocardial infarction and stroke, there is a considerable degree of uncertainty in this area. Factors which have been inconsistently incriminated are glucose intolerance, blood lipids, elevated haematocrit and cigarette smoking. A variety of environmental factors have similarly been incriminated, but their importance is uncertain: these include diet, obesity, soft water, alcohol, physical activity and climate. Further epidemiological investigation concerning the different stroke syndromes are discussed later.

PATHOLOGICAL MECHANISMS

There are four possible mechanisms by which disease of the cerebral blood vessels may injure the brain:

1. The wall of a cerebral artery may be thickened, with resulting narrowing of the lumen or even occlusion leading to impairment of blood supply to a particular portion of the brain. This may result in ischaemic changes in the brain, depending on collateral circulation and, if severe enough, may produce ischaemic necrosis; the term for this is infarction.
2. The wall of a cerebral artery may be weakened leading to rupture and haemorrhage into the tissue of the brain or over the surface of the brain.
3. A vessel may enlarge or dilate (aneurysm) and compress adjacent brain tissue.
4. A common concomitant of infarction is cerebral oedema, which itself may produce pathological changes.

The commonest form of stroke is cerebral infarction resulting from impairment of circulation within the territory of a particular artery; this may occur as a result of a number of separate processes:

1. Arterial wall disease, e.g. atheroma, hypertensive arteriosclerosis, granulomatous disease
2. Block of the arterial lumen by an embolus: either thrombotic, tumourous or infected
3. Failure of blood flow may occur as a result of sludging, due to either a circulatory defect, or to a haematological abnormality such as polychythaemia
4. The blood vessel may become narrowed as a result of a vasospasm

In this chapter the following categories of stroke will be considered:

1. Atherosclerotic cerebrovascular disease
2. Non-atherosclerotic causes of stroke, including cerebral embolism of cardiac origin
3. Hypertensive cerebrovascular disease, including primary intracerebral haemorrhage and lacunar infarcts
4. Subarachnoid haemorrhage (including arteriovenous malformations).
5. Cerebral venous thrombosis

ATHEROSCLEROTIC CEREBROVASCULAR DISEASE

We decided to use this term to cover all forms of cerebral infarction resulting from atheromatous disease of the arteries supplying the brain and within this we encompass the terms cerebral thrombosis and thromboembolic infarction. For many years there has been debate about the mechanism whereby atherosclerosis of the cerebral arteries results in cerebral infarction. Traditionally it was thought that in situ thrombosis of the intracranial cerebral arteries was one of the common mechanisms resulting in cerebral infarction. Currently it is felt that, in many cases, patients previously thought to have suffered cerebral thrombosis have in fact been examples of embolic infarction resulting from atheromatous disease in the proximal arteries supplying the brain.

Figure 11.7 is a diagrammatic representation of the sequence of events that are thought to be the mechanisms of arteriosclerotic cerebral infarction.

PATHOLOGY

Atherosclerosis is typically found in the large elastic arteries and the muscular distributing arteries which have a wall consisting of three layers—intima, media and adventitia. The intima consists of an inner single layer of endothelial cells and a peripheral fenestrated sheath of elastic fibres. The endothelial cells are linked together by highly interdigitated margins and form a barrier to the passage of blood constituents into the arterial wall. Between the two layers are various components of extracellular connective tissue and occasional smooth muscle cells which increase in amount and number with age. The media consists of diagonally orientated smooth muscle cells surrounded by variable amounts of collagen, small

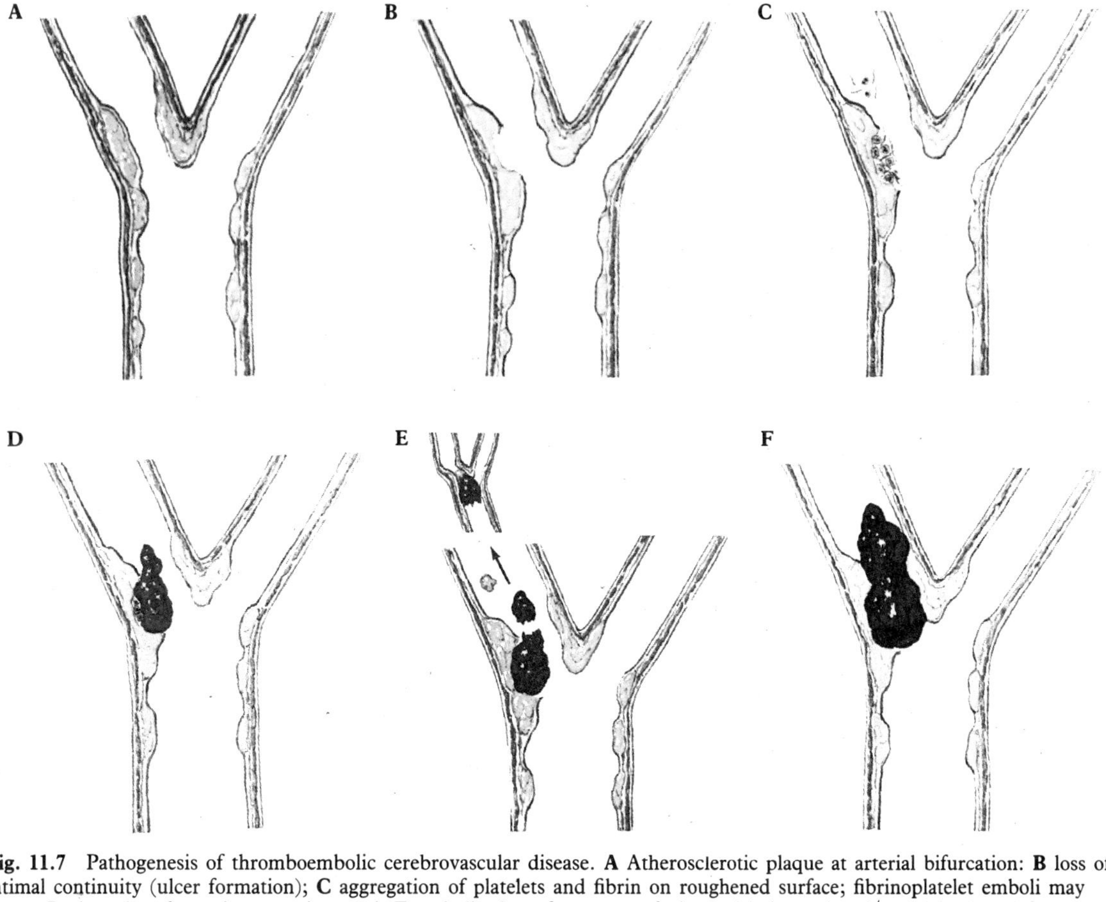

Fig. 11.7 Pathogenesis of thromboembolic cerebrovascular disease. **A** Atherosclerotic plaque at arterial bifurcation: **B** loss of intimal continuity (ulcer formation); **C** aggregation of platelets and fibrin on roughened surface; fibrinoplatelet emboli may occur; **D** thrombus formation superimposed; **E** embolisation of contents of plaque (cholesterol and/or calcium) and fragments of organised thrombus; occlusion of blood vessels distally in arterial tree; **F** thrombus causes total arterial occlusion. (After 1973 Ciba Pharmaceuticals Clinical Symposia, Vol 25, with permission.)

elastic fibres and proteoglycans; the proportion of elastic tissue is greater in elastic arteries such as the aorta and carotid arteries. Fibroblasts are not present and the morphology of the media does not alter with age. The adventitia consists of fibroblasts, smooth muscle cells, bundles of collagen and proteoglycans. The arteries of the nervous system have a very thin adventitia and lack a definitive external elastic lamina which elsewhere usually separates media and adventitia.

Types of atherosclerotic plaques

Atherosclerosis primarily affects the intima, although the media may be secondarily affected. Three different categories are recognised:

1. The fatty streak
2. The fibromusculoelastic plaque
3. The complicated lesion.

The fatty streak commonly seen in the aorta of young persons consists of focal accumulations of relatively small numbers of intimal smooth muscle cells, containing and surrounded by deposits of lipid (cholesterol and cholesterol esters).

The fibromusculoelastic plaque consists principally of a subendothelial accumulation of proliferated, intimal, smooth muscle cells laden with lipid (cholesterol and cholesterol esters). The complicated lesion is a fibromusculoelastic plaque containing intramural haemorrhage and/or collections of atheromatous debris with superficial serration or luminal thrombus.

Mural thrombus

There is evidence that, in at least a proportion of atherosclerotic lesions, the plaques have enlarged by the incorporation in them of mural thrombus. The exact nature of the process which initiates atherosclerosis in the human is not yet certain, although there is increasing evidence to suggest that damage to endothelial cells is the key factor resulting in adherence and aggregation of platelets to the cells.

Although atheroma occurs principally in late middle-age and old age, it is now recognised that its early manifestations may be seen in individuals in their 20s and 30s. It is a generalised process and involvement of the cerebral blood vessels parallels a similar process in the aorta and coronary arteries. The process may occur in a patchy fashion and it shows a predilection for certain vessels. In relation to the cerebral blood supply one of the commonest sites is at the bifurcation of the carotid artery.

Evolution

The lesions develop and enlarge gradually over a matter of 20 or 30 years and usually clinical effects become manifest only as a result of secondary thrombotic complications. The plaques of atheroma may narrow the lumen of the artery, causing stenosis, but complete occlusion occurs only when there is in situ thrombosis. The thrombus which forms is called the primary thrombus. If this occludes the lumen of the vessel, secondary thrombus develops in an anterograde and (usually shorter) retrograde fashion, in the now stagnant columns of blood. Secondary thrombus will usually fill the artery as far as the first collateral branch. In the case of the internal carotid artery this usually will be the ophthalmic artery.

The relationship between actual thrombosis within an atheromatous vessel and occlusion either of that vessel or a distal vessel and the occurrence of infarction, is complex. Collateral circulation is clearly an important factor and many others as yet undetermined are thought to influence the end result.

CLINICAL PICTURE

The evolution of symptoms in thromboembolic stroke may be variable: usually there is a single attack of sudden onset with preserved consciousness and, not infrequently, headache; occasionally the deficit may persist over a few hours and one characteristic of thromboembolic stroke is that the deficit may be intermittent or stutter over a period of hours or days. In some instances there is a fleeting deficit followed by the completed stroke and in at least 10% of patients who suffer an acute stroke there are preceding 'little strokes' (so-called transient ischaemic attacks).

A preceding history of transient ischaemic

attacks is of considerable importance in establishing the diagnosis of thromboembolic cerebral infarction (see below). In the absence of such a history, it may be difficult on clinical grounds to differentiate cerebral infarction from cerebral haemorrhage. Thromboembolic stroke often occurs during the night when the patient is asleep; he wakes to discover a hemiplegia. Sudden collapse to the ground with a hemiplegia is more common in cerebral haemorrhage or cerebral embolism of cardiac origin.

NEUROVASCULAR SYNDROMES

Specific clinical pictures may result from occlusion of particular arteries supplying the brain. As it is important, particularly in relation to the management of transient ischaemic attacks, to be able to recognise the arterial territory of an ischaemic event, the typical syndromes of the major arteries are described below.

Internal carotid artery

The area of supply of this artery is shown in Figure 11.3. Total occlusion may often be silent, owing to the efficiency of the circle of Willis. In other instances, however, there may be massive infarction involving the whole of the anterior two-thirds of the cerebral hemisphere. Most common of all, however, is a clinical picture mimicking that of a middle cerebral artery occlusion (see below). Anomalies of the circle of Willis may produce almost any pattern of deficit as a result of an occluded internal carotid artery. Progressive obliteration of the lumen by atheroma and thrombus often produces the picture of a stuttering stroke. There is a gradually progressing contralateral hemiparesis and hemisensory disturbance and there may also be transient ipsilateral visual impairment due to retinal ischaemia. Unilateral frontal headache may be an accompanying symptom and the end result may be a dense neurological deficit.

Carotid territory transient ischaemic attacks may produce similar transient deficits of which amaurosis fugax (see below) is the most characteristic.

Clinical clues supporting a diagnosis of disease of the internal carotid artery are a bruit at the angle of the jaw, a lowered ipsilateral retinal arterial pressure and the changes in the pulses over the face and scalp. In internal carotid artery occlusion the facial and scalp pulses on the affected side may be more prominent than those on the contralateral side. In total occlusion of the common carotid artery, the facial and scalp pulses may be impalpable.

The anterior cerebral artery

The area of supply of the anterior cerebral artery is shown in Figure 11.3. A proximal block of the anterior cerebral artery is associated with a contralateral hemiplegia and hemisensory loss affecting the foot and leg to a greater degree than the arm and usually sparing the face. Occlusion of the stem proximal to its connection with the anterior communicating artery may well be tolerated because of adequate collateral flow. When both arteries arise from one anterior cerebral stem there may be infarction of the medial parts of both hemispheres, resulting in paraplegia, incontinence and profound mental symptoms. Transient ischaemic attacks in the anterior cerebral artery territory may mimic any of the above syndromes and probably can be recognised clinically only when they present with transient ischaemic monoparesis of one or other leg.

The middle cerebral artery

The area of supply of this artery is shown in Figure 11.3. Obstruction of the artery at its origin causes contralateral hemiplegia and hemisensory loss, the weakness being most marked in the face, tongue and upper limb, with relative sparing of the legs. When the area of infarction involves the supply of the penetrating arteries then there is a deep wedge of infarction extending into the internal capsule, resulting in a profound contralateral hemiplegia, hemisensory defect and hemianopia.

As the middle cerebral artery supplies an extensive area of cortex on the lateral surface of the hemisphere, involving many specialised areas on the dominant and non-dominant side, there are often associated profound neuropsychological deficits. Total infarction of this area on the dominant side will produce global aphasia. Occlusion of distal branches may produce localised aphasic defects in the form of either Broca's aphasia or Wernicke's aphasia. The commonest cause of a middle cerebral artery occlusion is a thromboembolus.

Transient ischaemic attacks in the middle cerebral artery territory will produce transient deficits of the type described above; the most characteristic is a transient hemiparesis in association with dysphasia.

The posterior cerebral artery

The area of supply of this artery is shown in Figure 11.3. It is important to remember that the posterior cerebral artery supplies not only a considerable portion of the medial surface of the occipital lobe but also a considerable portion of the medial and under surface of the temporal lobe. Occlusion of the posterior cerebral artery results in infarction of the visual cortex with a contralateral hemianopia. The macular region of the blind field usually escapes (macular sparing) owing to overlapping of the posterior and middle cerebral areas of supply at the occipital pole. If the obstruction is proximal to the supply of the thalamus, a thalamic syndrome may be present. An embolus passing up the basilar artery may break up at the bifurcation into the two posterior cerebral arteries and occlude both of these; this may result in total bilateral blindness. Where the embolus lodges in the distal branches of the posterior cerebral artery there may be ischaemic damage to both medial temporal lobes, resulting in an amnestic syndrome. The syndrome of transient global amnesia may be caused by a transient ischaemic attack within this territory.

The basilar artery (Fig. 11.4)

Occlusion of the main trunk of the basilar artery results in extensive infarction of the brain stem and cerebellum, and is rapidly fatal. Progressive thrombosis within the basilar artery produces the characteristic syndrome of a stuttering brain stem stroke which, if recognised clinically, merits anticoagulation (see below). A variety of named syndromes have been described over the years, resulting from local areas of infarction within the brain stem and cerebellum; these have often been thought to have resulted from occlusion of specific branches of the basilar artery: for example, the lateral medullary syndrome has been thought to result from occlusion of the posterior inferior cerebellar artery. It is now recognised that these pictures may result from partial occlusion of the basilar artery or occlusion of proximal arteries such as one vertebral artery. The use of the eponyms should probably be abandoned as, clearly, almost an infinite combination of neurological symptoms and signs may result from localised infarction in such a complex structure as the brain stem (see p. 77).

The vertebral artery (Fig. 11.4)

Occlusion of the vertebral artery may be asymptomatic when the opposite vertebral artery is able to maintain a collateral circulation. However, the variability in the size of the vertebral arteries occasionally means that occlusion of one artery deprives the basilar artery of almost its total supply; there will then result the clinical picture of basilar artery occlusion. One specific arterial syndrome occuring within the territory of the vertebrobasilar system is the so-called subclavian steal syndrome. Although this is well recognised and known to most neurologists, it is, in fact, extremely rare. The clinical picture is of recurring transient ischaemic attacks within the vertebrobasilar system, occurring either spontaneously or following exercise of one or other arm. The syndrome results when there is stenosis of either the left subclavian artery or the innominate artery before the take off of the vertebral artery. Either spontaneously, or following exercise of the ipsilateral arm, there is a steal of blood *down* the vertebral artery, which may be demonstrated radiologically at the time of an angiogram (Fig. 11.8). The syndrome may be suspected clinically in a patient with vertebrobasilar transient ischaemic attacks by the absence of a pulse or by a difference in blood pressure between the two arms. The absence of a difference in pulse or blood pressure between the two arms excludes a diagnosis of subclavian steal syndrome (see above).

INVESTIGATIONS

In many cases of cerebral infarction where the diagnosis is not in doubt, no specific neurological investigations are required. The definitive investigation to demonstrate cerebral infarction is the CT scan. The indications to perform a CT scan are that the diagnosis of stroke is in doubt, or to differentiate cerebral infarction from cerebral haemorrhage. In the early stages of cerebral infarction, the CT scan appearance differs from that seen some weeks later (Fig. 11.9). As there

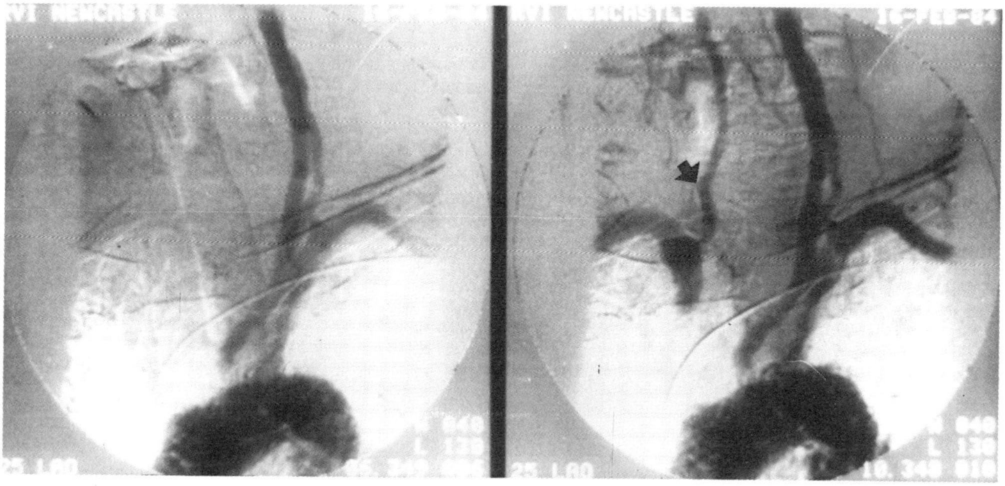

Fig. 11.8 Arch aortagram showing a vertebral steal syndrome. In the left-hand radiograph no filling of the right subclavian or vertebral arteries is seen. The later radiograph on the right shows reversed flow down the right vertebral artery in order to fill the right subclavian.

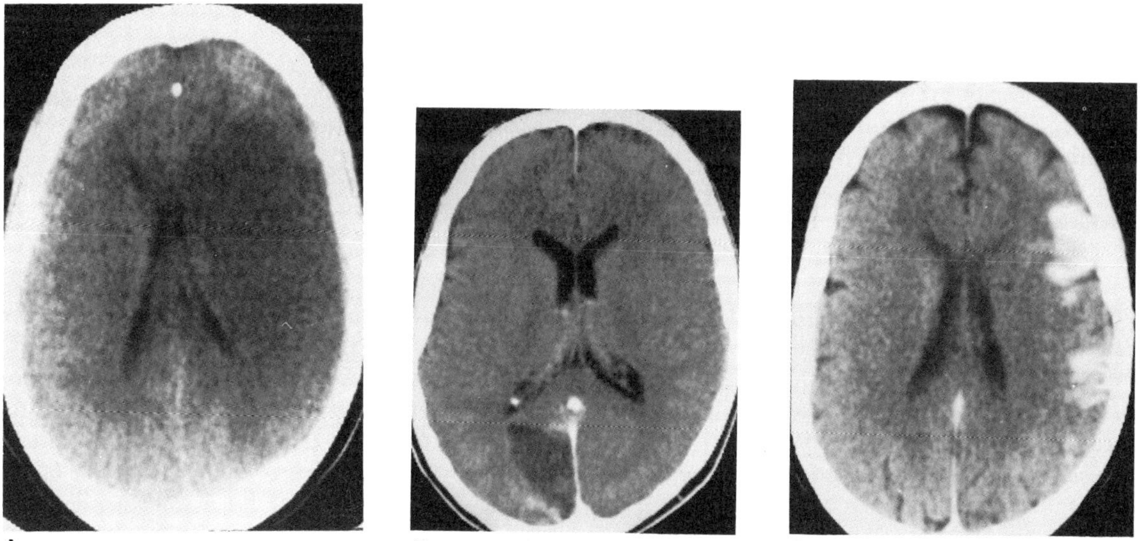

A **B** **C**

Fig. 11.9 CT scans showing differing appearances of cerebral infarction. **A** Early massive hemisphere infarction with diffuse low density of the right hemisphere with some hemisphere swelling and shift, **B** left occipital infarction showing low density with some peripheral enhancement following the administration of contrast, **C** right hemisphere infarction showing dramatic enhancement following the administration of contrast 10 days after infarction.

is some evidence to suggest that contrast-enhanced scanning may have a deleterious effect, this should probably be avoided in the acute stages.

Lumbar puncture is of limited value in the assessment of a patient with suspected cerebral infarction. The c.s.f. pressure is usually normal unless there is a massive infarct with associated cerebral oedema. The c.s.f. protein may show a mild elevation and, where the infarct extends to the surface, then there may be a c.s.f. pleocytosis. Serum cholesterol or triglycerides are elevated in some cases and because of the associated presence of hypertension and diabetes relevant abnormalities from these disorders may be noted.

The electroencephalogram will invariably show an abnormality in a patient suffering hemispheric infarction, but is of limited value in differentiating infarction from haemorrhage. Radionuclide scans are of very limited value. Arteriography in the acute stages of stroke is of no diagnostic help and, because of its risk, should not be undertaken unless there are other indications.

Table 11.4 Complications of stroke

Early (0–48 h)	Cerebral oedema	Leads to deterioration of neurological deficit and in some instances raised intracranial pressure and rostrocaudal herniation resulting in death
	Myocardial infarction	Common cause of sudden death in the early stages of stroke
Short-term (1–14 days)	Pneumonia	Results largely from immobility
	Myocardial infarction	
	Pulmonary embolism	Tends to develop 7–14 days after stroke, often when patient is becoming mobilised
	Recurrent stroke	May develop at any stage
Long-term (> than 14 days)	Recurrent stroke	May develop at any stage
	Myocardial infarction	Commonest cause of death following a stroke
	Other vascular problems	e.g. peripheral vascular disease

MANAGEMENT

The patient who has suffered a complete stroke, with infarction of a large portion of one hemisphere with contralateral hemiplegia, hemisensory loss and hemianopia, requires simple basic medical and nursing care and nothing more in the acute stage. A variety of complications may develop and the timing of these shows significant variation (Table 11.4). A proportion of such patients will develop cerebral oedema and over the next 24 hours or so this may result in rostrocaudal herniation of the brain, leading to impairment of consciousness, coma and death. There is currently nothing that can be done to influence either the early or the late prognosis in patients with this form of cerebral infarction. Avoidance of dehydration, treatment of chest infections and general maintenance of the body's homeostasis is all that can be done. Specific attempts to treat the cerebral oedema by corticosteroids or dehydrating agents have not been shown to be of value. It has recently been suggested that a raised haematocrit, or that even minor degrees of hyperglycaemia in acute cerebral infarction, may have an adverse effect on prognosis and this requires further study.

PROGNOSIS

The long-term prognosis of a deficit in the early stage is difficult to predict. In general, the longer the delay before recovery begins the poorer the prognosis and, if at the end of the first week there is no recovery of motor activity or speech, then it is unlikely that these functions will return completely. Hemianopia which persists for more than a week will usually be permanent and the presence of non-dominant parietal lobe deficits usually indicate that rehabilitation will be difficult. Deficits resulting from brain stem infarction usually have a better prognosis than deficits from cerebral hemisphere dysfunction. Although recovery may continue for up to a year, and in the case of aphasia for up to two years, any paralysis persisting at six months will usually not recover.

In a massive stroke, the paralysed muscles are usually initially flaccid, although occasionally they may show extensor tone with so-called decerebrate responses. Gradually over the next few weeks spasticity develops and the tendon reflexes become brisk. The arm and leg then adopt a characteristic posture with the arm adducted at the shoulder and flexed at the elbow and wrist. The leg typically is extended at the hip and knee and the foot is plantar-flexed. The gradual development of this posturing usually indicates that functional recovery will be poor. Even in patients who show little functional recovery walking will be achieved. Failure to achieve independent walking usually results from either profound impairment of comprehension, severe disturbance of body image or neglect, memory loss or impairment, or loss of confidence or depression.

Prevention of progression

Progressive strokes are uncommon; however, in patients seen at an early stage after the onset of stroke, where the deficit is not profound, it is natural to wish to attempt to minimise further progression. The patients who present with a mild hemiparesis, within 24 hours either may have recovered or may have become hemiplegic; the prediction of this is impossible. In general, it is recommended that patients should remain horizontal in bed and minor degrees of hypertension should not be treated. In patients with lower blood pressure it might be advisable to attempt to increase this; anaemia should be corrected and polycythaemia, if severe, treated appropriately.

A number of specific measures have been tried in an attempt to prevent deterioration of patients with minor or progressive strokes. Cerebral vasodilators, thrombolytic agents and surgery in the acute stage have not been shown to be of value. The use of anticoagulants in this situation remains controversial and before their use in cerebral infarction it is mandatory to be sure about the diagnosis. At the very least, c.s.f. examination should be performed and ideally a CT scan to exclude cerebral haemorrhage. The use of anticoagulants in this situation may be considered in a number of different clinical situations.

The patient with a minor stroke with residual deficit

Some patients with thromboembolic infarction present with a single episode resulting in a minor deficit such as a hemiparesis. In this situation it is uncertain in the early stages whether the deficit will resolve or progress. If there is progression then it is not unreasonable (in the absence of a contraindication such as hypertension) to consider treating with intravenous heparin in an attempt to prevent progression of the deficit from partial to complete hemiplegia.

The patient with an evolving, progressing or stuttering stroke

The patient with a stuttering or progressing hemiplegia presents a difficult management problem. A CT scan is necessary to exclude a tumour or a haematoma and in some cases it may then be justifiable to treat with intravenous heparin in an attempt to prevent progression. The situation where this has been shown to be of most benefit is in the syndrome of progressive basilar thrombosis, where there are progressive or stuttering symptoms of brain stem ischaemia (see below); intravenous heparin is thought to halve the mortality rate, which otherwise is at least 90%.

Completed cerebral infarction

The patient with a total hemiplegia and a large area of infarction of one cerebral hemisphere will not benefit from anticoagulants and these should be avoided because of the potential risk of haemorrhage.

TRANSIENT ISCHAEMIC ATTACKS

Transient ischaemic attacks are defined as focal transient neurological deficits persisting for less

Table 11.5 Pathophysiology of transient focal cerebral ischaemic attacks

1. Large artery atherosclerosis with ulceration
2. Intracranial artery atherosclerosis with or without ulceration
3. Haemodynamic dysfunction associated with intracranial or extracranial arterial stenosis or occlusion
4. Disease of small arteries or arterioles (hypertension)
5. Migraine (vasospasm?)
6. Arterial dissection
7. Inflammatory arterial disease
8. Cardiac disease—valvular disease, arrhythmia, congestive failure, or recent myocardial infarction

than 24 hours. We have already pointed out that when transient ischaemic attacks precede a stroke they clearly indicate that the stroke has been thromboembolic in origin. It is extremely rare for patients who suffer cerebral embolism or cerebral haemorrhage to have preliminary symptoms. Transient ischaemic attacks are, in general, caused by the same mechanisms as thromboembolic stroke and the bulk of evidence now suggests that the majority are embolic in origin (Table 11.5). Hypoperfusion of a particular area of the brain above a narrowed vessel may in some instances produce transient deficits, but this is now thought to be relatively uncommon. In the majority of cases the neurological deficit in a transient ischaemic attack persists for only a matter of seconds or minutes and it is uncommon for such attacks to persist for more than 30 minutes. The clinical features depend upon the territory of arterial involvement.

Carotid territory transient ischaemic attacks

In these there will be either contralateral motor sensory disturbance, ipsilateral visual disturbance, or both. Transient ischaemic attacks in the territory of the ophthalmic artery produce the characteristic syndrome of amaurosis fugax. In a typical attack there is sudden impairment of vision in one eye. Often the visual loss begins as a curtain descending from above, ascending from below or crossing vision horizontally. Patients usually can identify the visual loss as monocular by covering one or other eye and the visual impairment persists at most for a few minutes and then clears gradually. Occasionally it is possible to examine such a patient during an attack and in some instances an embolus may be seen blocking the central retinal artery (Fig. 11.10); as the vision improves the embolus appears to break up and the fragments move distally along the branches of the central retinal artery. The importance of amaurosis fugax is that it is a marker of carotid territory ischaemia

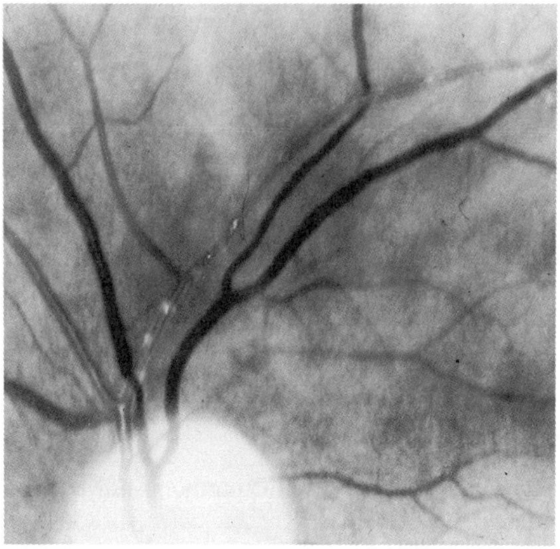

Fig. 11.10 Fundal picture showing the presence of cholesterol emboli within a retinal artery.

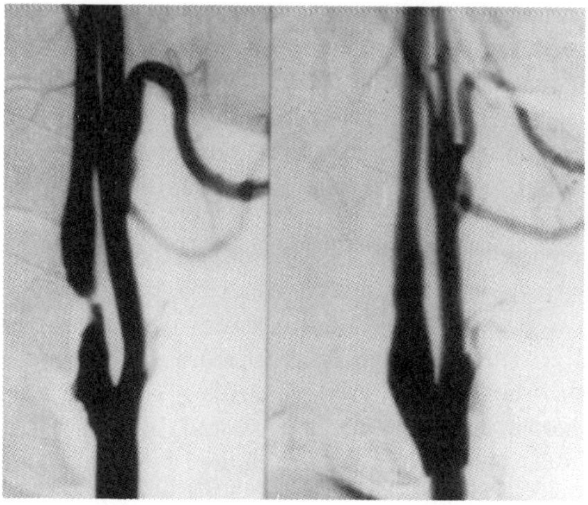

A B

Fig. 11.11 **A** Carotid angiogram showing a severe stenotic lesion of the internal carotid. **B** Radiograph of the same vessel following carotid endarterectomy.

and in the majority of cases indicates carotid artery stenosis (Fig 11.11).

Vertebrobasilar transient ischaemic attacks

These show a diverse pattern. Dizziness, diplopia, dysarthria and weakness or sensory disturbance affecting one or other or both limbs may occur singly or in combination. Unsteadiness, impairment of vision and dysphagia are less common, and memory lapses, confusion, transient unconsciousness and hearing impairment are rare manifestations. Vertebrobasilar transient ischaemic attacks are difficult to diagnose and a variety of other conditions are often misdiagnosed as such attacks; perhaps the commonest is that of dizziness in isolation. In general, an isolated symptom such as dizziness or diplopia should not be diagnosed as a vertebrobasilar transient ischaemic attack unless it is accompanied by other symptoms suggesting a transient brain stem disturbance.

Transient ischaemic attacks of uncertain vascular territory

Isolated hemiparesis or hemisensory loss, which is thought to be vascular in nature, may occur either as a result of carotid or vertebrobasilar territory ischaemia; other clinical evidence may be necessary to help in diagnosing the arterial territory.

The importance of transient cerebral ischaemic attacks is that they indicate that the patient is at risk for stroke, i.e. the 'little stroke' may become a big stroke. About 10% of patients who suffer a completed stroke will have suffered transient ischaemic attacks in the preceding weeks or months. The risk of stroke in a patient presenting with transient ischaemic attacks is of the order of 30% over the next 5 years. There is some evidence to suggest that the risk of stroke is maximal within the first six months and the greatest risk may be within the first few weeks.

Management of transient ischaemic attacks

Sensory seizures, syncope, vertigo of labyrinthine origin and migraine all may be mistaken for transient ischaemic attacks. The differentiation of these is usually possible on clinical grounds, but in some instances it may be necessary to exclude these by appropriate investigations such as electroencephalography or CT scan. There is now good evidence to suggest that treatment of transient ischaemic attacks may reduce the risk of stroke, but the precise therapy to apply in any individual case remains controversial.

General management

Patients with transient cerebral ischaemia should undergo a number of routine investigations to exclude anaemia, polycythaemia and other general medical disorders that might affect the cerebral circulation. Hypertension and diabetes, when present, should be treated and patients should be urged to stop smoking. The general aims of the assessment of the patient are, first, to determine the territory of the ischaemic attacks and, second, to attempt to determine the pathogenesis.

Determination of the arterial territory

The practical importance of this is that carotid territory transient ischaemic attacks may be attributable to arterial disease which is surgically accessible. Vertebrobasilar transient ischaemic attacks are seldom caused by arterial disease that may respond to surgical interference; this means that the patients with such attacks are likely to be treated medically. The one exception is the patient with innominate artery or left subclavian stenosis with the subclavian steal syndrome. Clinically, it is usually possible to detect this form of arterial disease as the appropriate radial pulse will be of less volume on the affected side and the blood pressure will be significantly lower; patients with vertebrobasilar transient ischaemic attacks with this pattern of signs should be considered for arteriography.

The patterns of symptoms which suggest either vertebrobasilar or carotid territory transient ischaemic attacks are given above. It is important to emphasise that the presence of a bruit over a carotid artery does not necessarily indicate that the transient ischaemic attacks are occurring within the territory of that artery.

Determination of the pathogenesis

A number of different mechanisms may produce transient cerebral ischaemic attacks and these are listed in Table 11.6. In practice the commonest cause is thromboembolism and if, on clinical grounds or as a result of investigations, the other causes can be excluded, then patients with transient cerebral ischaemia should be assumed to have thromboembolic episodes.

Management of carotid territory transient ischaemic attacks

Patients with these attacks may be managed either medically or surgically and in most instances the choice of treatment will be determined by the physician's own prejudices. In some instances no specific treatment may be justified: for example, a patient who has suffered from amaurosis fugax for over a year without any residual deficit can probably be safely left untreated; similarly, a patient who has suffered a single transient ischaemic attack some six months before presentation can also be left uninvestigated and untreated.

Medical treatment. General treatment such as management of hypertension, correction of hyperglycaemia and hyperlipidaemia may in some instances be all that is required. In patients who are too old for surgery or anticoagulants, or in whom antiplatelet drugs are contraindicated, general treatment may be all the physician can offer.

Anticoagulants. The use of these in transient cerebral ischaemia remains controversial, although there is a body of opinion that suggests that the use in the first six months following the first transient ischaemic attack may halve the risk of stroke. If used, they should be continued for only a limited period and at most for six months.

Antiplatelet agents. There is now increasing evidence that the use of aspirin or other antiplatelet drugs may reduce the risk of stroke or sudden death in patients with transient ischaemic attacks. The side effects are relatively mild and more patients are now being prescribed these drugs. Aspirin is probably the best, though there is some debate as to the most appropriate dose. One 300 mg tablet daily is probably the best compromise.

The investigation of patients with suspected arterial disease with a view to surgical treatment

There is a wide diversity of opinion among neurologists concerning the indications for the investigation of suspected arterial disease in patients with carotid territory transient ischaemic attacks. This diversity of opinion stems from the varying views concerning the risks of angiography, carotid endarterectomy, and the benefits of such surgery.

There are now a number of non-invasive techniques that can be employed to help in the detection of arterial disease. Doppler ultrasonography can detect marked degrees of stenosis or carotid occlusion and the technique of digital subtraction angiography appears to be a safe technique for detecting arterial disease. Ultimately, however, the decision has to be made as to whether or not the patient should undergo formal angiography which, even in the best hands, has a risk of death or disability of the order of 1%.

Carotid endarterectomy. Carotid endarterectomy is now performed increasingly frequently in North America and yet in the United Kingdom it remains a relatively uncommon operation. It clearly is attractive to perform a carotid endarterectomy in a patient with carotid territory transient ischaemic attacks and carotid artery stenosis. However, it should be remembered that in the long term the commonest cause of death in patients who have suffered transient cerebral ischaemic attacks is myocardial infarction and not stroke. The evidence that carotid endarterectomy reduces the long-term risk of stroke is only slight and the operation itself carries a significant mortality and morbidity. There is, furthermore, the risk of investigation by arteriography to demonstrate a putative carotid stenosis.

A number of questions remain unanswered in relation to this clinical dilemma:

1. What are the indications for arteriography in patients with carotid territory transient ischaemic attacks?

2. Which patient should undergo endarterectomy?

3. What are the long-term benefits (or otherwise) of carotid endarterectomy?

In some patients with transient ischaemic attacks in the carotid territory, the appropriate internal carotid artery is found to be completely occluded. Increasingly, there has been interest in such patients with a view to treating them by the operation of extracranial–intracranial anastomosis: in this operation a branch of the superficial temporal artery is anastomosed to a branch of the middle cerebral artery in an attempt to bypass the carotid occlusion. The technical results of this operation appear to be quite good, but a large multicentre study has recently shown that it has no beneficial effects.

Management of vertebrobasilar transient ischaemic attacks

The decisions in this type of transient ischaemic attack revolve around which particular form of medical treatment to give. There is some evidence to suggest that vertebrobasilar transient ischaemic attacks have a better prognosis than carotid territory attacks and it is not unusual to encounter patients who have suffered from regular but infrequent attacks for many years without residual deficits. The medical treatment otherwise is the same as that for carotid territory attacks.

THE MANAGEMENT OF PRESYMPTOMATIC CEREBROVASCULAR DISEASE (the asymptomatic carotid bruit)

There has been increasing interest in the last few years concerning the treatment of patients who have cerebrovascular disease, but who as yet are asymptomatic. For example, how should patients with isolated carotid bruits be managed? What should be the management of a patient who is known to have carotid stenosis but who is asymptomatic? Should such patients who are undergoing coronary artery bypass, valve surgery or other major forms of surgery have prophylactic carotid endarterectomy? The answers to these questions are uncertain: there is no evidence to suggest that patients with asymptomatic carotid stenosis are more liable to have a stroke at the time of surgery than otherwise normal patients; furthermore, the risks of carotid endarterectomy are not inconsiderable. It is in this area that there is an apparent difference in management between neurologists in this country, who take a conservative view, and neurologists and neurosurgeons in North America where a more aggressive approach is followed.

MULTI-INFARCT DEMENTIA

Some patients with severe atherosclerotic cerebrovascular disease have multiple strokes resulting in extensive cerebral damage and dementia. These patients most often have a clear history of repeated strokes and have signs of bilateral damage with weakness, spasticity and speech abnormalities. Dementia in the absence of other neurological signs as a result of arteriosclerotic cerebral arterial disease is uncommon.

NON-ATHEROSCLEROTIC CAUSES OF STROKE

CEREBRAL EMBOLISM OF CARDIAC ORIGIN

We are here referring to cases in which the embolic material has not originated from an arterial source. Most commonly, the embolic material is a thrombotic fragment which has broken away from a larger thrombus within the heart. The causes of cerebral embolism are listed in Table 11.6.

The embolus may lodge in any artery and results in ischaemic infarction. The infarct may be pale, haemorrhagic or mixed; haemorrhagic infarction is a characteristic of embolism. The territory of the middle cerebral artery is most frequently involved, presumably because of flow phenomena, but large masses may block even the carotid arteries in the neck. Cerebral embolism should be suspected in a patient with a sudden onset of a cerebral infarct with no other manifestations of atherosclerotic vascular disease, in the context of known cardiac disease, or where accompanied by other evidence of emboli to systemic organs.

Table 11.6 Causes of cerebral embolism (After Adams R D, Victor M 1981 *Principles of Neurology*. McGraw-Hill, New York, with permission.)

Cardiac origin
Atrial fibrillation and other arrhythmias (with rheumatic, atherosclerotic, hypertensive, congenital or syphilitic heart disease)
Myocardial infarction with mural thrombus
Acute and subacute bacterial endocarditis
Heart disease without arrhythmia or mural thrombus (mitral stenosis, myocarditis, etc.)
Complications of cardiac surgery
Valve prostheses
Non-bacterial thrombotic (marantic) endocardial vegetations
Prolapsed mitral valve
Paradoxical embolism with congenital heart disease
Trichinosis

Non-cardiac origin
Atherosclerosis of aorta and carotid arteries (mural thrombus, atheromatous material)
From sites of cerebral artery thrombosis (basilar, vertebral, middle cerebral)
Thrombus in pulmonary veins
Fat, tumour, or air
Complications of neck and thoracic surgery

Undetermined origin

The commonest cause of cerebral embolism is chronic atrial fibrillation in association with atherosclerotic or rheumatic heart disease. The mural thrombus is within the atrial appendage and changes in rhythm are one of the causes of disruption of the thrombus, resulting in embolism. Intermittent atrial fibrillation may act in a similar manner. A mural thrombus overlying the damaged endocardium in continuity with an area of myocardial infarction is another important source of cerebral emboli.

Clinical picture

The hallmark of cerebral embolism producing stroke is the rapidity of onset of the stroke. There are usually no warning signs or symptoms and the patient collapses to the floor, hemiplegic yet conscious. The abruptness of onset of the symptoms might suggest a primary intracerebral haemorrhage, but headache in cerebral embolism is unusual. Embolic material may enter the vertebrobasilar system and, if arrested at the junction of the vertebral arteries, produces a devastating stroke resulting from brain stem infarction. More commonly the embolus is arrested at the upper bifurcation of the basilar artery, producing unilateral or bilateral visual disturbances. The diagnosis of cerebral embolism should always be considered in a patient who suffers a sudden stroke for which there is no other obvious cause. In such patients the non-atherosclerotic causes of stroke should be excluded (see below) and of these the most important is an embolic stroke from a cardiac source.

Investigations

A CT scan will confirm that the stroke has resulted from infarction and may show evidence of haemorrhagic infarction which is seen in 30% of infarcts resulting from cerebral embolism; appropriate c.s.f. changes may be seen. In the septic embolism which accompanies bacterial endocarditis, a c.s.f. pleocytosis may be seen with a combination of red and white cells. Appropriate cardiac investigations may show electrocardiographic or echocardiographic abnormalities.

Prognosis

The immediate prognosis depends on which artery is occluded: most patients who have suffered a carotid territory embolus will survive; occlusion of the basilar artery is almost always fatal. Certain forms of cerebral embolism have a better prognosis than others: cerebral air embolism, for example, usually has a fairly good prognosis.

Treatment

The treatment of patients who have suffered a cerebral embolus, other than prophylaxis, should follow the same lines as that for a patient who has suffered thromboembolic infarction. The main decision to be reached is in relation to the institution of anticoagulant therapy.

There is now good evidence that the long-term use of anticoagulants is effective in the prevention of embolism in cases of atrial fibrillation, myocardial infarction and valve prosthesis. The prophylactic use of anticoagulants in such patients before they have suffered any embolic phenomena is a controversial topic. Once cerebral embolism has occurred, the time of institution of anticoagulant therapy must be decided. In patients who have suffered a haemorrhagic cerebral infarct there is, clearly, a risk of producing intracranial haemorrhage and there is a theoretical risk that, in a patient who has suffered a white cerebral infarct, this might be converted to a haemorrhagic infarct with a subsequent risk of bleeding. In practice, if the infarct can be shown on a CT scan not be haemorrhagic, or if the c.s.f. is not bloodstained, then it is usually safe to proceed with anticoagulants. If the c.s.f. is bloodstained, or if the scan shows a haemorrhagic infarct, then it is probably safer to wait a minimum of a few days or more realistically 7–10 days, until the haemorrhagic areas have resolved. In patients who have suffered septic embolism resulting from bacterial endocarditis, anticoagulant therapy is contraindicated.

In the long term, the development of cerebral embolism in a patient with cardiac valvular disease should raise the question as to whether the cardiac abnormality should be treated surgically.

Table 11.7 Non-atherosclerotic causes of stroke

Cardiac causes
Cerebral emboli from prosthetic valves, intracardiac clot, intracardiac tumour
Air or fat embolism
Foreign body embolism
Haematological causes
Disorders associated with increased tendencies to thrombosis
Polycythaemia
Sickle cell disease
Thrombotic thrombocytopenic purpura
Thrombocytosis
Vascular causes
Arterial causes
Vasospasm (migraine)
Trauma
Miscellaneous arterial disease
Fibromuscular dysplasia
Postradiation damage
Arteritis
Meningovascular syphilis
Arteritis secondary to meningitis
Collagen vascular disorders
Dissecting aortic aneurysm
Venous causes
Cerebral thrombophlebitis

NON-ATHEROSCLEROTIC CAUSES OF STROKE IN CHILDREN AND YOUNG ADULTS

The occurrence of hemiplegia in infants, children and young adults without evident atherosclerosis is a well recognised phenomenon. Both thrombotic and embolic occlusions may be demonstrated in these cases, although often there is no obvious cause. The spectrum of disorders which may produce these syndromes is shown in Table 11.7. Some of these conditions have been described in other sections of the book or of this chapter and are readily excluded by appropriate investigations. It is perhaps appropriate to note that in the majority of such cases *no obvious cause* will be found. In the majority, the episode is non-fatal and non-recurrent.

Moya moya disease (Fig. 11.12)

'Moya moya' is the Japanese word for a cloud of smoke or haze and is used to describe the extensive basal cerebral rete mirabile, which can be demonstrated on angiography of such patients. It results from major arterial occlusion to the brain and is an anastomotic leash of vessels. The presenting symptoms are sudden strokes in young children, although occasionally in adults presenting features are those of subarachnoid haemorrhage. There is debate as to whether the rete mirabile represents a congenital vascular malformation or a rich collateral circulation.

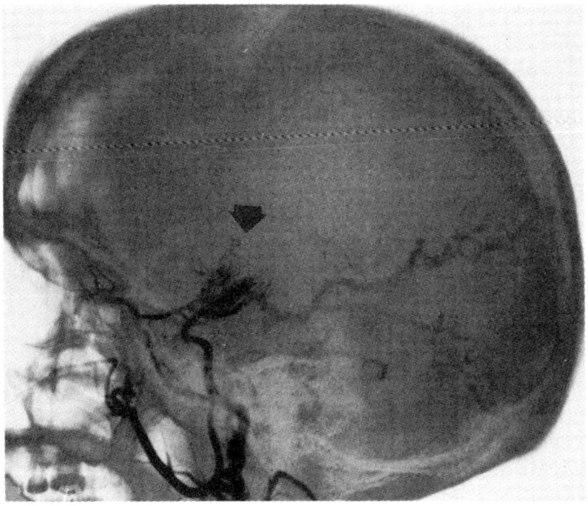

Fig. 11.12 Carotid angiogram showing leash of vessels (arrowed) in moya-moya disease.

HYPERTENSIVE CEREBROVASCULAR DISEASE

Hypertension may affect the cerebral vasculature in a variety of ways: one of the most common effects is the acceleration of atherosclerosis; another common and lethal complication is cerebral haemorrhage. There are many causes for this (Table 11.8), but the most important is hypertension.

PRIMARY INTRACEREBRAL HAEMORRHAGE (hypertensive intracerebral haemorrhage)

This is rare in the absence of hypertension and in most instances at presentation the diastolic blood pressure is in excess of 100 mm of mercury. The haemorrhage occurs within the parenchyma of the brain and it is believed that the haemorrhage originates from damaged arterioles as a result of chronic hypertension. Miliary (Charcot–Bouchard) aneurysms are commonly found on the intracranial arterioles in patients with hypertension and there is some evidence to suggest that intracerebral haemorrhage results from rupture of these small aneurysms, which are quite distinct from the aneurysms that produce subarachnoid haemorrhage. Charcot–Bouchard aneurysms and, indeed, primary intracerebral haemorrhage, most frequently occur in the following sites:

1. The putamen and adjacent internal capsule
2. Different parts of the central white matter
3. Thalamus
4. Cerebellar hemisphere
5. Pons

The extravasated blood forms a local mass which disrupts the tissue as it expands and compresses adjacent brain substance. In major haemorrhages there is displacement of midline structures and in haemorrhage in the cerebral hemispheres there is often rostrocaudal herniation. Rupture or seepage in the ventricular system occurs in 90% of cases with resulting blood-staining of the c.s.f. There is rarely haemorrhage outwards through the cortex of the brain into the subarachnoid space.

In patients who survive, the mass of blood gradually decreases in size over a matter of a few months and very often evidence of a previous cerebral haemorrhage is found at the time of autopsy as an orange-stained cleft deep in the cerebral substance. Because of this tendency of the haemorrhage to resolve, in patients who survive the prognosis for the neurological deficit is often quite good. There is now good evidence to suggest that prophylactic treatment of hypertension may prevent the development of intracerebral haemorrhage.

Table 11.8 Causes of intracranial haemorrhage (including intracerebral, subarachnoid, ventricular and subdural)

Primary (hypertensive) intracerebral haemorrhage
Ruptured saccular aneurysm
Ruptured arteriovenous malformation
Trauma
Haemorrhagic disorders
Haemorrhage into brain tumours
Ruptured mycotic aneurysms
Haemorrhagic cerebral infarction
Secondary to arterial or venous inflammatory disorders
Rare causes Severe hypertension Following angiography In association with severe encephalitis
Undetermined cause

Clinical features

Occasionally there may be prodromal symptoms of headache and dizziness, but this is uncommon. In the majority of cases the symptoms develop when the patient is active, and onset during sleep is rare. Occasionally onset of symptoms occurs during violent physical exercise or during sexual intercourse. The symptoms usually develop over a matter of minutes, or occasionally hours, and headache is a prominent feature. Typically a patient suffering an intracerebral haemorrhage will collapse to the ground as if felled by a blow.

Capsular haemorrhage

The most common haemorrhage develops deep in the hemisphere in relation to the internal capsule.

A rapidly evolving hemiparesis develops and often thereafter the patient becomes stuporose, comatose, and then develops signs of rostrocaudal herniation leading to death within a matter of hours.

Thalamic haemorrhage

A haemorrhage into the thalamus may produce a similar picture but, as a thalamic haemorrhage may extend medially and compress the upper brain stem, a variety of ocular manifestations are seen as the symptoms evolve: these include particularly vertical and lateral gaze palsies. Most common is forced downward deviation of the eyes, but other signs of an upper brain stem eye movement abnormality may be seen, including absent convergence, retraction nystagmus and lid retraction.

Pontine haemorrhage

Pontine haemorrhage usually is associated with early onset of coma in association with tetraplegia, bilateral small pupils and extensor motor responses. There may be ocular bobbing with absent horizontal reflex eye movements: prognosis is poor.

Cerebellar haemorrhage

Cerebellar haemorrhage accounts for 10% of all forms of primary intracerebral haemorrhage and has a characteristic clinical picture. Symptoms usually progress over a matter of hours and vomiting and dizziness are the earliest complaints. Inability to walk and headache usually become prominent symptoms and compression of the brain stem by the swollen cerebellum often produces paralysis of conjugate gaze to the affected side. Vertical eye movements are usually retained. A whole variety of ocular abnormalities suggesting a localised brain stem disturbance may be seen but nystagmus and ataxia of the limbs are uncommon. Impairment of consciousness is not an early feature but, as the syndrome progresses, patients may become unconscious as a result of brain stem compression.

Small haemorrhages

It is now recognised that much smaller haemorrhages may occur and produce a clinical picture of hemiballismus or even discrete brain stem syndromes as a result of haemorrhages measuring less than a centimetre in diameter. The detection of these has resulted from the more widespread use of the CT scan in stroke syndromes, as previously these were almost certainly misdiagnosed as localised areas of cerebral infarction.

In intracerebral haemorrhage at any site the prognosis is poor as the haemorrhage usually is massive and results in coma; smaller haemorrhages are compatible with survival. Clinically, it may be impossible to differentiate a restricted intracerebral haemorrhage from an area of cerebral infarction: headache and neck stiffness are useful signs supporting the diagnosis of haemorrhage but may be absent. Subhyaloid haemorrhages may occur where blood tracks into the subarachnoid space but are less common than in primary subarachnoid haemorrhage.

Investigations

The CT scan has now proved to be the most reliable method of differentiating cerebral haemorrhage from infarction: even small previously unsuspected haemorrhages may now be shown accurately and associated complications of cerebral oedema and hydrocephalus may also be demonstrated. One of the difficult problems is to decide who should have a CT scan when suspected of having a possible intracerebral haemorrhage; the following are some of the indications:

1. Deteriorating level of consciousness
2. Persisting fixed deficit
3. Persisting impairment of consciousness
4. Persisting headache
5. Development of seizures
6. Neck stiffness.

Examination of the spinal fluid will usually reveal haemorrhage in most cases of massive cerebral haemorrhage. In smaller haemorrhages, however, the spinal fluid may be normal in the early stages and show a degree of xanthochromia only later. The investigation is not without risk in a patient with a massive hemisphere haemorrhage, as it may aggravate rostrocaudal herniation. Radiographs of the skull and the electroencephalogram are rarely of diagnostic help. The peripheral blood white cell count often rises significantly, as does the ESR.

Prognosis

Overall the mortality rate is 80% and the majority of patients die within a few days. In patients with smaller haemorrhages, survival certainly may occur and the prognosis for recovery of function is surprisingly good. Second rebleeds are exceptional and patients may survive for some time, only to succumb to the other complications of hypertension, such as myocardial infarction.

Management

The general management is the same for patients with intracerebral haemorrhage as for those with any acute stroke syndrome. Surgical removal of the clot in the acute stage, either by evacuation or by aspiration, seldom proves beneficial. The following are some of the indications for surgery:

1. The patient who survives the initial ictus but who remains densely hemiplegic after the first week. At this stage the clot is beginning to liquefy and it may be possible to aspirate some of the blood from the cavity and reduce the deficit.

2. The patient with an intracerebellar haematoma. Because it is possible to gain access to these haematomas readily and leave little in the way of neurological deficit, early surgery in these patients is often advised.

3. In patients with superficial haematomas (lobar haematomas) it is often possible to remove the haematoma without making the deficit worse. Such patients should have angiography, looking for a small underlying arteriovenous malformation.

The major contraindication to surgery is the fact that most haematomas within the cerebral hemispheres occur deep in relation to the internal capsule. It is often possible surgically to remove the haematomas, but the removal usually damages the patient. General medical measures, such as lowering the blood pressure, the use of dehydrating agents to reduce cerebral oedema, or artifical hypothermia, have little to offer in the acute stages. It is worth noting that in some patients an intracerebral haemorrhage may be a manifestation of a small arteriovenous malformation. In patients with haematomas that are in unusual sites, consideration should always be given to performing carotid angiography to detect such angiomas.

THE LACUNAR STATE

Early in the twentieth century Pierre Marie described multiple small cavities deep in the cerebral substance and referred to them as 'état lacunaire'. It is now believed that those small cavities result from occlusion in small penetrating branches of the cerebral arteries resulting in localised areas of infarction. Fisher and Adams have now suggested, and produced evidence to support, the view that lacunar infarcts are due to occlusion of small arteries, 50–150 μm in diameter. These lacunes tend to be situated in similar sites to the so-called Charcot–Bouchard aneurysms of cerebral haemorrhage; they are found in the caudate and lenticular nuclei, the thalamus, the internal capsule, the pons and the cerebral and cerebellar white matter.

Clinical features

Affected individuals usually have the combination of hypertension and atherosclerosis and the lacunae are common incidental findings at autopsy in people over the age of 70. Miller Fisher has described a number of individual symptoms resulting from such lacunae. The size of the lacunae, however, is such that in some instances there may be just a transient deficit or they may occur in the absence of symptoms. Some of the syndromes described by Miller Fisher are a pure motor hemiplegia resulting from an internal capsule lacuna, a pure hemisensory defect resulting from a thalamic lacuna, or the dysarthria/clumsy hand syndrome resulting from a basis pontis lucune. In patients with severe and uncontrolled hypertension, multiple lacunar infarcts may develop, producing the clinical picture of dementia, pseudobulbar palsy and difficulty in walking. Such patients show a step-wise deterioration and usually it is possible to elicit a history of repeated transient episodes associated with deterioration of their condition. The term arteriosclerotic parkinsonism is sometimes mistakenly applied to patients who show this clinical picture.

HYPERTENSIVE ENCEPHALOPATHY

This syndrome became generally recognised and described in the 1920s and 1930s as the combination of extreme hypertension, headache, seizures and states of altered consciousness. It was thought to result from spasm of the cerebral arteries secondary to an abrupt rise in blood pressure and brain oedema.

It is now recognised that this is a relatively rare phenomenon and is identical clinically with eclampsia of pregnancy. Unquestionably, increasing use of antihypertensive agents has prevented the development of severe hypertension, leading to the virtual extinction of the syndrome. There remains considerable doubt concerning the roles of cerebral oedema and vasospasm in the pathogenesis of the syndrome, but in those rare cases that are seen the treatment is straightforward and that is to reduce the blood pressure to normal levels as soon as possible.

BINSWANGER'S DISEASE

This used to be thought to be a rare complication of severe hypertension and a pathological curiosity. Increasing use of the modern imaging techniques of the brain have shown that this disorder is more common than was previously thought. Pathologically the patients have multifocal areas of abnormality in the subcortical white matter and a variety of clinical presentations may be seen. In some the patients present with a progressive dementia and gait disturbance and in some with a clinical picture of the lacunar state. The condition may be recognised on computed tomography or magnetic resonance imaging (Fig. 11.13).

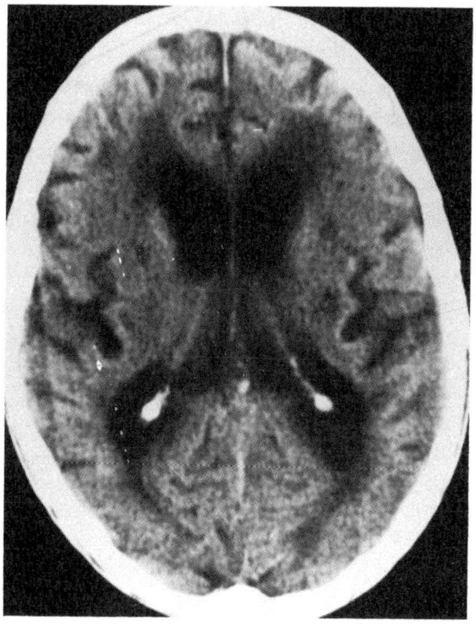

Fig. 11.13 CT scan showing cortical atrophy and white matter low attenuation in a hypertensive patient with progressive dementia, difficulty in walking, and incontinence.

PAPILLOEDEMA

For many years it has been recognised that papilloedema may be found in patients with severe hypertension. It has now been clearly demonstrated that the papilloedema in most instances occurs at a time when the c.s.f. pressure is not raised and in most instances the papilloedema occurs with other profound changes of a hypertensive retinopathy (grade IV retinopathy).

Although the c.s.f. pressure is not raised, the c.s.f. protein may show a moderate elevation in hypertension, possibly due to increased capillary permeability.

CRANIAL NERVE PALSIES

Cranial nerve palsies are not uncommon in hypertension. Facial palsy, mimicking a Bell's palsy, is a well-recognised complication of malignant hypertension and probably results from occlusion of the vasa nervorum secondary to the hypertensive changes in the arterioles. A third nerve palsy occurring on a similar basis is also not infrequent and shows clinical features similar to those of the third-nerve palsy seen as a complication of diabetes.

SUBARACHNOID HAEMORRHAGE

Haemorrhage into the subarachnoid space most commonly is arterial in origin and results either from rupture of an aneurysm of one of the major cerebral vessels, or as a result of rupture of one of the vessels of an arteriovenous malformation. Other causes are listed in Table 11.9.

Table 11.9 Causes of subarachnoid haemorrhage found in an autopsy series*

Causes	No. of cases	%
Craniocerebral trauma	193	30
Neurosurgical operations	49	8
Cerebromeningeal haemorrhages	141	22
Arterial aneurysms	57	9
Other vascular abnormalities	6	1
Inflammatory disorders	48	7
Haemorrhagic diathesis	39	6
Tumours	28	4
Intoxications	25	4
Embolism	12	2
Pregnancy and puerperium	5	1
Undiagnosed	43	6
Total	646	100

* Reproduced from Heidrick R 1972 Subarachnoid haemorrhage, Table 1. In: Vinken Bruyn (ed) *Handbook of Clinical Neurology*, vol 12. North Holland Publishing Company, Amsterdam, ch. 5, with permission.

ANEURYSMAL SUBARACHNOID HAEMORRHAGE

The aneurysms which are associated with subarachnoid haemorrhage are quite different from those which cause hypertensive intracerebral haemorrhage. The aneurysms, often called berry aneurysms, take the form of small thin-walled blisters protruding from the arteries of the circle of Willis or its major branches. For the most part the aneurysms are located at bifurcations or branches of the arteries and are thought to be the result of a developmental defect in the media and elastica; the common sites are shown in Figure 11.14. Because of the local deficiency in the vessel wall, the intima bulges outward covered only by the adventitia and the sac gradually enlarges until finally it ruptures. The aneurysms vary in size from 2 mm up to 3 cm in diameter, with an average size of approximately 1 cm, and may vary greatly in shape.

In routine autopsies the incidence of unruptured aneurysms is 2% and the incidence appears to increase with age. Therefore, although based on a congenital abnormality, the development of the aneurysms appears to depend on other factors and of these the most well recognised is hypertension. Very occasionally the aneurysms are familial and

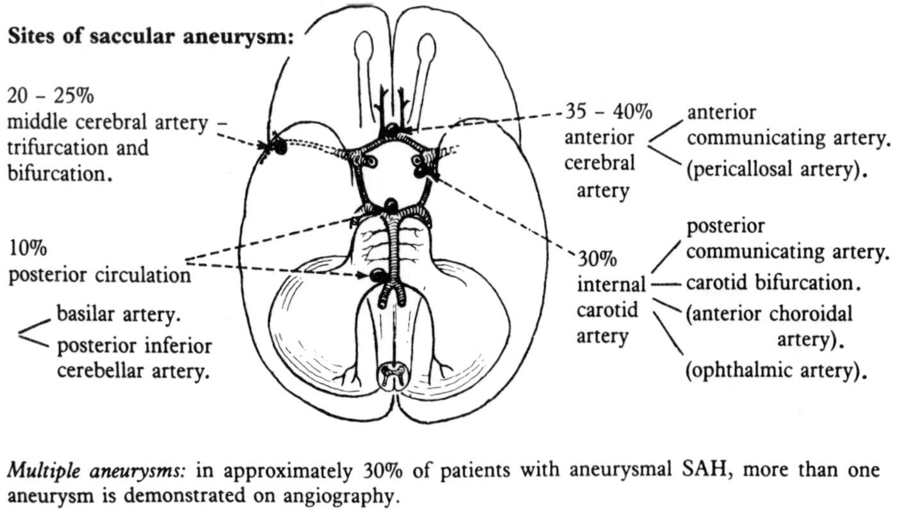

Fig. 11.14 Common sites of aneurysms of the intracranial vessels. (Reproduced from Lindsay K W, Bone I, Callander R 1986 *Neurology and Neurosurgery*, Churchill Livingstone, Edinburgh, with permission.)

there is an increased incidence in congenital polycystic disease of the kidney and coarctation of the artery.

Prerupture symptoms

The aneurysms are usually asymptomatic before they rupture. Occasionally they may be associated with symptoms of migraine or epilepsy but this is uncommon. In certain sites the aneurysms may become quite large and compress the intracranial structures, producing a variety of neurological signs: ophthalmic artery aneurysms may compress the optic nerves or chiasm; posterior communicating arteries may compress the third nerve, and large saccular aneurysms may develop on the carotid and basilar artery, producing a very characteristic pattern of signs. These giant aneurysms rarely rupture.

Aneurysms of the carotid artery developing within the cavernous sinus (intracavernous aneurysms) may compress the third, fourth, fifth and sixth cranial nerves and present with the clinical picture of a painful ophthalmoplegia. A similar type of aneurysm developing on the basilar artery may produce a mixed pattern of signs, attributable to compression of the lower cranial nerves in association with compression or ischaemia of the brain stem.

Clinical features

When the aneurysms rupture, blood at arterial pressure exits into the subarachnoid space and produces an immediate headache. The suddenness of onset of the headache is such to make patients feel as if they have been struck on the head. If arterial bleeding continues for more than a few seconds, then consciousness will be lost because of the rapid increase in intracranial pressure and, if the bleeding continues, death will occur within a matter of hours. Although such bleeding may be a cause of sudden death, it is rare for patients to die within minutes. In some cases blood is forced into the cerebral substance, producing focal signs such as hemiparesis.

The factor determining the early outcome is the extent of the bleeding and this appears to be related to the speed with which vasospasm develops. Blood in the subarachnoid space very rapidly is associated with arterial vasospasm, although the causes of this protective mechanism are ill understood. Where vasospasm develops early, there may be only headache and mild impairment of consciousness, with no more obvious deficit. In such cases the headache will usually persist for one to two weeks, as will the neck stiffness.

In some patients the initial headache and drowsiness is followed by progressive impairment of consciousness and the development of focal signs such as hemiparesis, hemianopia or aphasia. In these cases it is thought that the developing neurological deficit is occurring as a result of the protective vasospasm which has resulted in cerebral infarction. At autopsy in such cases, ischaemic infarction distal to the aneurysm (and the vasospasm) is the usual finding. Another cause of progressive impairment of consciousness after the initial bleed is the development of communicating hydrocephalus.

The clinical combination of a sudden collapse in association with a violent headache in the absence of other signs is diagnostic of a subarachnoid haemorrhage due to a ruptured aneurysm, and in most instances the site of the aneurysm cannot be determined on clinical grounds. However, occasionally there may be clinical clues: the patient with a subarachnoid haemorrhage who has developed a third nerve palsy is likely to have a posterior communicating aneurysm; hemiparesis or aphasia, either as an early or late sign, suggests an anterior communicating or middle cerebral artery aneurysm; unilateral blindness suggests an ophthalmic artery aneurysm; signs of a brain stem disturbance suggest an aneurysm on the basilar artery.

Unilateral predominance of headache may be helpful in localising the aneurysm to one side or the other and the presence of a preretinal haemorrhage on one side again is of lateralising value.

Signs

The hallmark of subarachnoid haemorrhage is the presence of neck stiffness. Occasionally this may be absent and in the deeply comatose patient neck stiffness may be difficult to detect. Preretinal (subhyaloid) haemorrhages, when present, indicate blood in the subarachnoid space leaking forwards along the optic nerves. Rarely these haemorrhages may rupture into the vitreous (Terson's syndrome). Other non-specific signs are extensor plantar responses and a mild confusional state. Fever often develops within the first week as a non-specific reaction and transient glycosuria and hyperglycaemia may occur. In the acute stage there is often a transient rise in the blood pressure.

Investigations

The diagnosis of a subarachnoid haemorrhage is confirmed by finding bloodstained cerebrospinal fluid; the amount of blood in the c.s.f. is proportional to the degree of haemorrhage. Even within hours of a subarachnoid haemorrhage there will be blood in the lumbar theca and the differentiation of spontaneous haemorrhage into the subarachnoid space and a traumatic lumbar puncture may be made from the presence of xanthochromia. This will usually develop within six hours of a spontaneous subarachnoid haemorrhage and is due to the lysis of the red cells and release of haemoglobin. Within a few days this is converted to the bile pigments and produces the very characteristic deep yellowness of the fluid. Following a subarachnoid haemorrhage frankly bloodstained c.s.f. gradually becomes replaced by xanthochromic c.s.f. within three to five days. Persistence of xanthochromia for at least a week is the rule and usually a faint yellowness of the fluid will be present for up to two weeks. When the spinal fluid is examined a few days after a subarachnoid haemorrhage there will usually be a brisk white cell pleocytosis; the protein level usually is raised and occasionally the sugar level is low.

There is some suggestion that performing a lumbar puncture in the acute stages following a subarachnoid haemorrhage may be dangerous. Certainly in a case where the diagnosis is not in doubt there is little point in performing the investigation; however, where the diagnosis is in doubt and where it is important to differentiate a subarachnoid haemorrhage from, for example, meningitis, there should be no hesitation in performing the lumbar puncture.

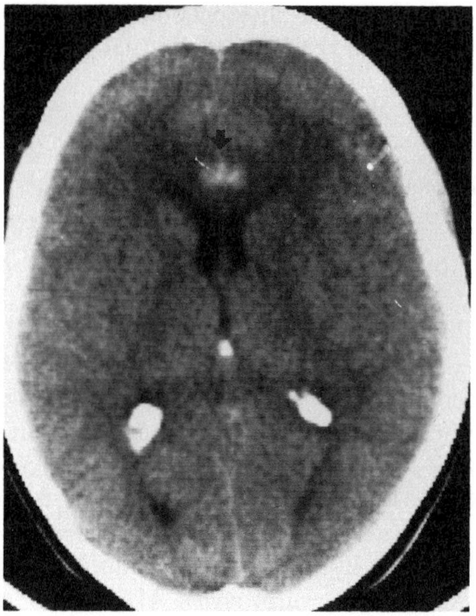

Fig. 11.15 CT scan in a patient with subarachnoid. Blood is present anteriorly in the inter-hemispheric fissure (arrowed).

Increasingly now the CT scan is used in the acute stage, both to confirm the diagnosis by finding evidence of intracranial haemorrhage and to provide clues as to the site of bleeding. Localised haemorrhage into the interhemispheric fissure suggests an anterior communicating artery aneurysm and this may be seen on the CT scan (Fig. 11.15). Blood selectively tracking into the sylvian fissure suggests a middle cerebral artery aneurysm. The CT scan may also show evidence of coexistent hydrocephalus. Because of these advantages the CT scan has virtually replaced the lumbar puncture as the technique of choice in centres where this investigation is available.

Radiographs of the skull and the electroencephalogram are of little value in the assessment of the patient with subarachnoid haemorrhage. The definitive investigation is angiography to demonstrate the aneurysm.

Prognosis

As many as one-third of the patients who suffer an aneurysmal subarachnoidal haemorrhage will die of the first bleed. Of the survivors, as many as one-half will rebleed and of these a significant proportion will die. Rebleeding may occur at any time following the original haemorrhage, although most commonly it occurs between the second and sixth week. Early rebleeding probably occurs as protective vasospasm wears off and may also be related to naturally occurring mechanisms of clot lysis within the aneurysm. The crux of management of the patient with aneurysmal subarachnoid haemorrhage is to attempt to prevent the recurrent haemorrhage.

Management

The general management is as for the acute stroke syndrome, or the patient with impairment of consciousness. Traditionally patients are kept in bed in an attempt to decrease arterial pressure, and avoidance of constipation is usually advised. The duration of bed rest is not based on any observations and is arbitrary. In the early stages analgesics and antiemetics may be required.

There has been much interest in the use of antifibrinolytic agents to prevent clot lysis within the aneurysm and therefore at least theoretically, to reduce the risk of rebleeding. Their use remains controversial and there is good evidence to suggest that patients given such drugs may develop thrombotic episodes with focal neurological signs. A variety of drugs have been tried in an attempt to prevent vasospasm but their use remains experimental.

Surgery

The specific treatment is surgical attack upon the aneurysm. A variety of procedures have been developed and the most satisfactory treatment is to occlude the neck of the aneurysm with a clip. The timing of investigation by arteriography and surgery is crucial. Angiography in the acute stages, when there is intense vasospasm, is known to be hazardous and usually arteriography is delayed for an arbitrary period of time until it is thought that vasospasm has abated. The best clinical guide to the presence or absence of vasospasm is the patient's conscious level. The patient who is normal from the time he is first seen, or one who recovers consciousness within a matter of a few days should be considered for angiography at an early stage. The patient who remains comatose for a week or longer should undergo angiography only if and when he recovers.

The presence of vasospasm is also a relative contraindication to surgery as an operation undertaken in the presence of intense vasospasm often will be followed by a pronounced neurological deficit due to an extensive cerebral infarction. There are now large series in the literature of operations on aneurysms in various sites with remarkably low mortality; there are, however, no control studies to show the benefit of such surgery in unselected patients presenting with aneurysmal subarachnoid haemorrhage. One common complication of subarachnoid haemorrhage is communicating hydrocephalus; this may develop early in some patients and be associated with decreasing conscious level. The diagnosis is made by CT scan and the hydrocephalus may require treatment with an appropriate drainage procedure.

ARTERIOVENOUS MALFORMATIONS

These consist of abnormal tangles of dilated vessels creating abnormal communications between the arterial and venous systems; in reality they represent an arteriovenous fistula. They begin as a developmental abnormality representing the persistence of an embryonic pattern of blood vessels. With time the blood vessels enlarge (although they may be enormous even at the time of birth). It has now been shown clearly that over a matter of years there is gradual enlargement of these anomalies in adult life. The term angioma is synonymous with arteriovenous malformation and these may vary in size, from a small anomaly a few millimetres in diameter lying on the surface of the cortex or within the white matter, to a huge mass of tortuous channels comprising a shunt of sufficient size to produce cardiac failure. The blood vessels are abnormally thin and readily rupture.

Clinical features

The malformations occur in all parts of the central nervous system including the cerebral hemispheres, the brain stem and the spinal cord, and they may occur on the surface or within the parenchyma of the nervous system. The largest malformations are found in the posterior parts of the cerebral hemispheres. Overall they are more common in men than in women and occasionally they appear to be familial. They may present as epileptic seizures, headache, a subarachnoid haemorrhage or a sudden focal deficit such as a hemiplegia.

Occasionally a migrainous type of headache is a presenting feature and the malformation is discovered only by the presence of a cranial bruit. Bruits are present in approximately 60% of malformations and the larger the malformation the more likely it is that a bruit will be present. In the case of spinal malformations a spinal bruit may be heard.

When rupture occurs into the subarachnoid space as a result of a malformation, then a clinical picture is produced similar to that of aneurysmal subarachnoid haemorrhage. In some instances the onset of the headache is not quite as acute and the term low pressure subarachnoid bleed is sometimes applied to the clinical syndrome which results. The first bleed from a malformation is rarely fatal and the long-term prognosis is much better than with aneurysmal subarachnoid haemorrhage. It is worth noting that in some patients with arteriovenous malformations these first come to light during pregnancy; in such an instance it is important that delivery is by caesarian section.

Investigations

The diagnosis of a malformation may be suggested by the typical linear calcification which is seen on the skull radiograph, but the definitive investigation is arteriography (Fig. 11.16). CT scan may show a pattern of abnormalities highly suggestive of a malformation (Fig 11.16).

Treatment

Surgical attack upon malformations is feasible when the malformation is of limited size and over the surface of the brain. Malformations around the brain stem or within the substance of the cerebral hemisphere are not suitable for surgical treatment and a variety of other treatments have been applied, including artificial embolisation and proton beam radiation.

CEREBRAL VENOUS THROMBOSIS

Thrombosis of the intracranial venous sinuses most commonly occurs as a result of infection of

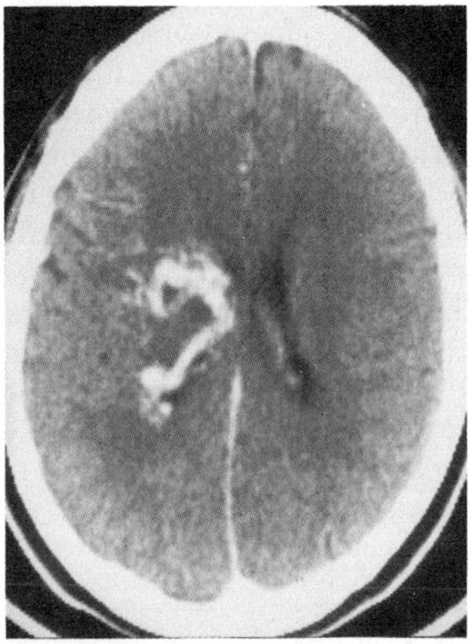

A

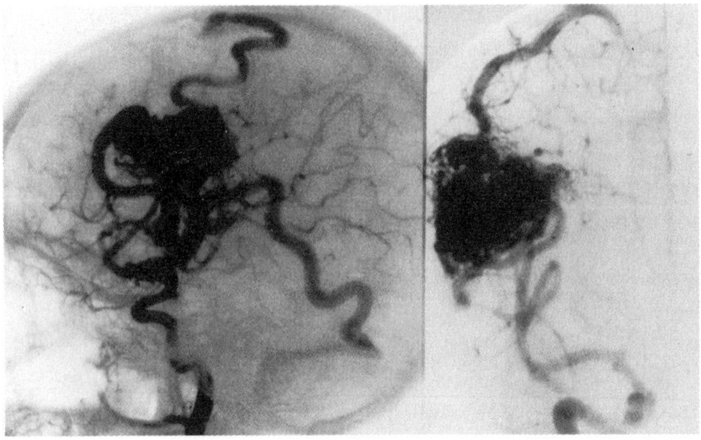

B

Fig. 11.16 **A** Contrast enhanced CT scan showing an arteriovenous malformation, **B** carotid angiogram showing abnormal circulation through an arteriovenous malformation.

the middle ear and mastoid air cells, paranasal sinuses, or the skin around the upper lip, nose and eyes. These cases are often associated with other evidence of intracranial infection such as meningitis, cerebral abscess or extradural and subdural empyema. Direct trauma to a sinus associated with fracture of the skull is a rare cause of thrombosis.

Primary or aseptic sinus thrombosis is rare and occurs most frequently at the extremes of life. It occurs in wasted, debilitated and dehydrated individuals, especially children, and may be a complication of congenital heart disease. In adults it is most common in women and is seen in the postpartum and postoperative states, in blood dyscrasias associated with a thrombotic tendency such as polycythaemia, or in women taking the contraceptive pill.

LATERAL SINUS THROMBOSIS

This usually follows chronic infection of the middle ear, mastoid or petrous bone and is characterised in such a patient by the symptoms of headache and the signs of papilloedema. If the thrombophlebitis spreads to other sinuses, such as the superior sagittal sinus, then focal neurological signs may develop and seizures are a prominent feature. Fever in such cases is invariable. The diagnosis should be considered in an patient with chronic middle ear disease who develops fever and headache.

CAVERNOUS SINUS THROMBOSIS

This usually is secondary to infection of the ethmoid, sphenoid or maxillary sinuses or of the skin around the eyes and nose. It presents with high fluctuating fever, headache and local signs around the orbit. These include gross oedema of the eyelids and cornea in association with proptosis, extraocular muscle pareses and papilloedema. Although usually unilateral at onset cavernous sinus thrombosis may readily become bilateral because of spread of infection to the opposite side. It may be difficult to differentiate cavernous sinus thrombosis from orbital cellulitis or from mucomycosis. Cavernous sinus thrombosis usually results from a mixed infection, although often staphylococci predominate.

In all types of infective thrombophlebitis the treatment is by high-dose antibiotics. As the infecting organisms are mixed, it is usually appropriate to give a combination of broad-spectrum antibiotics.

SAGITTAL SINUS THROMBOSIS

This is usually associated with rapidly developing raised intracranial pressure in association with unilateral focal seizures and hemiplegia. Focal signs may predominate in the leg or legs but usually more widespread signs are present. This syndrome most commonly occurs spontaneously as a form of primary aseptic sinus thrombosis; in such cases the cerebrospinal pressure is raised and there often is a degree of haemorrhage demonstrable in the spinal fluid, resulting from the haemorrhagic infarct which is a consequence of venous thrombosis. The definitive diagnosis may be made on angiography, which demonstrates non-filling of the appropriate sinus.

TREATMENT

Treatment of aseptic thrombosis of the intracranial sinuses is controversial. There is a body of thought which supports the view that anticoagulants should be used in the acute stage to try to prevent the thrombosis from spreading; this clearly is risky in the presence of a haemorrhagic infarct. Correction of dehydration and of associated haematological abnormalities, and symptomatic treatment with anticonvulsants should be instituted regardless of whether or not anticoagulants are used.

DIFFERENTIAL DIAGNOSIS IN CEREBROVASCULAR DISEASE

Here we need to deal with two separate problems:

1. Vascular disease needs to be differentiated from other types of neurological disorders.

2. The different types of vascular disease need separation one from another.

The diagnosis of a vascular disorder depends very much on the recognition of one of the stroke syndromes, without which the diagnosis is in doubt. The diagnosis of stroke depends on two main criteria: (a) the time course of development of the clinical syndrome and (b) the focal nature of the clinical syndrome.

The deficit in stroke almost invariably is of sudden onset. The deficit is usually maximal at the beginning or shortly thereafter and stabilisation of the deficit followed by improvement is the usual evolution; an adequate history is essential to obtain this information.

Almost no other neurological disturbance produces this characteristic evolution of symptoms. In trauma, naturally enough, a sudden insult occurs, but usually the cause is all too obvious. A sudden deficit may occur in migraine, but there is usually the preceding history and the age of the patient to help differentiate from stroke. Occasionally in demyelinating disease there may be a relatively abrupt onset of symptoms but, again, the age group of patients is against the diagnosis of stroke.

A previous history of transient ischaemic attacks is of considerable value in the diagnosis of thromboembolic stroke. Vertebrobasilar transient ischaemic attacks, in particular, may be difficult to differentiate from other transient neurological disturbances such as syncope or labyrinthine vertigo. Occasionally it may be difficult to differentiate a transient ischaemic attack from a seizure, but in general a TIA manifests itself as negative symptoms (such as weakness or numbness), whereas a seizure manifests itself as positive symptoms (such as movements of the limb or positive sensory disturbances).

The stuttering or progressive stroke may be difficult to differentiate from an expanding intracranial lesion such as a tumour, abscess or granuloma and in many instances this differentiation can be made only with the help of a CT scan.

The focal deficit characterising a stroke, in itself does not allow differentiation from other focal pathologies such as a tumour. On the other hand, deficits that are non-focal, such as confusion, should rarely be diagnosed as being due to cerebrovascular disease. Other points to bear in mind are that headache is common in stroke, both haemorrhage and infarction; seizures may occur as an early manifestation in stroke, yet loss of consciousness is rare other than in aneurysmal subarachnoid haemorrhage or basilar artery insufficiency.

The most common conditions to be misdiagnosed as stroke are subdural haematoma and brain tumour. A history of trauma is often absent in the patient with a subdural haematoma and the combination of headache, drowsiness and hemiparesis may all too easily be diagnosed as a small stroke. The clinical evolution of the symptoms is often suggestive of a stuttering stroke and the c.s.f. may be bloodstained or xanthochromic. The hallmark of a subdural haematoma which should allow clinical differentiation from a stroke is the presence of drowsiness as a more prominent feature than the focal deficit; that is to say, the patient might have only a mild hemiparesis but is very drowsy. In the stroke patient, drowsiness will usually be seen only in the patient with a very profound deficit.

In our own hospital as many as 1% of patients with an admission diagnosis of an acute stroke are subsequently shown to have a tumour. Sudden deficits developing in such a patient are thought to result from haemorrhage into the tumour. Pathologically, such haemorrhages are relatively rare and sudden deficits in tumour patients most commonly result from infarction of the tumour with oedema and local swelling. A detailed history will usually reveal symptoms prior to the onset of the sudden deficit. The presence of papilloedema in a patient with hemiparesis is more likely to be due to a tumour than to a cerebral infarct, *whatever* the evolution of the initial symptoms; when in doubt, a CT scan usually will allow the differentiation to be made.

THE DIFFERENTIATION OF CEREBRAL INFARCTION FROM CEREBRAL HAEMORRHAGE

It should be stated immediately that it may be impossible to differentiate, clinically, a primary intracerebral haemorrhage from a cerebral infarct of thromboembolic origin. In each case there may be symptoms of sudden onset accompanied by headache with, thereafter, a profound neurological deficit such as a hemiplegia. In some restricted intracerebral haemorrhages there is no extension of the blood into the subarachnoid space and no neck stiffness. In these cases the differentiation of the two depends on the CT scan.

The following are helpful in indicating that a stroke is likely to be of thromboembolic origin:

1. Previous history of TIAs
2. Intermittent or step-wise onset of neurological deficit
3. Relative preservation of consciousness
4. Normal c.s.f.
5. Evidence of atherosclerosis elsewhere
6. Age of the patient
7. Headache of only moderate severity
8. Carotid bruits
9. Clinical evidence of internal carotid artery occlusion (retinal artery pressures, facial pulses).

The following are clues to the diagnosis of hypertensive cerebral haemorrhage:

1. Absence of prodromal symptoms
2. Hypertension
3. Headache, often severe
4. Progression of deficit for minutes or hours after onset
5. Bloodstained c.s.f.
6. Early onset of stupor or coma
7. Onset during waking hours.

FURTHER READING

Barnett H J M, Stein B M, Mohr J P, Yatsu F M 1986 Stroke: pathophysiology, diagnosis and management. Churchill Livingstone, London

Ross-Russell R W 1983 Vascular disease of the central nervous system, 2nd edn. Churchill Livingstone, London

12

Infections of the nervous system

INTRODUCTION

C.n.s. infection is an important and often eminently treatable cause of what may otherwise be an acute life-threatening neurological illness. The introduction of antibiotic therapy for bacterial infections has revolutionised their incidence and outcome and for these reasons clinicians need to recognise and treat conditions early which they may now see rarely (e.g. tuberculous meningitis). A high index of suspicion remains essential.

While our abilities to treat viral infections remain limited, newer, less toxic, antiviral drugs are becoming available and our understanding of the unusual relationships between viruses and the nervous system continues to increase.

BACTERIAL INFECTIONS

PYOGENIC INFECTIONS

Acute meningitis

The incidence of acute pyogenic meningitis is difficult to ascertain and probably varies from one country to another. An incidence of 4–5 in 100 000 has been quoted for the United Kingdom. The risk is low even for carriers of the common pathogens: thus the risk to a carrier of meningococcus is approximately 1 in 1000; that for carriers of pneumococcus (20–40% of population) is 1 in 10–50 000.

Clinical features

The clinical features of pyogenic meningitis are fever and meningism. Meningism has been fully discussed in Chapter 8, but is characterised by symptoms of severe headache, photophobia, nausea and vomiting, which are associated with increasing drowsiness, confusion and declining conscious level, indicating a variable parenchymal cerebral involvement. Occasionally partial or generalised seizures may occur, most commonly in children. Patients show marked neck stiffness which is evident on anteroposterior movement of the head, but not usually on lateral head movement (this serves to differentiate meningism from neck stiffness due to cervical spondylosis).

The time course of pyogenic meningitis is usually acute and will bring patients to the attention of their physician within a day or two of onset. Sometimes a fulminating picture is seen with sudden collapse after a very short history. On occasion a more subacute course may be seen, particularly if inappropriate or inadequate doses of antibiotics are allowed to complicate the picture.

These classic symptoms and signs are those seen in older children and adults, but may be absent at the extremes of age. In the newborn, fever, irritability, vomiting and a bulging fontanelle may be the presenting symptoms, and in slightly older children meningitis may present with febrile convulsions. Similarly, in the elderly, signs and symptoms of meningism may be less marked and the diagnosis must be suspected in patients showing rapid onset of confusion and behaviour disturbance.

In addition to the signs and symptoms of meningitis itself, it is important to scrutinise both the history and the examination for other clues. There may be other marked systemic disturbance: for instance, in meningococcal meningitis there may be a characteristic purpuric rash (rashes may be seen with organisms other than meningococcus); with pneumococcal meningitis there may be evidence of a pneumonic process, or a localised infection of the ears or sinuses. Full cardiological examination is important to detect acute or subacute bacterial endocarditis. More obvious may be a recent head injury and skull fracture, or the presence of a ventricular shunt.

A full history is of major importance, and concurrent malignancy, chemotherapy, collagen vascular disorders or other causes of disturbed immunity greatly increase the risk of opportunistic infections.

Pyogenic meningitis is usually a monophasic illness; however, on occasion patients with recurrent meningitis are encountered, and in such patients exhaustive investigation of a number of possibilities must be undertaken. Some patients with c.s.f. rhinorrhoea as a result of head trauma or chronic hydrocephalus, may be prone to recurrent episodes of meningitis, as may patients with spina bifida with a communicating sinus between skin surface and the subarachnoid space. Very occasionally, no cause is found for recurrent meningitis; some such patients have recurrent acute episodes of meningitis with polymorphonuclear leucocytes but sterile culture of c.s.f. This condition has been termed 'Mollaret's meningitis', but whether this represents a discrete clinical entity is debatable.

Aetiology

The commonest bacteria causing meningitis are listed in Table 12.1. It will be seen that differing bacteria occur in different age groups. In the newborn period, Gram-negative organisms, including *E.coli*, *Klebsiella* and streptococci, are most common whereas in childhood, *Haemophilus influenzae* becomes the commonest cause of meningitis. *Pneumococcus* (commonly) and *Listeria* (rarely) cause meningitis at any time between childhood and old age. *Meningococcal meningitis* is most commonly seen in sporadic cases, but sometimes occurs in an epidemic form in closed communities. Staphylococcal meningitis is somewhat less common and is particularly associated with septicaemia and bacterial endocarditis and is often complicated by brain abscess. More unusual organisms may be found following trauma, neurosurgical procedures and in immunosuppressed patients. An important group of patients are those in whom no organisms can be identified: these may account for up to 25% of cases seen in specialist units.

Bacteria gain access to the subarachnoid space via haematological or local spread. Extension from the ears and paranasal sinuses is most common and is frequently due to *Pneumococcus*. However, chronic middle-ear infection may result in meningitis with a mixed flora of organisms which sometimes include anaerobes.

Table 12.1 Causes of pyogenic meningitis

Organism	Neonates %	Children (1 month–15 years) %	Adults %
Streptococcus pneumoniae	<5	15	40
Neisseria meningitis	1	30	30
Haemophilus influenzae	2	50	2
Other streptococci	30	2	5
Staphylococci	5	1	10
Listeria	10	1	5
Gram-negative bacilli (commonly *E. coli*)	50	1	<10

Investigation of the patient with meningitis

The single most important investigation of meningitis is spinal fluid examination. In general, too many patients with neurological disease are subjected unnecessarily to lumbar puncture. However, where the possibility of pyogenic infection is present, lumbar puncture is obligatory, the only exception being those cases in which there are grounds for suspecting the presence of a complicating cerebral abscess (i.e. localising neurological signs in the presence of progressive impairment of consciousness or bacterial endocarditis).

C.s.f. pressure is consistently elevated in meningitis, often to apparently alarming levels. C.s.f. may be turbid and microscopy will most commonly show the presence of large numbers of polymorphonuclear leucocytes. Immediate *Gram staining* may well display the presence of pneumococci, meningococci or *Haemophilus influenzae*. C.s.f. protein is universally elevated and it is common to find that c.s.f. sugar is depressed.

Cultures of spinal fluid are mandatory, as are blood cultures, which will prove positive in 40–60% of patients. It may often be helpful to obtain swabs from ears and pharynx, and radiographs of the chest, skull and sinuses should be undertaken routinely.

Particular problems may arise in the detection and culture of some more unusual pyogenic organisms and in patients who have been subjected to inadequate or inappropriate antibiotic therapy. In such cases, radioimmunoassay for specific bacterial antigens in the c.s.f. may be of value in diagnosis.

The place of specialised neuroradiology is limited in uncomplicated meningitis. CT scanning becomes necessary in patients showing poor clinical response to therapy, or those developing focal neurological signs (to exclude abscess formation), or showing late deterioration of conscious level (in whom hydrocephalus may be developing). In uncomplicated cases few changes in the CT scan are evident, although contrast enhancement of the linings of the ventricular cavities may be seen.

Differential diagnosis (Table 12.2)

The major differential diagnosis of acute bacterial meningitis is *viral aseptic meningitis*. The two will usually be differentiated on c.s.f. examination, patients with viral meningitis having larger numbers of lymphocytes in the c.s.f., less marked elevation of c.s.f. protein, and hardly ever any alteration in c.s.f. glucose concentration. However, partly treated pyogenic meningitis may produce c.s.f. changes indistinguishable from viral meningitis. Where genuine doubt exists, it will always be best to give an adequate course of broad-spectrum chemotherapy. Partly treated pyogenic meningitis must also be differentiated from other causes of chronic meningitis, the most important of which is tuberculous meningitis because of its therapeutic implications.

Table 12.2 Differential diagnosis of pyogenic meningitis

Other infections
Viral meningitis
Tuberculous meningitis
Fungal meningitis
Subarachnoid haemorrhage
Chemical meningitis
Intrathecal contrast or drugs
Dermoid tumours
Migraine

Migraine can occasionally cause diagnostic confusion, particularly as a mild c.s.f. lymphocytosis can be seen.

The clinical picture of subarachnoid haemorrhage may become confused with that of pyogenic meningitis and on occasions chemical aseptic meningitis may be caused by the injection of intrathecal contrast media or anaesthetics. It is, however, remarkably uncommon to see meningitis following diagnostic lumbar puncture.

Treatment of bacterial meningitis

Suggested antibiotic regimes are summarised in Table 12.3. Bacterial meningitis constitutes a medical emergency and therapy must be started immediately, often before the causative organism can be identified. Immediate Gram staining may display pneumococci or meningococci, in which case therapy may be started with penicillin at a dose of 2–4 megaunits 4-hourly. Where the

Table 12.3 Treatment of pyogenic meningitis

Before results of culture and sensitivity		Following identification of organism		
Patient	*Therapy*	*Organism*	*First choice*	*Alternative*
Neonates	Ampicillin + gentamicin	*Pneumococcus*	Penicillin	Erythromycin
Children	Penicillin + chloramphenicol	*Meningococcus*	Penicillin	Chloramphenicol
Normal adults	Penicillin (+ chloramphenicol)	*Haemophilus*	Chloramphenicol	Ampicillin
Adults with immunosuppression	Flucloxacillin + ceftazidime	*E.coli*	Ampicillin	Co-trimoxazole
		Staphylococcus	Flucloxacillin	Vancomycin
		Listeria	Ampicillin + gentamicin	Chloramphenicol

initial picture is less clear it is wise to combine this with chloramphenicol (100 mg/kg/day by intravenous infusion). This regime will usually be effective in infections attributable to the commoner organisms *Pneumococcus, Meningococcus* and *Haemophilus*. Ampicillin (1–2 g 4-hourly i.v.) is an alternative to the combination of penicillin and chloramphenicol. Where other Gram-negative organisms are suspected, gentamicin (5 mg/kg/day) should also be administered, and where there is evidence suggesting staphylococcal infection, high-dosage flucloxacillin and fucidic acid should be administered.

The increasing incidence of *Bacteroides* infections from spread from chronic middle-ear disease should be covered by treatment with metronidazole, where that is indicated.

Once a causative organism and its sensitivities have been identified, appropriate therapy will be necessary, usually as suggested in Table 12.3. Where no positive culture is obtained, a wide spectrum of antibiotic cover must be given and maintained: this would usually include penicillin, chloramphenicol, gentamicin and metronidazole. Chemotherapy must be administered intravenously for a full 14 days: progress during this time must be monitored carefully, not only clinically but by regular c.s.f. examination; at such times intrathecal penicillin, where appropriate, may be administered, although there is no very firm evidence that this procedure is of major benefit.

Although the administration of steroids may be necessary in occasional patients developing the Waterhouse–Friderichsen syndrome with meningococcal meningitis, there is no evidence that routine administration of steroids improves outcome, either by reducing liability to subarachnoid adhesions and subsequent complications, or by reducing cerebral oedema.

Course and prognosis

Overall, the prognosis of pyogenic meningitis is good. Patients will usually respond to treatment with antibiotics by rapid resolution of fever and gradually improving conscious level. Headache and neck stiffness may persist for some time, and serial c.s.f. examination will show a gradual reduction in total white-cell count in c.s.f., with a change to the mononuclear cells which may persist for a considerable period. A rise in c.s.f. glucose is one of the earliest signs of improvement.

Recurrence of fever, the development of seizures or localising neurological signs should prompt reinvestigation and reconsideration of the antibiotic regimen. In these circumstances CT scanning will become obligatory in order to exclude the presence of complicating cerebral abscess or hydrocephalus.

The mortality from pyogenic meningitis varies between 15% and 25% and is determined by a number of factors. The causative organism is important: mortality with *Haemophilus influenzae* and meningococcal meningitis is relatively low (5–15%); that for pneumococcal meningitis is considerably higher (up to 50%) and staphylococcal meningitis and meningitis due to non-

Table 12.4 Complications of meningitis

Immediate
Vascular
Cortical thrombophlebitis
Sinus thrombosis
Arachnoid
Cranial nerve palsies
Hydrocephalus
Parenchymal
Abscess
Delayed
Epilepsy

Haemophilus Gram-negative organisms may be associated with a even higher mortality.

A disproportionate number of deaths (50%) occur at the extremes of age, where there may be difficulty in making a diagnosis. The conscious level of the patient at presentation is also important and coma carries a very adverse prognostic significance (up to 50% mortality). The presence of other systemic disorders (endocarditis, immune disorders) all worsen the prognosis as undoubtedly do delayed diagnosis and therapy.

Patients who survive meningitis seldom develop long-term complications (Table 12.4). Acute complications include the development of abscess, vascular complications of phlebitis and major venous sinus thrombosis leading to seizures and hemiparesis; arachnoiditis may cause cranial nerve palsies (most commonly resulting in optic atrophy or deafness); communicating hydrocephalus may develop with time. Epilepsy is rare following meningitis, unless this has been complicated by thrombophlebitis or cerebral abscess. The precise incidence of such complications remains uncertain, but there is little doubt that neonates and infants run the greatest risk of intellectual and neurological damage.

Intracranial abscess

Intracranial abscesses are most commonly intracerebral but can be subdural or extradural. The overall incidence is difficult to determine, but they are becoming more uncommon as the prevalence of chronic middle ear disease declines. In the Mersey region, with a catchment population of 3 million, 60 cases have been identified in the last decade compared with 177 in the 1950s.

Cerebral abscess

Clinical features

Headache is the most common initial symptom of cerebral abscess, often associated with progressive *drowsiness* and *confusion*, *focal seizures* and localising neurological signs. The evolution is more rapid than that associated with cerebral tumour, and the usual time course of the history is perhaps no more than 1–2 weeks. *Fever* and other signs of systemic disturbance are helpful when present, but their absence by no means excludes the diagnosis of cerebral abscess.

It must be noted that a number of patients are at high risk of developing cerebral abscess and the diagnosis must always be suspected in such patients (Table 12.5). The evolution of symptoms and signs due to cerebral abscess may occasionally be complicated by inappropriate or inadequate antibiotic therapy; the recurrence of fever or worsening neurological state in a patient with a recognised sinusitis, middle ear infection or meningitis must always alert the physician to the possibility of cerebral abscess.

Particular primary sources of infection give rise to abscesses at differing sites. Abscesses resulting from haematological spread may well be multiple. Paranasal sinus infection is most commonly associated with frontal abscess, in which general

Table 12.5 Aetiology and treatment of intracranial abscess

	Frequency	Treatment
Otitic	38%	Ceftazidime + penicillin + metronidazole
Paranasal sinuses	16%	Penicillin + chloramphenicol + metronidazole
Septicaemia	22%	
Pulmonary disease (abscess & bronchiectasis) Cardiac disease (endocarditis & cyanotic)		Penicillin + (chloramphenicol + metranidazole)
Unknown	19%	
Cranial trauma	5%	Fusidic acid + lincomycin

impairment of attention and mental function are prominent; such patients frequently develop hemiparetic signs with or without dysphasia and motor seizures. Abscesses of the temporal lobe usually result from a spread from middle ear disease; these may produce less prominent localising symptomatology, but may result in visual field disturbance or dysphasia. Cerebellar abscesses are uncommon and present with ataxia with the rapid onset of headache and declining conscious level because of raised intracranial pressure; they usually complicate middle ear infection. Abscesses may, of course, occur at sites of complicated skull fracture.

In the patient with suspected cerebral abscess, considerable care must be taken to isolate the source of the infection in order to institute appropriate treatment: this will usually involve examination of the ears and sinuses, the chest and the heart; the skin should be examined for evidence of recent infection. On occasions, dental pathology and surgery may be complicated by the development of subsequent cerebral abscess.

Investigations

Blood cultures are essential, as are appropriate cultures from middle ear or sinuses. Plain radiographs of the chest and skull are obligatory to identify pulmonary and sinus infection and mastoid disease. The definitive diagnostic investigation for cerebral abscess is CT scanning. This should be undertaken in all suspected cases before resort to lumbar puncture. The appearance illustrated in Figure 12.1: there is usually severe surrounding cerebral oedema with an enhancing capsule surrounding a necrotic area; however, preceding cerebritis may be evidenced only by an area of relative low density, and the finding of one CT scan that is normal should not preclude the rescanning of a patient after a short period as, in some instances, the presence of an abscess may declare itself in the interim. Other neuroradiological studies are now rarely necessary.

In patients without evidence of raised intracranial pressure or shift on the CT scan, c.s.f. examination may be considered, particularly if it is not planned to aspirate material from an abscess.

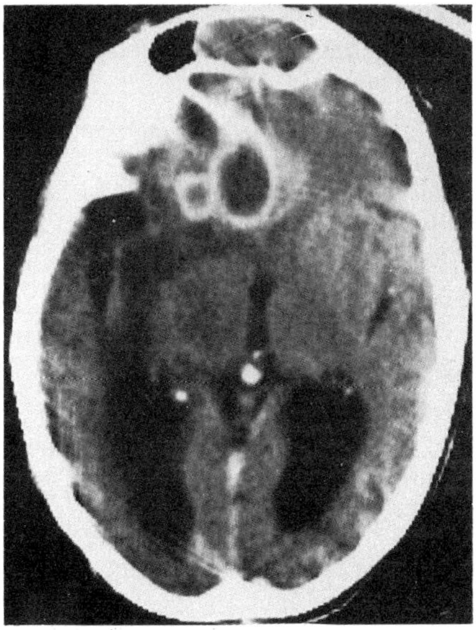

Fig. 12.1 CT scan (enhanced) of bilocular frontal abscess. Frontal sinus opacification is also present, indicating source of primary infection.

Differential diagnosis

The major differential diagnosis of cerebral abscess is from glioma, the CT scan appearance of which may be indistinguishable. Clinical history is of most value in differentiating between these two; where doubt exists, burr hole biopsy and aspiration is essential. More rarely, subdural haematoma may present a diagnostic problem. With more acute histories it may be difficult to differentiate cerebral abscess from haemorrhagic encephalitis, such as that caused by herpes simplex.

Treatment

Treatment of cerebral abscess has three arms:

1. It necessitates adequate and sustained *antibiotic therapy* given parenterally for 4–6 weeks. A regime of penicillin, chloramphenicol, gentamicin and metronidazole will provide cover against the mixed organisms which be present in an otitic abscess. Penicillin alone may be satisfactory for abscesses complicating sinus infection. Where multiple abscesses are present, suggesting haematological spread, then the possibility of a staphylococcal abscess is high and treatment with fucidin

and flucloxacillin will be necessary. These initial choices may be modified on the basis of results of culture and sensitivity.

2. The *surgical management* of abscess is usually by repeated aspiration, which is undertaken once there is clear evidence of capsule formation and central necrosis. However, early aspiration may be necessary in order to differentiate abscess from glioma, or to provide material for culture. In some centres, excision of the abscess and its capsule is undertaken.

3. Adequate *therapy for the primary infection* is necessary: this may involve surgical treatment of sinus or middle ear infection, or cardiac surgery for infected valves or prostheses.

The introduction of CT scanning has modified the management of multiple cerebral abscesses in that it may be possible to treat the abscesses with antibiotics and to perform serial CT scans in order to ensure resolution of the abscesses.

Prognosis and complications

Cerebral abscess continues to carry a high mortality (20–30%). This represents a considerable improvement from earlier figures, but emphasises the serious nature of the condition. Bronchogenic abscess carries the highest mortality (up to 70%), and abscess complicating head injury the least (10–20%). Improvement in mortality may in part be due to the decreasing proportion of the former and increasing proportion of the latter that has occurred with the passage of time. Patients in coma have an adverse prognosis.

In addition, cerebral abscess carries a considerable morbidity with neurological handicap in up to 50% of cases. The commonest problems are due to hemiparesis, dysphasia and visual field disturbance. The long-term risk of epilepsy is considerable and virtually all patients develop epilepsy, although the onset of seizures may be considerably delayed. There is no evidence to suggest that early antiepileptic treatment influences the subsequent development of seizures.

Subdural empyema

Subdural empyema most commonly occurs as a complication of paranasal sinus infection (and rarely as a complication of meningitis) and is approximately one-fifth as common as cerebral abscess. Less commonly, infection spreads to the subdural space from the middle ear, and superficial thrombophlebitis or venous thrombosis may intervene between this and the development of subdural empyema.

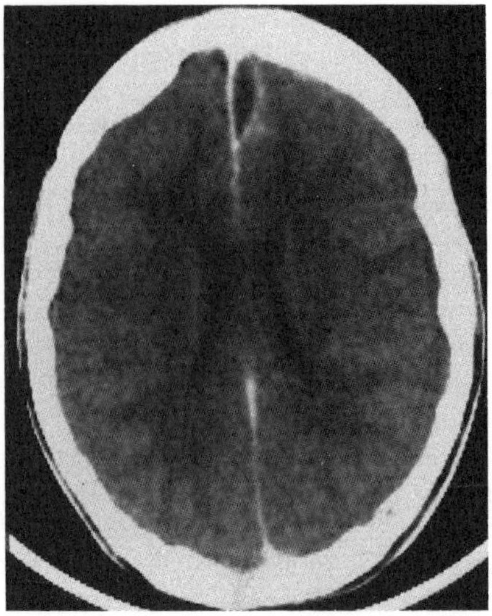

Fig. 12.2 CT scan (enhanced) of subdural empyema resulting from frontal sinusitis.

Streptococci are most commonly isolated, but on occasion staphylococci or anaerobic Gram-negative organisms are isolated.

The clinical features are similar to those of cerebral abscess but, as subdural empyema is most commonly frontal or subfrontal, patients develop hemiparesis at an early stage and often have focal motor seizures. The c.s.f. findings, diagnostic investigations and treatment are as described for cerebral abscess. CT scanning shows the presence of encapsulated surface collections (Fig. 12.2).

Extradural abscess

This condition is rare and usually results from osteomyelitis of the cranial bone secondary to surgical procedures for ear or paranasal infection.

The condition presents with localised pain and tenderness with induration in the frontal or periauricular regions associated with fever; neurological signs are rare; c.s.f. is usually clear or contains scanty lymphocytes. Treatment consists of appropriate antibiotic therapy and excision of any diseased bone.

Superficial thrombophlebitis and venous sinus thrombosis

These conditions, which can be considered together, are most commonly seen as an intervening complication of intracranial pyogenic infection, following spread from the ear or paranasal infection or meningitis. Very occasionally, superficial thrombophlebitis and sinus thrombosis may occur as the result of hypercoagulation states: post partum, postoperatively, in high-viscosity syndromes, and as a complication of carcinoma (p. 290).

Clinical features

Clinical features vary with the distribution of venous occlusion.

Superficial thrombophlebitis and *superior saggital sinus thrombosis* usually present with rapidly progressive hemiparesis and focal motor seizures which may often be continuous; localised pain and headache may occur. As thrombosis spreads to involve the superior saggital sinus, signs may become bilateral, and very often there is resulting paraparesis because of involvement of the lower-limb representation of the cortex; in addition, patients may have signs of hemianopia, aphasia and papilloedema.

Lateral sinus thrombosis most commonly complicates middle ear infection. Localised pain and tenderness are succeeded by the development of headache and papilloedema; frequently there are no other neurological signs but seizures are not uncommon.

Cavernous sinus thrombosis is usually secondary to infection of the ethmoid, sphenoid or maxillary sinuses, face or eye. Patients develop localised headache related to the original pathology and associated toxaemia followed by a progressive, initially unilateral proptosis, chemosis and induration around the eye. Retinal veins rapidly become engorged with papilloedema and third, fourth, sixth and first division of trigeminal nerve involvement. Thrombosis rapidly spreads to the opposite side, and bilateral symptoms and signs develop.

Investigation

Investigation will usually be directed towards the initiating pathology, and full radiology and appropriate bacteriological investigation of the ear, sinuses and mastoids are essential. C.s.f. examination may be helpful, showing polymorphonuclear cells with elevated protein. CT scanning should be undertaken to exclude the development of any complicating abscess. C.s.f. pressure may also be significantly elevated in lateral sinus thrombosis.

The EEG is often of considerable value in superficial thrombophlebitis, showing a very marked irritative disturbance with localised (at times, continuous) spike-wave discharge. Arteriography may show lack of filling or delayed filling during the venous phase.

Differential diagnosis

Differential diagnosis will vary according to the sinus involved. Lateral sinus thrombosis can present a picture very similar to benign intracranial hypertension, while sagittal sinus thrombosis will most commonly be confused with cerebral abscess or herpes simplex encephalitis.

Causes of aseptic thrombophlebitis must be differentiated from other causes of stroke syndromes.

Treatment

Treatment will be directed towards the underlying cause, whether this is infective (see treatment of cerebral abscess, etc.), or due to a hypercoagulable state. There is little evidence that anticoagulant therapy is helpful in the management of patients with venous thromboses. Patients with chronic lateral sinus thrombosis and persisting elevation of c.s.f. pressure may require treatment with corticosteroids or diuretics and, on occasion, lumboperitoneal shunting (see management of benign intracranial hypertension). It is important to identify any complicating cerebral abscess at an early stage and to treat it appropriately. The outcome will largely be determined by the aetiology of the syndrome but surviving patients may well be left with considerable neurological handicap.

Spinal abscess

Spinal abscesses are epidural in two-thirds of cases, subdural, or very rarely intramedullary. The condition is much rarer than intracranial abscess. Approximately one-half of cases result from haematogenous spread of infection, commonly from skin or urinary tract, and the other half from direct spread from vertebral osteomyelitis. *Staphylococcus* is the most common organism isolated, followed by Gram-negative organisms such as *E. coli* and *Proteus*.

Clinical features

Most run an acute course with preceding systemic illness followed by the onset of severe localised spinal pain, sometimes with a radicular element. Signs of cord compression develop rapidly to cause paraplegia when the abscess is thoracic (as is most common); cauda equina compression can occur. There is intense local tenderness and induration. Less commonly a more chronic presentation is seen, usually following local spread from vertebral disease.

Investigation

Blood cultures, plain radiographs of the spine to detect vertebral disease or a paravertebral mass, and exhaustive investigation to detect the source of primary infection are necessary. Myelography must be undertaken as soon as possible, in order to expedite surgical decompression. Examination of c.s.f. obtained at myelography shows leucocytosis and elevation of protein levels. C.s.f. culture may reveal the causative organism, but material obtained peroperatively will usually do this more satisfactorily.

Treatment

Spinal abscess demands immediate surgical decompression, and any delay considerably increases mortality and morbidity. Full parenteral antibiotic therapy is required for 4–6 weeks: prior to identification of the organism it is wise to give flucloxacillin and gentamycin to cover staphylococci and Gram-negative organisms. Associated vertebral osteomyelitis may require additional surgical treatment.

Prognosis

Mortality is 20–30%; there is also considerable morbidity. Although complete recovery may occur if decompression is undertaken before or within 24 hours of the onset of paresis, any delay beyond this has a grave outlook and paraplegia, once established, is rarely reversible.

CHRONIC AND GRANULOMATOUS INTRACRANIAL INFECTION

Mycobacterium tuberculosis may result in a subacute or chronic meningitic syndrome or tuberculoma; these may, on occasions, be associated.

Tuberculous meningitis

Tuberculous meningitis (TBM) has become much less common over recent decades, and its clinical features also appear to be altering. It is more common in the UK in immigrant communities, but overall has an incidence of approximately 0.2 in 100 000.

Clinical features

Classically, patients give a history of prodromal illness followed by typical meningitic symptoms with headache, confusion, fever and neck stiffness as prominent signs. The evolution of these symptoms is usually slower than those of pyogenic meningitis.

Other neurological signs are frequently present. These arise for two pathological reasons:

1. The development of an adhesive arachnoiditis may lead to cranial nerve palsies and hydrocephalus
2. Localised vasculitis and subsequent caseation may give rise to focal parenchymatous signs and seizures.

Frequently, at presentation or during the course of the disorder, cranial nerve palsies develop.

Ocular motor palsies are most common, but facial weakness and deafness can occur. More rarely, radicular signs or spinal cord compression are seen. Papilloedema and declining consciousness are ominous signs which may indicate the development of hydrocephalus.

There may be symptoms and signs of active tuberculosis elsewhere, usually in the lungs. TBM may also be seen as part of miliary tuberculosis. In the past it was uncommon for tuberculous meningitis to occur without systemic involvement; however, recent data suggest that active pulmonary disease accompanies only 20% of cases of TBM.

Up to 20% of cases present with non-specific symptoms, and little meningism or focal neurological signs. With a declining incidence of the disease, it is of the utmost importance that a high index of suspicion be maintained concerning the diagnosis.

Investigation

The primary investigation will be c.s.f. examination. Whereas in very early cases minimal c.s.f. changes may be found, there is most commonly a consistent rise in the number of leucocytes in the c.s.f. (50–500) and, although a proportion of these may be polymorphonuclear, with the passage of time a lymphocytic predominance develops. C.s.f. protein is almost always elevated to between 1–2 g/l and c.s.f. sugar is usually reduced. Ziehl–Nielsen staining of the c.s.f. may display the presence of acid-fast bacilli, but unfortunately it is more common for final confirmation of the diagnosis to be delayed until culture or inoculation proves positive.

Evidence of systemic infection should be actively sought with radiography of the chest, sputum culture and urinary examination. Tuberculin testing is a helpful procedure and it is uncommon for tuberculous meningitis to be associated with negativity. The presence of complicating signs of cord compression will require plain radiographs and myelography to define the site of the block and to aid active consideration of decompressive surgery. Declining conscious level will call for CT scanning to determine whether or not hydrocephalus is developing.

Differential diagnosis

Whereas tuberculous meningitis used to be the most common chronic meningitic syndrome, this would no longer seem to be the case in the United Kingdom, except possibly amongst patients from ethnic minorities. The classic picture of tuberculous meningitis may now more commonly be mimicked by carcinomatous meningeal infiltration and less commonly by lymphomatous meningitis. Other rarer causes of chronic meningitic syndromes similar to tuberculous meningitis are listed in Table 12.6.

The difficulties in obtaining early confirmation of the diagnosis mean that treatment may have to be started on the presumption of the clinical diagnosis.

Treatment

The treatment of choice for tuberculous meningitis is a combination of isoniazid (5 mg/kg/day), rifampicin (600 mg/day), and ethambutol (15 mg/kg/day). Isoniazid may cause pyridoxine deficiency and consequent neuropathy and more rarely seizures: thus it is usual to give pyridoxine. Alternative drugs include PAS, ethionamide, pyrazinamide and streptomycin, the latter having the advantage of being available for parenteral and intrathecal treatment of more fulminating infection. The use of these alternatives will usually be determined by the sensitivity of the cultured organism.

There is no evidence that treatment with corticosteroids prevents any of the complications of tuberculous meningitis. Anti-tuberculous treat-

Table 12.6 Differential diagnosis of TBM

Other infections
Partially treated pyogenic meningitis
Syphilis
Fungal infections
Toxoplasma
Malignant
Carcinoma
Lymphoma
Leukaemia
Other
Sarcoidosis

ment will have to be continued for between 18 months and 2 years, but it may not be necessary to maintain triple therapy throughout this time.

Complicating hydrocephalus carries a high mortality and ventricular shunting may be required. More rarely, surgical treatment of cord compression or tuberculoma may be necessary.

Course and prognosis

Untreated tuberculous meningitis is invariably fatal. Mortality in treated patients in the UK is probably between 20% and 30%. Presentation in coma, the development of hydrocephalus, and delay in diagnosis are important prognostic factors.

Some morbidity occurs in 30–40% of survivors: this is usually severe enough to cause functional disability and results from the complications of arachnoiditis and focal parenchymatous disease already discussed (see above).

Tuberculoma

Tuberculomas are space-occupying masses of granulomatous tuberculous tissue forming within cerebral tissue. These lesions will usually present as a cerebral tumour and, in third world countries, these may constitute a high proportion of intracranial mass lesions. Biopsy of lesions often may be required to differentiate tuberculoma from tumours in this country. Where a firm diagnosis can be made, medical treatment is to be preferred as surgical treatment can be complicated by sinus formation.

More rarely, symptoms of cord compression may develop from tuberculoma or tuberculous disease of the vertebrae, leading to gibbus and cord compression.

Neurosyphilis

The incidence of neurosyphilis has declined dramatically since the introduction of antibiotics; however, the condition remains important as a treatable cause of serious neurological disability. Furthermore, the incidence of early syphilitic infection has increased during the past decade, particularly among male homosexuals.

It is important to maintain a high diagnostic suspicion of neurosyphilis, particularly as its manifestations are protean, and may frequently mimic other common neurological disorders. For this reason it is important that all c.s.f. specimens taken for whatever reason, should be tested routinely for treponemal antigens and antibodies.

Aetiology

Syphilis is caused by a spirochaetal organism, *Treponema pallidum*. It is transmitted only by sexual contact or across the placenta and invades the central nervous system within 3–24 months of primary infection. It is estimated that, in the absence of adequate treatment of a primary infection, c.n.s. infection will occur in 25% of cases.

Clinical features

A variety of clinical manifestations of neurosyphilis are seen, which are largely time-related to the primary infection. The incidence of various types of neurosyphilis is noted in Table 12.7. Tertiary forms of syphilis are becoming less common.

All forms of neurosyphilis start as a meningitis, but this is frequently *asymptomatic*. The only clinical evidence of syphilitic infection in such early stages is c.s.f. abnormalities. Adequate treatment at this stage of infection virtually eliminates

Table 12.7 Incidence of clinical manifestations of neurosyphilis

	%
Asymptomatic	31
Tabetic	30
Paretic	12
Taboparetic	3
Meningovascular	18
Optic atrophy	3
Spinal	4
Eighth cranial nerve	1
Others	1

any possibility of development of later complications of neurosyphilis.

Meningeal neurosyphilis may occur at any time following infection, but is most common within the first 2 years, at the time of the development of a secondary skin rash. Most commonly it will present as an apparent aseptic meningitis with headache and neck stiffness. The condition must always be considered in the differential diagnosis of viral meningitis.

In *meningovascular syphilis* the primary pathology includes an inflammatory endarteritis as well as a meningitis. Most commonly the syndrome presents as stroke in younger patients: this may occur at any time within the first 10 years of infection, but is most common 5–7 years after the primary infection. Patients frequently have pupillary abnormalities at this stage of the disorder. Rarely, meningovascular syphilis may involve the spinal cord, causing acute spastic paraparesis or a hypertrophic cervical meningitis and syphilitic amyotrophy (wasting and lower motor neurone signs of the upper limbs with spastic paraparesis). Another rare complication of meningovascular syphilis is the development of hydrocephalus and raised intracranial pressure.

Paretic neurosyphilis is a late complication of nervous system infection developing some 15–20 years after a primary infection. The most characteristic syndrome is one of dementia. However, a number of characteristics may suggest a syphilitic aetiology: patients with paretic neurosyphilis are said to show tremor of the hands and tongue, muscle jerks and seizures; there may be a characteristic dysarthria and associated pyramidal tract signs with Argyll Robertson pupils; on occasions the dementia may appear patchy, with particular emphasis on the development of aphasia and apraxia. Classically, the mental state has been described as being one of megalomania, with delusions of grandeur; the frequency of such changes is, however, uncertain.

Paretic neurosyphilis should be considered and excluded in every case of presenile dementia.

Tabetic neurosyphilis represents another, now rare, late complication of neurosyphilis. The prime characteristics are symptoms of lightning pains, ataxia and incontinence with signs of pupillary abnormalities, ophthalmoplegia and ptosis. There is evidence of absent knee and ankle jerks and impaired posterior column sensation.

The pupils are abnormal in over 90% of cases and, in half of these, classic Argyll Robertson pupils are seen. The ankle jerks are absent in over 90% of patients and lightning pains occur in approximately 75%: these are brief sharp stabbing pains which are most frequently felt in the legs and may occur in bouts lasting several hours or days.

Patients have a relatively pure sensory ataxia with profound proprioceptive loss in the lower limbs. The bladder becomes insensitive and hypotonic with the development of overflowing incontinence; similarly, constipation and megacolon may occur. Rarer phenomena include the development of Charcot joints due to pain insensitivity, and of visceral crises, the most common of which are gastric: these are characterised by acute epigastric pain, nausea and vomiting which may persist for several days at a time; intestinal crises cause colic and diarrhoea.

Neurosyphilitic gumma of the central nervous system is extremely rare but will present as a space-occupying lesion of either the brain or spinal cord.

Other rare forms of neurosyphilis include syphilitic optic atrophy and nerve deafness, which may occur as late complications of a neurosyphilis in isolation from other symptomatology. Both of these phenomena are, however, seen as part of paretic or tabetic neurosyphilis. It should always be remembered that syphilitic infection may be congenital and that in such circumstances meningovascular, paretic or tabetic neurosyphilis may occur at an early age.

Investigations

The prime diagnostic procedure in neurosyphilis is c.s.f. examination. This will be abnormal in all cases of active neurosyphilitic infection, reflecting the fact that meningeal pathology is always present in neurosyphilis. The prime abnormalities are a pleocytosis of up to 200 or 300 cells, which are predominantly lymphocytes or other mononuclear cells. C.s.f. protein is usually elevated (up to 200 mg per 100 ml). There is an abnormal increase in c.s.f. IgG concentrations, which may be reflected

Table 12.8 Serological tests for neurosyphilis

Test	Antigen	Value
Wassermann	Cardiolipid	Screening
VDRL	Cardiolipid	Screening
Fluorescent treponemal antibody absorption (FTA-abs)		Specific
Treponemal haemagglutination (TPHA)		Specific

in classic colloidal gold abnormalities. However, the prime diagnostic procedure in neurosyphilis will be serological demonstration in the serum and c.s.f. of a non-specific reagin antibody, or specific treponemal antibodies. The serological tests available are summarised in Table 12.8.

If the c.s.f. is normal in a case of suspected neurosyphilis, it can safely be assumed that any prior syphilitic infection is burnt out. However, specific antibody tests may remain positive for some time after adequate treatment, but the absence of increased cellular content or protein concentration in the c.s.f. will exclude active neurosyphilis in patients with progressive neurological disease.

Treatment

Procaine penicillin or *benzyl penicillin* should be administered at up to 1–2 mega units per day over a course of 2–3 weeks. *Erythromycin* is a suitable alternative in patients sensitive to penicillin. Antibiotic treatment may be combined with steroids to avoid the dangers of a Herxheimer reaction. Lightning pains may respond to carbamazepine or phenytoin; antibiotic treatment is, of course, still required to prevent further progression, even in late cases. In all cases it is wise to follow the resolution of c.s.f. changes after treatment with regular follow-up examinations until c.s.f. cellular and protein content return to normal.

OTHER BACTERIAL DISEASE

Brucella

Brucella abortus and *melitensis* remain rare infections in the UK. Infection arises from domestic animals after an incubation period of between one week and several months: this is characterised by undulant fever and malaise and may be complicated by a variety of neurological disorders, the most common of which is a sub-acute or chronic meningoencephalitis which may rarely be associated with cranial nerve palsies. Myelopathy may occur, either as a result of constrictive arachnoiditis or secondary to vertebral disease. Vascular involvement can occur, leading to thrombotic stroke or subarachnoid haemorrhage from mycotic aneurysm. Psychiatric disturbance, most commonly depression, is frequent; radiculitis and Guillain–Barré syndromes occur rarely.

The diagnosis is dependent on appropriate serological testing and culture of the organism. The c.s.f. is usually abnormal with mononuclear pleocytosis, and elevated protein. The organism is usually sensitive to tetracycline, gentamycin and streptomycin.

Leptospirosis

The spirochaete *Leptospira* usually causes infections of domestic animals, but human infection may occur in veterinarians, farmers, and in those swimming in infected water. The disease usually begins with high fever, muscle pain and conjunctivitis, with a subsequent development of jaundice, nephritis or meningitis; the c.s.f. findings in the latter case are not dissimilar from those of viral meningitis. The association of conjunctivitis and jaundice should alert the clinician, and penicillin therapy is indicated.

Lyme disease

This is caused by a spirochaete *Borrelia burgdorferi*, which is transmitted by bites of deer tic. Increasing numbers of cases are being reported, characterised by rash, polyarthritis, low-grade fever and a meningoencephalitis; the latter results in headache and quite commonly cranial nerve palsies. The c.s.f. shows increased white cells with mixed polymorphonuclear cells and lymphocytes. A rising titre of antibodies to the organism confirms the diagnosis. There is usually a good response to erythromycin or tetracycline.

Mycoplasma infections

This unusual organism (a bacterium lacking a cell wall) is a common cause of atypical pneumonia. The disorder is associated with the development of cold agglutinins in blood and occasionally haemolytic anaemia, arthralgia and rashes. Neurological complications may develop approximately one week after the onset of respiratory illness and manifestations may encompass aseptic meningitis, encephalitis, Guillain–Barré syndrome, acute cerebellar ataxia, and transverse myelitis. The c.s.f. usually shows some degree of pleocytosis and elevation of protein level with a normal sugar level. The course of neurological complications tends to be benign. The organism is sensitive to antibiotics, tetracycline or erythromycin.

DISORDERS DUE TO BACTERIAL TOXINS

Tetanus

The spores of *Clostridium tetani* are widely distributed and may infect wounds. Resulting tetanus is rare, but important, because lack of adequate intensive care results in a high mortality. The clinical syndrome is caused by a bacterial endotoxin which blocks inhibitory interneurones in the spinal cord; toxin may enter the spinal cord via local spread along ventral roots to produce local symptoms, or more commonly it enters the nervous system more diffusely to produce a generalised syndrome.

Clinical features

The incubation period may vary from a few days to 3–4 weeks. Patients usually develop early symptoms of trismus, neck stiffness and facial spasms; generalised rigidity becomes evident, on which are superimposed acutely painful spasms which occur in response to sensory stimuli or disturbance; these lead to opisthotonic posturing in the presence of preserved consciousness. Profound autonomic disturbance is not uncommon: this can include hyperpyrexia, tachycardia and lability of blood pressure. If the condition is untreated, death occurs from exhaustion, dehydration, pneumonia or respiratory arrest. More rarely, symptoms remain localised to a limb or the head, depending on the site of injury and infection. Similar but localised spasms are seen which, when the head is involved, may also be accompanied by facial or ocular paresis.

Diagnosis should not present major problems where the history of antecedent injury is apparent. Acute dystonic reactions to antipsychotic drugs are most likely to be confused with tetanus.

Treatment

Prevention by the routine use of tetanus toxoid has greatly reduced the incidence of the disorder. When the diagnosis is made, human globulin antitoxin should be given in doses of up to 100 000 units intravenously. Penicillin therapy should be started, and any necessary wound débridement undertaken.

Tracheostomy must be undertaken at an early stage. In patients with milder forms of the disorder, sedation with chlorpromazine and nursing in quiet surroundings may suffice. However, for most patients muscle relaxants and ventilation are required with full supportive care in an ITU. Mortality may still remain as high as 50% at the extremes of life.

Botulism

The syndrome is attributable to an exotoxin produced by *Clostridium botulinum*, a food-borne pathogen; the toxin interferes with release of acetylcholine at neuromuscular junctions, leading to profound weakness and fatiguability.

Clinical features

Nausea, vomiting and diarrhoea may occur within a few hours of the ingestion of contaminated food; in other patients, constipation may occur because of intestinal paresis. The first neurological symptoms are usually those of blurred vision with dilated pupils and subsequent diplopia and ptosis due to extraocular involvement. Bulbar palsy, sometimes associated with vertigo and deafness, usually precedes respiratory depression, trunk and limb weakness. The main diagnostic problems arise in differentiation from the Guillain–Barré syndrome and myasthenia.

Treatment

The condition may last for some weeks, and the mainstay of treatment during this time is respiratory support. Antisera to varieties of botulinus toxin are usually given and guanidine may have some effects in reducing weakness in a similar fashion to its effects in the Eaton-Lambert syndrome. Before the advent of modern intensive care the condition carried a high mortality, but this should not now be the case.

Diphtheria

Because of a successful programme of immunisation this disease is now rare; however, up to 20% of cases are complicated by the development of neurological complications due to the production of an exotoxin. Bulbar muscles are usually involved first, with palatal paresis occurring after 5–10 days; other cranial nerves may subsequently be affected including the hypoglossal. External ophthalmoplegia is rare, but ciliary paralysis leading to blurred vision is common. Subsequently, peripheral neuropathy may occur, which may be mild, or sufficiently severe to mimic the Guillain–Barré syndrome.

Treatment consists of antibiotic therapy, with the early administration of antitoxin. The severely affected patient may require all the supportive therapy needed by patients with bulbar palsy.

VIRAL INFECTIONS OF THE NERVOUS SYSTEM

The specific interaction between virus particles and neurones gives rise to a wide variety of clinical syndromes and presents one of the more puzzling aspects of neurology. In recent years our understanding of virus-induced disease has increased greatly, and with it has come the realisation that virus-like particles can produce some chronic neurological disorders.

CLASSIFICATION OF VIRUSES

Viruses are entities whose genomes are elements of nucleic acid that replicate inside living cells using the cellular synthetic machinery and causing the synthesis of specialised elements that can transfer the virus genome to other cells'. Thus, viruses contain nucleic acid, DNA or RNA and a surrounding protective coat of polypeptide in either an icosahedral or helical formation, with or without a surrounding envelope derived from the cellular membrane of the host cell. Viruses may thus be classified according to the nucleic acid content, polypeptide structure and type of envelope. A brief classification of viruses which are important in human neurological disease is given in Table 12.9.

THE PATHOGENESIS OF C.N.S. VIRAL INFECTION
(Fig. 12.3)

The most extensive barrier to entry of viruses is the skin. Some opportunistic method of crossing it may be required, such as a bite by insect or animal or by human intervention in vaccination, or transfusion of blood; other viruses gain access via the exposed mucous membranes of the respiratory, gastrointestinal or genitourinary tracts. These surfaces are protected, not only by IgA immunoglobulin, but also by cilia and mucus. In spite of this, a large number of viruses, including

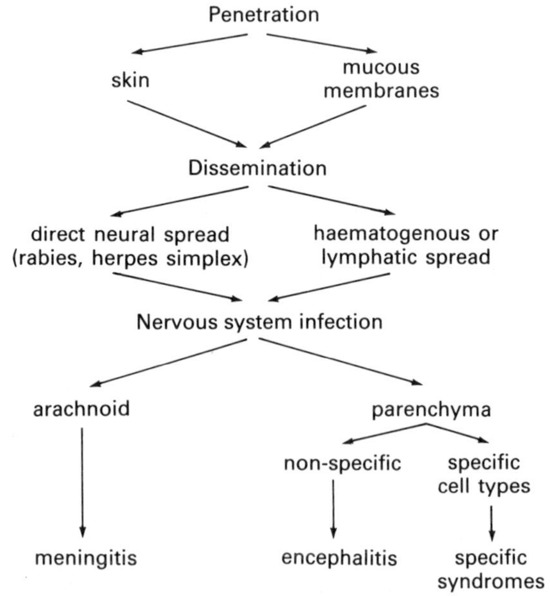

Fig. 12.3 Pathogenesis of viral neurological disease.

Table 12.9 Viruses and neurological disease

	Size (nm)	Nucleic acid*	Envelope	Human syndrome
Herpes viruses	100–200	DNA(ds)	+	
Simplex				Encephalitis
Zoster				Shingles
Cytomegalovirus				Encephalitis
Epstein–Barr				Encephalitis
Adenoviruses	70–90	DNA(ds)	–	Meningo-encephalitis
Papovaviruses	45–55	DNA(ds)	–	
JC virus				Progressive multifocal encephalopathy
Simian virus 40				
Paramyxoviruses	150–300	RNA(ss)	+	
Parainfluenza				} Meningo-encephalitis
Mumps				
Measles				
Orthomyxovirus	80–120	RNA(ss)	+	
Influenza				Meningo-encephalitis
Rhabdovirus	60–80	RNA(ss)	+	
Rabies				Rabies
Retrovirus	100–120	RNA(ss)	+	Tropical spastic
HTLV I				paraparesis
HIV				AIDS
Arenaviruses	50–300	RNA(ss)	+	
Lymphocytic choriomeningitis				Aseptic meningitis
Bunyaviruses	90–100	RNA(ss)	+	Various arthropod-borne enchephalitides
Togaviruses	40–70	RNA(ss)	+	
Alpha and flaviviruses				Various arthropod-borne encephalitides
Rubella				Congenital infection
Picornaviruses	24–30	RNA(ss)	+	
Polioviruses				Poliomyelitis
Coxsackie viruses				} Meningo-encephalitis
Echoviruses				

*Double (ds) or single-stranded (ss)

enteroviruses, adenoviruses and parvoviruses may gain entry by this route.

Once penetration has occurred, viruses may reach the central nervous system by a variety of mechanisms. Direct invasion of the c.n.s. via peripheral and cranial nerve routes is of limited importance in neurological disease. There is experimental evidence for four possible pathways of spread by neural routes: these include direct axonal transport, spread via perineural lymphatics, or via the tissue spaces between nerves, and via Schwann cells; rabies and herpes simplex viruses may gain entry to the c.n.s. by these routes.

The majority of viruses gain access to the c.n.s. via a haematogenous route. In such instances initial viral replication occurs at the port of entry, usually the respiratory membrane or gastrointestinal mucosa. There are a considerable number of mechanisms acting as barriers to a further spread: viruses will usually be phagocytosed by macrophages, which then transport intact or degraded virus particles to the local lymphatics where an immune response is initiated; viruses that survive cause viraemia, but the blood–brain barrier still presents a major barrier to viral entry: the tight junctions of cerebral capillary vessels are relatively impermeable to viral passage. Some viruses may be capable of infecting capillary endothelial cells (poliovirus); others may infect glial elements in a manner similar to that by which colloid particles can cross endothelial cells in pinocytotic vesicles. Alternatively, some virus particles may be carried across the endothelial cells by infected lymphocytes.

The ultimate expression of c.n.s. viral disease, however, will be determined by spread of virus infection within the c.n.s. itself. The cerebrospinal fluid in the subarachnoid space presents few barriers to the spread of viral infection and meningitis is a common, relatively non-specific viral syndrome. In other instances the manifestation of c.n.s. neural disease may be determined by an apparent selective vulnerability of cell populations to viral infections. Some viruses are capable of producing only a meningeal syndrome, without causing parenchymal infection and encephalitis. Anterior horn cells seem to be favoured selectively by polioviruses, while varicella has a clear preference for primary afferent neurones. Rabies localises in neurones of the limbic system sparing the neocortex, whereas selective infection of oligodendrocytes may lead to demyelinating responses to viruses.

Immune responses to viruses in the c.n.s.

The central nervous system is relatively isolated from the general immune system: it lacks any intrinsic system for antibody production, there is no lymphatic system and few, if any, cells are present that can actively phagocytose particles. Immunoglobulins in normal c.s.f. are solely derived from blood.

In acute viral infections of the c.n.s. one of the early findings is of perivascular round-cell infiltration: this appears to be made up of populations of short-lived cells from the blood, and of non-dividing circulating mononuclear cells. The latter begin to undergo rapid division once they cross the vascular endothelium. It is these cells that appear to represent a specific cell clone sensitised to the infecting virus.

Initially, impairment of the normal blood brain barrier may allow a transudate of serum proteins to enter the c.n.s. After the first week, however, plasma cells migrating into the c.n.s. will start intracerebral immunoglobulin synthesis of a specific nature, as shown by distortions in the spinal fluid : serum ratios of immunoglobulins. The clearance of virus particles from the c.n.s. seems wholly dependent on this immune response.

Failure of these mechanisms due to immunological tolerance, to defects in the host immune response, or to the strategy of the virus, may allow persisting viral infection, which can result in delayed or chronic neurological disease.

CLINICAL SYNDROMES OF VIRAL NEUROLOGICAL DISEASE

An acute infection with viruses most commonly results in one of two non-specific clinical syndromes: aseptic meningitis or acute encephalitis. Many viruses are capable of causing these syndromes, the most common being Coxsackie B, echoviruses, and mumps virus. Other viruses appear to have more specific neurotropic effects which are manifested in more specific clinical syndromes: such viruses include poliomyelitis, herpes zoster, herpes simplex and rabies. Non-specific syndromes are described below and specific virus-related syndromes are subsequently discussed in sections pertaining to the individual causative virus.

Acute encephalitis

The clinical features of acute encephalitis are altered conscious level with drowsiness, confusion and possibly coma, frequently associated with seizures and pyrexia. Seizures may be either partial or generalised. Very frequently there is associated meningeal infection resulting in mild to moderate signs of meningism and, indeed, there is a continuum between the clinical syndromes of aseptic meningitis and acute encephalitis. Occasionally aphasia, hemiparesis, abnormal eye movements and myoclonic jerks may occur; these neurological symptoms may be preceded by symptoms due to local entry and replication of virus (upper respiratory tract infection or gastrointestinal disturbance) and subsequent viraemia with influenza-like symptoms. Death may occur in between 5% and 20% of patients with acute viral encephalitis and persisting neurological deficit may be present in up to 20% of patients. These figures are, to a large extent, dependent on the causative organism (herpes simplex encephalitis has a particularly high mortality and a large percentage of those surviving have persisting neurological disability—see below). It must also be recognised that some patients with less severe illnesses may never be admitted to hospital.

Investigations

The diagnosis of acute encephalitis remains a clinical one. The EEG is usually helpful in showing a usually gross generalised disturbance of cerebral activity with continuous moderate—to high-amplitude delta activity. In most instances these changes are generalised but focal fronto-temporal changes may be seen in herpes simplex encephalitis, with the development of periodic discharges. CT scanning is of no specific value, although it may be helpful in excluding cerebral abscess. Most commonly, diffuse cerebral swelling is present with compression of the cerebral sulci and ventricles. C.s.f. examination is helpful in displaying a lymphocytic pleocytosis, sometimes with a slightly raised c.s.f. protein. Rising titres of c.s.f. antibodies may be of value in determining the causative organism and, on occasion, the virus may be cultured from c.s.f. Sometimes c.s.f. may be normal in acute encephalitis and this finding does not exclude the diagnosis.

Aetiology

A wide variety of viruses may give rise to an encephalitis syndrome and in the majority of cases the causative organism is not easily identified. Important causes of encephalitis include herpes simplex virus, measles, mumps, infectious mononucleosis, Coxsackie viruses and echoviruses.

Differential diagnosis

The main differential diagnoses are from acute encephalopathies due to drugs and other metabolic disturbance such as hepatic and renal failure, as well as encephalopathies associated with systemic infection, such as septicaemia and typhoid. Other non-viral infective agents of the c.n.s. may be confused with acute viral encephalitis and, in particular, bacterial meningitis and cerebral abscess must be excluded.

Treatment

Most viral encephalitides require nothing other than symptomatic treatment to control fever, seizures and confusion. Specific antiviral therapy is discussed below in those sections dealing with specific groups of viruses. Although there is little objective evidence, high doses of corticosteroids are frequently given to patients with acute viral encephalitis in the belief that suppression of cerebral swelling and oedema may be beneficial.

Aseptic meningitis

Clinical features

The syndrome consists of fever, headache and other signs of meningism following a prodromal illness; there is a lymphocytic pleocytosis of the c.s.f. with a raised c.s.f. protein. A variable, though usually minor, degree of drowsiness and confusion may occur as there is a continuum between this syndrome and acute encephalitis: indeed, many cases are more aptly termed meningoencephalitis. Not infrequently there may be an associated erythematous papulomacular rash or exanthemata.

Aetiology

The most common viruses causing aseptic meningitis are mumps, echo and Coxsackie viruses, adenoviruses and lymphocytic choriomeningitis virus.

Differential diagnosis

A number of conditions may be mistaken for viral meningitis clinically or because they show similar c.s.f. abnormalities. Partly treated pyogenic meningitis is one of the most important entities to be confused with viral meningitis, and low-grade bacterial meningitis resulting from sinusitis or mastoid infection can also be confused; estimation of c.s.f. sugar may be important in this differentiation. Other specific bacterial disorders including syphilis and tuberculous meningitis must be considered. Leukaemias, lymphomas and carcinoma give rise to a lymphocytic pleocytosis and headache, but are usually associated with a slower evolution of symptoms, and show a more marked predisposition to be associated with cranial nerve palsies and radicular signs.

Prognosis

Symptomatic treatment is usually all that is required in lymphocytic meningitis, and the prognosis is excellent, with resolution of symptoms within a few days with little risk of any residual neurological disturbance; indeed, the syndrome is in every way benign.

Transverse myelitis

The syndrome of acute transverse myelitis has most commonly an indirect viral aetiology—a post-infectious process leading to spinal cord demyelination without direct viral invasion of the cord. In these circumstances the picture may be accompanied by an encephalopathy (encephalomyelitis). Rubella, measles, mumps, influenza and vaccination may cause such a syndrome.

Direct viral invasion of the spinal cord occurs as part of the specific syndromes poliomyelitis and rabies and extremely rarely may occur with herpes zoster, when an atypical transverse myelitis may result. Opportunistic viral myelitis may occur in AIDS.

SPECIFIC VIRUSES AND C.N.S. DISEASE

Picornaviruses are non-envelope RNA viruses. Over 70 human types are recognised, including poliovirus, Coxsackie viruses and echovirus. Transmission is usually by faecal contamination.

Poliomyelitis

The incidence of poliomyelitis has been dramatically reduced by programmes of immunisation. Up to the 1950s it occurred in epidemics, most frequently in summer or autumn, but now it represents an uncommon illness. This disorder is caused by infection with one or all three antigenically distinct types of poliovirus; very rarely, similar syndromes may be seen with other viruses.

Clinical manifestations are simply a sore throat, gastrointestinal upset, or influenza-like illness in the majority of patients infected by poliomyelitis. The virus usually fails to invade the c.n.s. but where this occurs, initial symptoms are those of listlessness, headache and neck stiffness. At this time an active aseptic meningitis is disclosed by c.s.f. examination; again, the course of the illness frequently aborts at this stage without the development of a paralytic stage. In paralytic poliomyelitis the patient develops a monoplegia or occasionally (particularly in older patients), involvement of two or more limbs. This is accompanied by the development of arreflexia and fasciculation in affected muscles with the progressive development of muscle atrophy. On occasion, bulbar involvement is seen independent of, or in addition to, spinal involvement and this presents particular dangers in view of the disturbances of respiration, vasomotor control and swallowing.

Treatment

The management of poliomyelitis is supportive with positive pressure ventilation and tracheostomy for bulbar involvement, symptomatic treatment of meningism, and the prevention of contractures.

Prognosis

The overall mortality is between 5% and 10% and rises strikingly with age, older patients appearing to be more susceptible than children to more widespread paralysis during the course of poliovirus infection. Some recovery of muscle strength usually occurs in the first few months after infection due to the enlargement of motor units by reinnervation from damaged or partly damaged nerve cells. Late complications include a very slowly progressive wasting and weakness which may be confused with motor neurone disease.

Prevention

Initial progress towards prevention came with the introduction of a killed vaccine (Salk). This has largely been replaced by an attenuated live vaccine which is administered orally (Sabin). This includes the three antigenically distinct subtypes and has the advantage that attenuated virus may also be spread to others to confer immunity. In the UK this is administered during infancy and childhood and booster doses during adult life are advisable.

Herpes virus infections

Herpes viruses are DNA viruses consisting of five specific human forms: *herpes simplex viruses (1 and 2); varicella-zoster virus; Epstein–Barr virus*; and *cytomegalovirus*. Frequently, initial infection with these viruses is asymptomatic, but all share the ability to reactivate to cause acute neurological illness. The mechanism of latency of herpes virus infections probably involves the integration of viral DNA into chromosomal DNA in either neural cells (herpes zoster and varicella) or haemopoietic cells (Epstein–Barr virus and cytomegalovirus).

Although herpes simplex viruses type 1 and 2 are antigenically related and difficult to differentiate in the laboratory, they cause an entirely different spectrum of human disease.

Type 1 virus is ubiquitous. Spread is usually by salivary or droplet infection and primary infection is usually asymptomatic. Very occasionally, primary infection may lead to widespread cutaneous lesions in immunosuppressed patients. It seems likely that the virus establishes latency in sensory ganglia, most commonly the trigeminal nerve ganglion. Up to 25% of the population suffer reactivation of herpes simplex type 1 virus in the form of cold sores.

Herpes simplex encephalitis

This syndrome may occur due to primary infection, reinfection or reactivation of type 1 herpes simplex virus. The mechanism by which it leads to localised inflammation, necrosis and inclusion body formation in the unique distribution affecting the inferior surfaces of the frontal and temporal lobes is controversial. Earlier suggestions that the virus spread might be via the olfactory route now seem less likely than the possibility that spread occurs from the trigeminal ganglia to the meninges of the anterior middle fossa.

Herpes simplex encephalitis is the commonest cause of fatal human encephalitis and its early recognition and differentiation from other more diffuse viral encephalitides is necessary because of the possibility of response to specific antiviral agents.

Clinical features

The encephalitis may occur at any age but is most common in childhood. The lowest incidence is between 20 and 40 years. Fever and headache are prominent early symptoms and sometimes bizarre behaviour and hallucination may lead to psychiatric admission. These early signs are, however, usually followed by the development of declining levels of consciousness associated with focal neurological signs. Hemiparesis occurs in one-third of patients and usually affects the face and arm more than the leg. Aphasia is not uncommon and upper-quadrant field defects may also occur. Repeated focal seizures with or without secondary generalisation are common.

Investigation

Investigation will usually reveal marked changes in the c.s.f. with a lymphocytic pleocytosis of up to 1000 cells/ml, occasionally associated with some xanthochromia or excess red cells; protein content will usually be somewhat elevated; on occasion, however, the c.s.f. may be relatively normal. The EEG may be particularly helpful in showing marked focal changes in frontotemporal regions and periodic discharges from these regions are particularly characteristic of herpes simplex encephalitis (but are not specific) (Fig. 12.4). CT scanning most frequently shows diffuse cerebral swelling, but on occasions localised necrotic change in one of the temporal lobes with accompanying shift and contrast enhancement may occur.

A

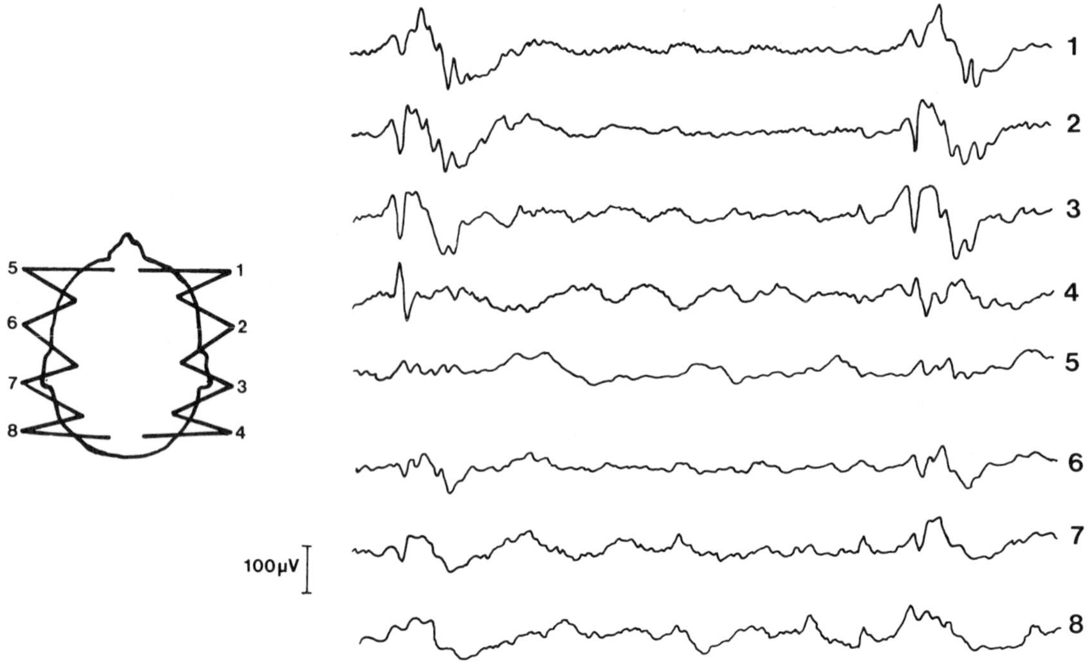

B

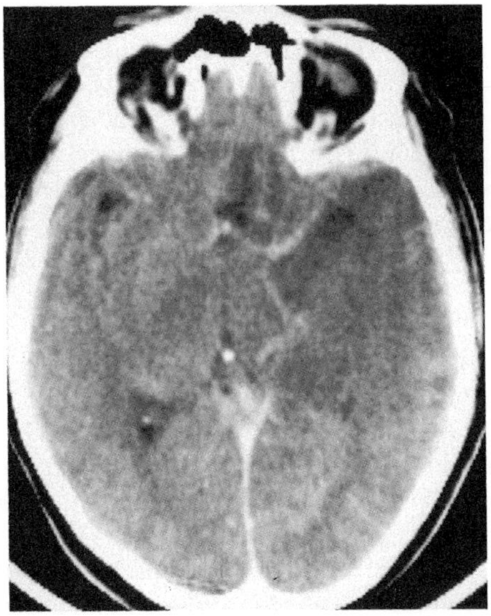

Fig. 12.4 **A** An EEG in herpes simplex encephalitis showing periodic complexes over the right hemisphere. **B** A CT scan showing right temporal swelling and low density in the same patient.

Whereas all these investigations may be helpful in giving substantial supporting evidence to the diagnosis of herpes simplex encephalitis, definitive diagnosis may be more difficult. In the past this has necessitated cerebral biopsy, but because of the localised nature of the infection it is always possible to obtain false negative biopsies. A diagnosis by detecting rising titres of antibody takes too long to be of clinical value. Earlier optimism that detection of fluorescent antibody for herpes simplex virus on mononuclear cells in the c.s.f. would be helpful, have not been upheld: for these reasons the diagnosis remains a clinical one. The advent of less toxic antiviral agents means that it is now reasonable to treat on clinical suspicion, before the diagnosis is proved.

Prognosis

It is difficult to be certain of the overall mortality and morbidity of the condition as it is possible that milder cases of herpes simplex encephalitis are not accurately diagnosed. However, it would seem that approximately 50% of patients with herpes simplex encephalitis die, and the majority of those who survive are left with severe neurological disturbance including hemiplegia, aphasia and severe memory disturbances of a Korsakov's type. Conscious level at the start of treatment, and the age of the patient, are important prognostic factors.

Treatment

Studies have been undertaken using vidarabine in biopsy-proven herpes simplex encephalitis, and this agent appears to reduce mortality from 70% to 40%. Acyclovir (30 mg/kg/day) for 10 days appears to be superior, reducing mortality to 28% and also reducing morbidity; the latter drug is less toxic and is now the treatment of choice for herpes simplex encephalitis. Its low toxicity should obviate the need for cerebral biopsy to provide a specific diagnosis, and should allow early treatment on clinical suspicion.

It is usual to combine a specific antiviral drug with high-dose corticosteroid treatment, with the aim of reducing cerebral oedema and intracranial pressure.

Herpes simplex type 2 virus

This virus is spread either by sexual contact, or in utero. The majority of infections occur in the third and fourth decades of life and the virus appears to become latent in the ganglia of the sacral roots; when it is activated, genital herpes is produced.

Herpes simplex type 2 virus may cause disseminated herpetic infection and a diffuse encephalitis in both the newborn and in immunosuppressed patients. On occasion, the occurrence of genital herpes may be associated with pain and dysaesthesiae in a radicular distribution, occasionally severe enough to simulate zoster infection.

Varicella zoster virus

This virus probably infects only man. Spread is via the respiratory route and most children will be infected during the early years of life and develop the typical illness of chickenpox. Rarely, this may be complicated by a postinfectious encephalomyelitis, acute ataxia or Guillain–Barré syndrome (see p. 240).

Delayed zoster infection occurs because of spread of the virus into sensory ganglia centripetally along sensory nerves from skin lesions of varicella. Herpes zoster is a common syndrome that increases in incidence with age. One-quarter of cases will occur over the age of 40 and as many as one-half of the people surviving to the age of 85 will have suffered at least one attack of shingles. The severity of the clinical syndrome increases with age and, unfortunately, one attack of shingles does not confer immunity to a second attack.

Shingles

The clinical syndrome of shingles begins with the development of malaise and fever, with segmental pain and paraesthesiae in an appropriate segmental distribution. The characteristic vesicular rash develops 4–5 days after the onset of symptoms. Any sensory dermatome may be affected, but thoracic dermatomes are more frequently involved (60% of cases) with the next commonest site being the ophthalmic branch of the trigeminal nerve (10–15% of cases). The facial nerve is more rarely involved, resulting in facial weakness and vesicles on the fauces and at the external auditory meatus (Ramsay Hunt syndrome). Disturbance of hearing and vertigo may accompany this syndrome, giving clinical evidence of the pathological findings of brain-stem involvement.

Although the radicular symptoms are almost invariably sensory, on occasion motor involvement does occur, not only in the Ramsay Hunt syndrome but with cervical or lumbosacral disturbance. Rarely, urinary retention may occur, with involvement of sacral dermatomes. It is also possible that typical pain and sensory disturbance of zoster may occur without the development of typical vesicles.

A rare complication of herpes zoster ophthalmicus has recently been recognised. Some patients develop an associated contralateral hemiparesis often associated with confusion and even coma, and occasionally with ipsilateral ophthalmoplegia. The pathological basis seems to be a cerebral angiitis caused by zoster, which causes a high mortality in the elderly patients in which it is seen. Treatment with acyclovir is indicated, but the results are uncertain.

A rare syndrome of fulminating zoster encephalitis, with or without myelitis, is now recognised in immunosuppressed patients. It may be that the use of specific antiviral agents, such as vidarabine or acyclovir, may be helpful in the treatment of this condition.

The most common problem of management of patients with zoster is that of a postherpetic neuralgia, the incidence of which increases with age. Although the incidence may be reduced by prompt treatment with an antiviral agent (acyclovir), once established it appears unfortunately to be refractive to most treatment. Some patients may benefit from treatment with carbamazepine or tricyclic antidepressants.

Epstein–Barr virus

This virus, causing glandular fever, is restricted to humans and most infections are asymptomatic and occur in childhood. Later infections give rise to a subacute illness with fever, laryngitis and lymphadenopathy. Splenomegaly and hepatomegaly are seen and 90% of patients have abnormal mononuclear cells in the peripheral blood and a heterophil antibody to antigens of sheep or horse red cells which will lyse them.

A variety of neurological complications may occur in patients with Epstein–Barr virus infection: these include the Guillain–Barré syndrome, facial palsy and a meningoencephalitis; more rarely, transverse myelitis or isolated cranial nerve palsies or retrobulbar neuritis occur.

Cytomegalovirus

This is another ubiquitous virus which establishes latency in haematogenous cells. It is an important cause of intrauterine infection, and infection during later life may either be asymptomatic, or give rise to a glandular-fever-like illness; it is a rare cause of aseptic meningitis and encephalitis in healthy individuals. It may also be associated with a Guillain–Barré syndrome and may cause a fulminating encephalitis in immunosuppressed patients.

Rabies virus

This RNA virus of the rhabdovirus group is a worldwide virus for which dogs, foxes and other mammals form the major reservoir. It has fortunately been excluded from populations of such animals in Great Britain.

For human infection to occur, the virus must be inoculated directly into human muscle by a bite. Spread to c.n.s. occurs via motor and sensory fibres, with subsequent rapid dissemination within the c.n.s. particularly to neurones of the limbic system. The incubation period for man can be anything between two weeks and a year, depending on the distance between the site of entry and the brain. There may be prodromal symptoms of malaise, headache and fever with the subsequent development of delirium, seizures, rigidity of the neck and a period of hyperexcitability. Pharyngeal spasms when drinking or seeing fluid may occur in up to one-half of the cases (hence the old name, hydrophobia).

Although some patients have recovered, the disease is almost invariably fatal. The major treatment for rabies is to prevent spread of virus to the c.n.s. in patients who have been bitten by a rabid animal. Local treatment and toilet of wounds reduces the risk, but vaccination is essential: it is usually undertaken with a combination of active and passive immunisation. Immunoglobulins will provide immediate passive immunity but active immunity may be stimulated with inactivated virus grown in human diploid cell cultures. The use of earlier neural tissue vaccines was complicated by a relatively high incidence of acute disseminated encephalomyelitis and Guillain–Barré syndromes.

DISEASES OF POSSIBLE VIRAL AETIOLOGY

Epidemic neuromyasthenia

There have been approximately 20 outbreaks recorded of this bizarre disease, most often affecting hospital staff; it has also been known as the Royal Free disease (after the hospital of that name). The disorder begins with headache and myalgia, sometimes associated with cervical lymphadenopathy and fever. Some degree of muscle weakness may develop, but this occurs in the absence of muscle wasting or hyporeflexia. Sensory symptoms are common but objective signs are rare. The results of laboratory investigations, including spinal fluid examination, are usually normal. The disease runs a prolonged course, but recovery is usual within three months. Relapses with further weakness and emotional disturbance are by no means uncommon.

The viral aetiology of this condition remains somewhat suspect, but the stereotyped nature of outbreaks detracts from the alternative aetiological theory of mass hysteria.

Cat scratch disease

This unusual disease, which develops after cat scratches and results in a red papule at the site of the scratch with low-grade fever and painful lymphadenopathy, is very occasionally complicated by a mild meningoencephalitis.

POSTVIRAL DISORDERS

As well as causing neurological disease by direct invasion of the nervous system, viruses are potent and frequent precipitants of delayed, presumably immunologically mediated, disease. Indeed, in many situations it is controversial how much of viral-induced neurological disease is caused by direct invasion of virus and how much by immunological reaction. The spectrum of such disorders is wide and is summarised below:

1. Acute haemorrhagic leucoencephalitis
2. Acute disseminated encephalomyelitis
3. Transverse myelitis
4. Neuralgic amyotrophy
5. Guillain–Barré syndrome
6. Combination syndromes.

These disorders are discussed in detail in chapters dealing with demyelinating diseases (Ch. 16), and peripheral nerve disease (Ch. 10).

The differential diagnosis of viral diseases

It is important to recognise and differentiate a number of other infective conditions that may on occasions be confused with viral disorders because of their ability to produce a meningoencephalitis and other neurological complications allied to similar c.s.f. changes; these bacterial, fungal and protozoal infections are summarised in Table 12.10 and are considered later.

SUBACUTE AND CHRONIC NEUROLOGICAL DISEASE DUE TO VIRUSES

INFLAMMATORY DISEASE

Subacute sclerosing panencephalitis (SSPE)

This disorder has been estimated to have an incidence of approximately one case per million children per year. Onset may be anywhere between 2 and 30 years, but median onset is at approxi-

Table 12.10 Diseases that may be confused with viral c.n.s. disease

Bacterial
Neurosyphilis
Tuberculosis
Mycoplasma
Brucella
Partly treated pyogenic meningitis
Abscess
Rickettsia
Typhus
Fungi
Cryptococcus
Candida
Parasites
Toxoplasma
Malaria

mately 7–8 years; males are three times more likely to be affected than females.

Aetiology

It is now accepted that SSPE is caused by a persisting chronic measles virus infection. The mechanisms of this are complicated and multifactorial: there may be some necessary host immune defect, the disease being more frequent in children who contract measles before the age of 2 years; this might imply some necessary tolerance on the part of the host in order to allow persisting infection. In addition, there is clear evidence of an abnormality of the measles virus within neurones of the brain in patients with SSPE. In normal replication of measles virus, RNA and glycoproteins are organised in buds or membranes derived from the host cell wall; a specific M protein is necessary for this to occur. Whereas all other elements of mature measles virus are present in the neurones and glia of patients with SSPE, the M protein seems to be lacking or greatly reduced; in consequence, normal budding and spread of the virus is inhibited, which may account for the chronic nature of the disorder.

Clinical features

The clinical progression of the disorder has been described in a number of stages. The first stage is that of insidious intellectual decline and behaviour disturbance and the second one of increasing motor disturbance, with the development of myoclonic jerks and ataxia with extrapyramidal rigidity and abnormal movements, seizures and visual impairment, which may be due either to cortical disturbance or retinopathy. In the third stage the child becomes rigid and bed-bound and enters what is almost a persistent vegetative stage. Death usually results 2–3 years after the onset; occasional prolonged survival or even improvement has been reported.

Investigations

In the early stages the EEG shows non-specific high-voltage slowing but, with disease progression, periodic complexes (see p. 102) are seen, consisting of spike and polyspike–wave and slow-wave disturbances of high amplitude occurring at approximately one-second intervals between which the EEG is isoelectric. The c.s.f. usually shows normal total protein and no excess of cells, but there is an increase in IgG content. Oligoclonal bands can be detected and there are very high titres against measles virus in both the serum and spinal fluid. The ratio of serum to spinal fluid concentrations of antibody titres compared with those against other viruses would indicate production of measles antibody within the c.n.s.

Pathology

Lesions are found involving the white matter of the hemispheres and brain stem with neuronal loss and swelling. There is perivascular cuffing with round cells and inclusion bodies are found in the cytoplasm and nuclei of neurones and glial cells. Staining techniques of viral antigen show the presence of measles virus in neurones and glial elements.

Treatment

There is no effective treatment for this condition. It may be that measles vaccination has a significant effect in reducing the incidence of the disease. Cases of the disease following vaccination are well documented, but seem to occur at approximately one-tenth of the rate of SSPE following natural measles infection.

Subacute measles inclusion body encephalitis

Immunosuppressed patients may develop a subacute illness associated with measles inclusion bodies, leading to more rapidly progressive neurological disease. There is usually a history of antecedent measles infection within the previous six months. The disorder runs a subacute course characterised by seizures, progressive neurological deficit with declining conscious level resulting in death within a few weeks. Little inflammatory change is found within the brain, and elevation of measles antibody levels is often lacking.

Progressive rubella encephalitis

This appears to represent an analogue of SSPE related to rubella, but is rarer. The disorder may develop after congenital or acquired rubella. The onset of deterioration can be in the first or second decade of life with progressive dementia and ataxia; motor signs, dysarthria and myoclonus may develop late and there may be a choroido-retinitis. The progress of the condition seems generally to be slower than that of SSPE.

Progressive multifocal leucoencephalopathy

This is a rare untreatable disease which most commonly occurs in immunosuppressed patients, particularly those with chronic lymphocytic leukaemia or lymphoma. It is characterised by dispersed demyelinating lesions throughout the white matter of the hemispheres and brain stem.

The disorder usually presents with rapidly advancing hemiparesis, quadriparesis, visual field defects progressing to cortical blindness, dementia and coma; death occurs 3–6 months after the onset of the disorder. The c.s.f. is normal and perhaps the most striking indication of the diagnosis may be obtained from CT scanning, where low-density lesions in the white matter of the hemispheres are seen.

The presence of papovaviruses within affected oligodendrocytes has been demonstrated by electron microscopy and subsequently two differing viruses have been isolated from cases of the disease: these are an SV40 virus and a so-called JC virus (derived from the initials of the patient from whom it was initially isolated); the latter virus seems the more common.

Multiple sclerosis

The implication of viral infections in the aetiology of multiple sclerosis is a large and controversial subject which is discussed in the chapter on demyelinating diseases (Ch. 16).

AIDS and its neurological complications

Retroviruses were not thought to be pathogens in man; however, it now appears that acquired immunodeficiency syndrome (AIDS) is caused by infection by a retrovirus (human immunodeficiency virus—HIV). This causes a severe defect in T cell function, particularly a reduction in helper T cells, which leaves patients at risk of a wide variety of opportunistic infections and tumours; the virus is also neurotopic and c.n.s. infection may first occur around the time of seroconversion resulting in an atypical aseptic meningitis or myelopathy. Transmission may be by sexual (mainly male homosexual) contact, or by blood products. High-risk groups include homosexuals and their partners, drug addicts, haemophiliacs and children born to AIDS sufferers.

Clinical features

AIDS causes a wide variety of systemic symptoms, but up to 40% of sufferers have neurological disorders: these are summarised in Tables 12.11 and 12.12; c.n.s. disorders are five times more common than peripheral disorders. Specific opportunistic infections are described below, but some syndromes which appear to be due to HIV itself demand further description.

Subacute encephalitis (AIDS dementia). This (presumed virally induced) disorder presents with progressive dementia, in which frontal damage

Table 12.11 C.N.S. features of AIDS

	* %
Direct HIV viral syndromes	
Subacute encephalitis/vacuolar myelopathy	17
Atypical aseptic meningitis	6
Specific viral syndromes	
Herpes simplex encephalitis	3
Progressive multifocal leucoencephalopathy	2
Viral myelitis	1
Non-viral infections	
Toxoplasma gondii	32
Cryptococcus	13
Other fungal infection	3
Mycobacterial infection (tubercular + atypical)	3
Neoplasms	
Primary c.n.s. lymphoma (microglioma)	5
Spread from systemic lymphoma	4
Metastatic Kaposi's sarcoma	1
Stroke	3
Undefined c.n.s. disorders	8

* % of 320 patients with AIDS and neurological disorders (after Levy et al 1985).

Table 12.12 Peripheral nervous system involvement in AIDS

	* %
Cranial nerve syndromes	
Multiple cranial nerve palsies	
Due to chronic inflammatory polyneuropathy	10
Due to lymphoma	10
Bell's palsy	10
Peripheral nerve syndromes	
Chronic inflammatory polyneuropathy	24
Distal symmetrical polyneuropathy	26
Zoster radiculitis	12
Muscle syndromes	
Myalgias	4
Myopathy	4
Polymyositis	2

* % of 51 patients with peripheral nervous system disorder in AIDS (after Levy et al 1985).

and motor signs are prominent; myoclonus and seizures occur; CT scanning often shows marked atrophy, but c.s.f. shows an elevated protein level, sometimes with a lymphocytosis. The disorder appears increasingly frequent with prolonged survival and is rapidly progressive and fatal. Autopsy shows in grey and white matter changes, but with an absence of inflammatory cells. HIV particles can be recovered from the brains of patients with this syndrome.

Vacuolar myelopathy. This chronic or subacute disorder causes ataxia and incontinence with usually symmetrical sensory disturbance and pyramidal motor weakness of the lower limbs.

Atypical aseptic meningitis. The atypical features of this illness are chronicity, tendency to relapse, and a relatively high incidence of cranial nerve and long-tract signs in what otherwise appears to be an aseptic meningitis.

Chronic inflammatory polyneuropathy. This syndrome is usually accompanied by fever, malaise and night sweats. It can present the picture of a mononeuritis multiplex or a distal asymmetrical neuropathy. Biopsy shows a chronic inflammatory picture without evidence of vasculitis.

CHRONIC DEGENERATIVE NEUROLOGICAL DISEASE DUE TO VIRUS-LIKE PARTICLES

The discovery of particles capable of transmitting spongiform encephalopathies (Fig. 12.5) has been one of the most remarkable developments of the last 20 years. It now seems that the animal diseases of scrapie in sheep and transmissable mink encephalopathy, the human diseases of kuru in the Fore district of New Guinea and the more widely dispersed, though rare, Creutzfeldt–Jakob disease, may all be due to a group of particles that will pass through filters through which viruses will not pass, are highly resistant to heat and formalin and to ionising and ultraviolet radiation. The particles are stable between wide ranges of pH and resistant to lipid solvents and detergents.

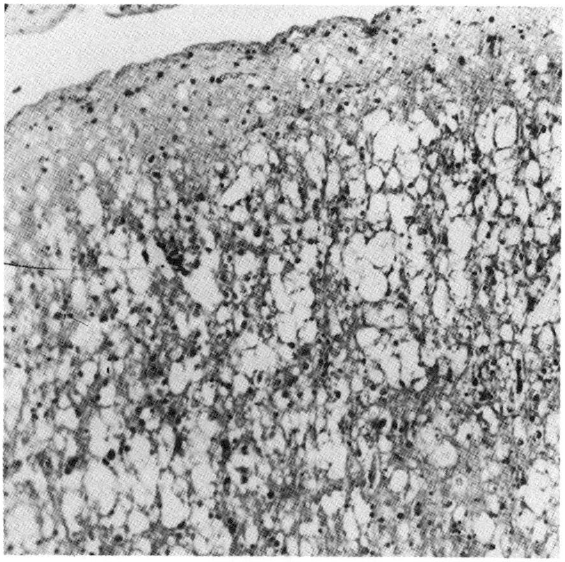

Fig. 12.5 Microscopy of spongiform cortical change in patient dying with Creutzfeldt–Jakob disease.

Creutzfeldt–Jakob disease

This disorder presents as a rapidly progressive presenile dementia. True incidence figures are difficult to obtain but are probably of the order of one per million per year. Between 10% and 15% of cases may occur within familial pedigrees.

Aetiology

Transmission of spongiform encephalopathy to the chimpanzee was first achieved in 1968 and it has now been successfully transmitted to a number of species including Old and New World monkeys, cats, guinea pigs and mice; the mode of natural transmission, however, remains uncertain. Infectivity seems to be extremely low and only two conjugal cases have ever been reported. However, iatrogenic transmission has certainly occurred: one patient developed the disorder 18 months after receiving a corneal implant from a patient who had died of the disease, and the disorder has also been transmitted by the reuse of stereo-EEG electrodes previously implanted in a patient with the disease. The possibility that neurosurgery can transmit the disease was raised by the finding that three patients subsequently developing the disease had been operated upon by the same neurosurgeon within a period of 8 months.

Clinical features

The disease presents with intellectual change and dementia, sometimes associated with behaviour disorder, hallucination and illusion which may lead to psychiatric referral. However, the development of motor symptoms and signs occurs quickly; these may be very varied, but the commonest element is the occurrence of myoclonus of a stimulus-sensitive variety: this can be precipitated by sudden loud noises, flashing lights, and sensory stimuli to the extremities. Approximately 80% of patients with this condition will show myoclonus at some stage of the disease; in addition, pyramidal signs, chorea and dystonia, ataxia and wasting with fasiculation may all occur. Death occurs in 80% of patients within 12 months of onset, although occasional prolonged survival has been recorded.

Investigations

The c.s.f. is always normal and the most helpful investigative tool is usually that of electroencephalography: this displays the characteristic pattern of periodic complexes, similar to those seen in SSPE.

OTHER NON-VIRAL CNS INFECTIONS

On rare occasions, other organisms may invade and infect the central nervous system. In the United Kingdom such infections are most usually opportunistic, occurring in patients with immune suppression due to intercurrent diseases such as leukaemia, lymphoma and carcinoma, or due to treatment with wide-spectrum antibiotics, corticosteroids or other immunosuppressant drugs.

Rickettsial diseases

Rickettsia are intracellular parasites which differ from viruses in that they maintain their own cellular integrity. They cause a variety of diseases in man, including typhus and Q fever, the usual source of infection being ticks. Their course may be complicated by an encephalitis which may be difficult to differentiate from viral encephalitides.

The c.s.f. shows few changes, but the diagnosis may be supported by the detection of antibodies which agglutinate strains of *Proteus vulgaris* (the Weil–Felix reaction). This is an adequate screening test, but definite diagnosis requires specific serological testing. Rickettsial infections are usually responsive to tetracycline or chloramphenicol.

Fungal infections

Fungi may give rise to a variety of neurological syndromes, but they most commonly present with a subacute meningitis, which is not dissimilar to tuberculous meningitis; however, thrombophlebitis and cerebral abscess may complicate the picture. Predisposing factors to fungal c.n.s. infection include general debilitation due to malignancy, alcoholism or organ failure, parenteral nutrition, AIDS or broad-spectrum antibiotic or immunosuppressive therapy. The most common fungi associated with c.n.s. infection in the UK are *Cryptococcus*, *Nocardia* and *Candida*. A rare syndrome is seen with mucormycosis in patients with diabetes; infection arises in the paranasal sinuses and spreads to the retro-orbital tissues and brain resulting in proptosis, ophthalmoplegia and haemorrhagic cerebral infarction.

The diagnosis of fungal meningitis must be suspected in patients with immunosuppression; it will be confirmed by c.s.f. examination, which shows changes typical of chronic meningitis with polymorphonuclear leucocytosis, increased protein and the demonstration of fungal cells either on routine Gram staining or by demonstration with

Indian-ink staining. Special techniques may be necessary to culture the organisms.

Treatment is possible with a variety of antifungal agents. *Amphotericin B* has been available for many years and this may also be administered via an intrathecal route. Newer agents such as *5-fluorocytosine* and *miconazole* may be used as alternative or adjunctive treatment. Particular care must be taken with amphotericin in view of its ability to cause renal damage.

Fungal c.n.s. infection carries a high mortality and morbidity, even allowing for the fact that most patients developing such disorders have serious underlying systemic disease.

Protozoal c.n.s. infection

Toxoplasma

Toxoplasma gondii is an intracellular parasite which occasionally causes infection which is most commonly congenital, but occasionally acquired and opportunistic; it is the commonest opportunistic c.n.s. infection in AIDS. It may present with a diffuse skin rash, encephalitis, myocarditis and polymyositis associated with seizures, confusion, coma and focal neurological signs. The c.s.f. shows a lymphocytic pleocytosis and increased protein and multiple ring lesions of encysted *Toxoplasma gondii* may be seen with CT scanning. A diagnosis may be made using a toxoplasma dye test in serum or c.s.f.; however, this may be unreliable in the AIDS syndrome, where presumptive treatment or cerebral biopsy may be necessary. Sulphadiazine in combination with pyrimethamine may be used as treatment.

Malaria

Cerebral malaria is occasionally imported into the UK. With increasingly rapid air travel, clinicians must maintain a high level of suspicion concerning the diagnosis.

Cerebral malaria almost always results from infection with *Plasmodium falciparum*. Approximately 2% of patients with such infections develop the complication, most commonly those with severe infestation (more than 5% of red cells in peripheral blood showing evidence of parasitisation). Incubation is from 8 to 14 days, but relapse may occur after periods of several months following initial infection.

The pathology of the condition seems largely vascular, the cerebral capillaries being filled with malarial parasites, giving rise to areas of surrounding necrosis. Clinical features consist of preceding typical fever and malaise, followed after 2–3 weeks by the rapid development of headache, seizures and coma; more rarely there may be focal manifestations with hemiplegia and aphasia. The diagnosis is dependent on the demonstration of parasites in a thick film of peripheral blood. C.s.f. examination will usually be necessary to exclude pyogenic meningitis, but shows normal protein, glucose and a minimal increase in white cells.

The condition carries a high mortality. Quinine is the most satisfactory treatment, but must be used in conjunction with full supportive care to prevent renal failure, dehydration and hypoglycaemia, which may complicate the illness. Seizures must be controlled, but there is no evidence that steroids have any major protective effects against the development of cerebral oedema.

FURTHER READING

Anderson M 1984 Bacterial meningitis. In: Matthews W B, Glaser G H (eds) Recent advances in clinical neurology, vol 4. Churchill Livingstone, London

Bateman D E, Newman P K, Foster J B 1983 A retrospective survey of proven cases of tuberculous meningitis in the Northern Region, 1970–80. Journal of the Royal College of Physicians of London 17: 106–110

Bradley P J, Shaw M D M 1983 Three decades of brain abscess in Merseyside. Journal of the Royal College of Surgeons of Edinburgh 28: 223–228

Johnson R T 1982 Viral infections of the nervous system. Raven Press, New York

Levy R M, Bredesen D E, Rosenblum M L 1985 Neurological manifestations of the acquired immunodeficiency syndrome (AIDS): experience at UCSF and review of literature. Journal of Neurosurgery 62: 475–495

13

Raised intracranial pressure and cerebral tumours

INTRODUCTION

Unlike any other organ in the body the brain is enclosed within the box of the skull. The contents of the skull are the 1500 g brain, the blood and cerebrospinal fluid of approximately 100 ml each. A change in the volume of any of the three constituents must be countered by an equal and opposite change in one or other of the two remaining compartments. Thus, in the elderly patient, as the brain atrophies, the volume of cerebrospinal fluid tends to increase in the condition of 'hydrocephalus ex vacuo'. The corollary is that if any one of the three compartments within the skull increases beyond that stage at which compensation can occur in the other compartments, then the pressure inside the head will increase resulting in the syndrome of raised intracranial pressure. The role of the physician, when presented with a patient who has raised intracranial pressure, is to identify the cause of the increased pressure and to apply the appropriate therapy.

MECHANISMS OF RAISED INTRACRANIAL PRESSURE

CEREBROSPINAL FLUID

The physiology of the cerebrospinal fluid

Cerebrospinal fluid is formed, predominantly by the choroid plexuses of the lateral, third and fourth ventricles, at the rate of approximately 25 ml per hour. The total volume of c.s.f. is of the order of 100 ml and therefore the total circulation of c.s.f. is achieved between four and six times a day. The cerebrospinal fluid flows from the lateral ventricles through the foramen of Monro into the third ventricle and thence via the aqueduct into the fourth ventricle. It leaves the fourth ventricle via the foramina of Magendie and Luschka into the subarachnoid space where it circulates around the hemispheres and down the spine. It is absorbed through the arachnoid granulations, predominantly over the superior surfaces of the cerebral hemisphere and around the base of the brain and the spinal nerve roots. Absorption from the arachnoid granulations is into the venous

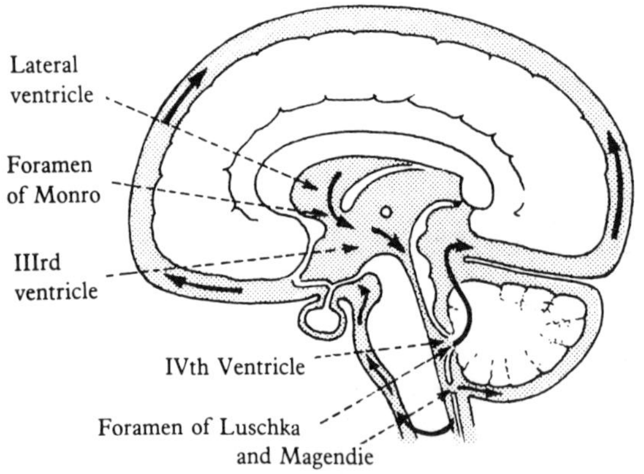

Fig. 13.1 The circulation of the cerebrospinal fluid. (From Lindsay K W, Bone I, Callander R 1986 *Neurology and Neurosurgery Illustrated*. Churchill Livingstone, Edinburgh, with permission.)

sinuses. The flow of c.s.f. is probably encouraged by the intermittent arterial pulsations within the head and the consequent variations in intracranial pressure (Fig. 13.1).

The cerebrospinal fluid acts as a protective cushion for the brain and spinal cord and it has been suggested that when the brain, which is predominantly water in content is suspended in c.s.f. its effective weight is only of the order of 50 g; this, therefore, protects it from potentially injurious blows. The c.s.f. also acts as a route whereby waste products from the brain may be excreted into the blood, but it should not be regarded as being a purely passive reservoir, but rather as an active system which determines the rate and concentration of ions, molecules, proteins and drugs which are allowed to enter the fluid from the blood or interstitial tissues of the cerebrum. Anything which blocks the flow of cerebrospinal fluid, prevents its resorption or results in its excessive production will cause hydrocephalus and may result in raised intracranial pressure.

Increase in c.s.f.

An increase in the cerebrospinal fluid results in the phenomenon of hydrocephalus, which is described later. Such an increase may occur either as a primary abnormality or as compensation for loss of other intracranial tissues. In the former instance, an excessive production of cerebrospinal fluid may be seen very rarely in patients with choroid plexus papilloma; a reduced absorption may be seen in conditions in which the arachnoid granulations are blocked and any cause of interruption to the normal circulation of cerebrospinal fluid will tend to result in an increase proximal to the block. Compensatory hydrocephalus will occur where there is cerebral atrophy and being compensatory there will be no increase in intracranial pressure. Excessive production, reduced absorption or a blockage will result in raised intracranial pressure.

CEREBRAL OEDEMA

Cerebral oedema may be divided into two major types: vasogenic, or inflammatory, oedema and cytotoxic oedema. The two forms of oedema may coexist, but their causes are distinct and their reactions to therapy differ (Fig. 13.2).

Vasogenic oedema

Vasogenic or inflammatory oedema is intercellular oedema in which there is increased permeability of the capillary endothelial cells which allows plasma to enter the extracellular space. Whether this increased permeability is due to defects in the tight endothelial cell junctions of the capillaries or to increased active transport across the endothelial cells is uncertain but this form of oedema, which is most commonly seen around tumours, abscesses and the plaques of multiple sclerosis, is predominantly confined to the white matter. The intercellular oedema has a high protein content and this, together with the local pressure, disrupts conduction within nerve fibres.

Cytotoxic oedema

This form of oedema, which is predominantly intracellular, is the typical oedema seen in cerebrovascular accidents and hypoxic brain injury. The oedema is almost certainly due to ischaemic damage to the ATP dependent sodium pump

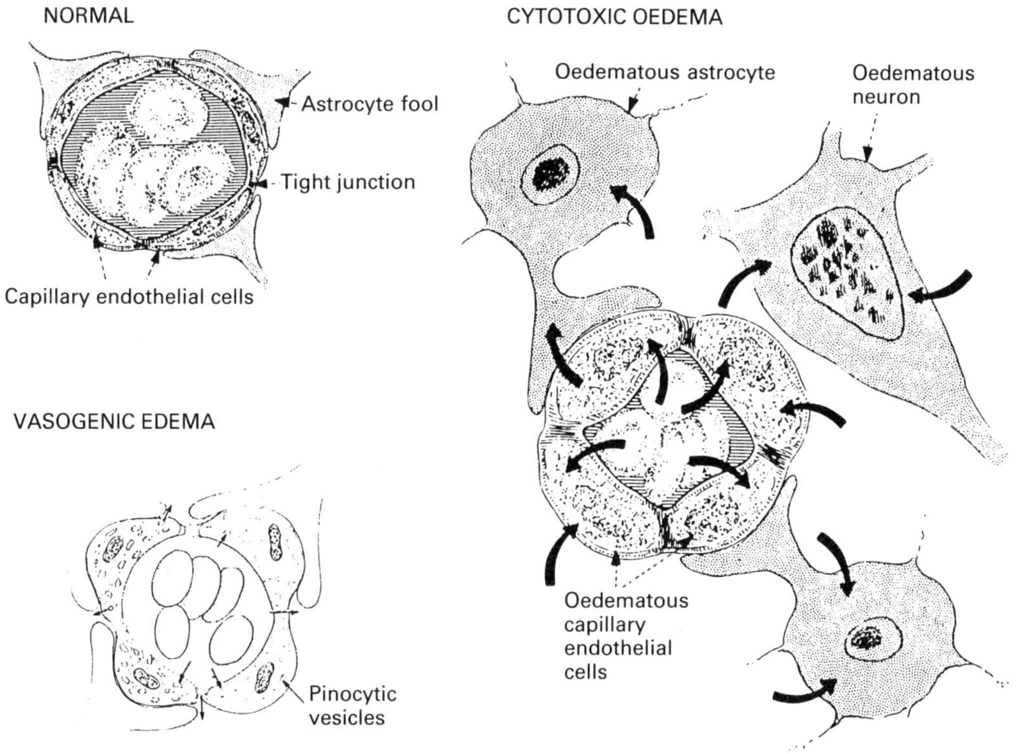

Fig. 13.2 Representation of capillary endothelial cells and astrocytes in the normal situation and in vasogenic and cytotoxic cerebral oedema. (From Fishman R 1980 *Cerebral Spinal Fluid in Diseases of the Nervous System*. Saunders, Philadelphia, with permission.)

resulting in the accumulation of sodium, calcium and water within the cell. Cytotoxic oedema is not confined to the white matter but involves all cell types within the brain. It is most commonly seen in the presence of hypoxia, but can also occur with disequilibrium syndromes in renal dialysis, dilutional hyponatraemia and in inappropriate secretion of ADH.

It is apparent that both forms of oedema may be seen together in that a cerebral tumour may cause intercellular oedema in the area around which a relative ischaemia occurs due to the increased pressure, and consequent cytotoxic or cellular oedema occurs as well. The importance of differentiating between the two types of oedema is that, whereas vasogenic or interstitial oedema is readily responsive to treatment with steroids, mannitol or dehydration with diuretics, cytotoxic oedema is relatively resistant to all these therapies and much more difficult to control.

Whatever the cause of cerebral oedema it will tend to result in raised intracranial pressure and may then be self-perpetuating.

INCREASE IN BLOOD

In the resting physiological state the volume of blood within the cranium is of the order of 100 ml, but vasodilatation occurring in response to physiological stimuli, such as increased $P\text{CO}_2$, or in the pathological situation of a hypertensive encephalopathy, can result in an increase in this compartment of the intracranial contents and a consequent rise in intracranial pressure. Much more commonly the volume of blood inside the cranium will increase in conditions of cerebral haemorrhage, particularly parenchymal and extraparenchymal haematoma when the situation may be complicated by the development of local cerebral oedema.

SPACE-OCCUPYING LESIONS

Apart from changes in the three normal constituents of the cranial cavity, namely cerebrospinal fluid, brain and blood, there may also arise space-occupying lesions within the cranial cavity and consequently raised intracranial pressure. Haematoma, which has been mentioned in the preceding paragraph, is one such example, and cerebral tumours, cerebral abscesses and fluid-containing cysts within the cranium in the form of porencephaly or arachnoid cysts may all cause increased intracranial pressure.

The development of a cerebral tumour or a cerebral abscess may be associated with a degree of cerebral oedema so that the raised intracranial pressure will be caused partly by the space-occupying lesion itself and partly by the consequent, predominantly intercellular, oedema.

EFFECTS OF RAISED INTRACRANIAL PRESSURE

Raised intracranial pressure will cause two important clinical phenomena: the effect of raised intracranial pressure within the cranium itself and consequent brain shifts, which may occur due to an asymmetrical effect of the pressure.

THE CLINICAL SYNDROME OF RAISED INTRACRANIAL PRESSURE

Headache

As described in Chapter 8, the headache of raised intracranial pressure is recognised by the fact that it is usually occipital and tends to occur when the patient is lying down, frequently waking the patient from sleep early in the morning. The headache may, however, vary considerably and can occasionally, when dural involvement of the causative tumour is prominent, be localised to the site of the pathology. The characteristic headache is periodic and bioccipital, with radiation to the frontal region which tends to awaken the patient during the night, or is present early in the morning and is relieved by adequate analgesia and by adopting the erect posture. It is made worse by those manoeuvres which raise intracranial pressure, such as coughing, sneezing, straining and bending.

Changes in mental function

The majority of patients with raised intracranial pressure will show evidence of alteration in mental function. This may vary from a mild and unusual irritability, a degree of emotional lability or lack of insight and extend to forgetfulness, specific memory defects and reduced ability to handle conceptual thought and occasionally to a frank dementia. In many of the patients it is necessary to take a history from a member of the family or a friend who can document this change in the patient's character and it is important to recognise that such changes may be incorrectly attributed to worry or anxiety which the patient may be suffering.

The raised intracranial pressure will also tend to cause a degree of drowsiness or retardation in the patient and his or her own description of symptoms at this stage may consist of complaints of fatigue or lethargy, alteration in sleep pattern and difficulty in pursuing their normal daily occupation or undertaking their routine chores.

Vomiting

Although most commonly seen in patients with tumours in the posterior fossa, vomiting may be a feature with any cause of raised intracranial pressure. It is common for the patient to vomit without feeling nauseated and the vomiting may be unexpected, forceful and projectile. Vomiting is occasionally most prominent with the early morning headache and patients may comment that the headache is relieved somewhat when they have been sick.

Dizziness

Symptoms of light-headedness or dizziness are common in patients with raised intracranial pressure, though true rotational vertigo is uncommon except when the lesion lies in the posterior fossa. The symptom of dizziness is presumably a reflection of brain stem pressure and is more frequently described as a light-headedness or mild unsteadiness, being usually unaccompanied by any significant physical signs.

Visual difficulties

The most frequent visual symptom is of blurring of vision, which may occasionally become frank diplopia. The cause for blurring of vision is often difficult to establish, it may represent the beginning of a sixth nerve palsy though there is some evidence that distortion of the globe itself may occasionally be the cause of this symptom. The more dramatic symptoms of visual obscuration, when vision is lost momentarily whilst bending, is seen only in those patients with frank papilloedema.

Seizures

Although epilepsy may occur in more than one-third of patients with cerebral tumours, it is more commonly a reflection of the irritative effect of the tumour than of the raised intracranial pressure per se. Patients with hydrocephalus may present with seizures which are usually non-focal and tonic-clonic in type.

The clinical signs which are apparent on examination in patients with raised intracranial pressure may be remarkably few, but there are certain features which represent typical findings in raised intracranial pressure:

Papilloedema

This, the cardinal sign of raised intracranial pressure, may be an unexpected finding in someone presenting with a minor headache or may serve simply to confirm the suspicion of raised intracranial pressure in someone with a more typical story. The stages of papilloedema are described as an initial blurring of the optic disc margins with filling of the veins and an important early sign may be the loss of the normal spontaneous venous pulsation seen on the disc. Later, grossly distended venules will be apparent together with the presence of pericapillary haemorrhages, areas of retinal infarction and, ultimately, gliotic scarring of the disc. It may be difficult to identify early papilloedema in patients with some loss of clarity of the disc margin, when the use of retinal fluoroscein angiography should be considered to show whether or not there is late leakage of dye from the vessels. The differential diagnosis of papilloedema is from papillitis, in which condition there is usually reduced visual acuity—unlike papilloedema where the acuity will remain normal although the size of the blind spot may be enlarged on visual field testing (Fig. 13.3). The absence of papilloedema does not exclude raised intracranial pressure and cannot, alone, be taken as evidence for the safety of lumbar puncture in a patient with other symptoms of raised intracranial pressure and focal signs.

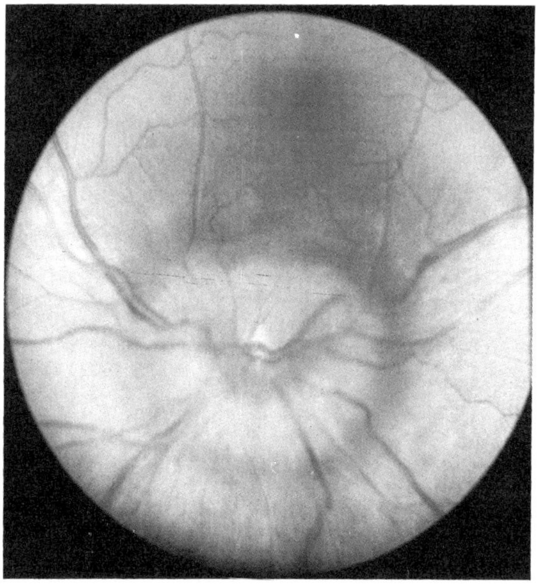

Fig. 13.3 Fundus photograph showing papilloedema.

Neck stiffness

Raised intracranial pressure will frequently cause tension upon the meninges in the posterior fossa and ultimately herniation of the cerebellar tonsils through the foramen magnum. The symptom of pain on neck movement is therefore not uncommon and patients may show discomfort on attempted neck flexion. The differential diagnosis is then from meningitis, though the latter, unlike the former, should be accompanied by a positive Kernig's test on straight-leg raising.

Hyper-reflexia

In general, increased intracranial pressure will result in generalised hyper-reflexia and, although this must be differentiated from anxiety or other significant pathology, it can be a useful indication of the possibility of raised intracranial pressure.

False localising signs

Although the symptoms and signs which suggest the presence of raised intracranial pressure, together with those which indicate a focal pathology are important in identifying the site of an intracerebral space-occupying lesion, there are problems in that certain cranial nerve signs and some long tract signs may arise as false localising signs due to the pressure on, or distortion of, structures distal to the original lesion. The most classic example of a false localising sign is the sixth nerve palsy, since this, the longest intracranial nerve, is commonly compressed or distorted with raised intracranial pressure. There will be failure of abduction of one or both eyes, indicating damage to the abducent nerve and, although it is important to exclude the possibility of a local pathology, it is an important sign of raised intracranial pressure.

Other cranial nerve palsies may also occur: third cranial nerve palsies are seen with distortion of the brain stem; lower cranial nerve palsies are less commonly seen as false localising signs, but tumours in the posterior fossa may cause contralateral cranial nerve palsies due to distortion of the pons or medulla. Pressure on the midbrain from suprasellar tumours may cause compression of the contralateral cerebellar peduncle and therefore result in hemiparesis which is, misleadingly, ipsilateral to the side of the tumour. This is particularly common with extra-axial swellings such as meningiomas and subdural haematomas.

These non-specific symptoms and signs of raised intracranial pressure are important in that they may be the only clue to the physician that there is an intracerebral pathology, such as a mass lesion or hydrocephalus. Similar symptoms may, however, occur in other conditions. Benign intracranial hypertension, occurring classically in young women, may present with precisely the same symptoms and signs. The relatively uncommon hypertensive encephalopathy can also mimic non-specific symptoms of cerebral tumour, but should be differentiated by evidence of more diffuse changes in the fundi, the elevation of blood pressure and the findings of other stigmata of vascular problems. Hypercapnoea, particularly occurring in patients with episodic apnoea, can be much more difficult to differentiate from non-specifically raised intracranial pressure though the assessment of the $P\text{CO}_2$ is obviously diagnostic. Chronic meningitis may rarely cause many of the symptoms and signs described above and this may be a diagnosis of exclusion since lumbar puncture is not indicated until one is sure that there is no asymmetrical increase in intracranial pressure. Cerebral or cortical venous thrombosis may occasionally present similar problems, as can some of the rare endocrine disturbances such as Addison's disease. It is important to bear in mind the possibility of such other pathology in patients presenting with syndromes of raised intracranial pressure, but it must be recognised that in many instances it will be necessary to undertake investigations of the cerebrum, usually with CT scan, and then to identify other possible causes.

BRAIN HERNIATION

When intracranial pressure rises, due to the growth of a tumour with surrounding oedema, haemorrhage, abscess or other cause of focal brain swelling the importance of the division of the cranial cavity into separate compartments becomes evident. The falx between the hemispheres and the tentorium cerebri separating the posterior from the middle fossa form potential barriers penetrated by holes which connect the spaces occupied by the right and left hemispheres and the cerebellum beneath them. As a tumour grows in any compartment the pressure may force brain tissue from one side to the other in a subfalcine herniation, or through the tentorium in a tentorial herniation. Tumours in the posterior fossa may cause upward herniation through the tentorium or result in the more common and potentially lethal foraminal herniation, where the tonsils of the cerebellum are pushed into the foramen magnum. All of these herniations are important and increase

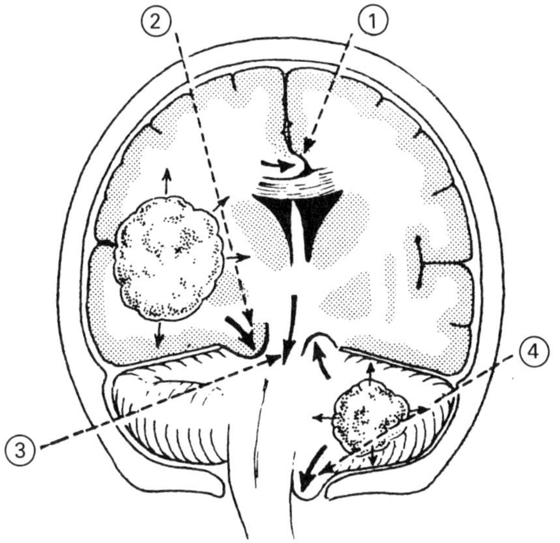

Fig. 13.4 Cerebral herniation showing 1 subfalcine herniation, 2 uncal herniation, 3 diencephalic herniation, 4 foramen magnum herniation.

the damage caused by the original lesion (Fig. 13.4).

Subfalcine herniation

A tumour in either hemisphere will tend to cause that hemisphere to be compressed beneath the falx and, although this herniation is frequently seen radiologically or at autopsy, signs of it are relatively uncommon.

Tentorial herniation

Cerebral hemisphere lesions may also cause pressure downwards through the tentorium, compressing either the ipsilateral uncus of the temporal lobe, or compressing the diencephalon centrally through the tentorial hiatus. Clinically, the former type of herniation causes pressure on the ipsilateral third nerve resulting in ptosis and pupillary dilatation and later ophthalmoplegia; on occasion a contralateral third nerve palsy may be seen as a false localising sign. In addition, pressure on the contralateral cerebral peduncle causes hemiplegia ipsilateral to the tumour. Central herniation causes flattening of the midbrain and a rostrocaudal progression of deterioration of

Table 13.1 Features of tentorial (uncal) herniation

Pathology	Clinical signs
Crushing of ipsilateral oculomotor nerve between uncus and petroclinoid ligament	Ptosis and pupillary dilatation—later ophthalmoplegia
Displacement of midbrain, pressing contralateral cerebral peduncle against tentorium (Kernahan's notch)	Hemiplegia ipsilateral to herniation (false localising)—later bilateral corticospinal signs
Crushing of midbrain and haemorrhages around arterioles (Duret haemorrhage)	Cheyne–Stokes respiration, stupor and coma, bipyramidal signs, extensor rigidity, dilated and fixed pupils, loss of oculovestibular and oculocaloric responses
Infarction of occipital lobes due to compression of posterior cerebral artery against tentorium	Homonymous hemianopia (unilateral and bilateral)—may not be detectable in coma
Increased intracranial pressure due to distortion of aqueduct	Increasing coma, rising blood pressure and bradycardia

respiration, motor signs and conjugate upward gaze, problems resulting ultimately in declining consciousness and coma. The posterior cerebral arteries are compressed against the tentorium and this results in a unilateral or bilateral occipital infarct and homonymous hemianopia. Pressure at this site of the brain stem may also result in compression of the aqueduct, causing a block in the flow of c.s.f. resulting in an obstructive hydrocephalus (Table 13.1).

Foramen magnum pressure cone

This consists of downward displacement of the cerebellar tonsils through the foramen magnum. It may occur with tumours of the posterior fossa or be due to more generally increased intracranial pressure with massive tumours above the tentorium. The effects are due, not to the pressure on the tonsils themselves, but rather to the consequent pressure upon the medulla resulting in brain stem distortion and petechial haemorrhages called Duret's haemorrhages in the pons and medulla. Clinically there is tonic extension of the limbs, which may resemble seizures, changes in respiration and cardiac irregularities with increasing blood pressure. Neck pain is often the first and may be the only prominent symptom.

In addition, all of these herniations may be associated with decreasing consciousness due to the fact that the herniation affects the brainstem ascending reticular activating substance and the resulting hydrocephalus tends also to depress conscious levels.

HYDROCEPHALUS

AETIOLOGY

Hydrocephalus may be divided into those types due to a block of the normal flow of c.s.f., commonly called obstructive hydrocephalus, those due to disturbed absorption or secretion of c.s.f., so-called communicating hydrocephalus, and those secondary to cerebral atrophy, or hydrocephalus ex vacuo.

Obstructive hydrocephalus

Though the original definition of obstructive hydrocephalus as being due to the complete block of flow of c.s.f. is no longer tenable, the concept of an obstruction in the c.s.f. pathways resulting in the accumulation of fluid proximal to the block is a reasonable one. A tumour lying within the third ventricle such as a colloid cyst is likely to block the foramen of Monro causing unilateral or bilateral dilatation of the lateral ventricles. The narrowest site of the normal c.s.f. pathway, and therefore the place most liable to obstruction, is the cerebral aqueduct, which may be congenitally narrowed, impinged upon by granulations, occluded by tumours or distorted by shifts of the intracranial contents. In this instance the third and lateral ventricles will be dilated (Fig. 13.5) but the fourth ventricle will remain small. Obstructions at the level of the foramina of Luschka and Magendie, or of the basal cisterns, will result in dilatation of all four ventricles. This condition may be seen when there is meningeal scarring following meningitis, subarachnoid haemorrhage, or significant cranial trauma. It may also occur in congenital anomalies, such as the Dandy–Walker syndrome or the Arnold–Chiari malformation (Table 13.2).

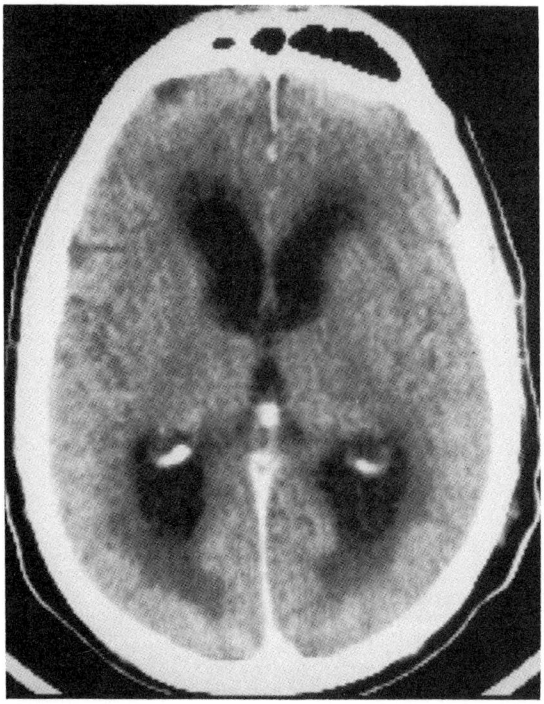

Fig. 13.5 CT scan showing dilatation of the lateral ventricles with periventricular low density (oedema) indicative of acute hydrocephalus.

Table 13.2 Causes of obstructive hydrocephalus

Congenital	Acquired
Aqueduct stenosis	Aqueduct stenosis due to adhesions or granuloma
Dandy–Walker syndrome	Intraventricular haematoma
Arnold–Chiari malformation	Intraventricular tumours
Vein of Galen aneurysm	Meningioma Colloid cyst Ependymoma
	Parenchymal tumours
	Pineal region Posterior fossa
	Abscesses
	Granuloma
	Arachnoid cysts

Communicating hydrocephalus

This condition will arise under two circumstances. The first, which is very rare, is due to over-

Table 13.3 Causes of communicating hydrocephalus

Leptomeningeial thickening
Infection
Subarachnoid haemorrhage
Trauma
Carcinomatous meningitis
Excess c.s.f. production
Choroid plexus papilloma
Increased c.s.f. viscosity
High protein content
Venous sinus thrombosis

production of c.s.f. which is seen occasionally with choroid plexus papillomas. The second, and by far the more common, is in those situations in which the arachnoid granulations have been damaged by previous meningitis, subarachnoid haemorrhage, or following cranial trauma and where they are no longer adequate to allow normal resorption of fluid from the c.s.f. In both cases the volume of cerebrospinal fluid will be increased, either by excess production or by inadequate absorption, resulting in hydrocephalus. It is a theoretical possibility that occlusion of the venous sinuses could likewise result in failure of the arachnoid granulations which feed into it to transport the normal quantities of c.s.f. but there is considerable doubt as to whether dural sinus thrombosis does in fact give rise to the syndrome of hydrocephalus, though it is recognised that it may cause cerebral infarction and is possibly responsible for cerebral oedema.

One form of communicating hydrocephalus is termed normal pressure hydrocephalus, which is described in the following section (Table 13.3).

Hydrocephalus ex vacuo

In generalised cerebral atrophy or localised under development of the cerebrum (porencephaly), the increase in cerebrospinal fluid will be compensatory and is termed hydrocephalus ex vacuo (Fig. 13.6).

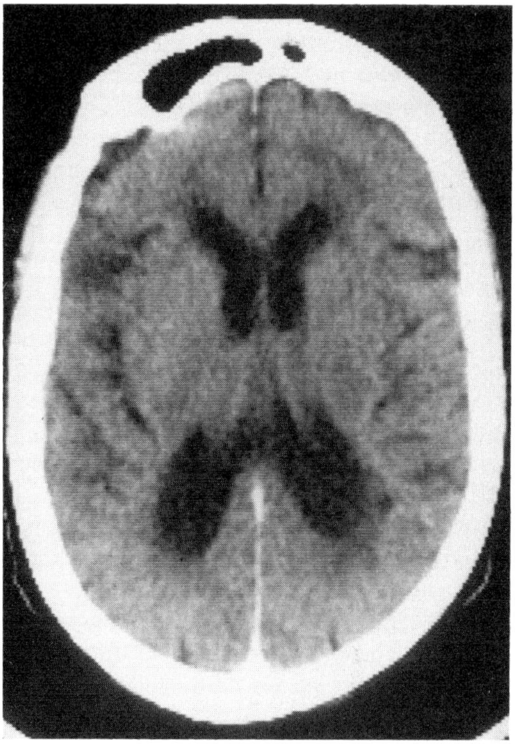

A

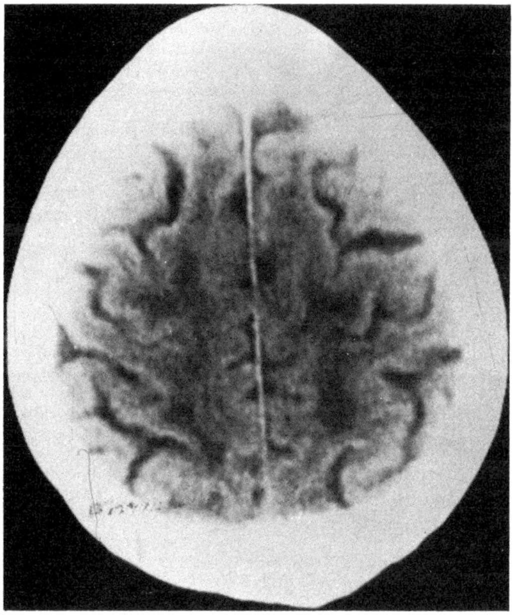

B

Fig. 13.6 **A** and **B** CT scan showing evidence of generalised cerebral atrophy with **A** ventricular dilation and **B** cortical atrophy.

CLINICAL FEATURES

The symptoms of hydrocephalus will depend upon the cause and also upon the age at which it develops. The two major syndromes are those of overt hydrocephalus, in which there is craniomegaly, and covert hydrocephalus, in which there is no such obvious physical stigma. Since the bones of the cranium fuse within the first two years of life, hydrocephalus must begin before this time to result in craniomegaly.

Infantile hydrocephalus

Hydrocephalus developing in the neonate and young child is usually due to the presence of a malformation such as the Arnold–Chiari malformation and the Dandy–Walker syndrome, or aqueductal stenosis or atresia and rarely due to cerebral haemorrhage or neonatal infection. The head will tend to enlarge rapidly with bulging of the fontanelle. The child gradually becomes drowsy and there is the classic appearance of the face with retraction of the lids and downturning of the eyes. There is also paralysis of upward gaze, the so-called 'setting sun' sign followed by the development of corticospinal tract signs, retardation and problems of mobility.

Non-communicating hydrocephalus

The increasing fluid within the cranium results in raised intracranial pressure, bifrontal and bioccipital headache and the development of a bilateral frontal lobe disorder. The symptoms of raised intracranial pressure which have been previously described will occur and, in addition, there is a deterioration in gait; there may be epileptic seizures and the enlargement of the third ventricle into the pituitary fossa can result in the presentation of pituitary dysfunction. Sphincters become involved and the patient develops bilateral papilloedema, primitive reflexes and a spastic tetraparesis which is more marked in the legs than the arms.

Normal pressure hydrocephalus

This is characteristically the picture seen in patients with communicating hydrocephalus in which there appears to be a compensation between the production of c.s.f. and the failure to resorb. There is a characteristic triad of clinical signs with a slowly progressive gait disorder, impairment of mental function and sphincter disturbance resulting in incontinence. The patient does not show papilloedema, but there will be signs of frontal lobe disturbance and frequently symmetrically brisk reflexes. This form of communicating hydrocephalus will follow subarachnoid haemorrhage, meningitis, chronic granulomatous meningitis and cerebral trauma. In some cases, no predisposing history can be determined.

INVESTIGATIONS

The advent of CT scanning has seen the ending of the great majority of investigations to determine the site and nature of obstruction in hydrocephalus. Skull X-ray may reveal changes suggesting the presence of hydrocephalus, including the 'copper beaten' appearance of the skull together with an enlarged pituitary fossa (Fig. 13.7). Flattened posterior clinoid processes and a relatively small posterior fossa may indicate the presence of aqueduct stenosis.

A CT scan, including contrast examination, will be likely to show which ventricles are dilated, and frequently the site and cause of the obstruction. If all ventricles are dilated then the possibility is of a communicating hydrocephalus. There is now little indication to proceed to other investigations, such as air encephalography, ventriculography or rhisa cisternography. Occasionally, intracranial pressure monitoring is used in patients with communicating hydrocephalus and may reveal that there are plateau waves of increased pressure, particularly during the sleeping hours, which may account for the development of the ventricular dilatation seen in normal pressure hydrocephalus.

THERAPY

The therapy for hydrocephalus consists essentially of removing the underlying cause, if this is possible, as in the case of colloid cysts of the third ventricle, intraventricular meningioma or other obstructive causes. Failing this the pressure can be relieved by the insertion of a ventriculoatrial or ventriculoperitoneal shunt. A valve on the

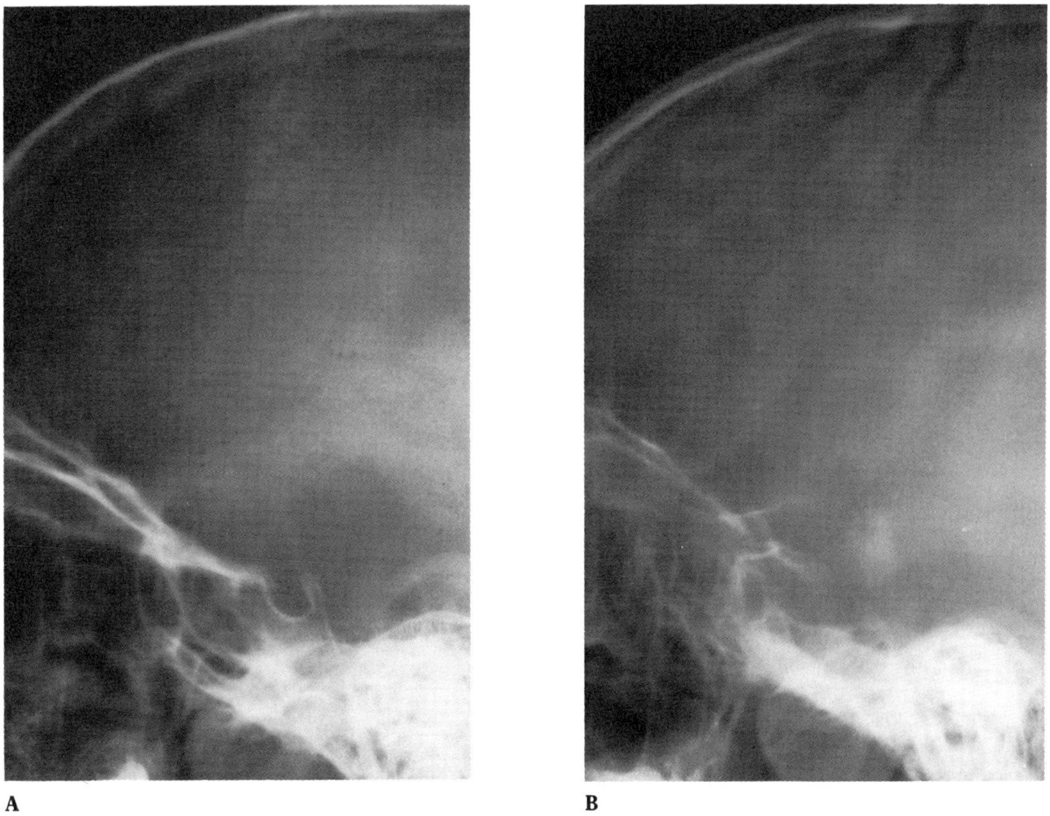

Fig. 13.7 **A** Normal appearance in 7-year-old. **B** Skull radiograph showing posterior clinoid erosion in a child with raised intracranial pressure. Suture diastasis and 'copper beating' are also seen.

shunt may be set at the appropriate pressure to allow c.s.f. to escape from the ventricle into the blood or peritoneal cavity. The risk of inserting shunts into patients with hydrocephalus is that the reduction of pressure within the cranium may result in collapse of the cerebral hemispheres away from the cranial wall and the consequent development of hygroma or subdural haematoma. If patients deteriorate after ventricular shunting they should always be investigated with a CT scan lest one or other of these complications has developed.

COMPLICATIONS

There are more long-term complications of the use of intra-atrial shunts, including the risk of infection, the need for repeated replacements in children as growth occurs and the possibility of fibrin and platelet emboli being released from the shunt into the bloodstream. For these reasons many surgeons are now electing to use ventriculo-peritoneal shunts, which have the advantage of being longer lasting and are probably freer from complications (Table 13.4).

Table 13.4 Complications of ventriculoatrial and ventriculoperitoneal shunts

Infection
Meningitis
Peritonitis
Subcutaneous
Bacteraemia
Subdural haematoma
Shunt obstruction
Low pressure state
Platelet fibrin emboli (VA shunts only)
Shunt nephritis
Thrombosis of internal jugular vein (VA shunts only)

BENIGN INTRACRANIAL HYPERTENTION (pseudotumour cerebri)

INCIDENCE

This is a rare syndrome occurring in approximately 2 patients per 100 000 per year. It is most commonly seen in obese young women with menstrual irregularities. It is used to describe a group of patients with raised intracranial pressure and no evidence for any mass lesion or hydrocephalus.

AETIOLOGY

In most patients no particular cause for the syndrome can be identified, other than that they are female, relatively young and often overweight. There are, however, certain recognised causes of benign intracranial hypertension (Table 13.5). It is seen as a complication of hypervitaminosis A and may occur with endocrine abnormalities, such as pregnancy, menarche, menstrual irregularities and Addison's disease. It has been reported in patients with iron deficiency anaemia and with polycythaemia rubra vera. It is recognised to occur in certain patients taking oral contraceptives, has been related to steroid withdrawal and occurs with tetracycline and nalidixic acid therapy. It was originally suggested to occur in patients who had lateral sinus thrombosis complicating middle ear infection, hence its alternative name of otitic hydrocephalus and there is evidence that some patients now may have venous sinus thrombosis when presenting with this syndrome.

The mechanisms of the syndrome are not fully established, though there appears to be generalised cerebral oedema which may be due both to excessive c.s.f. production and to reduced absorption.

Table 13.5 Causes of benign intracranial hypertension

Intracranial sinus thrombosis
Diet
Obesity
Hypervitaminosis A
Endocrine
Pregnancy
Menarche
Menstrual irregularities
Addison's disease
Haematological
Iron deficiency anaemia
Polycythaemia rubra vera
Drugs
Oral contraceptives
Steroid withdrawal
Tetracyclines
Nalidixic acid

CLINICAL FEATURES

The history usually suggests gradually increasing intracranial pressure over a period of weeks or months, giving rise to headache as the first symptom, occasionally with blurring of vision or even visual obscurations. Examination reveals gross bilateral papilloedema without any significant focal intracranial signs.

Rarely, other signs have been described in benign intracranial hypertension, in particular sixth nerve palsies and occasional lateralising long-tract signs, but when these are present they should always be regarded with grave suspicion.

INVESTIGATIONS

The diagnosis is one of exclusion and it is mandatory that patients be investigated with a CT scan to exclude the possibility of a structural cause for raised intracranial pressure, or to indicate the presence of hydrocephalus. In benign intracranial hypertension the CT scan will usually show normal or small ventricles without any evidence of structural space occupying lesions. C.s.f. pressure may then be measured at lumbar puncture, an important investigation to exclude the possibility of chronic meningitis. Lumbar puncture can be therapeutic in this syndrome in that the removal of c.s.f. will tend to result in the relief of symptoms.

Although it was not previously felt justified to investigate patients with angiography because of the risks of this procedure, the advent of digital subtraction angiography has made this investigation relatively safe. Such studies may show the venous phase of the intracranial circulation and some patients are found to have evidence of venous sinus thrombosis.

TREATMENT

Repeated lumbar puncture may be used to reduce the pressure and to alleviate the symptoms. Steroids tend to give symptomatic relief and diuretics may also be used to achieve a reduction in intracranial pressure. All of these measures are, however, temporary, but the disease is frequently self limiting and patients may show spontaneous recovery. It has been suggested that advice about diet is useful for those patients who are obese and may also help to bring about resolution of the symptoms.

In patients in whom visual obscurations become a problem, or in whom the other methods fail to give relief, the possibility of lumboperitoneal shunting should be considered, creating a persisting fistula between the lumba theca and the peritoneum and allowing the c.s.f. pressure to be reduced.

CEREBRAL TUMOURS

INTRODUCTION AND INCIDENCE

Tumours of the central nervous system account for only approximately 5% of all neoplasms in the body, but almost 20% of patients dying of other tumours will be shown to have intracranial metastases, about one-quarter of which are symptomatic. Thus approximately one-half of all patients presenting with cerebral tumours will have a secondary tumour rather than a primary brain tumour.

The incidence of primary brain tumours is difficult to assess and appears to vary in different countries. In the western hemisphere, for every 100 000 of the population there are approximately 10–15 patients presenting with primary brain tumours each year. The types of tumour also vary from population to population, but in Europe and North America the commonest are tumours of the glial cells, which account for 30% of all primary brain tumours, followed by meningiomas, 20%, and craniopharyngiomas and pituitary tumours which make up a little over 10%. The remainder of the tumours comprise other parenchymal growths, some of vascular origin, and a proportion, variously estimated at about 5%, which cannot be histologically identified (Table 13.6).

Table 13.6 The frequency of primary intracranial tumours

	Child (%)	Adult (%)
Neuroepithelial		
Medulloblastoma	25	5
Spongioblastoma	26	8
Oligodendroglioma	1	9
Astroglioma	3	7
Glioblastoma	<1	14
Ependymoma	12	<1
Choroid plexus papilloma	3	<1
Pinealoma	<1	<1
Mesodermal		
Meningioma	2	21
Angioblastic meningioma	<1	1
Sarcoma	3	4
Chordoma	<1	<1
Ectodermal		
Craniopharyngioma	6	4
Pituitary	<1	9
Glomus	<1	<1
Maldevelopment		
Dermoid/epidermoid	<1	2
Vascular		
Arteriovenous malformation	6	4
Other	7	7

The prevalence of different tumour types also varies with age: thus in the child medulloblastomas of the posterior fossa account for more than 50% of all cerebral tumours, whereas in the adult secondaries, gliomas and meningiomas are much more common. Of all secondaries, the most common are from primary tumours in the lung, followed by tumours in the breast and kidney. Some tumours, such as those from ovary and colon, virtually never metastasise to brain.

CLINICAL FEATURES

The presentation of a cerebral tumour will depend upon the site of the lesion and the speed of growth. It is possible to divide the symptoms with which the patient presents and the signs which may be discovered on examination into those which indicate the presence of raised intracranial pressure, those which are due to focal effects of the underlying tumour upon a particular area or areas of brain and those which are false localising signs.

The symptoms of raised intracranial pressure

These which have been detailed earlier in the chapter include headache, changes in mental function and alertness, vomiting, dizziness, visual difficulties and non-focal seizures. The signs which indicate raised intracranial pressure consist of papilloedema, neck stiffness, hyper-reflexia and a sixth nerve palsy (Table 13.7).

Focal symptoms and signs

The focal symptoms and signs necessarily depend upon the area of the brain in which tumour growth occurs. Their nature will depend to an extent upon whether the effect of the growth is irritative or destructive in nature. If the growth is irritating, then many of the symptoms will have the features of epilepsy and be 'positive' in nature. If destructive, then the consequent damage to the tissue will result in loss of function of the brain involved. In addition the focal presentation will depend upon the relative importance of the area of brain involved with the tumour. Thus, a tumour growing in the dominant frontal or parietal lobe will be more likely to present at an early stage due to problems with speech and communication than one growing in the right side of the brain. The most important focal symptoms which may occur with brain tumours are described in the following section and also in Chapter 6.

Table 13.7 Clinical features of cerebral tumours

Raised intracranial pressure
Headache
Vomiting
Papilloedema
Focal features
Focal epilepsy
Destructive symptoms
False localising signs
Sixth nerve palsy
Rarely other cranial nerve palsy
Long-tract signs

Frontal lobe

Tumours growing in or compressing the frontal lobe may cause evident changes in personality and frequently alter learned behaviour. Thus the patient may show evidence of disinhibition: there may be incontinence of sphincters and emotion and a general retardation. Such classic features of frontal lobe disturbance are seen more commonly when both frontal lobes are involved, usually with spread across the corpus callosum. Frontal lobe tumours may involve the motor pathways on one side and result in contralateral disturbances of motor function. If the tumour is irritative then focal motor seizures may ensue, spreading either with a Jacksonian march or rapid generalisation to give tonic-clonic seizures. Status epilepticus is a not uncommon presentation of frontal lobe tumours. Those tumours which are destructive will result in pareses, most commonly with spasticity and rarely flaccidity of the contralateral limbs and may rarely produce the syndrome of apraxia, in which no paralysis is apparent but the limb is no longer useful.

Examination will frequently reveal the development of primitive reflexes in such patients, bilateral damage giving rise to a pout reflex together with a brisk jaw jerk and unilateral damage to a palmar–mental reflex and a grasp reflex on the contralateral side. In addition, there may of course be changes in the deep tendon reflexes on the contralateral side and evidence of a significant paresis.

Patients with lesions in the dominant frontal lobe may also show evidence of dysphasia. Lesions in the frontal lobe will most commonly result in the so-called anterior or non-fluent dysphasia in that the production of words will be poor, but comprehension will be relatively normal.

Parietal lobe

Lesions in the parietal lobe will affect the sensory cortex and those which cause irritation will produce dysaesthesia, tingling and pins and needles in the contralateral limbs together with focal sensory epilepsy. Destructive lesions will tend to result in loss of sensation varying from subtle problems of agnosia to the more gross difficulties with anaesthesia and loss of awareness. In addition, patients will frequently show visual disturbances most characteristically in the form of a contralateral inferior quadrantanopia and they may also have difficulty with inattention in the contralateral field, a problem which may extend to involve sensation on the contralateral side of the body. Patients with non-dominant parietal lobe tumours will have problems of spacial orientation and may present with symptoms of dressing apraxia, topographical agnosia and constructional apraxia. Patients with dominant parietal lobe tumours may show difficulties with speech, most typically with a posterior dysphasia in that production of speech may be reasonably fluent but comprehension will be poor.

Temporal lobe

Lesions in the temporal lobe may be more difficult to identify clinically, although those on the dominant side will usually present with a posterior, or fluent dysphasia and difficulties in comprehension. A common presentation of tumours in the temporal lobe is with partial or secondary generalised seizures, the former causing olfactory or gustatory hallucinations, occasionally auditory aura and frequently psychomotor episodes in which the patient will see or hear organised hallucinations. Temporal lobe tumours may also present with difficulties with memory though, since this function is represented bilaterally, this is not invariable. Tumours in the non-dominant temporal lobe are particularly likely to be clinically silent, presenting with a syndrome of raised intracranial pressure.

Occipital lobe tumours

Lesions in the occipital lobe rarely present with focal or partial seizures, phenomena which take the form of flashes of light or spots and shimmering in the contralateral field, but more commonly produce hemianopia due to destruction of one or other calcarine cortex or the pathways subserving vision.

Cerebellar tumours

Tumours in the posterior fossa most commonly cause raised intracranial pressure early in their course due to the relative vulnerability of the aqueduct to pressure and consequent development of hydrocephalus. None the less, hemispheric cerebellar lesions may indeed present with unilateral ataxia, often associated with a degree of truncal ataxia and ocasionally with dysarthria. Cerebellar hemisphere lesions will cause ipsilateral clinical symptoms rather than the contralateral symptoms seen with cerebral hemisphere lesions.

Brain stem tumours

Tumours growing in the brain stem are also likely to cause hydrocephalus at an early stage of their development and therefore to present with raised intracranial pressure. They are also identifiable by their tendency to cause damage to cranial nerve nuclei, with or without involvement of the descending pathways passing through the brain stem. Patients thus tend to present with cranial nerve abnormalities but little in the way of long tract signs.

Intraventricular tumours

Midline intraventricular tumours, such as colloid cysts of the third ventricle or ependymomas of the fourth ventricle, may produce relatively little in the way of focal signs and simply present with intermittent hydrocephalus due to a valve-like effect. Meningiomas in the lateral ventricles most commonly present with a homonymous hemianopia on the contralateral side together with symptoms of raised intracranial pressure.

Other midline tumours

Pinealomas tend to present with raised intracranial pressure due to distortion of the posterior part of the third ventricle, and tumours of the sella and suprasellar region most commonly present with problems affecting vision, classically a bitemporal hemianopia.

SPECIFIC TUMOUR SYNDROMES

Metastatic carcinoma

Secondary tumours are the commonest form of space-occupying tumour within the cranium. They reach the brain by haematogenous spread; about one-third of them are secondaries from the lung and a little under 20% from the breast. Melanoma is the third most frequent metastasing tumour to the brain, followed by gastrointestinal tract neoplasms, urogenital neoplasms and lymphomas. Metastasis to the skull and dura also occurs from the breast, prostate and kidneys (Table 13.8). Secondary tumours may present in the context of a recognised and previously diagnosed primary tumour, but may also be the initial manifestation of neoplasia originating elsewhere in the body. The rate of growth of secondary tumours, and therefore the rate of clinical presentation, is typically rapid. The symptoms of raised intracranial pressure together with focal symptoms due to the particular site of the lesion develop within days or weeks. Epilepsy is a relatively common presenting sign of such tumours and in almost 50% of patients the lesions will be found to be multiple so that the presence of raised intracranial pressure, together with diffuse or multifocal clinical signs, should raise the possibility of metastatic carcinoma. Cerebellar metastases are particularly common and in adults a secondary tumour is the commonest space-occupying lesion in the cerebellar hemisphere. They tend to present with symptoms of ataxia and rapid development of raised intracranial pressure due to obstruction of the c.s.f. pathways.

Table 13.8 Common primary sites for cerebral metastases

Bronchus	Stomach
Breast	Prostate
Kidney	Testes
Thyroid	Melanoma

Secondary tumours may infiltrate the meninges causing chronic meningitis and resulting in the symptoms of chronic headache, raised intracranial pressure and multiple cranial nerve palsies. Carcinomatous meningitis may cause loss of reflexes due to spinal meningeal involvement.

If a primary tumour is already identified, investigation may not be warranted, but where doubt exists the investigation of patients with suspected metastatic tumour is by CT scan and the management will depend upon the site, nature and number of the tumours identified (Fig. 13.8). In patients in whom the primary is already identified, or can be identified at the time of presentation, management will depend upon the nature of the primary and the accessibility of a solitary secondary. In those patients in whom a secondary tumour is suspected but not proven, there may be an indication for biopsy or decompression to provide a tissue diagnosis and, rarely, to obtain relief of symptoms. There are certain occasions in which, even though the nature of the primary tumour is known, the fact that the cerebral tumour is seen to be solitary and easily accessible might indicate the desirability of surgical removal. Tumours in the posterior fossa are frequently treated by surgery simply to alleviate the devastating symptoms.

In most cases of cerebral metastasis the prognosis is very poor although, with identification of the particular type of tumour, it may be possible to undertake certain more specific therapies such as radiotherapy and chemotherapy, particularly in the case of intracerebral lymphoma or breast carcinoma. Radiotherapy without surgery may be used as palliative treatment for cerebral secondaries. The mainstay of palliative management for patients with cerebral secondaries is steroids, which will frequently give short-term benefit in such patients and result in dramatic resolution of symptoms. They are, however, merely palliative and terminal care with adequate analgesia will then become necessary.

In general, in patients with no other evidence of systemic cancer, the median survival period for patients with solitary metastasis treated by excision and radiotherapy is approximately two years after operation. In patients with other

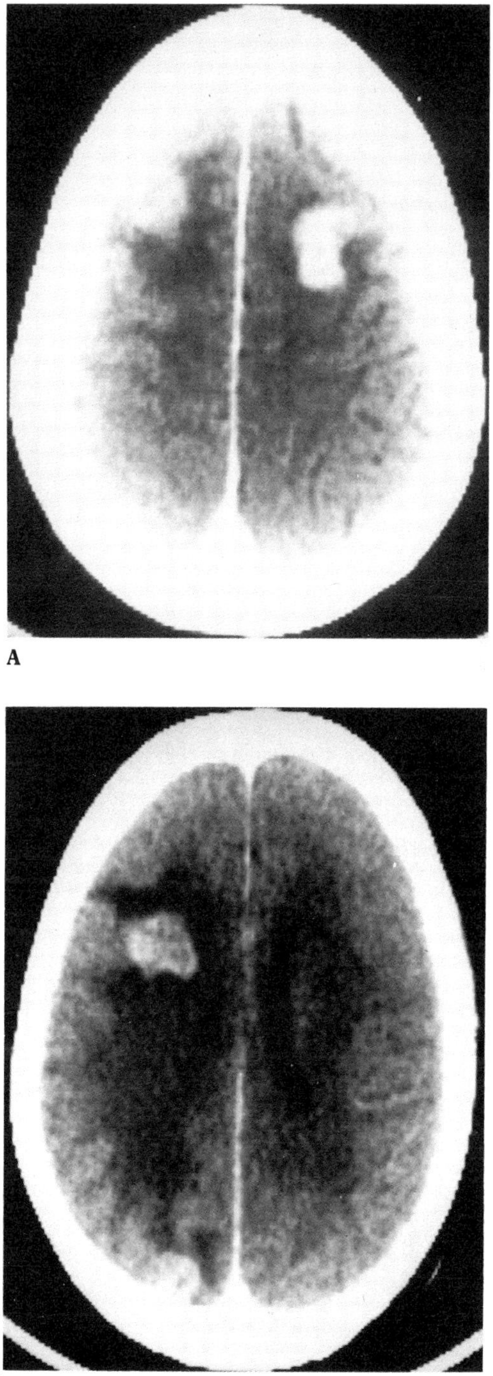

A

B

Fig. 13.8 **A** and **B** CT scans following enhancement showing the presence of multiple cerebral secondary deposits. In **B** note the presence of marked surrounding cerebral oedema (low density).

evidence of systemic disease the results of therapy are less good and the median survival is of the order of six months. In patients with multiple metastasis operative removal is seldom indicated and, if the possibilities of multiple abscesses or tuberculomata can be excluded, whole brain radiation may be used, but the prognosis may be measured in months.

Astrocytoma

The astrocytoma, which is the commonest primary tumour of brain, may occur at any age, but is most common between the ages of 40 and 60 years. It is twice as common in males as females. The tumours occur equally throughout the frontal, temporal and parietal lobes, but are uncommon in the occipital lobes. In children the juvenile astrocytoma is found in the optic nerve, hypothalamus and cerebellum.

Pathologically the tumours are divided by microscopic examination into four grades (Kernahan grades I–IV), but it is frequently difficult to identify precisely the grade of an individual tumour. It is more practically useful to describe the tumours in terms of those which are malignant, such as the glioblastoma multiforme (Kernahan grades IV), the malignant astrocytoma (Kernahan grade III–IV) and a separate group of low-grade astrocytoma (Kernahan grades I–II).

Malignant Astrocytoma

The more aggressive forms of malignant astrocytoma and glioblastoma multiforme constitute almost 50% of primary intracranial tumours. Their growth is rapid and they infiltrate widely into adjacent brain. At autopsy more than 75% can be shown to have microscopic spread to distant sites within the central nervous system and frequently to the contralateral hemisphere. There may occasionally be evidence, both histologically and on CT scan, for the tumour spreading across the corpus callosum as the so-called 'butterfly' astrocytoma.

Patients present with seizures, signs and symptoms of focal brain destruction and signs and symptoms of raised intracranial pressure. The evolution of symptoms tends to be over weeks or months. Sometimes patients will show sudden deterioration, possibly due to a haemorrhage inside a necrotic area of tumour, although pathologically this is a rare occurrence and it seems more likely that sudden deteriorations are due to the development of significant cerebral oedema.

The skull X-ray may show erosion of the dorsum sella or shift of a calcified pineal, but in general is of little help. A CT scan is the investigation of choice and malignant astrocytomas and glioblastoma multiforme will tend to show a plane of distinction between tumour and brain. There may occasionally be an area of surrounding low density due to cerebral oedema and frequently ventricular compression and midline shift are demonstrated (Fig. 13.9).

It may occasionally be difficult to differentiate a glioblastoma from a cerebral abscess and any doubts necessitate biopsy to establish the diagnosis and exclude a treatable lesion.

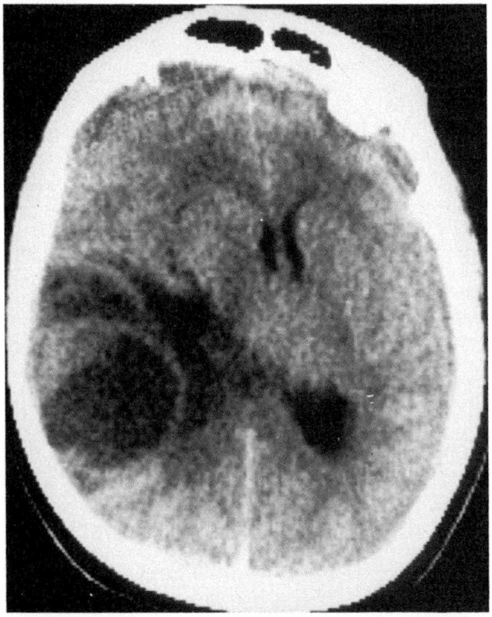

A

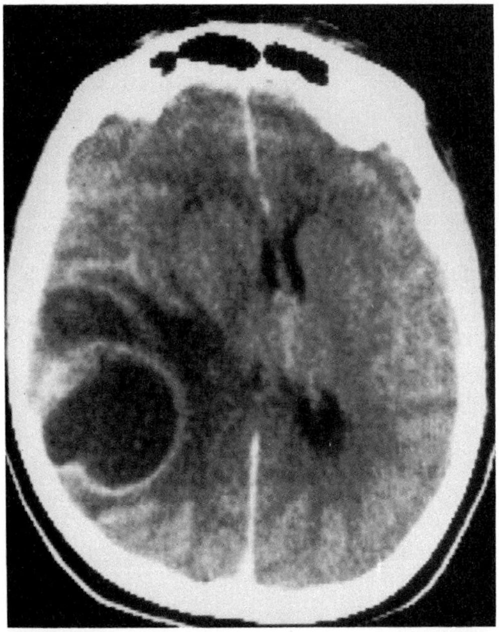

B

Fig. 13.9 **A** CT scan of right parietal cerebral glioma prior to the administration of contrast. **B** The same patient following the administration of contrast.

Low-grade astrocytoma

Low-grade astrocytomas are more common in children and in young adults, making up approximately 15% of primary intracranial tumours. They are the tumours identified as Kernahan grades I and II and are diffuse but slow growing, comprised histologically of astrocytes which may be identified as fibrillary, protoplasmic or gemistocytic. The fact that they are low grade should not be taken to indicate that they are benign, since they tend to infiltrate surrounding brain and have no definitive edge or capsule. Many of these tumours will show evidence of calcification which may be visible on skull X-ray. Again the investigation of choice is a CT scan, which may either show a low-density region giving no enhancement with contrast, or possibly a cystic lesion with an area of contrast enhancement.

Whilst the evidence of focal signs which show progression over weeks or months indicates the likelihood of a cerebral glioma, and the presence of raised intracranial pressure demands urgent investigation, it is also important to remember that patients who present with seizures, but whose control is difficult, may also be harbouring such a growth.

Management

Once a single and possibly primary cerebral tumour is identified by CT scan, management of the patient will then depend upon many individual factors. In those patients who have an apparently malignant tumour which crosses the midline and which could not be totally removed, it is reasonable to undertake palliative therapy with steroids and to consider radiotherapy and chemotherapy. The question as to whether or not a tissue diagnosis should be obtained is a vexed one. There is evidence that CT appearances may be misleading in up to 5% of patients with a clinical and CT scan diagnosis of glioma. This risk of missing benign pathology such as meningioma or abscess has lead most surgeons to recommend biopsy in all patients. The technique of burr hole biopsy has been commonly used, but is complicated by a significant number of patients suffering haemorrhage and deterioration at the time of biopsy. For this reason many surgeons favour open biopsy, although the newer techniques of sterotactic biopsy may reduce the risk of complication and improve the use of this technique.

In other tumours, which are assumed on CT scan appearances to be malignant but in which there is some doubt of diagnosis, or when the tumour is eminently accessible, decompressive surgery may be performed—though it is rarely possible to achieve complete excision of the tumour. In terms of surgical management of cerebral tumours, the older methods of suction excision of the tumour are being replaced to an extent by CT-guided surgery and even sterotactic surgery, particularly for the deeper tumours. When the diagnosis of the tumour is substantiated, consideration should be given to the use of radiotherapy and to cytotoxic therapy. The latter technique has been of little use to date in the management of patients with cerebral gliomas, but the newer techniques of tissue culture of tumours, followed by investigation of their responsiveness to various chemotherapeutic agents, provides a potential for improved chemotherapy in the future.

The more benign tumours may be excised completely and this is particularly true of astrocytomas in childhood. Again it is common to use radiotherapy after surgery in these patients, though the advent of CT scanning means that the progress of the patient after surgery may be monitored by non-invasive methods and radiotherapy may then be deferred.

A major problem exists in those patients who present with epilepsy but without focal signs, who have an evidently focal EEG and in whom a CT scan reveals a probable glioma. The vexed question arises as to whether the patient should be managed conservatively with anticonvulsant therapy and followed with repeated CT scans, or whether an attempted biopsy should be undertaken at the time of initial diagnosis and aggressive surgery and radiotherapy considered. Many factors, such as the age of the patient, the certainty of diagnosis and the accessibility of the presumed tumour, must be taken into acount before making such decisions.

Unfortunately the great majority of patients with cerebral tumours have a limited life expectancy: median survival is only three to four months, though more benign tumours may allow survival for many years even without aggressive treatment. Anti-seizure therapy is indicated and ultimately terminal care needs to be established, when palliation with steroids may help and adequate analgesia is essential. Patients with diagnosed cerebral tumours are ineligible to hold driving licences, even if they have not suffered seizures, and a decision as to how much information to give to the patient and relatives will depend upon individual circumstances.

Oligodendroglioma

These tumours of the oligodendrocytes are less malignant than astrocytomas and tend to occur in a younger age group, with the maximum incidence between 30 and 50 years. They are most commonly found in the frontal lobes and up to 40% will have calcification. They may occasionally involve the ependyma of the ventricle and cause seeding throughout the ventricular system. The presentation of such tumours is frequently with seizures, though they may occasionally present with slowly developing focal signs. The investigation is again with CT scan, which will show a well-demarcated tumour and frequently reveal areas of clacification (Fig. 13.10). They form only

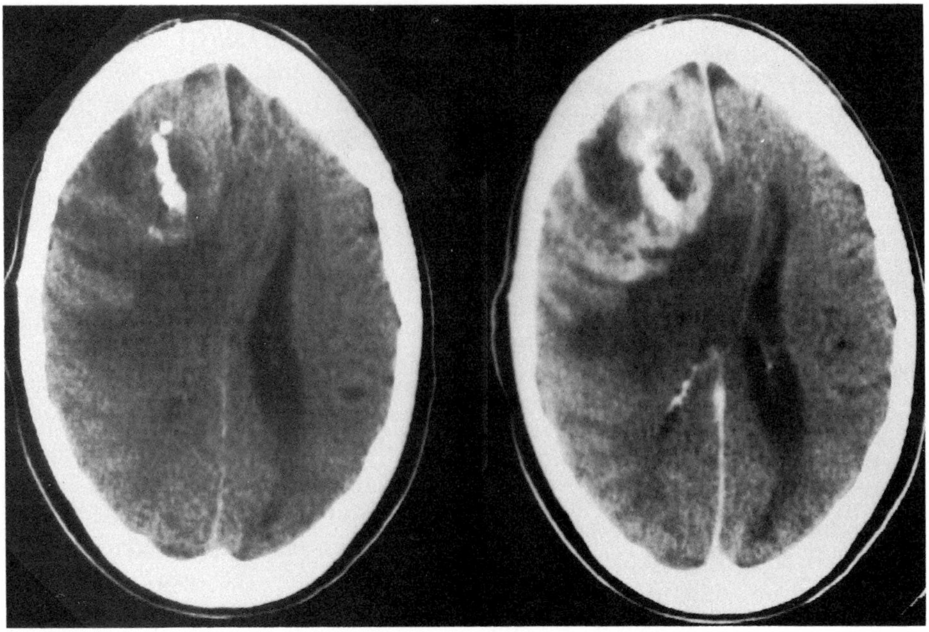

Fig. 13.10 CT scan of oligodendroglioma with calcification (left). Scan on right shows appearance following contrast enhancement.

approximately 10% of primary intracranial tumours and in view of their slow-growing nature the survival time is considerable. In most series, symptoms have been present for almost a decade before the diagnosis is made. Surgical excision is the treatment of choice since radiotherapy has doubtful effects and the long-term survival may reach as much as 20 years.

Ependymoma

This glial tumour arising from the ependymal cells is most commonly found in the fourth ventricle, though they may occasionally be seen in the third ventricle and in the caudal part of the spinal cord. They are most commonly found in the young and have a peak incidence in children and in the early 20s.

The tumours which present in the fourth ventricle tend to cause symptoms of intermittent raised intracranial pressure due to hydrocephalus, though they may cause cerebellar signs and symptoms of ataxia, vertigo and vomiting. The investigation of choice is a CT scan, which tends to show an isodense mass with or without calcification within the fourth ventricle and which usually shows enhancement with contrast. The management is surgical excision, though infiltration into the floor of the fourth ventricle often prevents total excision and postoperative radiotherapy is indicated.

Meningioma

These usually benign tumours are uncommon in childhood, but probably account for some 20% of primary intracranial tumours in adults. They arise from the arachnoid cells and are most common in the sylvian region, the parasagittal surface of the parietal and frontal lobes, the olfactory grooves, the lesser wings of the sphenoid, the tuberculum sellae and the cerebellopontine angle. They may occasionally invade and erode the cranial bones or cause an osteoblastic reaction of the skull, either of which phenomena might be visible on plain skull X-ray and give indication to the diagnosis. Small meningiomas are often found at autopsy in middle-aged and elderly people having been apparently asymptomatic throughout life. Many of those which are asymptomatic can be shown to have been present for some 10–15 years prior to diagnosis.

The presentation will depend upon the site of the tumour, though up to 25% of patients will present with focal epilepsy. In the remainder, focal neurological signs may occur related to the site of growth and the symptoms and signs of raised intracranial pressure are common.

Parasagittal meningioma

Meningiomas arising in the parasagittal region tend to irritate and compress the areas of the primary motor and sensory cortex relating to the lower limbs. They may cause motor seizures of the lower limbs or pyramidal weakness in both lower limbs which can mimic a paraparesis. More posterior parasagittal tumours can present with visual disturbances in the form of homonymous hemianopia and more anterior parasagittal tumours may impair memory and intellect and result in dementia.

Convexity meningioma

Meningiomas arising over the convexity of the brain most commonly present with focal seizures due to local irritative pressure on the frontal or parietal lobes. The attacks may therefore be motor or sensory in nature and will tend to result in focal motor or sensory deficits. Meningiomas arising in the temporal region will tend to cause epilepsy of temporal lobe type and on the dominant side may result in dysphasia. The symptoms may be intermittent and can occasionally mimic transient ischaemic attacks. It may be many years before more permanent disability ensues followed by raised intracranial pressure.

Olfactory groove meningioma

Meningiomas arising on the olfactory groove will cause anosmia and may then compress the optic nerve, producing visual impairment with a central scotoma or other field defect. Optic atrophy is frequently present and when the size of the tumour results in raised intracranial pressure it may show the Foster-Kennedy syndrome of optic atrophy in one eye with papilloedema in the other.

Sphenoidal ridge meningioma

Meningiomas growing on the lesser wing of the sphenoid bone expand medially to involve the wall of the cavernous sinus, anteriorly to involve the orbit and laterally into the temporal bone. They are most common in women and the age at onset is usually over 50 years. The classic clinical features are of slowly developing exophthalmos, bulging of the bone in the temporal region and radiological evidence of thickening or erosion of the lesser wing of the sphenoid. Such tumours may occasionally account for the development of a painful eye or the evolution of blindness and optic atrophy in the eye. They may also cause seizures beginning in the temporal lobe as uncinate fits and ultimately will cause raised intracranial pressure. The involvement of the cavernous sinus may cause ptosis and impaired eye movements (third, fourth and sixth nerve palsies), together with facial pain and anaesthesia in the first division of the trigeminal nerve.

Tuberculum sellae meningioma

Meningiomas in the region of the tuberculum sellae will cause chiasmal compression and visual field defects similar to those seen with pituitary tumours. The differential diagnosis from a pituitary tumour may be difficult, but the presence of a meningioma can be suggested by the finding of hyperostosis of the tuberculum sellae on plain X-ray and confirmed by angiography.

Cerebellar pontine angle meningioma

Meningiomas growing in the cerebellar pontine angle will produce symptoms and signs similar to those of an acoustic neuroma. There may be loss of hearing in the ipsilateral ear, together with tinnitis and occasionally vertigo, a lower motor neurone seventh nerve palsy and altered sensation on the face ipsilaterally. The loss of a corneal reflex on the affected side is a common finding and growth of the tumour will result in ataxia on the ipsilateral side and, due to brain stem shift and compression of the contralateral cerebral peduncle, may also cause ipsilateral or contralateral pyramidal signs. Evidence of a progressing cerebellar pontine angle lesion in the absence of a hearing defect is more suggestive of a meningioma than of an acoustic neuroma.

Although most meningiomas are solitary, multiple meningiomas may occur and are particularly common in patients with the central form of neurofibromatosis.

Investigations

Plain skull X-ray may reveal features which indicate the likelihood of a meningioma, since 15% of these tumours will show areas of calcification within them (Fig. 13.11). In addition, there may be hyperostosis of the adjacent bone and meningiomas in the parasagittal or convexity regions can be associated with dilatation of the middle meningeal groove. There may of course be signs of raised intracranial pressure, demineralisation of the dorsum sella, but the pituitary fossa and internal auditory meati will appear normal.

The CT scan is the most important investigation and will typically reveal a well cirumscribed lesion of high density with surrounding low density due to cerebral oedema. Calcification may be seen on CT scan in up to 25% of cases (Fig. 13.12). When a meningioma is suspected, angiography should be undertaken to confirm the diagnosis and indicate the vascular supply of the tumour. It may be necessary to undertake four-vessel angiography in tumours in the posterior fossa. The angiogram will characteristically show a typical tumour blush and, because of the vascular nature of these tumours and the fact that they are usually supplied from the external carotid circulation, the possibility of selective catheterisation with embolisation has been suggested to reduce tumour vascularity and consequently reduce operative risks.

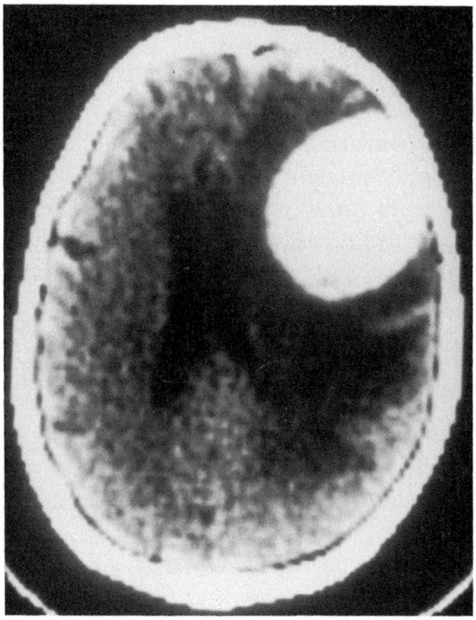

Fig. 13.12 CT scan of same patient as Figure 13.11 showing a subfrontal meningioma after the administration of contrast.

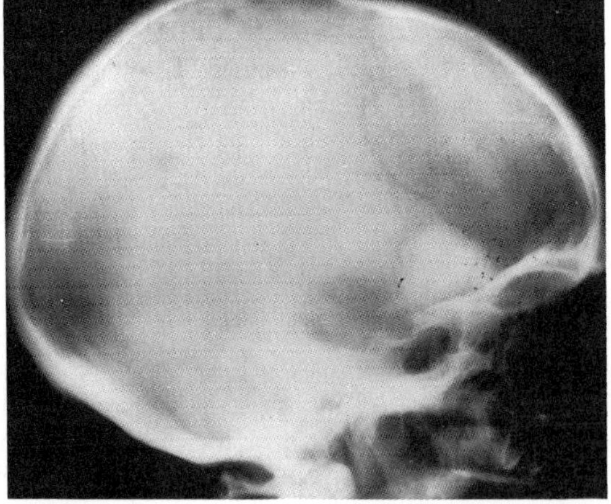

Fig. 13.11 Skull radiograph showing subfrontal calcification.

Management

The management of cerebral meningiomas depends to an extent upon the age of the patient and the accessibility of the tumour. Tumours in the elderly, or which are inaccessible and cause little in the way of symptoms, may be managed conservatively. In general the aim is to excise the tumour completely, though in the more malignant angioblastic meningiomas and those which have invaded the bone complete removal may not be possible. In terms of parasagittal meningiomas it is important to the surgeon to know whether or not the sagittal sinus is occluded before he undertakes surgery. Those tumours which have already occluded the sagittal sinus can be more safely removed than those which have not obliterated the sinus as surgical damage to the sinus can result in significant postoperative deficits.

When surgery is recognised to be incomplete, or where the site of the tumour prevents total excision, radiotherapy may be given though its value is unproven.

With modern techniques and the possibility of preoperative embolisation of feeding vessels the operative mortality should be of the order of 5% and the prognosis of survivors is good. Tumour recurrence will depend upon the completeness of removal and is seen in up to 30% of patients followed for more than 10 years. It is more common in tumours of the angioblastic type and in those which are evidently malignant.

Primary cerebral lymphoma (microglioma)

These diffuse parenchymal tumours of the nervous system can be both monofocal or multifocal in origin. They grow as rapidly as glioblastomas and tend to be much more diffuse: they are particularly common in immunosuppressed patients. Histologically they are due to primitive reticulum cells which have a perivascular distribution. The history from initial symptoms to presentation is usually short, of the order of three months, and the symptoms vary widely and are due to involvement of almost any part of the brain. Seizures, both focal and generalised, may occur together with evidence of focal cerebral disturbance.

The CT scan will tend to show either a poorly enhancing, low-density lesion, which may show some enhancement with contrast, the latter frequently being in the periventricular areas, or occasionally a strongly enhancing hyperdense lesion. Biopsy is essential for diagnosis once the presence of the tumour is suspected and radiotherapy may produce dramatic results, though the ultimate prognosis remains guarded. The possibility of chemotherapy, as in other forms of systemic lymphoma, can also be considered with both systemic and intrathecal chemotherapy.

Medulloblastoma

This tumour, which is confined to children, arises from embryonic tissue in the posterior part of the cerebellar vermis. It is one of the few intracranial tumours which may metastasise either within the cranium or into the spinal cord and give rise to seedlings of tumour, probably via the c.s.f. pathways. It is most commonly found between the ages of 4 and 8 years and is approximately twice as common in boys as in girls. The most common presentation is with listlessness, vomiting and early morning headache followed by the development of unsteadiness, falls and double vision. Examination will reveal the presence of paralytic strabismus together with ataxia, papilloedema and nystagmus. There is frequently neck stiffness due to tonsillar herniation caused by the tumour.

Diagnosis is by CT scan, which will show an isodense midline lesion in the cerebellum compressing and displacing the fourth ventricle and showing marked contrast enhancement (Fig. 13.13). There will also be the presence of hydrocephalus and there may be signs of c.s.f. tumour seeding within the ventricles. Angio-

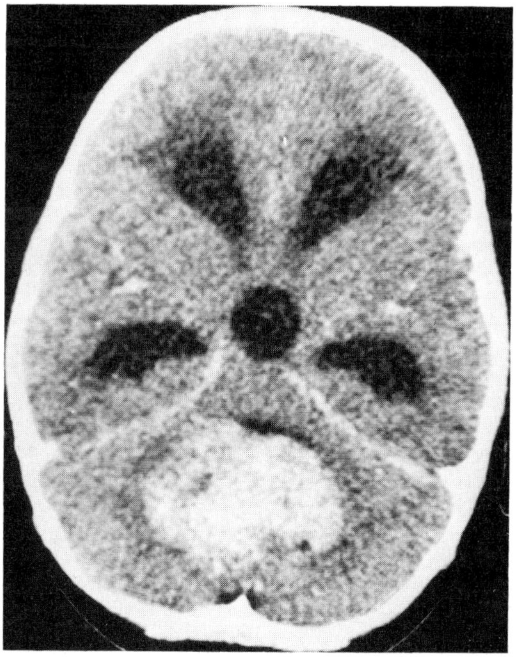

Fig. 13.13 CT scan of medulloblastoma following the administration of contrast.

graphy is occasionally indicated to identify the nature of the tumour.

The therapy is essentially surgical, possibly with a preoperative ventriculoperitoneal shunt although this provides a further potential route for tumour seeding and may carry the risk of an upward cerebellar cone. The tumours are highly radiosensitive and the patient should be subject to craniospinal irradiation to treat any undetected c.s.f. seeding. Chemotherapy does not yet have a part to play in the management of this tumour, but with radiotherapy the 5-year survival can be extended to as high as 70%.

The neuroblastoma which is discovered in young children is of a similar origin to the medulloblastoma, but when it metastasises to the cranium it tends to remain extradural in site. It is a tumour of the adrenal gland which may show wide spread metastases.

Hemangioblastoma

These tumours of vascular origin occur in young and middle-aged adults causing a cystic swelling in one or other cerebellar hemisphere. They may occasionally be multiple, occurring in the retina and spinal cord, and can be associated with polycythaemia due to the production of erythropoietin. In some families they are associated with cystic lesions in other tissues such as kidney and pancreas (von Hippel–Lindau disease). The typical history is of a rapid evolution of a cerebellar disturbance together with raised intracranial pressure. Occasionally subarachnoid haemorrhage may occur. It is slightly more common in males, but in female patients is one of the tumours which is more likely to present in pregnancy.

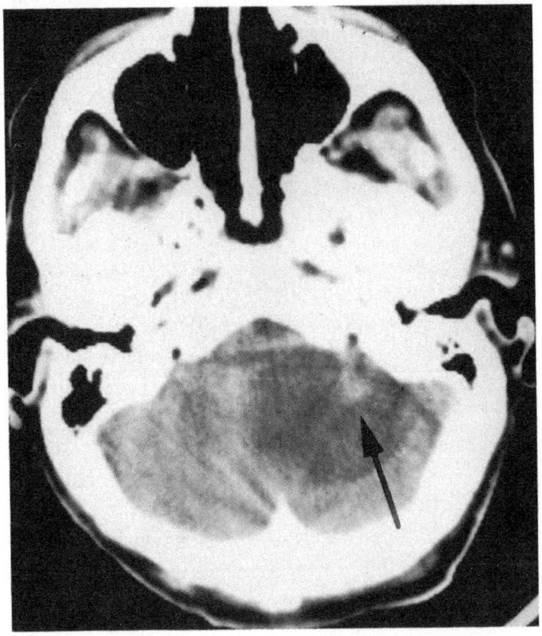

Fig. 13.14 CT scan following enhancement showing a cerebellar haemangioblastoma. A small enhancing nodule within the posterior fossa cyst is arrowed.

A CT scan may reveal a cystic lesion in the cerebellum with a small enhancing nodule in the wall (Fig. 13.14). There may occasionally be multiple lesions present, when the differentiation from metastases is vital. Angiography is indicated and will help to differentiate hemangioblastoma from secondary tumour.

The treatment is by operative removal, although recurrences, either at the same site or elsewhere, will occur in approximately 20%.

Pinealoma

The pinealoma is usually a teratoma rather than a tumour of the pineal gland itself. There are a variety of differing pathological types originating from the posterior part of the third ventricle. Histologically, teratomas with well-differentiated tissues, germinomas resembling seminomas of the testes, pinealcytomas and pinealblastomas of truly pineal origin and glial cell tumours, both astrocytomas and ependymomas, may occur at this site.

They most commonly present during the first three decades of life and cause hydrocephalus and the symptoms of raised intracranial pressure due to obstruction at the posterior part of the third ventricle. The characteristic clinical finding is of a patient with bilateral papilloedema and complete inability to elevate the eyes, together with dilated pupils with impaired response to light and accommodation (Parinaud's syndrome). The tumour sometimes shows spread around the third ventricle and may then be associated with hypothalamic disturbances including diabetes insipidus, hypophagia, precocious puberty, hypopituitarism and visual field defects.

The investigation is by CT scan, which shows a mass lesion projecting into the posterior aspect of the third ventricle with associated hydrocephalus. Pinealomas themselves may occasionally be calcified and all of the tumours may show enhancement (Fig. 13.15). C.s.f. cytology may reveal the presence of malignant cells and can indicate the tumour type. In some patients with germinomas there may be elevated levels of human chorionic gonadotrophin and alphafetoprotein in the serum and cerebrospinal fluid.

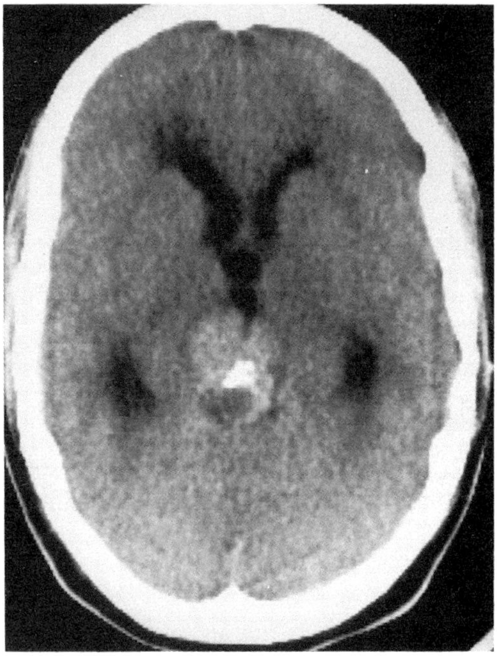

A

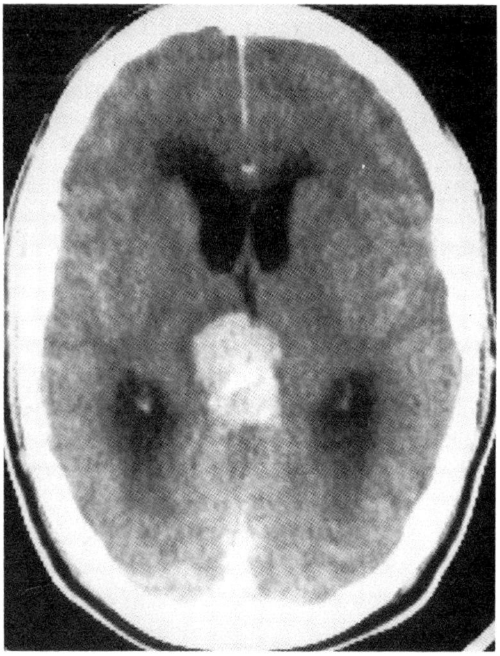

B

Fig. 13.15 CT scan of a pineal tumour, **A** before and **B** after the administration of contrast.

The treatment of these tumours frequently requires emergency surgery with ventriculoperitoneal shunt. In large tumours which extend anteriorly, there may be obstruction of the foramen of Monro, in which case bilateral lateral ventricular drainage is necessary. The site of pineal tumours makes surgery both difficult and dangerous and the majority of these tumours are treated, with or without histological evidence of their nature, with radiotherapy. Many tumours are radiosensitive and show rapid response, but for those which do not direct exploration or stereotactic surgery is indicated. The mean survival following radiotherapy is of the order of 5 years.

Colloid cysts

These benign cysts are believed to develop from the ependymal cells of the anterior portion of the third ventricle between the intraventricular foramina. They are almost certainly congenital, but rarely present until adult life when they cause intermittent blockage of the anterior part of the third ventricle and produce obstructive hydrocephalus. The history is of intermittent headache occasionally with episodes of loss of consciousness, sometimes precipitated by changes in posture and associated with mental change, frontal lobe incontinence and unsteadiness or sudden weakness of the legs.

A CT scan will show a small round mass of usually increased density lying at the anterior portion of the third ventricle and associated with bilateral lateral ventricular dilatation (Fig. 13.16). The treatment of choice is excision of the tumour, ideally performed prior to ventricular shunting through the dilated right ventricle. Occasionally presentation is as an emergency when bilateral ventricular shunting may be required but this creates increased difficulty for the surgeon when attempting total removal through the foramen of Monro. The prognosis after surgery is good, but some patients dying a sudden death are discovered to have this undiagnosed condition.

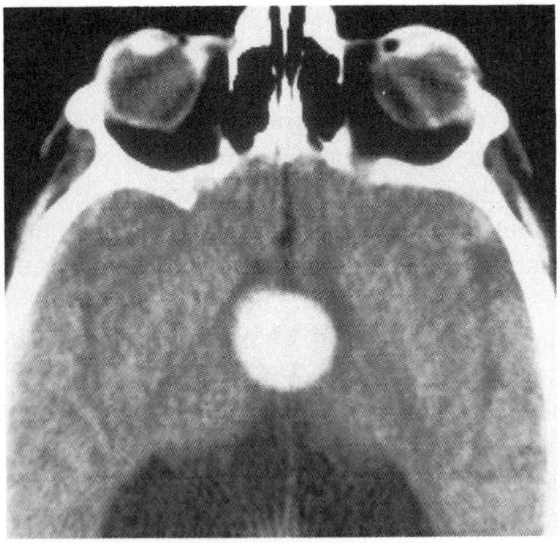

Fig. 13.16 CT scan of a colloid cyst of the third ventricle following the administration of contrast.

Craniopharyngioma

This tumour, which is believed to originate from remnants of Rathke's pouch at the junction of the infundibular stem and pituitary gland, is a cystic lesion lying above the sella turcica and depressing the optic chiasm. Such tumours consist of squamous epithelium, calcified debris and cystic regions containing cholesteatomatous fluid. They constitute approximately 3% of all primary intracranial tumours and are most commonly seen in children and young adults, though may be discovered later in life. They are benign tumours, but owing to their site may present with derangement of the hypothalamic–pituitary axis or the optic chiasm resulting in symptoms varying from delayed physical development to visual disturbance. Classically the visual disturbance will begin as a bitemporal inferior quadrantinopia and become a bitemporal hemianopia. The tumours may rarely present with hydrocephalus due to obstruction of the flow of c.s.f. at the third ventricle.

Plain skull X-ray will show calcification lying above or within the pituitary fossa in 80% of cases. A CT scan will show a lesion of mixed density containing both solid and cystic components in the suprasellar region. Pituitary function studies should be undertaken and may frequently reveal evidence of endocrine abnormality (Fig. 13.17).

Ideally, therapy consists of complete excision of the tumour, though this may not always be possible. Alternatives are partial removal of the tumour followed by radiotherapy, and drainage of the cystic areas of the tumour followed by external radiotherapy, or the implantation of radioactive yttrium. The operative mortality and morbidity is high and may reach 30% with residual defects in pituitary function and vision. Recurrence is common and may then require further radiotherapy.

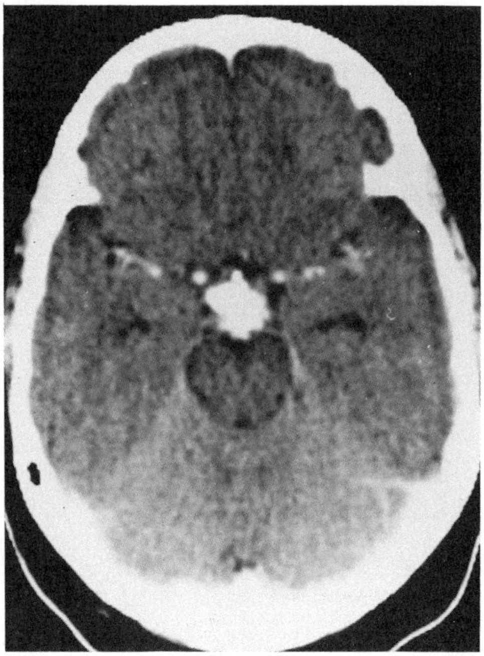

Fig. 13.17 CT scan of a patient with calcification in a craniopharyngioma.

Pituitary adenoma

Tumours arising in the pituitary gland account for between 5% and 10% of intracranial tumours and may present symptoms related to their endocrinological effects or neurological disturbances. The original histological identification of tumour types included eosinophilic adenoma, basophilic adenoma and chromophobe adenoma, but the more recent development of immuno chemical techniques together with the improvement in endocrinological studies differentiates tumours into prolactinoma, growth hormone secreting tumours, ACTH secreting tumours, and the rarer TSH and FSH secreting tumours. Some tumours are endocrinologically inert—the true chromophobe adenoma.

The clinical presentation can be of two types: those resulting from large tumours, which produce a local mass effect and compression of adjacent brain structures, together with compression of the normal pituitary gland resulting in hyposecretion of pituitary hormones; smaller tumours are more likely to present with an endocrinological effect due to hypersecretion of a specific hormone. Both forms of tumours can result in panhypopituitarism. The symptoms of local mass effect which are most commonly seen with prolactinomas are those of headache and visual field defect due to pressure on the inferior aspect of the optic chiasm. The resulting visual field defect is initially a superior temporal quadrantanopia progressing to bitemporal hemianopia. There may also be lateral extension of the tumour into the cavernous sinus, resulting in ophthalmoparesis due to pressure on the third, fourth and sixth nerves and occasionally sensory abnormalities in the first two divisions of the trigeminal nerve. More rarely, erosion through the wall of the sphenoid sinus will result in the symptom of c.s.f. rhinorrhea.

One rare but important presentation of pituitary tumour is apoplexy due to infarction or haemorrhage. This presents acutely with headache, visual impairment, and ophthalmoplegia with confusion or coma. It necessitates steroid cover and early surgery.

The most common endocrinological abnormality is probably that due to hyperprolactinaemia which, in the female, results in symptoms of infertility, amenorrhoea and galactorrhoea and, in males impotence and loss of libido. Such tumours are diagnosed by measurement of serum prolactin, but it must be remembered that other causes of hyperprolactinaemia can occur and must be excluded, i.e:

1. Stress
2. Pregnancy
3. Drugs—dopamine antagonists
4. Hypothyroidism
5. Renal disease
6. Hypothalamic lesions
7. Stalk section.

Those factors which suggest the presence of a prolactin secreting tumour are loss of the normal diurnal fluctuation in prolactin levels, the failure of TRH to induce a reduction in prolactin secretion and the failure of metaclopramide to stimulate release of prolactin. Prolactin is produced from the anterior pituitary under tonic inhibitory control from the hypothalamus and, therefore, lesions of the hypothalamus or pituitary stalk will, due to a deficiency in prolactin inhibitory factor, produce a rise in serum prolactin.

Many prolactinomas are small and do not cause a significant enlargement of the pituitary gland; however, they may be shown with contrast CT scanning. Some tumours are large and are visualised with conventional CT investigation (Fig. 13.18). The management of prolactinoma is initially with bromocriptine, which causes a dramatic reduction in the level of prolactin in the blood and has been shown to result in reduction in size of some tumours. In those patients whose tumours are large and causing pressure effects, the possibility of surgery should be considered early, though it is reasonable to undertake a trial of bromocriptine first and monitor the size of the tumour by CT scan.

The transphenoidal approach to pituitary tumours has led some neurosurgeons to suggest that transphenoidal microsurgery is the treatment of choice for small prolactinomas and the question

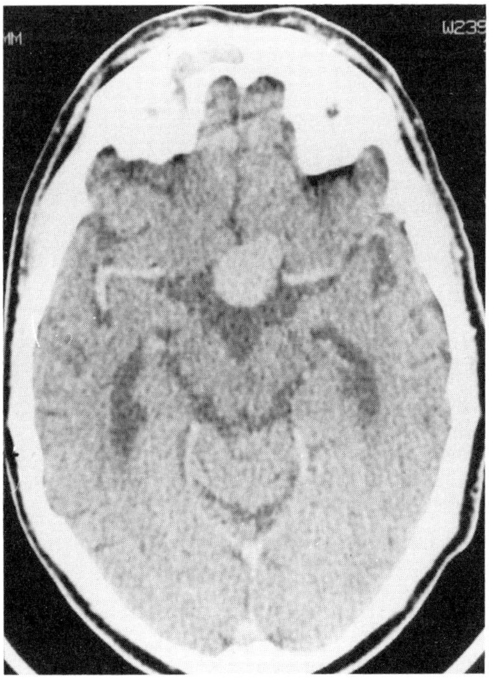

Fig. 13.18 CT scan of a pituitary adenoma following the administration of contrast.

as to whether medical or surgical therapy is to be preferred remains controversial.

The second most common endocrinological abnormality with pituitary tumours is the finding of panhypopituitarism. This may, in children, result in pituitary dwarfism with retarded sexual development and episodes of hypoglycaemia, but in adults more commonly causes amenorrhoea, infertility and loss of libido together with generalised muscle weakness and fatigue and secondary hypothyroidism. In the puerperal female failure of lactation may also be a clue. The standard endocrinological tests of TRH injection, gonadotrophin-releasing hormone injection and insulin tolerance tests can confirm the presence of hypopituitarism though the latter is, of course, dangerous in patients with significant disease who may suffer dangerous hypoglycaemia (Table 13.9).

The presence of panhypopituitarism may be seen with large tumours of the pituitary gland but can also occur with the 'empty sella' syndrome, when the pituitary gland appears to be absent. CT scan will identify the difference between these two conditions, the former showing a contrast enhancing lesion within the pituitary and extending above it and the latter a low density c.s.f. filled cavity in the pituitary fossa. It is usual to undertake angiography in these patients to exclude the rare but important complication of an aneurysm within the dilated sella, following which the management depends upon the findings. In the empty sella syndrome pituitary replacement therapy is usually adequate though occasionally tension on the optic chiasm from the arachnoid bulging into the diaphragma sellae may require a transfrontal surgical approach and decompression of the chiasm.

When tumour is detected, trans-sphenoidal surgery is indicated unless the tumour is so large that a subfrontal approach has to be undertaken.

Growth hormone excess may be seen with pituitary tumours of eosinophilic type and results in the syndrome of gigantism in the child, or of acromegaly in the adult. Growth hormone levels are usually increased in the serum and the measurement of growth hormone levels during a glucose tolerance test will reveal lack of the normal suppression of growth hormone secretion. The management of these patients is by trans-sphenoidal surgery and tumour excision.

ACTH secreting pituitary tumours are relatively rare and will result in the development of Cushing's syndrome. The diagnosis is established by demonstrating elevated plasma cortisol levels with a loss of normal diurnal variation and a failure of suppression with dexamethasone administration. The ideal treatment for pituitary driven Cushing's syndrome is trans-sphenoidal surgery to the pituitary gland. Occasionally, patients with idiopathic Cushing's disease due to adrenal tumour and subjected to bilateral adrenalectomy may develop Nelson's syndrome with increased ACTH secretion, enlargement of the pituitary and skin pigmentation.

TSH, FSH and LH secreting tumours are extremely rare but will be diagnosed by the relevant endocrinological tests. In general, pituitary tumours may be suspected from the clinical examination and confirmed by plain X-ray of the skull, which will frequently reveal ballooning of

Table 13.9 Clinical presentations of pituitary tumours.

Endocrine
Oversecretion
Hyperprolactinaemia
Acromegaly/gigantism
Cushing's syndrome
Thyrotoxicosis
Undersecretion
Hypopituitarism
Myxoedema
Pituitary dwarfism
Addison's disease
Combinations of above
Structural
Visual syndromes
Bitemporal hemianopia
Progressive visual failure
Cranial nerve syndromes
Oculomotor palsy
Abducens palsy
Trochlear palsy
Ophthalmic division of trigeminal nerve
Cerebral syndromes
Complex partial seizures
Generalised seizures
C.s.f. rhinorrhoea
Pituitary apoplexy

the pituitary fossa with asymmetrical erosion of the floor and also confirmed by CT scan with contrast enhancement. High definition CT scanning with axial and coronal views of the pituitary fossa are particularly helpful. It is occasionally necessary to undertake a basal cisternogram in which contrast, either radio-opaque or air, is introduced to the lumbar or cisternal theca and allowed to flow forwards over the region of the diaphragma sellae.

The management of pituitary tumours depends upon the age of the patient, the clinical presentation and the definition of the nature of the tumour. The possible methods of therapy available are endocrinological, operative via either a trans-sphenoidal or a subfrontal route, and radiotherapy. The prolactinoma, as has been previously described, can be treated with medical therapy even when there is a mass lesion present, though careful clinical monitoring of the patient is essential and surgery may be necessary in the absence of a satisfactory clinical and radiological response. In general, patients with mass lesions require decompression followed by radiotherapy and correction of endocrine abnormalities and those with microadenomas need treatment of the underlying hormonal disturbance. It should be remembered that many patients with pituitary tumours will require steroid cover during surgery and all should be subject to repeat endocrinological investigation after surgery to assess the need for long-term replacement.

Acoustic neuroma

The neurofibroma or neurolemmoma of the eighth cranial nerve may occur in isolation or as part of the central form of von Recklinghausen's neurofibromatosis. They are the commonest of infratentorial tumours and comprise approximately 5% of intracranial tumours. They most commonly present in midlife and are more common in women. They are benign, slow-growing tumours which usually develop on the vestibular division of the eighth cranial nerve and are frequently found at the internal auditory meatus within the cerebellopontine angle. Neuromas may rarely arise on the trigeminal nerve. A pathological distinction is made between the neurilemmoma, which arises from the Schwann cells and grows outwards from the surface of the nerve trunk, and the neurofibroma, which also arises from the Schwann cells but which diffusely expands the nerve trunk.

The clinical presentation may rarely include the symptom of pain over the mastoid process on the side of the tumour with, more commonly, a gradually progressive sensorineural deafness which is rarely associated with vertigo or tinnitus. As the tumour grows there may be pressure on the trigeminal nerve resulting in facial pain, numbness and paraesthesia and, ultimately, pressure on the seventh cranial nerve will result in ipsilateral lower motor neurone facial weakness. In addition, distortion of the cerebellum and brain stem may cause a degree of ataxia and compression of the aqueduct can result in hydrocephalus.

Clinically, the finding of a sensory neural hearing loss together with an absent corneal reflex and a mild facial weakness strongly suggests the presence of a lesion in the cerebellopontine angle and the most important distinction is between an acoustic neuroma and a meningioma. When the tumour is large enough to displace the brain stem there may also be features of ataxia, ipsilateral incoordination and nystagmus. Damage to the pons and cerebral peduncle may produce a contralateral hemiparesis.

The investigations include both neuro-otological testing and radiography. The use of techniques including audiometry, tone decay, speech discrimination and brain stem auditory evoked potentials, possibly with electrocochleography, will help to differentiate deafness due to a retrocochlear lesion. Caloric testing will invariably show impairment of the response on the affected side. Plain radiography of the internal meati, sometimes enhanced by tomography of the meati, may show erosion and dilatation on the affected side. A CT scan may show little without contrast since acoustic tumours are often isodense (Fig. 13.19). With contrast, the tumour enhances strongly and may contain cystic areas of low density. There may frequently be compression of the fourth ventricle and dilatation of the third and lateral ventricles. Contrast scanning of the basal cisterns with either metrizamide or air may be helpful to outline small acoustic neuromas projecting from the internal auditory meatus which are less immediately apparent. If

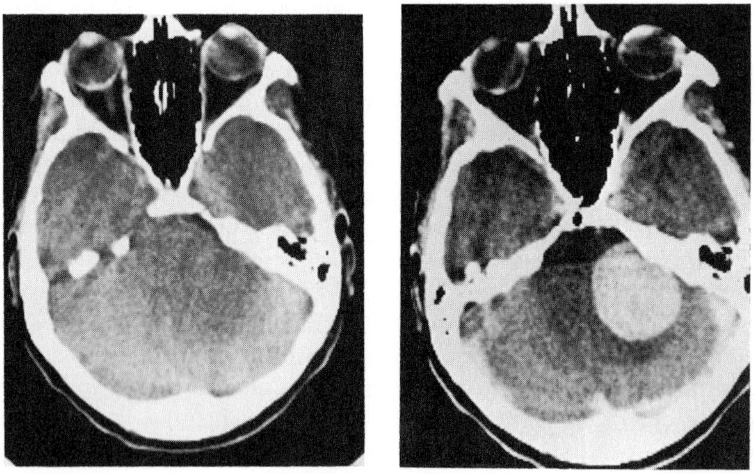

A B

Fig. 13.19 CT scan of an acoustic neuroma: **A** before and **B** after contrast administration.

this investigation is undertaken, the measurement of c.s.f. protein will often reveal grossly elevated levels.

The preferred treatment of acoustic neuroma is by surgical removal. Patients with large tumours may require ventriculoperitoneal shunting prior to surgery, though there is the theoretical risk of upward herniation of the contents of the posterior fossa. The mortality rates for surgery of acoustic neuroma relate to tumour size and can be up to 20% with large tumours. There is also a significant morbidity due to the pressure and consequent vascular disturbances affecting the brain stem. With small tumours direct and complete removal is advocated, but with larger tumours incomplete removal is frequently the only therapy which can be applied and there seems no role for radiotherapy. With modern techniques of microsurgery it is increasingly possible to preserve the facial nerve function at the time of operation and occasionally, particularly with neurilemmomas, it may be possible to preserve hearing in the affected ear.

Chordoma

These rare tumours arise from primitive notochord and are usually found either intracranially at the back of the clivus or in the sacral part of the spine. They are more common in males than females and are typically midline. They tend to present during the fourth decade of life and occasionally metastasise. In the cranial variety the presentation is usually with multiple cranial nerve palsies and occasionally nasal obstruction. The cranial nerve palsies may range from ophthalmoparesis to bulbar problems. There may also be chronic local pain due to bone erosion.

Plain radiology of the skull usually shows a soft tissue mass with an osteolytic lesion in the base of the skull and CT scan confirms the presence of a partly calcified mass causing bone destruction in the base of the skull. They should be differentiated from other tumours destroying the base of the skull, including meningioma, neurofibroma, carotid body tumour and carcinoma of the nasopharynx. Wegener's granulomatosis must also be excluded.
Wegener's granulomatosis must also be excluded.

Surgical treatment is extremely difficult for this form of tumour and total removal is impossible. Debulking operations, preferably via the transoral route, can be considered and radiotherapy is used, though it appears not to be particularly effective. Most patients die within 10 years of presentation.

Cysts

There are three major forms of benign cysts which can have a space-occupying effect within the cranial cavity. *Arachnoid cysts* are collections of c.s.f. like fluid which may communicate with the c.s.f. and which are typically found in the suprasellar region, the sylvian fissure or the convexity and may also occur in the cisterna magna of the posterior fossa. The cause of these cysts is unknown, although they may be related to local agenesis of brain. They are frequently asymptomatic, may occasionally be associated with epilepsy and are most commonly found coincidentally when a CT scan is undertaken for a different reason. Treatment is only required if there are symptoms related to the arachnoid cyst, such as raised intracranial pressure due to a valve-like effect allowing accumulation of fluid, and then consists either of marsupialisation of the cyst into the c.s.f. or a cystoperitoneal shunt.

Epidermoid cysts are pearly white tumours filled with cholesterol crystals and keratinised debris most commonly found in the posterior fossa and frequently in the cerebellopontine angle. They may cause multiple cranial nerve palsies and occasionally rupture into the subarachnoid space, causing a chemical meningitis. CT scan reveals them to be low-density lesions which show enhancement (Fig. 13.20).

Dermoid cysts are thicker walled than the epidermoids and contain hair follicles and glandular tissue. They are frequently in the midline of the posterior fossa and may connect to the surface of the skin through a bony defect which can be a potential source for infection and may cause an associated meningitis. They may be calcified on CT scan, but otherwise look identical to an epidermoid. The fact that these cysts tend to be adherent to adjacent structures makes their total removal impossible, but evacuation of contents is usually easy and gives adequate symptomatic relief. They may recur many years later.

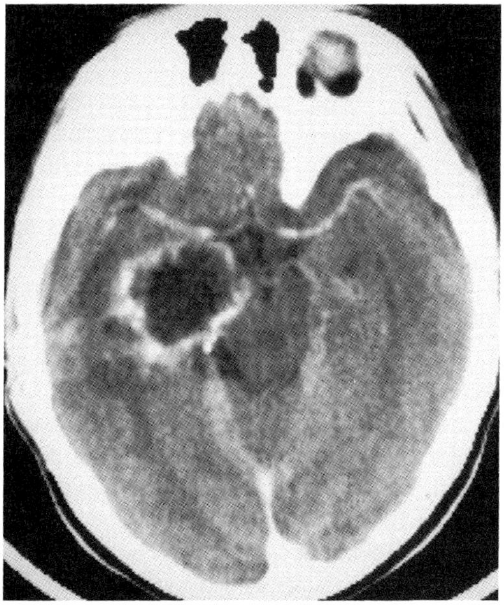

Fig. 13.20 CT scan showing an epidermoid cyst in the right middle fossa following the administration of contrast.

Glomus tumour

This highly vascular tumour is derived from non-chromaffin paraganglioma cells found in the jugular bulb lying immediately below the floor of the middle ear. There are also other potential sites of origin in and around the temporal bone. The cells of origin are part of the chemoreceptor system that includes carotid, vagal, ciliary and aortic bodies. The tumour extensively erodes the jugular foramen and petrous bone and presents with partial deafness, facial palsy, dysphagia and unilateral atrophy of the tongue, combined with a vascular polyp seen in the external auditory meatus and occasionally a palpable mass below and anterior to the mastoid eminence. A bruit is often heard over the mass. It may rarely cause phrenic nerve palsy, facial numbness, Horner's syndrome, and even cerebellar ataxia and temporal lobe epilepsy if it erodes the base of the skull. Women tend to be more commonly affected than men and it is most common in midadult life. The tumour grows slowly, often over more than 10 years, and diagnosis is by basal skull X-ray, which reveals an osteolytic lesion expanding the jugular foramen, and CT, which may show an enhancing lesion in this region. Angiography of the external carotid artery will usually show the presence of a vascular tumour, though occasionally vertebral angiography is required as well.

Treatment is best performed by radical mastoidectomy with removal of as much of the tumour as possible followed by radiation. Recently, the technique of selective embolisation of the external carotid artery supply may reduce the risk of direct surgery. Occasionally, radiotherapy alone is used as treatment.

The glomus jugulare tumour should be distinguished from the much rarer but potentially malignant tumour arising from the carotid body and presenting as a painless mass at the side of the neck below the angle of the jaw. They may implicate the sympathetic nerves in the neck together with the ninth, tenth, eleventh and twelfth cranial nerves. They have occasionally been reported to be associated with transient ischaemic attacks and they have been recorded in association with von Recklinghausen's neurofibromatosis. The treatment is with surgical excision, frequently after embolisation.

INVESTIGATIONS

The investigation of cerebral tumours is aimed to identify the presence and site of the growth and its probable pathology. Basic investigations may be haematological, revealing polycythaemia with a haemoangioblastoma, or evidence of leukaemia or lymphoma; or biochemical in tumours of endocrinological origin and to identify the possibility of a primary tumour in some other organ. Radiological techniques to identify the site of primary tumours may be used, as may both radioisotope and other scanning systems.

The more definitive investigations include skull X-ray and imaging techniques of the head. The skull X-ray may show signs typical of increased intracranial pressure (p. 115) and occasionally calcium may be seen on a lateral skull X-ray, or shift of the pineal on an AP film.

The investigation of choice for cerebral tumours is computerised imaging most commonly by CT scanning and, occasionally, and particularly with basal and posterior fossa tumours, with the technique of magnetic resonance imaging.

Many patients will require further investigation with angiography to attempt to differentiate between meningiomas, secondary tumours and gliomas and to exclude the possibility of arterio venous malformations or aneurysms. Prior to surgery, angiography may be important in identifying the site of blood supply to the lesion and indicating the possibility or otherwise of embolisation.

Air encephalography and ventriculography are now rarely indicated in the investigation of intracranial tumours and the final possibility of investigation is biopsy, either by a burr hole, stereotactic biopsy, or by open biopsy with decompression.

MANAGEMENT

The treatment of specific cerebral tumours has been detailed in the last section and depends upon the identification of their pathology. In general, where specific treatment is available as in the case of many pituitary tumours, this conservative therapy should first be applied. Benign tumours, in general, are best treated by surgery and the advent of microneurosurgery has improved the possibility of total excision of such tumours. There will, of course, be exceptions in the very elderly patient, the inaccessible benign tumour and the benign tumour which, because of its attachment to other structures, is irremovable.

In patients with malignant tumours the decision about management depends on many factors, including the definition of the histological type of the tumour, where possible, its site and the age of the patient, together with the known presence or absence of other disease or tumours. In general, the considerable peritumour oedema can be helped by the use of steroids such as dexamethasone and also by the use of diuretic agents or mannitol. The most difficult problem in management is the decision as to the timing of operation, or when to advise against operation in those patients with tumours, but with relatively little in the way of symptoms or signs. The advent of CT scanning and the possibility of repeated non-invasive investigations in this way makes it reasonable to continue the care of some patients conservatively and to use a surgical approach only when the tumour can be shown to be increasing in size or when symptoms and signs develop. The dilemma is always that without a biopsy of tissue, histological definition of the nature of the lesion is impossible and there remains the fear that one may be watching a relatively benign tumour which should be approached surgically sooner.

The question of radiotherapy and chemotherapy in cerebral tumours is a difficult one. There is some indication that in secondary tumours and in those large gliomas which are not being subject to operation, some palliation may occur with radiotherapy and there is also evidence that prognosis for the lower grades of cerebral glioma (Kernahan grades II and III) is enhanced by the use of radiotherapy postoperatively after decompression or biopsy. There is no good evidence that radiotherapy helps with grade IV glioma or glioblastoma multiforme and it should probably be withheld in this situation. Radiotherapy is of most use in patients with proven lymphoma of the nervous system and as palliation in secondary tumours.

Chemotherapy in the nervous system has so far been disappointing. The two agents CCNU and BCNU have been used, but evidence that they prolong life expectancy or will improve quality of life is currently lacking. One of the problems in using chemotherapeutic agents in cerebral tumours is that the blood–brain barrier prevents the passage of many agents from the systemic circulation into the cerebral parenchyma. There is always the possibility that the abnormal circulation within a tumour will allow the transport of such agents and there have been attempts to instil intraventricular chemotherapeutic agents in patients with ependymal disorders. The current hope is that new techniques of biopsy and culturing cerebral tumours will enable identification of which tumours are responsive to chemotherapy in much the same way that one can undertake this task with cultures of infecting organisms. But at present the role of radiotherapy and chemotherapy in prolonging life expectation in patients with malignant cerebral tumours is uncertain.

FURTHER READING

Fishman R A 1980 Cerebral spinal fluid in diseases of the nervous system. Saunders, Philadelphia.
Russell D S, Rubinstein L J, 1977
Pathology of tumours of the nervous system, 4th edn.
E Arnold, London

14

Trauma and the nervous system

INTRODUCTION

This chapter deals with trauma affecting the brain, the spine and the spinal roots. Peripheral nerve trauma is covered in the peripheral neuropathy section and in the section concerned with iatrogenic disorders.

EPIDEMIOLOGY

In accidents, fatal or otherwise, the commonest single site of injury is the head. In England and Wales approximately 100 000 patients with head injuries are admitted to hospital annually and similar numbers proportionately are hospitalised in most countries in the western hemisphere. Men outnumber women by almost 2 : 1 and more than half of those who are admitted to hospital are under the age of 20.

Mortality figures for head injury are appalling, accounting for no less than 70% of total accident fatalities. A higher proportion of deaths occur in people over the age of 40 and, of those, 30% die before reaching hospital and probably as many as a further 20% die in casualty departments.

It is perhaps worth noting that, in addition to the impact in terms of human suffering, there is a profound financial impact: it has been estimated that the annual cost of care for patients with head injuries in the United States is 3×10^9 US dollars.

HEAD INJURY

CAUSES

A variety of factors, including individual and environmental components, determine the cause of accidents—one of the most important factors being age. Children, particularly, may be injured by falls either at home or in the playground; young adults are especially prone to road traffic accidents; old people are prone to falls or accidents on the road as pedestrians. Overall, the commonest causes of head injury are road traffic accidents, accidental falls, work accidents, sports accidents and assaults.

MECHANISMS

The brain is highly protected within the bony skull, being surrounded not only by the meninges but also by the thin film of cerebrospinal fluid within the subarachnoid space. Further protection results from the compartmentalisation of the different parts of the brain by the falx cerebri and the tentorium. It is possible to recognise a variety of different mechanisms whereby the brain may be injured as a result of trauma.

Penetrating injuries (Fig. 14.1)

The damage done by penetrating injuries depends to a large extent on the area of the brain that is penetrated by the object. Missile injuries penetrating the brain may traverse the brain substance yet produce few after-effects. High-velocity missile injuries, however, may produce quite extensive damage because of the high velocity impact within the brain and the subsequent shock waves. Penetrating head injuries are uncommon in the United Kingdom but are more frequent in the United States, where gunshot injuries to the brain are an unfortunate feature of major city life.

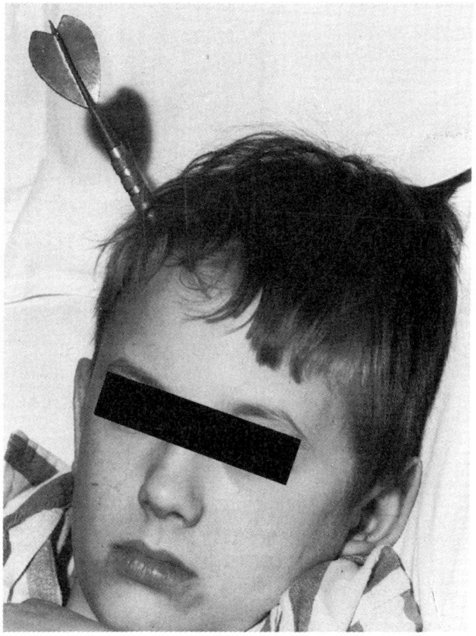

Fig. 14.1 Example of penetrating injury.

Crush injuries (Fig. 14.2)

Primary crush or compression injuries occur infrequently. An example is the tractor driver who is crushed when his vehicle tips over. Often, more damage is done to the skull than to the brain, although clearly this depends on the force of impact.

Accleration/deceleration injuries (impact head injuries) (Fig. 14.3)

This is the commonest type of head injury, where the head is hit by a moving object or the moving head hits an immobile object. At the moment of impact a temporary deformation of the skull occurs, associated with a sharp but transient rise of intracranial pressure. The crucial factor producing damage to the brain is movement of the head so that the semiliquid brain impacts against the hard unyielding surface of the skull. It is claimed that the rotational movement of the brain within the skull is that which is the most important in producing damage as it may result in tearing of intrinsic fibre pathways within the cerebral substance. Similarly, fibre tracts within the brain stem may be damaged, as may the

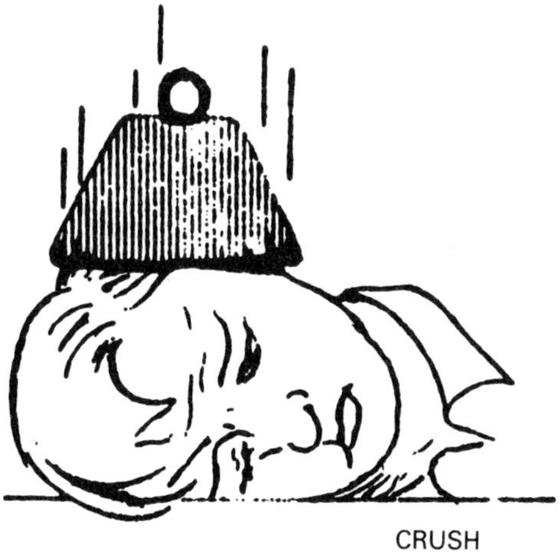

Fig. 14.2 Example of crush head injury.

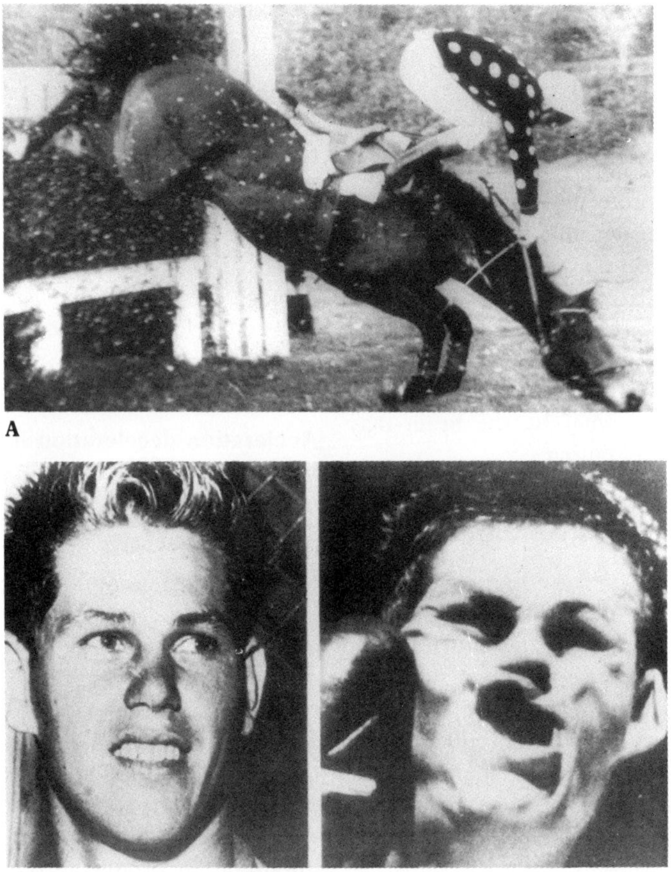

Fig. 14.3 **A** Examples of impact head injury. **A** Jockey being thrown from horse, **B** boxer being hit by blow from fist—before and after. (Reproduced from Unsterharuscheidt F J 1975 *Handbook of Clinical Neurology*, vol. 23 North Holland Publishing Company, Amsterdam, with permission.)

cranial nerves as they leave the brain stem through the base of the skull. Loss of consciousness is one of the hallmarks of an acceleration/deceleration injury and for many years it has been recognised that the abrupt movement of the head relative to the cervical spine is the important factor in determining loss of consciousness. Immobilisation of the neck by means of a collar is an effective means of preventing loss of consciousness in the monkey when given a 'knock-out' blow by a weighted pendulum.

We have deliberately omitted the use of the term 'concussion'. This term has been applied to loss of consciousness without any obvious structural cerebral damage: it is, therefore, a term used clinically to describe a pathological entity. It is now recognised that patients may suffer a minor head injury with loss of consciousness (concussion) yet pathologically show minor neuronal changes or fibre tears.

The final point to emphasise in relation to impact head injury is that the clinical effects result from brain injury and not skull injury and that the two may differ in degree and extent. For example, severe brain damage may occur in the absence of skull fracture, or skull fracture may occur without impairment of consciousness.

PATHOLOGY

It is important to differentiate between the primary and secondary effects of a head injury upon the brain.

Primary effects

The effect upon the brain of an acceleration/deceleration injury depends upon the rate of movement and the magnitude of the force acting upon the skull and hence the brain. Severe injuries are associated with widespread contusions and lacerations, particularly to the undersurface of the frontal and temporal lobes. Tearing of fibre tracts may be evident and the corpus callosum may be totally disrupted. Damage to the intrinsic substance of the brain may be associated with haemorrhage. The site of trauma to the skull may, in some instances, be mirrored by damage to the brain: a direct blow to a site will produce appropriate pathological changes in the form of contusions directly beneath that site. However, injuries in one site may be associated with so-called contrecoup contusions which occur in the cerebral substance directly opposite the site of local trauma (Fig. 14.4).

One of the hallmarks of acceleration/deceleration injuries is diffuse axonal injury. This shows itself pathologically by so-called axon retraction balls and microglial clusters. The numbers of these are closely correlated with the severity of brain damage; nevertheless, it has now been clearly established that they may be seen in patients who (at least clinically) were thought to have suffered a relatively minor head injury.

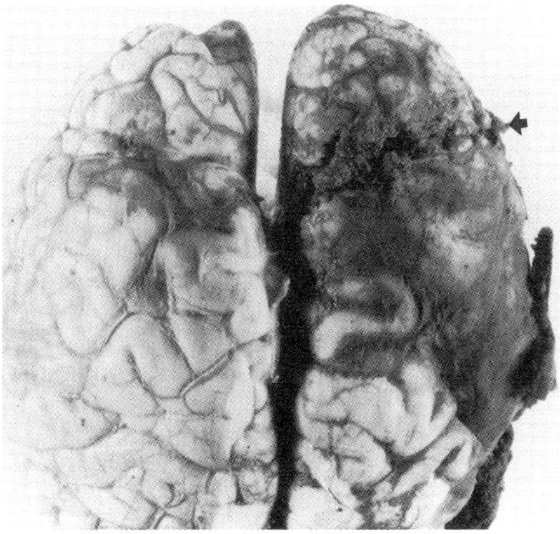

Fig. 14.4 Pathological specimen showing occipital laceration which occurred directly opposite site of trauma (contrecoup injury).

Secondary effects (Fig. 14.5)

Head trauma may induce a number of other pathological processes that may become manifest after some delay. Damage to the skull and blood vessels overlying the brain may produce subdural and extradural haemorrhage. Extradural haemorrhage is more a complication of skull injury than of brain injury and often results from damage to the middle meningeal arteries. Subdural haemorrhage is more often associated with damage to the surface of the cerebral hemispheres, with tearing of the superficial veins. Cerebral oedema is another common delayed effect, usually seen in cases of severe injury. Recently there has been interest in the problem of delayed vasospasm occurring in the cerebral blood vessels and producing secondary ischaemic change within the cerebral parenchyma.

One particular secondary effect which occurs in most moderate or severe head injuries is that of traumatic subarachnoid haemorrhage. This produces a characteristic series of symptoms and signs with headache, restlessness and confusion being prominent clinical features. In some instances this clinical constellation of physical signs may be confused with that of an aneurysmal subarachnoid haemorrhage and at times it is difficult to differentiate clinically the patient who has fallen and suffered a traumatic subarachnoid haemorrhage from the patient who has suffered an aneurysmal subarachnoid haemorrhage and has subsequently fallen and injured his head.

One other complication of head injury is infection. This occurs most commonly as meningitis

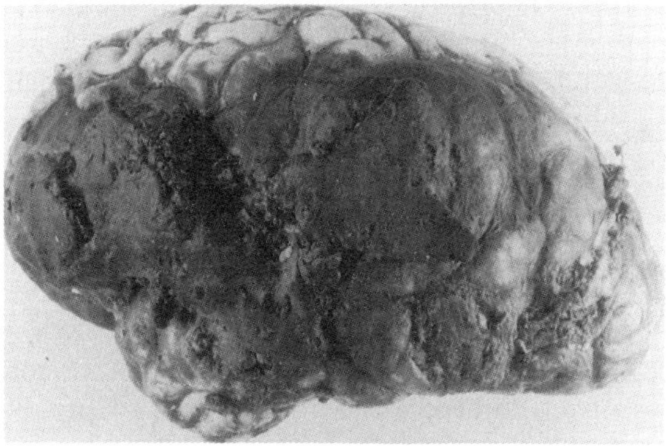

Fig. 14.5 Pathological specimen showing large subdural haematoma over surface of brain.

resulting from infection spreading intracranially as a result of a compound fracture.

MANAGEMENT

Discussion of the management of head injuries is beyond the scope of this book, but a few brief comments merit inclusion. Management may be considered under two separate components:

1. The management of coma
2. The management of secondary complications.

The management of acute head injury coma

Unfortunately, medical science has not yet reached the stage where the primary effects of trauma to the brain can be dealt with effectively. Accordingly, much of the management of acute head injury is concerned with treatment of the coma and with the necessary careful observation of such patients (p. 131). Two aspects of particular importance are care of the associated injuries that may manifest themselves only as shock, and the complications of hypoxia which may result from respiratory insufficiency. Anoxia resulting from a compromised airway is a common cause of impairment of consciousness in the head-injured patient: particular attention, therefore, should be paid to the posture of patients under these circumstances and to the maintenance of their airway. Shock in a head-injured patient should always be regarded as indicating another injury, as it is extremely rare as a manifestation of the head injury itself.

Once the patient's airway and circulation are under control, then an early and detailed assessment of the level of consciousness should be made so that this forms the baseline for further studies (see below). In addition, details of the external injuries should be recorded.

Management of secondary complications

It is of paramount importance that unconscious patients with head injuries are monitored carefully in the early stages: only in this way can secondary complications be treated appropriately; as some of these (such as extradural haemorrhage) are eminently curable, it is vital that they are not overlooked. It is important to look for a delayed deterioration in consciousness, the two most frequent causes of which are delayed cerebral oedema and the development of an intracranial haematoma.

Cerebral oedema

In many rapidly fatal injuries, massive cerebral oedema occurs almost immediately after the impact as a result of distension of the entire cerebral vascular bed. Although unconsciousness after head injury is not *always* accompanied by cerebral oedema, localised oedema often accompanies cerebral contusions and, clinically, the development of cerebral oedema shows itself as a deterioration in the level of consciousness. Treatment of cerebral oedema involves either the use of dehydrating agents such as mannitol, the use of corticosteroids, or the use of controlled ventilation.

Of the dehydrating agents, mannitol, in a dose of 1.5–2 g/kg given in a 20–25% solution is perhaps the most widely used agent. Cortiosteroids, although widely used, are not of confirmed value in cerebral oedema following head injury. Controlled ventilation has the dual benefit of maintaining the P_aO_2 and lowering the P_aCO_2: the latter change produces constriction in the reactive vessels in the unaffected areas of the brain, leading to a decrease in intracranial blood volume and intracranial pressure. This is now increasingly used with intracranial pressure monitoring, but the indications of which patients to monitor and which patients to treat, remain uncertain.

In the United States in particular there has come into widespread use the technique of intracranial pressure monitoring, controlled ventilation and the use of barbiturate sedative drugs. This has not found widespread favour in the United Kingdom.

Intracranial haematoma

Extradural haematoma (Fig. 14.6). An extradural haematoma is a rare, acute and eminently treatable complication of acute head injury which usually

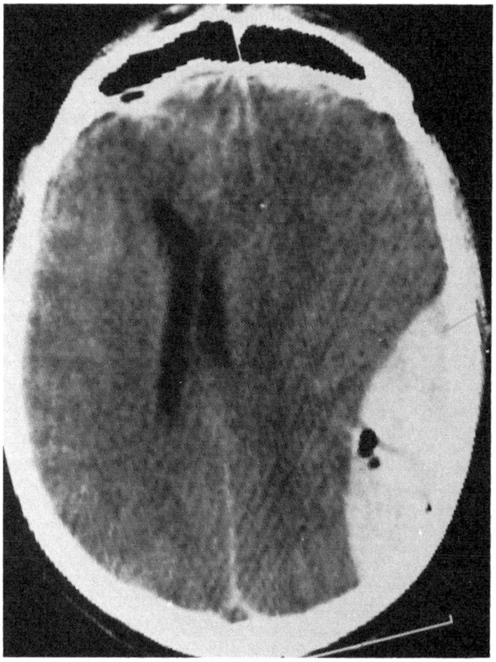

Fig. 14.6 CT scan showing typical appearance of extradural haematoma. Within the right-sided haematoma some air is seen, indicating communication via a fracture.

occurs in young people. It is a complication of skull rather than brain injury and the site of the haematoma is usually under the point of impact. The haematoma is often referred to as a middle meningeal haemorrhage, but the bleeding is not necessarily from the middle meningeal vessels. It is important to remember that the vascular marking on the inner table of the skull is caused by the middle meningeal vein which has a thin wall and which (unlike an artery) can rupture easily. This accounts for the fact that relatively trivial blows, especially to the side of the head, can precipitate an extradural haemorrhage. As many as 30% of patients with this potentially lethal complication have had a non-concussional head injury, although a fracture is commonly seen. As the dura becomes increasingly adherent to the skull with age, extradural haemorrhage is rare in patients over 40 years of age and more than half of those affected are under the age of 20 years. The haematoma usually shows itself clinically as a deterioration in the level of consciousness, which develops within 24 hours of the primary injury.

Acute subdural haematoma. Unfortunately this is an all-too-common complication of head injury with a mortality and morbidity far higher than that of an extradural haemorrhage; this is because there is often associated primary brain injury. Subdural haematomata occur at any age, but are particularly common at the extremes of life. Typically, the bleeding occurs from lacerations of the tip of the temporal lobe and of the undersurface of the frontal lobes. Different types of subdural haematoma may be recognised, the differences largely being attributable to the degree of associated primary brain damage and the rapidity of development of the haematoma. In such severe injuries there may often be accompanying intracerebral haemorrhage.

Chronic subdural haematoma The chronic subdural haematoma (Fig. 14.7) is typically seen in middle-aged and elderly patients in whom, even in retrospect, a history of head injury is the exception rather than the rule. The usual picture is that of a patient past the age of 50 years who presents with fluctuating confusion and drowsiness, neck stiffness, brisk tendon reflexes and extensor

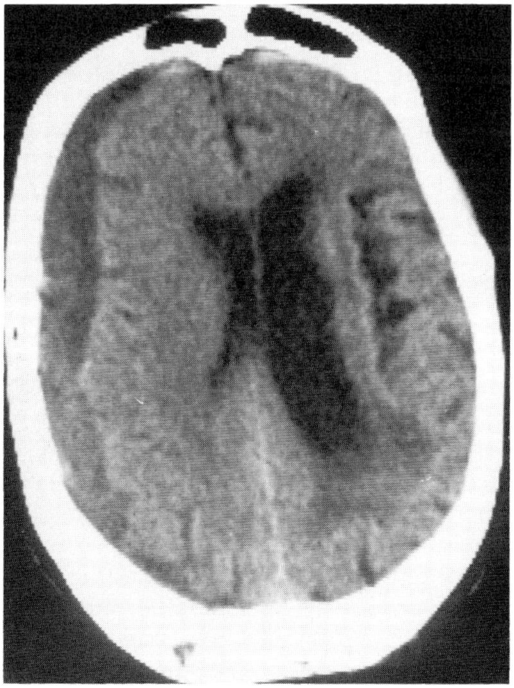

Fig. 14.7 CT scan showing typical appearance of chronic subdural haematoma.

plantar responses. These haematomata are generally fluid and, if detected and treated appropriately, have an excellent prognosis.

C.s.f. rhinorrhoea and the problem of compound fracture of the base of the skull

Bleeding from the ear, or bleeding from the nose following head injury suggest the possibility of a basal skull fracture with c.s.f. rhinorrhoea. Such patients should almost certainly receive prophylactic antibiotics to reduce the risk of meningitis; in most instances the c.s.f. leak heals spontaneously. Occasionally air may be sucked in through the fracture to produce the picture of a pneumoencephalogram, but this complication is unusual.

Compound skull fracture

Compound skull fractures are commonly overlooked, because it is easy to forget that a patient with a skull fracture may have a small laceration in the overlying skin. Similarly, patients with large lacerations of the scalp but no evidence of other damage should always have a skull radiograph to detect a possible fracture. Such a combination is potentially lethal and all such patients should receive prophylactic antibiotics because of the risk of development of meningitis.

INVESTIGATIONS IN HEAD INJURY

Skull radiographs should probably be taken at an early stage in the management of head injuries in all cases: however, these are of limited value and in many instances are taken merely for medicolegal purposes. It is probably a wise precaution to take radiographs of the skull of any patient who has suffered a head injury associated with loss of consciousness if the patient is to be sent home immediately.

The electroencephalogram has little to offer in the assessment of the head-injured patient. Echoencephalography is a safe bedside technique and, in the context of head injuries, is used to detect shifts of the supratentorial structures. It is, however, rather unreliable and has now been replaced by computerised tomography of the head.

The computerised tomogram may provide information which is very valuable in the management of acute head injuries. The indications for using CT scan in head injury vary from centre to centre. Its main use is to detect treatable conditions, such as intracranial haematomas.

Some of the common indications for performing a CT scan after head injury are:

1. The patient with progressively deteriorating consciousness
2. The patient with coma persisting for more than 6–12 hours
3. The patient who is in deep coma with extensor plantor responses and depressed brain stem reflexes.

THE SEQUELAE OF HEAD INJURIES

The most clearly defined and obvious after-effect of head injury is death; analysis of the mortality figures mirrors fairly accurately the general epidemiological profile of head injury.

The acute effects of injury

Here we consider the type of clinical effects that may accompany injuries of differing degrees of seriousness.

A knock-out blow to the head in boxing may result in the victim slumping to the ground inert. Within seconds he is able to get up and stagger around and at this stage may answer simple questions. It may be minutes before he returns to apparent normality and, later, it will be found that he has no memory for events immediately after the blow.

In more severe injuries the individual will fall to the ground and lie motionless, with temporary arrest of respiration and a few myoclonic jerks of the legs. A reflex dilatation of the pupils and an absent lash reflex may be a temporary finding. Respiration may resume immediately, with movement of the limbs and restlessness; this stage may be limited to a few minutes or may last a few hours and be associated with prolonged post-traumatic amnesia.

The more severe head injury is associated with loss of consciousness for 24 hours or more, and often will be followed by a prolonged period of post-traumatic delirium. Such patients may be irrational and difficult to manage and may then pass into a confused state which may last for some days. This degree of disturbance often is associated with a traumatic subarachnoid haemorrhage. As a general rule, the longer the period of unconsciousness the more prolonged are the stages of recovery. The really severe cases are those which show the features of a so-called primary brain stem injury. In such cases, immediate decerebrate rigidity may be apparent and this may persist up to the time of death. Abnormalities of respiration, eye movements and pupillary reflexes are common and many such patients die. These are the sort of patients who, if they recover, show severe disability, such as the persistent vegetative state.

The neurological sequelae of head injury

Loss of consciousness is the most obvious after-effect of head injury and there is considerable debate about the mechanism involved. The relative movement of the cerebral hemispheres and brain stem in relation to the spinal cord appears to be a crucial factor (see above) and this suggests that head injury coma results from a disturbance of the primary reticular formation. Memory disturbances are well recognised: these may be amnesia for events leading up to the moment of consciousness (retrograde amnesia), or amnesia that may follow a recovery of consciousness and considerably exceed the actual period of unconsciousness (post-traumatic amnesia).

Retrograde amnesia

This is defined as partial or total loss of ability to recall events that have occurred immediately preceding brain injury. In most head injuries the period of retrograde amnesia is only momentary, although in severe injury its duration is longer. Retrograde amnesia has one peculiar tendency of shrinking during the period of recovery. The explanation for retrograde amnesia is uncertain, although the most popular theory is that it is due to a disturbance of short-term memory before it becomes encoded as long-term memory.

Post-traumatic amnesia

This is defined as the time lapse between the accident and the point at which the functions concerned with memory are judged to have been restored. It is thus a retrospective determination which can be made only after recovery and, indeed, upon recovery to normality the period of post-traumatic amnesia may shrink. Post-traumatic amnesia is characteristically much longer than the period of unconsciousness and probably results from the failure of long-term registration of memory traces. Patients 'still in' post-traumatic amnesia may appear to be normal and it is easy to underestimate the extent of this period. Obliteration of memory during this period may not be uniformly complete and there may be islands of isolated memories.

The most important aspect of post-traumatic amnesia in closed head injuries is that it correlates well with the degree of severity. Patients with periods of post-traumatic amnesia of more than 12 hours are arbitrarily regarded as having suffered severe head injuries. It is worth emphasising that this is a clinical measure that can be assessed in retrospect and it is almost certainly the best clinical indicator of head injury severity; however, this correlation does not hold good in either penetrating or crush injuries.

Symptoms attributable to focal brain injury

Localised damage to cerebral function may result from either superficial damage to the cortex or from damage to fibre pathways. Motor defects after head injury, such as hemiplegia, are quite common and yet the prognosis for these is remarkably good. Aphasia after head injury occurs in 5–10% of hospitalised patients and, again, usually has a good prognosis. Dysarthria is usually a feature of more severe damage and has a poorer prognosis. Other focal deficits, such as hemianopia and hemisensory disturbances, are less common.

The recovery patterns for these types of deficits after head injury have now been mapped out and recovery curves can be predicted with reasonable degrees of accuracy. Improvement may continue for up to 2 years, although the most substantial recovery usually occurs in the first 6 months.

Cranial nerve injuries (Table 14.1)

At least 10% of all head injuries are complicated by damage to one or more cranial nerves.

Olfactory nerve. Anosmia resulting from head injury is the most common neurological deficit occurring in severe or minor and even in trivial head injuries. The highest incidence is in frontal and occipital injuries and anosmia may be partial or complete. Perversions of taste and smell may be apparent upon recovery.

Optic nerve. Damage to the optic nerve occurs in approximately 1–2% of hospitalised patients with head injuries and often results from local damage to the frontal region. Pathologically, in severe injuries, damage to the optic chiasm is not uncommon, but obvious clinical effects of this damage are only seldom found in patients who survive head injuries.

Third, fourth and sixth cranial nerves. Persisting abnormalities of the extraocular muscles occur in approximately 5% of cases. Such abnormalities are most common in association with servere injuries, but occasionally local injury to the orbit may produce impairment of eye movement (blow-out fracture). The prognosis for recovery of eye movement is good.

Table 14.1 Incidence of cranial nerve injuries in Newcastle Head Injury Study

Cranial nerve	Incidence	Prognosis
Olfactory	10%	Good, usually within 6 months
Optic nerve	1%	Poor, no recovery after 1 month
Oculomotor nerves (3rd, 4th and 6th cranial nerves)	1–5%	Good
Trigeminal nerve	Rare	Poor
Facial nerve	3%	Good, for both early and late
8th nerve	5–10%	Good
Lower cranial nerves (9th, 10th, 11th and 12th)	Excessively rare	—

Fifth cranial nerve. Damage to the fifth cranial nerve is uncommon. Peripheral branches of the fifth cranial nerve, such as the supraorbital branch, may be damaged by local injury and occasionally jaw fracture may result in damage to the inferior dental nerve. Symptoms from such injuries are rarely particularly disabling.

Seventh nerve. Facial paralysis is a relatively common sequel of head injury and often results from a fracture of the petrous part of the temporal bone. In about 50% of patients there is concomitant evidence of damage to the structures of the middle and inner ear and bleeding from the external meatus is common. Two types of facial nerve palsy may be recognised, each of equal incidence: immediate facial palsy is a direct result of the trauma and 75% of patients will recover; delayed facial palsy occurs after a few days and the prognosis is slightly better. The delayed type is thought to result from swelling or haemorrhage around the nerve and such patients often have evidence of a basal skull fracture with bleeding from the ear. It has been suggested that, in patients with such bleeding, ACTH or steroids should be given to improve the prognosis of delayed facial palsy.

Eighth cranial nerve. Loss of hearing after head injury occurs in 5–10% of patients. The prognosis for patients with nerve deafness is poor: nevertheless, as the hearing loss in a significant proportion of head-injured patients is conductive, and attributable to ossicular dislocation, it is important to recognise this complication because surgical treatment may improve the hearing loss. Damage to the vestibular apparatus is common (see below).

Lower cranial nerves. (9, 10, 11, 12) Damage to these cranial nerves is rare, but may result from penetrating head injuries.

Post-traumatic epilepsy

Epilepsy occurs in approximately 5% of hospitalised patients with closed head injuries. The crucial factor appears to be damage to the cerebral cortex: thus, penetrating injuries occurring as a result of missile injuries may be followed by epilepsy in as many as 50% of cases. It is convenient to divide post-traumatic seizures into early and late. A seizure in the first week after a head injury is important as a marker for the development of late epilepsy. For medicolegal purposes the prediction of the likelihood of epilepsy in an individual case of head injury is of considerable importance: predictive factors include early seizures, intracranial haematoma, depressed fractures, and more severe head injuries, as evinced by prolonged periods of post-traumatic amnesia. Epilepsy in the absence of these features is uncommon and, in the individual who develops fits after a minor injury, the injury should probably be regarded as irrelevant.

The majority of patients who are going to develop post-traumatic epilepsy will have their first seizure within 5 years of the injury, although there are a few recorded cases in which the time lapse has exceeded 5 years. There are certain differences between post-traumatic epilepsy in children and adults: early fits are more common in children, whereas they less commonly develop late epilepsy. Children appear to be particularly prone to a fit which occurs immediately after a head injury.

Recently, there has been interest in the routine prophylactic use of anticonvulsants after head injury, but no definite evidence of benefit has emerged and their routine use is not recommended.

Prolonged coma

One of the most tragic complications of a severe head injury is prolonged coma. Such patients often have shown decerebrate rigidity at an early stage after injury and they remain with their eyes closed for some weeks. They often then begin to show features of the vegetative state with eye opening but unresponsiveness. A variety of motor deficits may be seen, with rigidity and dystonic posturing. Lack of evidence of cognitive activity for more than a month is rarely associated with a good recovery. Such patients will usually require long-term care.

Psychiatric sequelae

This is one of the most controversial areas in the field of head injuries. The difficulty is that both psychological and physical determinants may influence the development of psychiatric sequelae and it is often difficult to determine the relative role of each in an individual.

The incidence of psychiatric sequelae is difficult to estimate, but prospective studies have shown that 30–50% of hospitalised patients with head injuries develop mental symptoms, the most common of which is the so-called post-traumatic neurosis.

Post-traumatic neurosis

This controversial area impinges on both the so-called postconcussional syndrome and the problem of simulation. It has been known for many years that there is no close correlation between the severity of the acute head injury and the severity of post-traumatic neurosis, which appears to be determined by psychosocial factors including pending litigation, continuing problems with compensation, occupational stress and persisting physical disability.

Post-traumatic psychosis

The incidence of this varies considerably, depending on the selection of cases and often on the severity of injury. In an unselected group of hospitalised head-injured patients the incidence is claimed to be 2–5%. In a study of 100 head-injured patients with post-traumatic amnesia exceeding 24 hours, 10 psychotic patients were found, all with dementia. Impairment of intellectual function resulting in an organic psychosis is very closely related to severity of injury. Functional psychoses may occur after head injury but are rare. Schizophrenic psychosis is excessively rare and such associations may be coincidental: however, endogenous depression is more common and may be a genuine after-effect of injury.

Natural history of psychiatric sequelae

Recovery patterns for neuroses after head injury are very variable and poorly documented in the literature; however, organic psychoses have been studied in depth. Although recovery curves are difficult to establish, it appears that maximum improvement occurs in the first six months. Personality and behaviour changes, which are not uncommon with severe injuries, may persist for a considerable time and may be permanent. Recovery from these often distressing after-effects is often impossible to predict, but middle-aged and elderly head-injured patients have a poorer prognosis for recovery from these sort of deficits than do younger patients.

Consideration of the psychiatric sequelae inevitably leads us to the thorny problem of postconcussional syndrome.

The postconcussional syndrome

It is with some reluctance that we retain the use of this term as we believe that this concept should be abandoned. The term was originally applied to patients who complained of headache, dizziness and a variety of psychological symptoms following head injury, and in whom the head injuries were often relatively minor. Much has been written about the physical and psychological determinants of the syndrome and, separately, about the question of simulation in the genesis of the symptoms. Incontrovertible facts about the syndrome are that it is more common in men, is rare in sporting injuries and most commonly occurs in those patients who are claiming compensation.

Headache after head injury is not uncommon. In the majority of patients it improves within a matter of days; prolonged headache may be seen in a patient who has suffered a traumatic subarachnoid haemorrhage, but headache persisting for more than a few months occurs in only about 20% of hospitalised patients with head injuries. The incidence of such headache is higher in patients who suffer minor or less severe head injuries. Headache is more common in patients who have other psychological symptoms such as anxiety and depression; the description of the headache varies, although typically it resembles a tension headache.

Post-traumatic dizziness is another common symptom. Recently it has been recognised that vestibular damage is common in head-injured patients and, indeed, may occur in those with relatively minor head injuries. Such patients often first notice the dizziness on turning in bed and any movement of the head may precipitate the symptom. The finding of positional nystagmus suggests that the damage is to the peripheral labyrinth. The prognosis for recovery is good, with the majority of patients improving within six months and virtually all recovering within two years.

The combination of headache and dizziness often occurs in the same patient. In some, the two symptoms are present from the time of injury; in others, one symptom is present from an early stage and the other develops at a later stage. In another group of patients both symptoms develop some time after the injury, usually after discharge from hospital. It is always useful to try to determine at what point after the injury the symptom developed, although sometimes this is impossible. As a rough guide, patients who have had symptoms from the time of their injury should probably be regarded as having an organic deficit. Patients whose symptoms have developed after a delay should be regarded as either simulating the deficit or suffering from an associated psychological disturbance such as depression. Many other combinations can exist, with one symptom having an organic basis and another developing as a result of associated depression. Thus, postconcussional symptoms show considerable variation in their nature, causation and independence and each individual case should be analysed in detail and assessed on its merits.

Medicolegal aspects

Some of the most difficult aspects in the management of head injury are the ensuing medicolegal problems. The case of a patient who is severely damaged and who is likely to have a shortened life expectancy is relatively straightforward and is not controversial: difficulties arise with the patient with no neurological abnormality but multiple neurological symptoms, as in the postconcussional syndrome. In many instances it is impossible to determine the pathogenesis of the symptoms and clinical judgement must be called into play. In the absence of any overt psychiatric disturbance it is usually fair to urge the lawyers not to prolong the case: in our experience it is a common finding that once the case is finished the symptoms will resolve. It is rare for a neurologist to be able to state *with certainty* that an individual is malingering, but there is often a *suspicion* of simulation or frank exaggeration, and this should be stated firmly.

Medical sequelae of head injury

Damage to the brain may be associated with a variety of medical problems, some common, some rare.

Neuroendocrine disorders

Damage to the pituitary and hypothalamus is common in patients with fatal head injury: abnormalities have been found in as many as 50% of such cases. Clinical manifestations of hypothalamic and pituitary dysfunction are, however, much less common. Diabetes insipidus occurs in less than 1% of hospitalised patients with head injuries and usually results from severe injury, although the prognosis may be good. Post-traumatic hypopituitarism is even less common and only isolated cases have been documented. Few studies, however, have examined hypothalamic and pituitary function in the acute stages after injury.

Cardiovascular disturbances

The commonest clinical vasomotor phenomenon associated with head injury is the so-called Cushing's response, in which rising intracranial pressure is associated with rising systemic blood pressure and a progressively slowing pulse rate. Electrocardiographic abnormalities are more common: it has been claimed that these may result from minor degrees of cardiac damage that may be found upon histological examination of the myocardium of patients with fatal head injuries. It has been suggested that these pathological changes result from the high catecholamine levels which may be found in the blood in conditions such as head injury where there is subarachnoid bleeding.

Gastrointestinal sequelae

Stress ulceration of the stomach has been recognised since the time of John Hunter, and Cushing first described ulcers in patients with brain injuries. Gastric acid secretion is increased in comatose patients with head injuries and the estimated incidence of stress ulcers in such patients has been put as high as 60%.

Respiratory abnormalities

Severe head injuries, not surprisingly, are associated with disordered integration of the neural influences controlling respiration, but these abnormalities are not seen in patients with minor head injuries. Neurogenic pulmonary oedema is also seen in patients with severe head injuries: experience with Vietnam combat casualties has shown that degrees of pulmonary oedema are seen in the majority of soldiers with fatal head injuries, even in those dying within minutes of injury.

Haematological changes

Any trauma may stimulate coagulation and fibrolytic systems and the degree of activation is said to be directly proportional to the severity of the trauma. Major coagulation changes may be seen after severe head injury, although the clinical importance of these changes is uncertain. Disseminated intravascular coagulation occurs very occasionally after acute brain injury.

PERINATAL INJURIES

During delivery the head is subjected to considerable force and the sudden release of the applied pressure in cases of rapid delivery is probably the major causative factor in infantile intracranial haemorrhage. This accounts for 10–20% of all neonatal deaths within two weeks; a lesser degree of damage may result in cephalhaematoma. This swelling is often parietal and unilateral and, when below the pericranium, is confined by the attachment of the periostium at the sutures. No specific treatment is required.

Skull fracture in the newborn is uncommon because the skull is elastic and may be distorted without fracturing. The newborn membranous skull when compressed may form a depression which is termed the 'ping pong' fracture.

Damage to the cranial nerves may occur at the time of delivery, the commonest nerve to be damaged being the facial nerve. The prognosis is usually quite good.

INFANTILE AND JUVENILE HEAD INJURIES

A number of important differences exist between head injuries in children and in adults. Postconcussional symptoms in children are uncommon; the prognosis for recovery after head injury is much better than that for adults and sequelae such as epilepsy are much less common. Skull fractures are frequent in the head-injured child and one particular type of fracture is unique to children: this is the so-called growing fracture where a linear fracture in the parietal region may be associated with disruption of the meninges, resulting in the development of a gradually expanding fluid-filled space between the brain and the arachnoid, giving a radiological appearance of an enlarging and widening fracture. Surgical repair is necessary.

THE PROBLEM OF REPEATED HEAD INJURIES

Increasingly it has been recognised that sports associated with repeated head injuries may result in a neurological picture with a characteristic constellation of physical signs. The syndrome was first recognised in boxers and became known as the 'punch drunk' syndrome. This typically occurs in boxers who have fought in more than 50 bouts and results in clinical symptomatology of intellectual impairment, dysarthria, ataxia and personality change. Such symptoms develop insidiously and may progress. Cerebral atrophy may be documented both radiologically and eventually pathologically. The recognition of this syndrome has led to changes in legislation for the control of boxing. Recently it has been recognised that a similar, if not identical, syndrome may be seen in National Hunt jockeys who have repeatedly fallen from their horses. It remains to be seen whether similar clinical and pathological findings will be detected in other sportsmen suffering similar injuries.

INJURIES OF THE VERTEBRAL COLUMN AND SPINAL CORD

EPIDEMIOLOGY

Although injuries of the spinal cord account for about 80–90% of acute or subacute interruptions of spinal cord conduction, detailed statistical data on the incidence of spinal cord injury are scanty. The only national statistics are those from Switzerland where the incidence of traumatic paraplegia and tetraplegia from all causes rose from 10 new patients per annum per million population in 1960 to 15 new patients per annum per million population in 1967. Even higher figures are reported from Australia: 19 patients per annum per million. The estimated figure for the United Kingdom is similar to the Australian figure, but the estimated figure for the USA is approximately 50 new cases per annum per million. Eighty per cent of injuries to the spinal cord are thought to occur as a result of motor vehicle accidents. Overall, the causes of closed injuries differ greatly between industrialised and non-industrialised countries: in the latter, falls from trees are a common cause; in the former, three main groups of causes are noted:

1. Road, rail and air traffic accidents account for the majority and most of these result from car, motorcycle, bicycle or pedestrian accidents
2. Industrial accidents account for a further proportion, although this has been on the decrease in recent years because of the declining numbers of mining accidents
3. The remaining proportion is largely made up of sporting accidents, with a smaller proportion of accidents in the home. Tetraplegia caused by diving into shallow water is increasingly common and cord damage may also result from falls from horses or from collisions during rugby football.

The majority of spinal cord injuries occur in the young and in males, aproximately 75% occurring in individuals under 40, 90% of whom are male. The relative proportions of paraplegics and tetraplegics vary: in most industrial and civilised countries the ratio is 1 : 1.

PATHOLOGY

Severe spinal trauma may result in injury to the bony elements of the vertebral column or to the neural elements of the spinal cord and spinal roots. Injury to the bone may occur without evident injury to cord or nervous elements; similarly, damage to the neural elements may be present without demonstrable injuries to the bone. More often, however, there is concurrent injury to both elements.

There is no constant quantitative relationship between the extent of injury to the bone of the spinal cord and the extent of injury to the spinal cord itself. Neurological signs following spinal trauma may be the result of four different pathological factors acting individually or in combination:

1. Oedema and 'concussion' of the cord
2. Haemorrhage into the cord
3. Compression of the cord by fractured or misaligned vertebrae
4. Transection of the cord by elements of the vertebral column.

Oedema of the cord

Oedema of the cord occurs in every major spinal injury which is severe enough to produce neurological symptoms and the cord may well swell to twice its normal size within a few minutes after such trauma. This is the most frequent cause of block in the subarachnoid space during the first 48–72 hours after trauma and it usually subsides after the third day.

Haemorrhage into the cord

Haemorrhage into the cord (haematomyelia) is an almost constant pathological consequence of major spinal cord trauma. A degree of haemorrhage into the cord is present whenever the cord has been damaged and haemorrhage in the epidural, subdural and subarachnoid spaces is not infrequent, though rarely sufficiently severe to cause compression of the cord.

COMPRESSION OF THE CORD BY FRACTURED OR MISALIGNED VERTEBRAE

Compression of the spinal cord by misaligned elements of the vertebral column may often contribute to the neurological symptoms and signs following trauma. Deformities of the vertebral column resulting from spinal injuries follow fairly fixed patterns which are determined by the character of the initial force and the spinal level at which the trauma was received.

Fracture of the odontoid process

This relatively rare type of fracture is produced by a direct blow to the back or front of the head, violently forcing the head either forwards or backwards and putting great stress on the articulation between the atlas and the axis. In this situation the transverse ligament of the atlas remains intact and the odontoid process of the axis is broken off.

Fracture dislocation of the cervical spine
(Fig. 14.8)

A primary function of the cervical spine is mobility: the head must be able to flex both in the AP and lateral plane, and to rotate. For this reason all the articulating facets of the cervical vertebra are shallow and predisposed to the common fracture dislocation of the cervical spine. This type of spinal injury occurs when the forward motion of the body is arrested while its long axis is at right angles to the direction of motion, e.g. when an automobile strikes a tree with the passenger sitting upright. Under these circumstances the weight of the head prolongs its forward motion and pulls forward the upper cervical vertebra; a forward dislocation of the upper vertebra upon the lower vertebra may thus occur. In such cases the forward dislocation is the primary lesion and the fracture of the articulating facets is secondary.

Compression fracture of the cervical spine

This type of fracture occurs when the forward movement of the body is arrested while the body is moving in the direction of its longitudinal axis, e.g. when a person diving vertically strikes the top of his head against the bottom of a swimming pool. In this situation, one of the vertebral bodies is usually severely comminuted and fragments may be forcefully projected into the spinal canal. These compression fractures usually inflict more

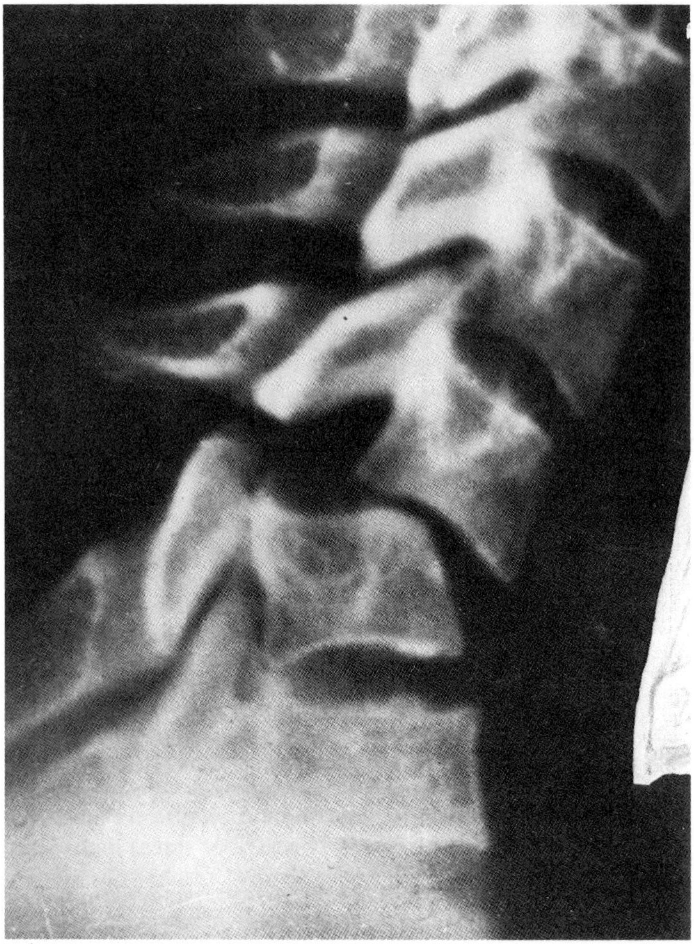

Fig. 14.8 Cervical radiograph showing fracture-dislocation

serious and permanent damage to the cord than fracture dislocation injuries and are often associated with the effects of head injury.

Fracture of the thoracic spine

The thoracic spine is so strongly reinforced by the overlapping of the spinous processes, by the articular processes and by the ribs, that fractures are seldom due to external injury except under conditions of exceptional violence. Whenever trauma of this degree of severity occurs it usually plays havoc with the vertebral column, fracturing, comminuting and dislocating a number of vertebra as well as adjacent ribs; such cases usually show extensive and irreparable damage to the spinal cord. Compression fractures of the thoracic spine may occur with lesser degrees of trauma and rarely cause cord damage.

Compression of the lumbar spine

By far the greatest number of compression fractures occur at the level of the twelfth thoracic or first lumbar vertebrae because of the anatomy this region. In the lumbar spine, strength and stability to support the great weight of the body are the prime functional objective. As a result, not only the bodies but also the articular processes of the lumbar vertebrae are strong and heavy, the articular facets are deep and the normal range of motion between any two vertebrae is slight. If the forward motion of the body is suddenly arrested, the inertia of the heavy thoracic cage tends to continue its forward motion. In the cervical region, as discussed above, fracture dislocations may occur, but in the lumbar region, because the articulations are so deep and strong, fracture dislocations are rare. Instead, the articulating facets act as a fulcrum and the force is transmitted in such a way as to compress the bodies of the vertebrae, resulting in a compression fracture. This may be accompanied by acute angulation of the spinal column, resulting in damage to the cord, conus or cauda equina.

TRANSECTION OF THE CORD

Complete anatomical transection of the cord following indirect trauma to the spine occurs with relative infrequency. It may be seen in penetrating injuries to the cord, such as high-velocity missile injuries or stab wounds. The signs of complete transection are indistinguishable from those of a temporary physiological interruption of spinal function. The exact state of the cord can be determined only by laminectomy and direct inspection, although this of course reveals only the external appearance and not the inner structure of the cord. Laminectomy for this purpose is not generally recommended.

SPINAL SHOCK

The term spinal shock was introduced by Marshall Hall to describe the transient suppression of nervous function below the level of transection of the spinal cord. The clinical manifestations of spinal shock are those of motor paralysis below the level of the lesion. The paralysis is at first flaccid and all cutaneous and tendon reflexes are abolished or greatly depressed. The modern concept of spinal shock is that the depression in segments below the transection is due to the sudden withdrawal of a predominantly facilitating influence of descending supraspinal tracts. Once the spinal shock begins to subside, afferent impulses arising from peripheral receptors begin to exert their excitatory influence on the neural elements. There then follows the development of the reflex automatism of the isolated cord with hyper-reflexia, rigidity and spasticity. Recovery from spinal shock in man may be delayed for some weeks. Occasionally, reflex activity of skeletal muscles may reappear within a matter of 3–4 days (particularly in children), but in adults this may be delayed for up to 6 weeks. Sepsis resulting from pressure sores or urinary infection may delay recovery from spinal shock. As a rule, reflex return is in a headward direction: the reflexes appearing first in man are the anal and bulbocavernous reflexes and the response to plantar stimulation. Upper limb reflexes return last.

SPECIFIC CLINICAL SYNDROMES

The cervical cord contusion syndrome

The mobility of the cervical spine, as indicated above, predisposes the cervical cord to damage. The end result of severe injuries is tetraplegia with a poor overall prognosis. In a complete lesion, that is to say a lesion associated with absence of any motor, sensory or automatic function, the prognosis is very poor if there is no evidence of recovery after a period of 24–48 hours; the prognosis in incomplete lesions is much better.

In routine clinical practice one of the commonest types of cervical cord injury is that called the cervical cord contusion syndrome. This most commonly occurs in old people and results either from fall backwards, or a fall forwards on the forehead, resulting in a hyperflexion or hyperextension injury. The damage is mediated in part by associated cervical spondylosis. Such patients may be tetraplegic from the time of their injury and anaesthetic below the neck. They usually show no bony abnormality other than cervical spondylosis and no fracture dislocations may be demonstrated. Recovery may begin within a matter of hours and the recovery pattern thereafter usually progresses, to leave only a mild or moderate deficit. Failure of improvement within 24 hours suggests a poor prognosis, as in other forms of cord damage. In such injuries, differing patterns of neurological deficit may be recognised, such as the anterior cord syndrome or the central cord syndrome.

The central cervical cord syndrome is characterised by disproportionately more motor impairment in the upper than the lower extremities and by varying degrees of sensory loss in the arms, particularly loss of pain and temperature sense (a syringomyelia-like syndrome). The syndrome is seen predominantly in hyperflexion injuries; the predominant localisation of the deficit in the central part of the cord may result from haemorrhage along the central canal of the cord.

The dorsal root ganglion syndrome

In recent years a specific syndrome thought to result from dorsal root ganglion damage has been recognised following cervical injuries. Such patients usually have suffered a hyperflexion or hyperextension injury and, from an early stage after the injury, complain of intense dysaesthetic pain in the upper limbs. Such symptoms are usually made worse by flexion or extension of the head and it is rare to find objective sensory loss. The prognosis for recovery is good and the symptoms are thought to result from contusion and haemorrhage in and around the dorsal root ganglia.

Whiplash injuries

Cervical cord and spine damage probably bear the same relation to whiplash injury as head injury bears to the postconcussional syndrome. Indeed, the medicolegal significance of whiplash injuries is now probably as great, if not greater than, the postconcussional syndrome. Whiplash injuries typically occur in motor vehicle accidents when a car is hit from behind by another vehicle. A typical whiplash injury patient suffers a rapid flexion-extension movement of the head and, from an early stage, complains of pain in the neck and of headache. Although such injuries may be associated with neurological damage to the cord, in the typical whiplash injury no such evidence is present and the main complaints are of pain. Subsequently dizziness and a variety of other symptoms may develop and the effects of litigation may make such symptoms assume enormous significance in the individual's day-to-day life. Although it is true that a whiplash injury may produce contusion and haemorrhage in the soft tissues of the neck, in most instances the persistence of such symptoms is attributable to either an associated affective disorder or to frank simulation.

ACUTE PARAPLEGIA

Acute paraplegia may result from damage either to the dorsal cord or to the cauda equina. The level of the damage is of crucial importance, as the prognosis for cauda equina injuries is much better than that for dorsal cord injuries: statistically (see above), the latter are more common than the former. Although the detailed management of acute paraplegia is beyond the scope of this chapter, some general comments follow.

Management of acute tetraplegia or paraplegia

First aid and transportation

The proper management of the patient with a spinal cord injury should start at the place of the accident: great skill is required in moving such patients, both in or out of hospital. It has now been shown indisputably that the best comprehensive management of a traumatic paraplegic or tetraplegic injury can be given only in a special spinal centre: at an early stage, consideration should be given to transporting such patients to one of these centres.

A detailed neurological assessment should be made at an early stage to assess the degree of motor paralysis, the presence or absence of spinal shock, and the degree of sensory loss.

Radiological studies

An early priority should be to obtain a radiological study of the entire vertebral column, although special diagnostic radiological procedures are rarely required. For example, myelography is indicated only in the acute stage of a spinal lesion when there is a considerable time lapse between the accident and the onset of paralysis, or when there is definite progression of paralysis.

Shock and associated injuries

It is always important in a case of spinal trauma to treat associated injuries and shock at an early stage. There should be careful monitoring of the patient's pulse and blood pressure and associated head, chest or abdominal injuries should be sought.

Immobilisation

Until the stability of the spine has been assessed, it is important that the whole spinal column should be immobilised. In unstable fracture dislocations of the spine, appropriate action must be taken: however, discussion of this is beyond the scope of this chapter. After the initial clinical appraisal, various stages of management ensue until the stage of rehabilitation is reached. The principles of such management are as follows:

1. Prevention of extension of damage (immobilisation)
2. Preservation of bladder and bowel function
3. Preservation of integrity of the skin
4. Management of complications:
   a. cardiovascular system
   b. respiratory system
   c. gastrointestinal system (stress ulcers)
   d. temperature regulation.

The principles of the management of chronic paraplegic and tetraplegic patients, including rehabilitation, are included in detail in Chapter 9.

LONG-TERM COMPLICATIONS

Post-traumatic syringomyelia

This syndrome has been recognised in recent years as a late after-effect of traumatic damage to the cord. Typically, the symptoms are of an increasing neurological deficit in a patient who has been stable for some time following spinal cord damage. Such symptoms rarely develop within a year of injury and may be delayed for many years. Most commonly, a patient who has been paraplegic for some years then becomes aware of an ascending sensory disturbance, with motor and sensory involvement beginning in the arms. The deficit results from an ascending central cord cyst which usually extends up from the level of the damage, although it may extend down the cord. The aetiology of the syndrome is unknown; without treatment, the cyst will usually continue to enlarge, with resulting increasing deficit. The only definitive therapy is to remove the distending fluid from the cavity; a variety of surgical procedures have been introduced to achieve this.

Arachnoiditis

Arachnoiditis may follow spinal cord damage; the clinical features of post-traumatic arachnoiditis are given in Chapter 9.

BRACHIAL PLEXUS AND CERVICAL ROOT INJURIES

Traumatic damage to the roots as they leave the spinal cord, and to the brachial and lumbosacral plexuses, are an increasingly common problem. The increase in incidence has been largely attributable to motor cycle accidents.

These injuries often occur in association with trauma to multiple systems, so that concern for preservation of life or limb may overshadow their presence. High-velocity injuries in motor cycle or automobile drivers are the commonest cause of brachial plexus injuries; the introduction of seat belts and motor cycle helmets has perhaps allowed the survival of such individuals, to be left severely damaged because of cervical root or brachial plexus trauma.

ANATOMY

The gross anatomy of the brachial plexus and the cervical root outflow is shown in Figure 14.9. For a thorough appreciation of the basic clinical aspects of the problem, various points must be borne in mind. The dorsal root ganglia which contain the cell bodies for the sensory nerves are located outside the cord, either within or near the intervertebral foramen. If the spinal roots are avulsed from the cord, the motor axons are disconnected from their cell bodies, the anterior horn cells, and undergo Wallerian degeneration. The sensory axons avulsed at the same level are still attached to their ganglia and do not degen-

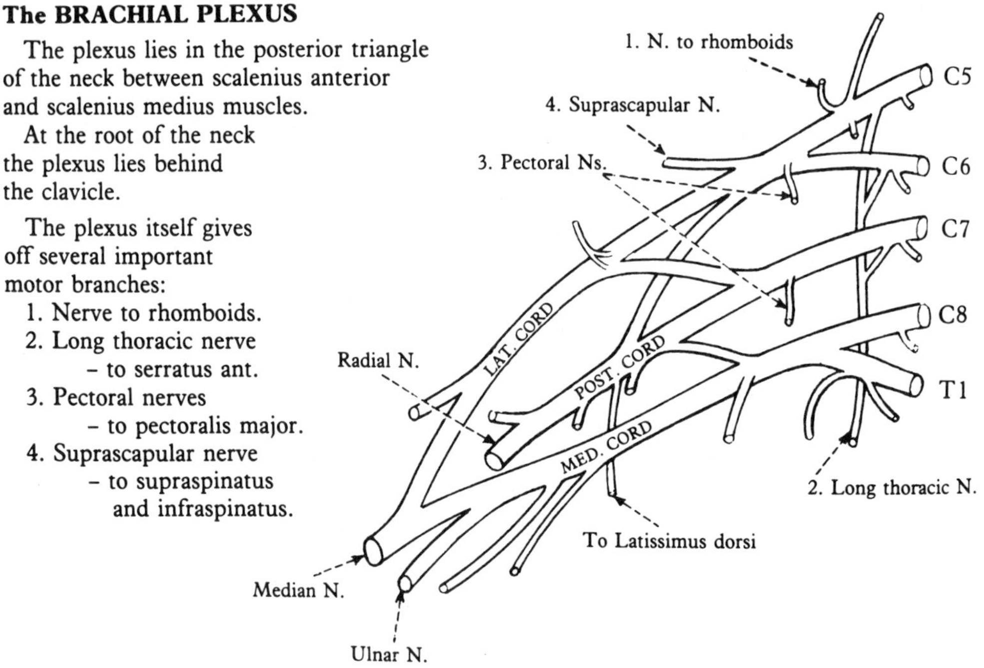
The BRACHIAL PLEXUS
The plexus lies in the posterior triangle of the neck between scalenius anterior and scalenius medius muscles.
At the root of the neck the plexus lies behind the clavicle.
The plexus itself gives off several important motor branches:
1. Nerve to rhomboids.
2. Long thoracic nerve - to serratus ant.
3. Pectoral nerves - to pectoralis major.
4. Suprascapular nerve - to supraspinatus and infraspinatus.
1. N. to rhomboids
4. Suprascapular N.
3. Pectoral Ns.
C5
C6
C7
C8
T1
LAT. CORD
POST. CORD
MED. CORD
Radial N.
2. Long thoracic N.
To Latissimus dorsi
Median N.
Ulnar N.

Fig. 14.9 Anatomy of the brachial plexus and cervical roots. (Reproduced from Lindsay K W, Bone I, Callander R 1986 *Neurology and Neurosurgery Illustrated*. Churchill Livingstone, Edinburgh, with permission.)

erate, but sensation is lost because the central connection from the dorsal root to the cord has been ruptured. Rupture of the root is described as a preganglionic lesion and the prognosis for recovery of function of that particular root is hopeless. Damage more distally, a so-called post-ganglionic lesion, may be associated with spontaneous recovery if the supporting structural elements persist despite axonal degeneration. In consideration of brachial plexus injuries the aim should always be to determine whether the problem is due to root avulsion or to damage within the plexus itself.

In the differentiation of root from plexus damage, it should be remembered that the deep cervical fascia invests the nerve roots and the cervical transverse processes; this may protect the plexus from traction injury, or the transverse processes may fracture, carrying with them the fragile nerve roots that are pulled from the cord. The phrenic nerve, which comes mainly from the fourth cervical root, is also augmented by fibres from the third and fifth cervical roots. Avulsion of the fifth cervical root is sometimes diagnosed indirectly by fluoroscopic demonstration of paralysis of the ipsilateral hemidiaphragm. Paralysis of the rhomboids after brachial plexus injury is also indicative of damage to the fifth cervical root, because the dorsal scapular nerve comes from this root soon after its exit from the foramen. The branches from the fifth, sixth and seventh cervical roots to the long thoracic nerve also arrive at this level before formation of the three trunks. If preservation of the above muscles can be demonstrated and there is paralysis of the lateral rotators of the humerus, the lesion can be located accurately to the region of Erb's point, where the fifth and sixth cervical roots join to form the upper trunk. The finding of paralysis of all of the above muscles would immediately indicate that the injury is supraclavicular.

MECHANISMS OF INJURY

The most common mechanism of injury to the brachial plexus is traction. This may be associated with bony injuries to either the clavicle, the humerus, or (more rarely) the scapula. Dislocation of the shoulder may be an associated injury. The energy imparted to the nerves will be determined by the violence of the trauma and the distribution of the damage is determined by the position of the arm in relation to the body at the time of the impact. If the arm is abducted, greater stress is expended on the lower roots whereas, if the arm is adducted, the reverse situation prevails. Compression is a far less common cause of the injuries of the brachial plexus. It may result from external factors such as the straps on knapsacks or from a figure-of-eight bandage used to immobilise a fractured clavicle. Acute open laceration of the plexus is relatively uncommon; in view of the close proximity of the great vessels, this may be a life-threatening injury. One other specific traction injury is occasionally encountered on the surgical ward after inappropriate positioning of an upper limb during a general anaesthetic; the incidence of this may be reduced by care during the anaesthetic procedure, but such traction injuries may be seen, for example, after a mastectomy.

Open injuries

These are uncommon: those that do occur are usually caused by sharp objects such as broken glass or knives, or by missiles, usually bullets. In this group of injuries, as distinct from traction injuries, the potential for direct surgical treatment by suture or graft may exist and immediate exploration is usually advised; however, the past results of surgical repair have not been favourable. The recent development of the operating microscope and refinements in techniques of nerve grafting may in time alter these results in carefully selected cases. The prognosis for *spontaneous* neurological recovery after an open wound has been shown to be considerably better in the upper trunk and its branches than in the lower.

Closed injuries

Mechanisms of nerve damage

A variety of different mechanisms of nerve damage may occur, depending on the severity of the traction injury.

Neuropraxia

In this injury, the axons are stretched but the axon sheath and nerve sheaths are preserved and there is no loss of continuity. Usually there is functional recovery within a matter of a few weeks.

Axonotmesis

In this injury there is loss of continuity of the axon sheath but the nerve sheaths are preserved. The axon will have to regrow by sprouting: it is thought that axons grow at a rate of approximately 1 mm/day. This usually means that there will be a good or reasonable prognosis in the proximal muscles supplied by the upper cervical roots, but a poor prognosis for the distal muscles, particularly the small hand muscles. Usually by the time the axons have regrown to reach the small hand muscles they have atrophied and fibrosed, and no recovery is possible.

Neurotmesis

In this injury there is complete loss of continuity of the nerve sheath. Such nerves or roots will not recover without surgery. The commonest site of traction injuries is to the supraclavicular portions of the plexus. Varying patterns of damage may be seen.

The C5, 6 or upper trunk lesion results in an adducted and medially rotated humerus that cannot be actively moved away from the side in any plane. There is paralysis of the deltoid and lateral rotators of the humerus, as well as the clavicular portion of the pectoralis major, with inability to flex the elbow or supinate the forearm. The prognosis for spontaneous recovery in these lesions is relatively good as they have the highest incidence of neuropraxis or nondegenerative lesions.

The more extensive the damage, the worse the prognosis: patients with involvement of C5, C6, C7, C8 and T1 have a bad prognosis, unless recovery of function starts within 6 weeks (suggesting neuropraxia).

Postoperative brachial plexus palsies, whatever their extent, usually recover completely.

METHODS OF EVALUATION

The patient with a brachial plexus injury must be systematically evaluated in order to arrive at an accurate prognosis for both neurological and functional recovery. The history of the type of injury must be obtained and a detailed physical examination performed. There should be a detailed neurological assessment, not only of the affected arm but also of other parts of the body. Spasticity of the ipsilateral lower extremity is highly suggestive of cord injury as a result of root avulsion. The presence of a Horner syndrome suggests a preganglionic lesion of the T1 root. Tapping over a peripheral nerve may be accompanied by a tingling sensation within the distribution of the nerve (Tinel's sign), and this indicates continuity of the affected nerve.

Radiographs of the cervical spine may provide important additional prognostic data in traction injuries of the brachial plexus. Avulsion of the cervical transverse processes suggests cervical root avulsion with a poor prognosis.

Electromyography is useful in the diagnosis and estimation of prognosis of brachial plexus injury. Electromyography performed after the period required for Wallerian degeneration can be used to determine motor activity or recovery too subtle to be detected by clinical examination. If the posterior cervical musculature is found to be denervated in a patient with a clinically observed plexus injury, the lesion for that segment can be said to be preganglionic because the posterior primary divisions arise from the main roots just lateral to the intervertebral foramina; the prognosis for that root can then be assumed to be hopeless. If the posterior musculature is spared, then the damage is likely to be postganglionic with a possibility of recovery. It is possible to perform nerve conduction studies across the plexus and find evidence of either loss or preservation of continuity of certain roots; assessment of the f waves may be helpful.

Assessment of the axon response may be a useful prognostic tool. If 1% Histamine acid phosphate is pricked into normal skin, a triple response consisting of local vasodilatation, formation of a weal, and then further vasodilatation (flare) occurs. In an anaesthetic area denervated by a preganglionic lesion, because the cell body is not seperated from the dendrite reaching the skin, the response will be unaltered; this will be a positive response and a poor prognostic sign. If, however, the damage is postganglionic the triple response is altered by elimination of the flare, and the possibility of recovery still exists. As the dermatomes are generally well delineated, the anaesthetic areas served by the roots in question can be tested.

Myelography may demonstrate the presence of traumatic meningoceles in the cervical myelograms of patients with root avulsion (Fig. 14.10). The presence of a meningocele indicates root avulsion and a hopeless prognosis for recovery of that root: unfortunately, the absence of a meningocele does not exclude the possibility that the root has been avulsed, as such meningoceles may be obliterated by fibrosis.

ASSESSMENT

To sum up, the assessment of the neurological prognosis should proceed as follows. The history, physical and neurological findings should be recorded initially in detail and radiographs of the cervical spine and shoulder girdle should be obtained. Repeated examination should be performed and electromyographic examination should be undertaken 4–6 weeks after injury. If at 3 months no recovery has taken place in a flail anaesthetic arm, then myelography should be performed, looking for signs of root avulsion. Traumatic meningoceles (Fig. 14.10), when present, indicate that the appropriate root has been avulsed; axon responses should be tested in anaesthetic areas. If at 3 months there is evidence of root avulsion, then there is no hope of recovery. If the damage is thought to be postganglionic and no recovery has occurred by 3 months, then surgical exploration, either to establish a prognosis or to consider nerve grafting, is justified.

There are well-documented histograms which enable a prognosis to be given for spontaneous recovery of damaged but unsevered nerves. For example, it is most unlikely that a paralysed deltoid will recover any noteworthy function if there is no evidence for a recovery either clinically

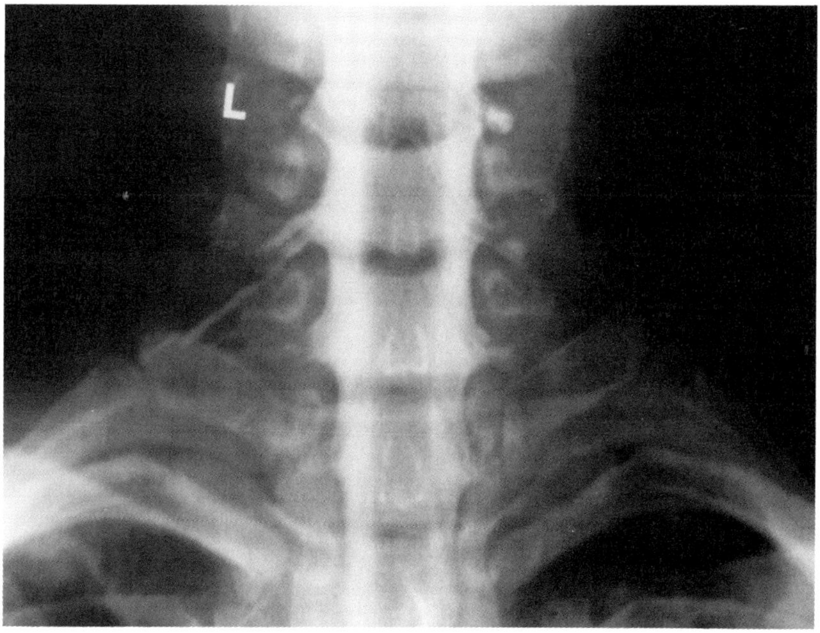

Fig. 14.10 Cervical myelogram showing traumatic meningocele in patient who suffered cervical root avulsion.

or electrically at one year; similar estimates may be made for other muscle groups. The worst prognosis is for the intrinsic muscles of the hand, because of their distal location and tendency to marked atrophy.

TREATMENT (Indications for surgery)

There is increasing interest in surgical intervention for patients who have postganglionic plexus damage: with the introduction of surgical techniques using the operative microscope, nerve grafting, resection and suture are now more feasible procedures. The timing of such operations varies from centre to centre and in some centres early operation is performed in order to establish the extent of root avulsion plexus damage.

UPPER LIMB REHABILITATION

Whatever the neurological evaluation, the overall potential for rehabilitation must be considered and appropriate action taken. A specific plan of passive and (where possible) active exercise should be undertaken on a daily basis from an early stage and appropriate splints applied to try to reduce contractures. For the patient with a flail anaesthetic arm there are a number of choices: first, he may retain the limb and be taught to act as a one-handed person; an alternative is the extensive surgical reconstruction of the limb, using the techniques of shoulder, elbow and wrist arthrodesis; the final means of dealing with such a limb is by amputation. In general, the first option is the one most commonly undertaken, usually in conjunction with the supply of appropriate mechanical aids.

COMPLICATIONS

One of the most feared complications of brachial plexus damage is that of intractable pain. This most commonly occurs in an anaesthetic paralysed arm and may begin immediately after the injury or after a delay. Typically it is burning, constant and interferes with everyday activities including sleep. There is unfortunately little effective treatment, although recently it has been claimed that percutaneous lesions to the dorsal root entry zones may be palliative (Nashold's procedure). Amputation of such an anaesthetic painful limb does not alleviate the pain.

LUMBOSACRAL PLEXUS INJURIES

Damage to the lumbosacral plexus is much less common than that to the brachial plexus because of the highly protected situation of the lumbosacral plexus within the pelvis. Occasionally, examples of damage to the lumbosacral plexus are encountered in patients who have suffered massive injuries to the plexus with multiple fractures of the pelvic bones. Penetrating injuries involving the lumbosacral plexus are similarly rarely encountered and are usually overshadowed by the massive injury to the other important organs situated within the pelvis. Direct traumatic damage to the lumbar plexus may be seen during retroperitoneal surgery, although with care this should be avoided. Traction on the lumbosacral plexus, and particularly upon the sciatic nerve, may occur during manipulation of the leg at the time of a hip joint replacement but, again, such damage is rare and, as with other postoperative plexus palsies, the prognosis is usually good.

THE FAT EMBOLISM SYNDROME

This important syndrome is one of the characteristic complications of major trauma.

PATHOGENESIS

It is important to recognise the distinction between fat embolism and the fat embolism syndrome. Up to 90% of patients who have suffered major trauma which includes bone injury can be shown at autopsy to have fat droplet deposits in the lungs and elsewhere, but only a small proportion develop this syndrome. The distinction between fat embolism and fat embolism syndrome is thought to be related to the total mass of fat which is released into the circulation from the traumatised tissues. The emboli are thought to block small arterioles and capillaries, after which they are coated with platelets; the fat embolism syndrome is typically associated with long-bone fractures. Some investigators believe that the fat emboli do not originate from bone marrow, but may be formed by the coalescence of fat chylomicrons.

CLINICAL FEATURES

Typically, these appear within 72 hours of a fracture of a long bone such as the femur or tibia. One of the most interesting features is that the syndrome has never been known to develop twice in the same patient, in spite of repeated orthopaedic manipulations of the original injury. Confusion, restlessness or coma with breathlessness are the most common presenting features. Grand mal seizures may occur and there is often an irritating cough, with or without haemoptysis. Occasionally, the syndrome may present as failure to regain consciousness following orthopaedic manipulations performed under general anaethesia. Focal neurological signs may be present but are unusual. Most patients with the fat embolism syndrome have haematuria, detectable by microscopy.

The neurological features of the syndrome result from embolic obstruction of arterioles or capillaries in the cerebral substance. It is uncertain how the fat passes through the pulmonary capillaries: one explanation is that a right-to-left shunt develops through a patent foramen ovale. However, only 25% of patients who die of the fat embolism syndrome have been found to have such an anomaly.

A variable degree of hypoxia is usually present and can be detected by analysis of the patient's blood gases. A rash may appear, often seen first on the anterior chest.

PROGNOSIS

The severity of the illness is largely related to the extent of the injuries: after very extensive fractures, patients may succumb within 24 hours of developing the syndrome. Death is usually from respiratory failure; there is usually a good prognosis for functional recovery from the neurological effects of fat embolism. Patients who die in the acute phase are usually found to have hundreds of petechial haemorrhages scattered through the cerebral white and grey matter. If the patient survives the immediate insult but dies days or weeks later, no gross areas of cerebral infarction are found.

TREATMENT

Hypoxia is the most dangerous feature of this condition and treatment of this should be instituted immediately the diagnosis is suspected. The fundamental principles of management include the maintenance of gas exchange, the prevention or treatment of fluid overload and pulmonary oedema, and the avoidance of potentially harmful agents.

FURTHER READING

Cartlidge N E F, Shaw D A 1981 Head injury. W B Saunders Company, Philadelphia

Jennet B, Teasedale G 1981 Management of head injuries. F A Davis Company, Philadelphia

Leffert R D 1974 Brachial plexus injuries. New England Journal of Medicine 291: 1059–1067

15

Inherited and degenerative disorders of the central nervous system

INTRODUCTION

A wide variety of conditions can loosely be considered together as being degenerative in nature. Although, in some of these conditions metabolic disorders have been clearly identified, the aetiology of most remains unknown. Many of these conditions have a genetic basis but can also occur in sporadic forms. In this chapter we have also included discussion of a number of conditions which are chronic or progressive, but which are not associated with definite pathological changes, such as torsion dystonia. We have not included a discussion of the many neonatal and early childhood neurological disorders which do not present to general physicians and adult neurologists, as these fall outside the scope of the book.

Few of the conditions are amenable to specific therapy, but the dramatic improvements in the symptomatic treatment of Parkinson's disease over the last two decades indicate that the search for such treatments is by no means hopeless. For many conditions, however, the most important clinical problem is that of offering a specific diagnosis as, in many cases, genetic counselling of affected families is of enormous importance. Nevertheless, it must be remembered that adequate symptomatic treatment and care can greatly improve the quality of life, both for sufferers and for their immediate family. The specialised problems presented by these patients needs considerable thought and the attentions of multidisciplinary teams, including physiotherapists, occupational therapists, nurses and speech therapists and social workers, as well as regular appraisal by a neurologist.

DEGENERATIVE DISORDERS IN WHICH DEMENTIA IS PROMINENT

The clinical features of dementia have been discussed in Chapter 6. Although degenerative disorders are the commonest causes of dementia, it must always be remembered that metabolic and other treatable causes of dementia, such as frontal meningioma and hydrocephalus, must actively be excluded by appropriate investigation.

Dementia is a common feature of a wide variety of degenerative disorders summarised in Table

Table 15.1 Classification of the degenerative dementias

Dementia alone	Dementia a prominent feature	Dementia a minor feature
Alzheimer's	Huntington's	Parkinson's
Pick's	Adreno-leucodystrophy	Wilson's
	Metachromatic leucodystrophy	Progressive supranuclear palsy
	Other storage diseases	Shy–Drager
		Striatonigral degeneration
		Hallervorden-Spatz
		Spinocerebellar degenerations
		Basal ganglia calcification

15.1. It is, however, necessary to differentiate normal ageing processes from degenerative dementia. Characterising normal ageing presents some difficulties: there are undoubted functional changes with age, which include slowed reaction, mild decline in intelligence, reduced short-term memory and slowed learning; brain weight and volume decline with increasing age, and there is a loss of cortical thickness, due to neuronal loss and increasing gliosis; pathological changes, in particular, differentiate normal ageing from the degenerative dementias.

ALZHEIMER'S DISEASE

The pathological changes in Alzheimer's disease are striking and specific and consist of amyloid (senile) plaques and neurofibrillary tangles, which may be quite diffuse, but most frequently predominate in cortical areas (Fig. 15.1); these are found both in presenile and senile dementias. One interesting feature of the pathology is its universal occurrence in those patients with Down's syndrome who survive into the fourth and fifth decades of life. Its incidence is very much age-related and over the age of 70 up to 4% of the population may be suffering from this disorder; it is 2–3 times more common in men than women. Approximately 10% of cases appear on a familial basis with an apparent autosomal dominant pattern of inheritance; in such instances the onset of the dementia is earlier than in non-familial cases.

Clinical features

The clinical features of the dementia of Alzheimer's disease are those of a cortical dementia. Onset is after 40 years, with increasing incidence in later decades. Memory disturbance usually appears first, together with increasing apathy, poor judgement and difficulty in reasoning; more profound disturbances of speech, praxis and personality follow; late in the disorder, progressive motor disturbances may be seen with development of both pyramidal and extrapyramidal signs; eventually, patients become bedbound. Myoclonic jerks may occur in up to 10% of patients late in the disease and occasionally seizures are seen. The rate of progression is variable, but the majority of patients die from the complications of immobility within 5–10 years of diagnosis.

Investigation

The investigation of patients with Alzheimer's disease reveals little that is specific and is largely undertaken to exclude other treatable causes of dementia. The CT scan usually shows atrophy of both grey and white matter, resulting in increase in size of both cerebral sulci and ventricles, respectively (Fig. 15.2). The c.s.f. is normal and the EEG shows only non-specific changes.

Treatment

No specific treatment for Alzheimer's disease is available. A variety of regimes aimed at increasing cerebral acetylcholine activity have been investigated, but none is effective.

PICK'S DISEASE

This represents a rare form of dementia (Alzheimer's disease is 10–15 times more common) and the diagnosis is rarely made during life. In essence, it is a pathological entity of

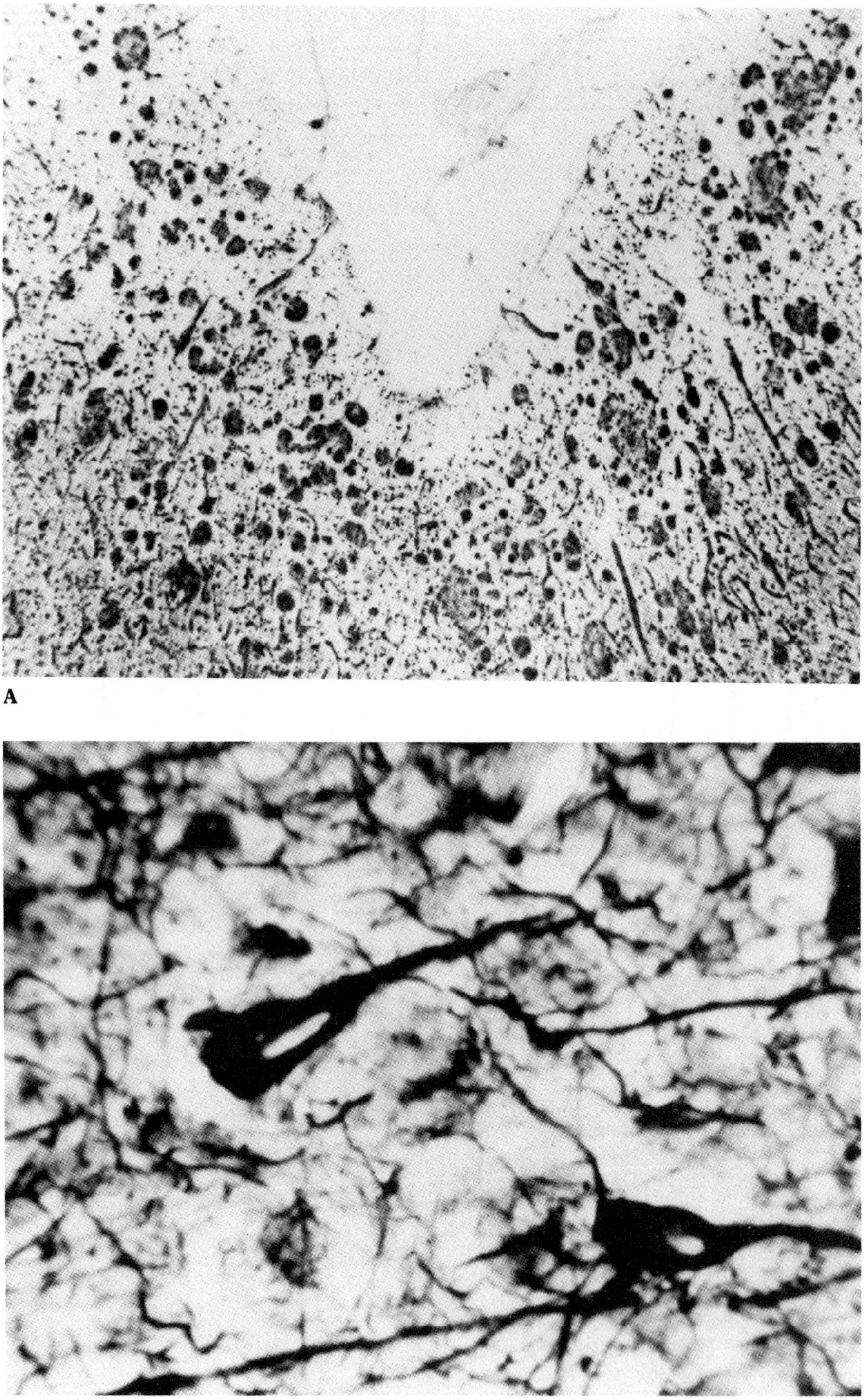

A

B

Fig. 15.1 Pathology of Alzheimer's disease. **A** Photomicrograph showing numerous argyrophilic plaques in cerebral cortex (Bielschowsky's silver method). **B** Photomicrograph showing neurofibrillary degeneration in neurones (Bielschowsky's silver method).

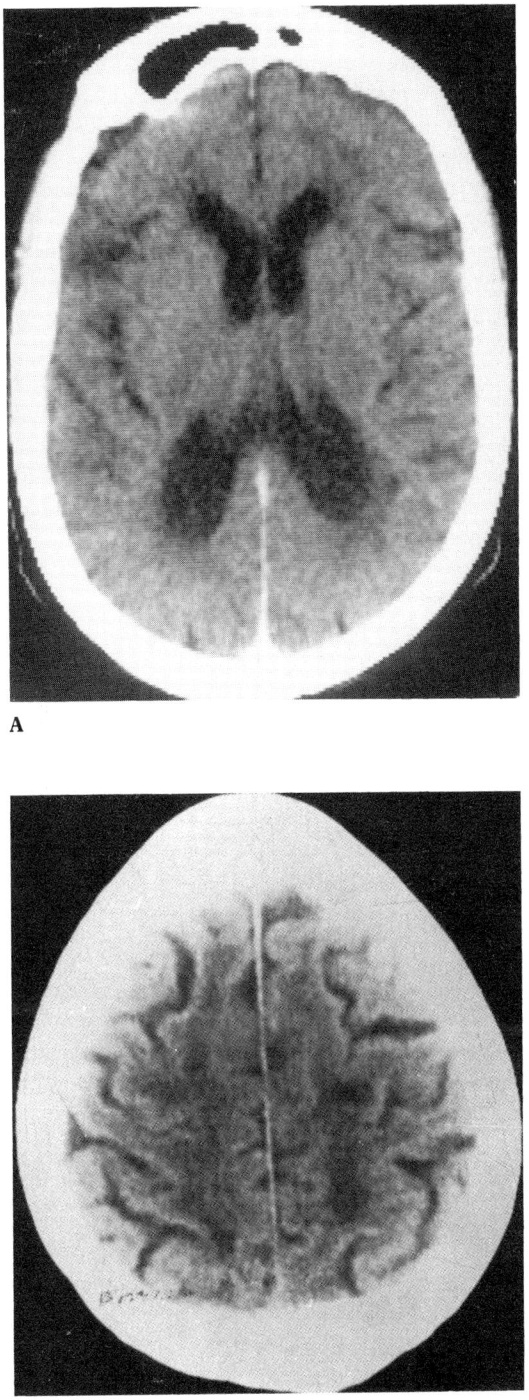

Fig. 15.2 Gross cerebral atrophy on two cuts of a CT scan in a patient with Alzheimer's disease. Note enlargement of ventricles and sulci.

unknown aetiology. Macroscopically there is gross focal wasting of grey and white matter of the frontal and temporal lobes. Histological changes are of loss of neurones with swelling of the cytoplasm of surviving cells which contain silver-staining bodies; this differentiates it from Alzheimer's disease.

Clinical features

Onset is usually between 40 and 60 years and it is more common in women. Although it is usually sporadic, 10–20% of cases may be familial. Patients with this cortical dementia are said to show more marked changes of personality than those seen in Alzheimer's disease, with increased apathy and disinterest as well as a high incidence of dysphasia with later impairment of memory. The Kluver–Bucy syndrome of emotional blunting, increased eating, oral exploration and inappropriate sexual activity, which was originally produced in monkeys by bilateral temporal lobe ablation, is said to be not uncommon in this condition. The ease with which these features distinguish the condition from Alzheimer's disease is questionable. The course of the disease is progressive, with survival for 10–15 years.

HUNTINGTON'S CHOREA

This represents perhaps the most striking of familial neurological disorders; it is certainly one of the most common, with a prevalence of 40–70 per million. The pathological changes are localised mainly in the caudate head and putamen of the basal ganglia, although there are more diffuse changes at cortical levels. There has been considerable recent interest in biochemical abnormalities in this disorder, as particularly low levels of GABA and acetylcholine have been found within the basal ganglia. This finding has not as yet borne any therapeutic fruit.

Clinical features

The syndrome presents as an autosomally dominant pattern of inheritance manifesting itself with subcortical dementia, personality and behavioural change and an associated choreic movement disorder; the psychiatric changes and dementia usually develop first. The peak onset is in the fourth and fifth decades of life, but symptoms may develop at any time from the first to the seventh decades: this has the unfortunate implication that many patients carrying the Huntington's gene will have passed through the reproductive years before the disorder declares itself.

The mental changes usually present with memory problems and disturbances of mood and behaviour. Choreic movements are often evident by this time; facial movement and distal limb chorea usually predominate. When Huntington's disease presents in early life (10–15%) the clinical features may be rather different: it may present as a rigid parkinsonian syndrome, sometimes with associated seizures; very occasionally a similar presentation is seen in adult life.

The disorder is progressive and results in death from the complications of immobility within 5–15 years of onset. Suicide is common (5–10% of cases).

The differential diagnosis does not present problems as long as a clear family history is evident; considerable effort is often necessary to unearth this. There is a low mutation rate, which may account for some cases without family histories, but it is said that a high incidence of an absence of family history in this disorder may be due to the trait manifesting itself in early life as sexual promiscuity. The main differential diagnosis is from other forms of chorea: Sydenham's chorea remains very rare, and an adequate history of drugs administered will usually help to exclude drug-induced choreas; there remain problems with patients with so-called 'senile chorea'—how real an entity this is remains debatable.

Investigation

Investigation of patients with Huntington's chorea rarely leads to the detection of specific abnormalities and the diagnosis remains a clinical one. In the late stages CT scanning is likely to show specific atrophy of the head of the caudate nucleus, but this feature is not useful or diagnostic in the early stages of the disease. In younger patients it is important to exclude Wilson's disease by estimation of serum copper and caeruloplasmin.

Treatment

No specific treatment is as yet available. The diagnostic importance is in the genetic counselling of affected families. Families must be aware that offspring of an affected individual have a 50% chance of inheriting the gene. In the absence of specific treatment it is more difficult to make use of tests which predict later development of the condition in an at-risk individual. The identification of a DNA sequence close to the Huntington's gene locus may shortly make such prediction possible.

The use of phenothiazines and haloperidol may reduce the chorea to a degree, at the expense of rendering the patient more rigid. In addition, behaviour may be modulated by these drugs. Tetrabenazine may also reduce chorea.

CREUTZFELDT–JAKOB DISEASE

This disorder with an apparently degenerative pathology has now clearly been associated with a transmissable agent. Clinical features of the condition are dealt with in Chapter 12 (p 320).

MULTISYSTEM DEGENERATIONS ASSOCIATED WITH DEMENTIA

Dementias are a not infrequent accompaniment of many multisystem degenerative disorders. They are, however, usually mild to moderate in severity and are overshadowed by other, usually motor, disorders.

Adrenoleucodystrophy

This is now recognised as a metabolic encephalopathy transmitted as an X-linked recessive trait, only males being affected. The full clinical picture comprises adrenal insufficiency and widespread hemisphere demyelination. The age of onset varies between 4 and 12 years, but adult cases are seen. Adrenal insufficiency or neurological disease may present first.

Frequently the first symptoms are those of intellectual deterioration, often associated with vomiting, syncope and other symptoms of circulatory disturbance; the skin becomes bronzed; patients develop progressive quadriparesis, dysarthria and dysphasia and pseudobulbar palsy; very often they go on to develop cortical blindness and ultimately become decorticate.

Investigation

The detection of biochemical abnormalities is most important in making the diagnosis. Classic findings are of low plasma sodium and chloride levels and elevated potassium. Serum cortisol levels are low, ACTH levels elevated, and there is no response to a synacthen stimulation test. C.s.f. protein levels are very often elevated. CT scanning shows white matter lucency.

Metachromatic leucodystrophy

This is a sphingolipid storage disease: there appears to be a deficiency or absence of aryl sulphatase A, which prevents the conversion of sulphatide into cerebroside. It is transmitted as an autosomal recessive gene and usually becomes evident within the first four years of life; however, it may occasionally present in adolescence or adult life. In adults the disorder results in prominent mental regression, pseudobulbar dysarthria, weakness and ataxia. The peripheral nervous system is involved, with neuropathy leading to paraesthesiae and areflexia. Blindness may occur, due to optic atrophy, and there are often signs of intention tremor and nystagmus; seizures occur on occasion. Very occasionally, the peripheral nervous system may be involved without c.n.s. involvement.

Investigations

Metachromatic material may be detected in the urine, but the diagnostic laboratory test is the finding of diminished aryl sulphatase A in urine, white blood cells and skin fibroblasts. No treatment is available and the disorder runs a rapidly progressive course. A number of other rare leucodystrophies (familial orthochromic leucodystrophy, Pelizaeus–Merzbacher and Cockayne's disease), which usually present in childhood, may declare themselves during adult life.

Very occasionally a number of other specific storage disorders may present in adult life with a prominent dementia, associated often with seizures, myoclonus and progressive spasticity and weakness. A full discussion is beyond the scope of this book, but some of these disorders are outlined in Table 15.2.

Table 15.2 Rare adult-onset storage disorders associated with dementia

Disorder	Cause	Stored material	Clinical features
GM2-gangliosidosis	Hexosaminidase A deficiency	GM2-ganglioside	Dementia Seizures Cranial nerve palsies Spasticity and ataxia
Gaucher's disease	Acid β-glucosidase deficiency	Glucocerebroside	Dementia Myoclonus and seizures
Fabry's disease	Ceramide trihexoside deficiency	Ceramide	Multi-infarct dementia Painful polyneuropathy Angiokeratoma corporis diffusum
Kufs' disease	Uncertain	Lipofuscin Membrane fragments Granular material	Dementia Myoclonus and seizures Spasticity and ataxia Visual failure
Cerebrotendinous xanthomatosis	Uncertain	Cholestanol	Dementia and psychosis Myoclonus Ataxia Xanthoma of tendons

DEGENERATIVE DISORDERS IN WHICH EXTRAPYRAMIDAL FEATURES ARE PROMINENT

PARKINSON'S DISEASE

Parkinson's disease is an extremely common cause of neurological disability. The disease predominantly affects patients over the age of 50, but much younger patients can develop the disorder. The prevalence of the disease rises progressively with age and above the age of 60 up to 1 in 100 of the population may be suffering from the disorder.

The cause of idiopathic Parkinson's disease remains uncertain. Recent evidence has focused research on possible toxic substances: a number of drug abusers using a synthetic opiate drug contaminated with MPTP (*N*-methyl-4-phenyl-1,2,5,6-tetrahydropyridine) have been shown to develop a condition that closely resembles Parkinson's disease in its clinical features, response to L-dopa and selective loss of striatonigral neurones; the metabolite MPP+ appears to possess marked neurotoxicity and it is possible that other polar substances could have similar effects.

The main pathological changes are loss of pigmented cells in the substantia nigra with the presence of Lewy bodies (Fig. 15.3). These cells appear to give rise to a discrete nigrostriatal tract, which largely terminates in the caudate nucleus; here it appears that there is a complex balance between dopaminergic and cholinergic functions. Thus, striatal dopamine deficiency or relative cholinergic overactivity produce lack of movement, rigidity and catalepsy, whereas increased dopaminergic activity or decreased cholinergic activity tend to increase movement and produce hypotonia of muscles. It is undoubtedly true that the severe striatal dopamine deficiency seen in Parkinson's disease is the single most important factor in producing the symptoms and signs of the disorder. However, other striatal neurotransmitters are abnormal in the condition: thus decreased concentrations of serotonin, GABA and catecholamines have been found. The role of these transmitter systems in the disability of Parkinson's disease is, however, considerably less certain.

Although most patients with Parkinson's disease have no family history, familial Parkinsonism does occur occasionally; in such instances the disorder tends to start earlier in life.

Clinical features

The cardinal features of parkinsonism have been described in Chapter 1. The most striking feature is the *bradykinesia*, which is the commonest cause of complaint in the parkinsonian patient. This may manifest itself in a variety of ways, including slowness of gait, difficulty in using—and clumsiness of—the hands, difficulty in writing, and alteration of facial expression. The earliest symptoms usually relate to use of the hands; patients with initial complaints about gait are unlikely to have Parkinson's disease. *Tremor* will be present in a varying proportion of patients with such symptoms: this is classically a 4–5 cycle per second rest tremor which most commonly affects the arms, resulting in a supernation-pronation or pill-rolling tremor; on occasion the tremor may be severe and the initial source of complaint. Some patients with Parkinson's disease also show varieties of action tremor or postural tremor, but these are much less common.

The characteristic plastic *rigidity* of Parkinson's disease (on which may be superimposed cogwheeling in patients with rest tremor) is rarely a source of symptomatic complaint. However, some patients with Parkinson's disease complain of muscle cramp and stiffness which is undoubtedly related to rigidity.

The early symptoms and signs of Parkinson's disease are frequently unilateral and this may lead to confusion in the inexperienced observer who may believe the patient to have a hemiparesis.

In addition to these cardinal features of Parkinson's disease, other changes can occur: the most striking of these are the alterations in posture leading to flexion of the trunk, neck, arms and legs. Some form of autonomic change is by no means infrequent in Parkinson's disease, including alterations in sweating and control of changes in blood pressure in response to postural stimuli. Extraocular movements are frequently impaired, with limited upgaze and convergence, although

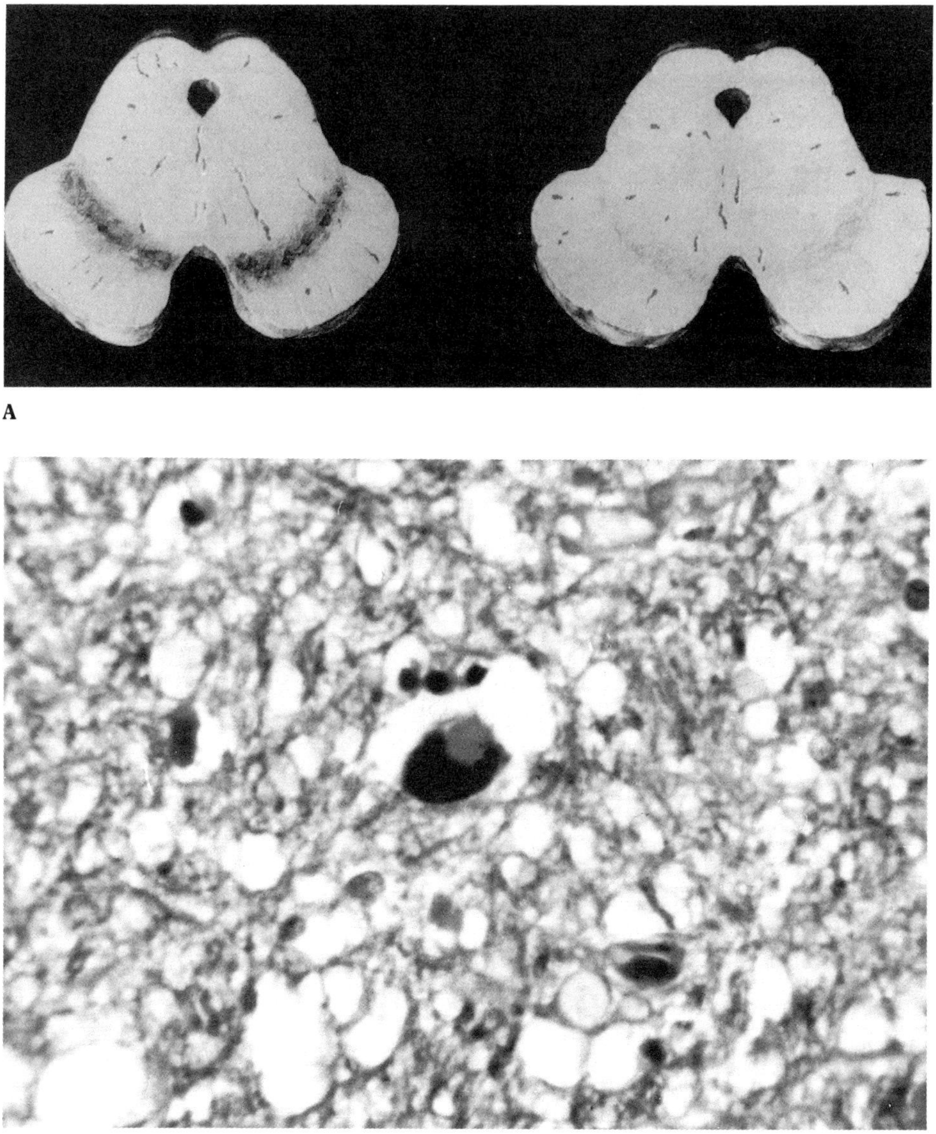

Fig. 15.3 **A** Substantia nigra showing normal pigmentation (left) and depigmentation in a specimen from a parkinsonian patient (right). **B** Photomicrograph showing an ovoid Lewy inclusion body within a pigmented cell (centre of field).

less markedly so than in progressive supranuclear palsy.

Twenty-five per cent to 50% of elderly parkinsonian patients show signs of dementia as the disorder progresses: the latter is of a subcortical type, usually with impaired and slow memory recall and slow problem solving; cortical disorders are rare.

Prognosis

In spite of improvements in treatment, the outlook for the patient is one of slow but relentless progression of the disease, with a spread of disability to the whole body and with an increasing incidence of dementia with the passage of time. Before the introduction of dopaminergic therapy, the death rate among patients with Parkinson's disease was three times the expected: average survival was some 8–10 years following diagnosis. The introduction of L-dopa and subsequent advances (see below) have led to a major change in this picture: life expectancy is now similar to, or very little worse than, that of the general population.

Diagnosis

The diagnosis of Parkinson's disease remains a clinical one. No specific investigations will confirm the diagnosis and further investigation of most patients presenting with parkinsonism is usually unnecessary. However, it remains important to differentiate primary Parkinson's disease from secondary parkinsonism. A classification of parkinsonism is contained in Table 15.3. Thus, before making the diagnosis of Parkinson's disease, it is important to exclude the possibility of drug-induced disease, and to consider the possibility of other rare treatable causes, such as Wilson's disease, in patients presenting with symptoms of parkinsonism at an early age. The presence of pyramidal or cerebellar signs will suggest the diagnosis of one of the multisystem disorders.

The condition which is probably most commonly misdiagnosed as Parkinson's disease is that of benign essential tremor (see below); the strikingly differing nature of the tremor and the absence of other signs of Parkinson's disease should, however, obviate any confusion on the part of an experienced observer.

It will be noted that arteriosclerotic parkinsonism has not been included in this discussion: the authors do not believe in the existence of this entity. Patients with multiple lacunar strokes exhibit some evidence of extrapyramidal disease, but also show striking signs of pyramidal disturbances and usually have a pseudobulbar palsy.

Table 15.3 Classification of parkinsonism

Primary
Parkinson's disease
Secondary
Infections (postencephalitic)
Toxins (manganese, carbon monoxide, MPTP)
Drugs (antipsychotic agents, reserpine)
Lacunar state
Tumour
Metabolic (hypoparathyroidism with basal ganglia calcification, chronic portosystemic encephalopathy)
Post-hypoxia
Multi-system disease
Progressive supranuclear palsy
Striatonigral degeneration
Olivopontine cerebellar degeneration
Shy–Drager syndrome
Alzheimer's disease
Wilson's disease
Hallervorden–Spatz disease
Juvenile Huntington's chorea

Treatment of Parkinson's disease

A wide range of drugs have been shown to have therapeutic effects in Parkinson's disease: these, together with suggested dosage regimes, are summarised in Table 15.4. Anticholinergic drugs and amantadine are mildly to moderately effective and are now less commonly used in the treatment of Parkinson's disease than in the past. All drugs have their most beneficial effects upon akinesia and rigidity. Dopaminergic compounds are also moderately effective in reducing tremor in the majority of patients; however, for a small group of patients with Parkinson's disease, tremor may remain incapacitating in spite of good control of other aspects of the condition. In this group of patients, particularly if the tremor is largely unilateral, it is still worth considering surgical treatment with stereotactic thalamotomy.

When to start treatment?

In some patients with Parkinson's disease the diagnosis may not necessitate immediate therapy. The most important consideration will be the patient's disability in relation to the demands of his existence: thus, relatively mild Parkinson's disease may require treatment in order to allow patients to continue with occupations demanding a high degree of manual dexterity.

There is, however, some controversy as to whether some of the late complications of Parkinson's disease relate to the duration of drug therapy; it is therefore not unreasonable to delay therapy with L-dopa until such time as patients are moderately disabled. In mildly disabled patients, active consideration can be given either

Table 15.4 Drug treatment of Parkinson's disease

Class	Drug	Dosage range (mg/day)	Doses/day	Adverse effects	Comment
Anticholinergics					
	Benzhexol	6–20	3–4	Blurred vision	Avoid in gluacoma
	Orphenadrine	150–400	3–4	Dry mouth Confusion	May precipitate urinary retention
Dopaminergics					
DA releaser	Amantadine	100–300	2–3	Confusion GI disturbance Peripheral oedema	
DA precursor	L-Dopa + benserazide or carbidopa	200–1000	3–8	GI disturbance Postural hypotension Dyskinesia Confusion	
MAO 'B' inhibitor	Selegiline	5–15	1–2	GI disturbance	Little effect alone Potentiates all L-dopa actions
DA agonist	Bromocryptine	10–100	3–4	GI disturbance Postural hypotension Dyskinesia Confusion	

to withholding therapy or, alternatively, to initiating therapy with anticholinergic drugs or amantadine. Ultimately, patients will require therapy with L-dopa plus a decarboxylase inhibitor.

Responses to dopaminergic therapy

L-Dopa plus a peripheral decarboxylase inhibitor (benserazide or carbidopa) represents the treatment of choice, and the mainstay of treatment for the vast majority of patients with Parkinson's disease.

Early experience with L-dopa given alone demonstrated marked peripheral side-effects (nausea, vomiting, diarrhoea, postural hypotension), which limited its use. The addition of a decarboxylase inhibitor, which prevents peripheral synthesis of dopamine but is unable to cross the blood–brain barrier to have a similar effect in the brain, has made patients' lives more tolerable and has greatly reduced the total dose of L-dopa required.

The early responses to treatment with L-dopa plus decarboxylase inhibitor are excellent in 70–80% of patients. The most satisfactory responses are seen in patients who are only mildly to moderately disabled at the time of initiation of therapy, but unfortunately in some 20–30% of patients there seems to be no major therapeutic response. It does not appear that such non-responders are likely to be helped by other dopaminergic drugs such as direct dopamine agonists (bromocryptine).

The duration of therapeutic response to L-dopa is initially prolonged. Thus, an individual dose will often produce a sustained benefit over a number of hours, and after a dosage change optimal therapeutic effect may take some 4–6 weeks to become fully established. These prolonged responses cannot be explained by the short half-life of L-dopa and imply some central pharmacodynamic interactions which are independent of the serum concentration. With the passage of time the sustained therapeutic response to L-dopa becomes less.

Early intolerance to treatment with L-dopa plus decarboxylase inhibitor is largely gastrointestinal and patients are likely to tolerate the drug if the dose is gradually increased by perhaps 100 mg of L-dopa per day each week up to an optimal starting dose of 300 mg per day. Thereafter, optimal dosage regimes must be tailored to the individual patient and it is of particular importance that patients and their families are encouraged to make sensible modifications to regimes to suit their own pattern of activities.

Patients do need warning, at an early stage, of the possible central dose-related effects of treatment with L-dopa plus decarboxylase inhibitor: these comprise confusional states, which are particularly common in elderly patients; this can encompass everything from mild confusion to frank psychosis with visual and auditory hallucination. Another problem is that of dopa-induced dyskinesias, which, in some patients, are simply dose-related. Sometimes this may erroneously be interpreted by patients as being due to their Parkinson's disease rather than its therapy, with a resultant increase in dosage and further exacerbation of their problems. These dyskinesias include both choreic movements (commonly orofacial dyskinesias) and a variety of dystonias.

The on-off syndrome

Long-term therapy with L-dopa is complicated by an increasing incidence of disabling fluctuations in the therapeutic response to drugs: thus patients 'swing'. This fluctuation may have a variety of causes related to the advancing Parkinson's disease itself or to the pharmacokinetics and receptor interactions of L-dopa. The percentage of patients showing some kind of response fluctuation increases so that, by 5–7 years after initiation of therapy, approximately 50% of patients may experience such fluctuations and this figure may have risen to 80% by 10–12 years after the initiation of therapy. For many patients, fluctuation in response becomes disabling and presents a major, and frequently insoluble, problem of management.

Fluctuations of response due to therapy. The most common cause of fluctuation of therapeutic response is *end-of-dose deterioration* in which the patient's disability increases before the next dose of L-dopa is due. This problem can frequently be improved by decreasing the interval between doses to three or two hours, or less. Smaller doses may need to be given on each occasion. With increasing periods of treatment, however, patients develop 'off' periods which are apparently unpredictable and which do not appear to respond to appropriate manipulation of dosing times. Ultimately, patients are seen in whom very dramatic and rapid oscillations occur over short periods, from being rigid and akinetic to being mobile with florid dyskinesia. These fluctuations occur frequently during the day in a way that can not easily be correlated with changing plasma levels of L-dopa.

Some improvement in such patients is achieved occasionally by additional dopaminergic manipulations. The first to be tried will usually be the addition of selegiline, a specific MAO inhibitor for subtype B. This has the effect of decreasing the rate of metabolism of dopamine, and thereby potentiating and prolonging the action of L-dopa. An alternative is the addition of a direct dopamine agonist, such as bromocryptine, which has a longer half-life than L-dopa and has an L-dopa-sparing effect. Nevertheless, ultimately the additional benefits produced by these manipulations are minor and transient for the majority of patients.

A variety of different patterns of dyskinesia are seen in the treatment of Parkinson's disease, the most common being *peak dose dyskinesia* of a choreic nature. The majority of patients with Parkinson's disease are able to tolerate moderate amounts of dyskinesia associated with mobility, a state which they prefer to rigidity and akinesia. However, for some patients peak dose dyskinesia can become a major problem, which may be helped by reducing the amount of individual doses.

More rarely, different patterns of dyskinesia are seen: some patients exhibit dystonia and chorea slightly before the onset of therapeutic action of an individual dose of the drug, and again when the action is disappearing; other patients experience dystonic posturing which occurs in the early morning preceding the therapeutic response to the first dose of L-dopa; an even smaller group of patients develop myoclonic jerking in response to L-dopa therapy; these latter dyskinesias are often refractory to any therapy.

One possible procedure which may be considered in patients with severe 'on-off' problems is a 'drug holiday'. The discontinuation of all therapy for a period of 5–7 days followed by its reinstitution may, on occasions, result in a more long-lasting therapeutic response to therapy, which may persist for some weeks.

The aetiology of the 'on-off' therapeutic phenomenon remains uncertain. Two different theories are advanced: the first, that it results from the effects of long-term dopaminergic stimulation—a direct drug effect; the second, that it results from progress in the underlying condition which affects drug responsiveness. Whatever the mechanism, the phenomenon continues to present major management problems. More recent attempted solutions include the administration of intravenous L-dopa or subcutaneous dopamine agonists. These may be of some value, and in the future slow-release formulations of L-dopa might offer some solutions.

Fluctuations due to Parkinson's disease. The pattern of response to therapy with L-dopa may be complicated by fluctuations that occur as a result of the disorder itself. The most common of these is episodic 'freezing' which most commonly results in patients suddenly coming to a halt, often in a doorway, and remaining static and immobile for several seconds before being able to move off again. It is apparent that the opposite can occur and that, particularly when parkinsonian patients are suddenly frightened, they may be able to produce a speed of movement of which they would not normally be considered capable.

Treatment of secondary parkinsonism

Parkinsonian syndromes which are symptomatic of identifiable cerebral disease generally respond much more poorly to conventional therapy than does the idiopathic condition. The notable exception is postencephalitic parkinsonism, in which remarkable responses are seen to very small doses of L-dopa. However, a short trial of L-dopa and decarboxylase inhibitors is warranted in many cases of secondary parkinsonism.

WILSON'S DISEASE (hepatolenticular degeneration)

This is a rare inherited metabolic disorder with an autosomal recessive pattern of inheritance. The incidence has been estimated at approximately 1 per 200 000 and a carrier rate of 1 per 140. The diagnosis is of great importance, not only as a potentially treatable cause of severe and progressive neurological disability, but also because of the implications for the family of an affected patient. Full and adequate screening of siblings and prophylactic treatment are necessary.

It has been suggested that the prime defect in Wilson's disease is an inability to synthesise caeruloplasmin (the copper-carrying plasma protein), leading to an excessive deposition of copper in tissues, particularly the liver, kidneys, cornea and basal ganglia. However, such a mechanism does not explain occasional cases in which serum copper and caeruloplasmin concentrations appear to be normal.

Clinical features

Perhaps the most useful diagnostic feature of the condition is the Kayser–Fleischer ring. This appears as a brown or greenish-brown pigmentation on the deep surface of the cornea; it may be visible as a ring extending around the margin of the iris, but at an early stage may be visible only on using a slit lamp, a form of examination which is obligatory in all patients suspected of this diagnosis.

Copper deposition in the liver leads to multilobular cirrhosis and splenomegaly. It is of interest that such cirrhosis usually presents within the first decade of life, whereas neurological presentations are most common in the second and third decades of life; the reasons for this are uncertain.

The neurological manifestations of Wilson's disease are extremely varied, but perhaps the most common presentation is one of a parkinsonian syndrome, often with particularly severe involvement of the oropharyngeal muscles, occurring at an early age. It is essential to screen all young patients with a parkinsonian syndrome for Wilson's disease. However, other patients may also show tremor of the head, postural and intention tremor of hands, and a wide variety of dyskinesias. Progressive flexion deformities develop and it is said a characteristic facies with drooling and facile grinning is common. Dyskinesias include wingbeating tremor, dystonia and myoclonus.

As well as extrapyramidal rigidity and akinesia, there are usually pyramidal signs with hyperreflexia and pseudobulbar palsy and frequently cerebellar signs are evident. Exceptionally, there may be intellectual change, with a psychiatric presentation due to an organic brain syndrome, usually with some features of dementia. Such patients present particular difficulties, as they may have received treatment with antipsychotic drugs so that extrapyramidal features may falsely be attributed to these.

Investigation

The classic findings in Wilson's disease are of a low serum caeruloplasmin concentration (<25 mg/100 ml), low serum copper and an increased urinary copper excretion. However, in some cases these investigations may show near-normal levels and perhaps the most satisfactory investigation is the estimation of copper as a percentage dry weight of liver obtained at biopsy. A high copper content in the liver biopsy is usually found, with levels greater than 250 μg copper per gram dry weight.

In addition to these pathognomonic findings, a degree of aminoaciduria is usually present, due to renal tubular damage, and liver function tests may show some alteration. Liver biopsy may show histological evidence of cirrhosis. Neuroradiological investigation of Wilson's disease is not of great benefit, although, in some cases, low-density lesions in the basal ganglia have been reported.

Treatment

The aim of treatment is to achieve a negative copper balance. Some form of dietary copper limitation may be helpful and certainly foods with a high copper content—such as liver, shellfish, chocolate, nuts and mushrooms—are best avoided. Copper excretion can be greatly increased by the administration of D-penicillamine in a dose of 1–2 g per day by mouth. Treatment should be monitored by estimation of serum copper concentration and of urinary copper excretion. Sensitivity reactions to D-penicillamine are common (rash, arthralgia, fever, leucopenia) and the drug may also cause lupus-like syndromes and a nephrotic syndrome. Occasional cases of myasthenia induced by penicillamine during the treatment of Wilson's disease have been documented. Such adverse drug reactions can very frequently be managed by reducing the dose of penicillamine and instituting steroid cover. Occasionally, patients are encountered who will not tolerate penicillamine: in such instances other chelating agents may be administered, e.g. triethylene tetramine.

Although there may be some initial deterioration in the neurological state of patients on starting therapy, it is said that the outcome will usually be excellent: severely disabled patients may eventually resume a normal existence. It is important to screen siblings for the condition and to institute prophylactic therapy.

PROGRESSIVE SUPRANUCLEAR PALSY
(Steele–Richardson–Olszewski syndrome)

This progressive degenerative condition of unknown aetiology is probably not as uncommon as was once thought and is certainly underdiagnosed. Most frequently it is confused with Parkinson's disease, or cases are attributed to diffuse cerebrovascular disease. The pathological changes comprise neuronal loss and gliosis with prominent neurofibrillary degeneration of residual cells, affecting periaqueductal grey matter, basal ganglia and oculomotor nuclei. The cerebral and cerebellar cortex appear to be relatively spared by the pathological process.

Clinical features

The primary clinical features are those of a striking eye movement disorder, disequilibrium of gait, with associated pseudobulbar palsy, pyramidal signs and dementia.

Onset is usually late in life, with peak incidence during the sixth decade. The most common presenting symptom is that of frequent falls: patients become very unsteady and particularly tend to fall over backwards; they appear unable to protect themselves during such falls and frequently injure themselves. At this stage patients show a degree of bradykinesia and slowness of movement which, to inexperienced observers, suggests a parkinsonian syndrome. However, patients will usually have a striking facial appearance (Fig. 15.4). The face becomes mask-like, but the eyes are fixed, staring and unblinking; they assume a startled expression and it will be noted that the patient turns his whole head and body to look at a point of interest to his side. Symptoms of a mild subcortical dementia are usually present, with an emphasis on psychomotor retardation and memory impairment, with relatively preserved cortical function.

Patients with progressive supranuclear palsy are remarkable for the wide variety of neurological signs that they show: the striking facial expression has already been noted. Patients show a very characteristic supranuclear gaze palsy: initially this results in a limitation of voluntary vertical eye movements, but when the patient is allowed to fix on an object and a doll's head movement is undertaken, then an increased range of eye movement is usually possible; lateral eye movements are affected later but eventually a complete ophthalmoplegia may result. Before this occurs, lateral eye movements lack a smooth pursuit movement and become jerky and saccadic. Optokinetic nystagmus in vertical directions, and subsequently in the lateral direction, is impaired. The striking eye movement disorder becomes so pronounced that the experienced observer should not confuse the diagnosis with that of other neurological degenerative conditions.

Patients will usually have signs of a pseudobulbar palsy and have brisk tendon reflexes and extensor plantar responses. They show a marked

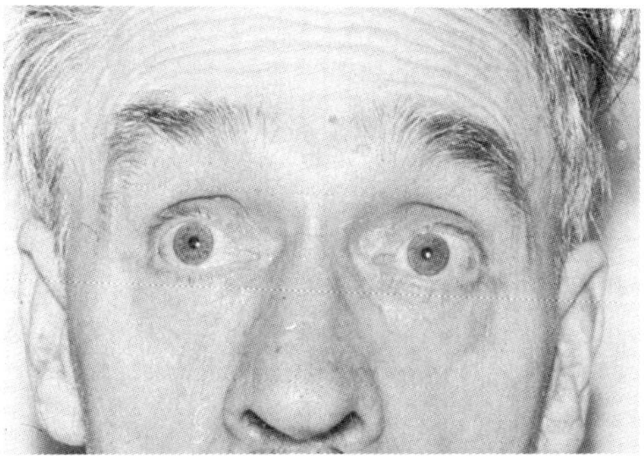

Fig. 15.4 The characteristic facial expression in a patient with progressive supranuclear palsy. The eyes are staring and unblinking, and there is great difficulty with upward gaze.

axial rigidity with extrapyramidal akinesia, but without significant tremor.

Unfortunately no treatment appears to be effective, although on occasions L-dopa plus a decarboxylase inhibitor, or amantadine, may have some minimal effects on extrapyramidal symptoms. The disorder is progressive, with the patient ultimately becoming chairbound and bedbound. Death usually occurs between 5 and 10 years after diagnosis, often due to aspiration and pneumonia because of profound pseudobulbar disturbance.

SHY–DRAGER SYNDROME

The syndrome of progressive autonomic failure has already been described (p. 97). However, on occasion, autonomic disturbance is seen in association with multisystem degeneration (Shy–Drager syndrome). Degenerative changes are found affecting autonomic neurones throughout the c.n.s., particularly the lateral and intermediolateral columns of the spinal cord. In addition there may be atrophy affecting the basal ganglia, cerebellum and brain-stem.

The clinical features are of severe postural hypotension, disturbance of sweating, impotence, bladder and bowel dysfunction associated with evidence of a parkinsonian syndrome with mild pyramidal and cerebellar signs and in some instances a mild dementia.

The cause of this syndrome is unknown, but in some rare cases may be familial. Treatment is largely symptomatic: α-fludrocortisone and sympathomimetic drugs such as ephedrine may be helpful; blocking the bed during sleep to achieve a head-up tilt can help maintain blood pressure; eventually the wearing of a G-suit may become necessary.

STRIATONIGRAL DEGENERATION

The definition of this condition is difficult, and it is certainly uncommon. Most cases appear to be clinically indistinguishable from Parkinson's disease, with the possible exception that more profound autonomic disturbances are seen in this condition.

The diagnosis can only be made at postmortem examination, which reveals not only neuronal loss from the zona compacta of the substantia nigra, but also striking degenerative changes in the putamen and caudate nucleus; these are not seen in Parkinson's disease.

It may be that this condition contributes to that proportion of patients diagnosed as having Parkinson's disease who fail to show response to dopaminergic therapy.

HALLERVORDEN–SPATZ DISEASE

This is an autosomal recessive inherited disorder, with onset of symptoms usually in late childhood or early adolescence. It is rare, and the pathology is that of a pigmentary degeneration of the basal ganglia (globus pallidus, substantia nigra and red nucleus), with an associated deposition of iron within the basal ganglia. No biochemical abnormality has been identified in this condition.

The clinical features are those of progressive motor disorder with marked pyramidal tract signs (pseudobulbar palsy and spastic quadriparesis) with, in addition, extrapyramidal disorder with rigidity, dystonia and chorea. Very often there is evidence of dementia and, in some instances, the predominant presentation has been one of ataxia or myoclonus.

Onset is usually within the first two decades of life, occasionally later. The condition is rapidly progressive with death within a few years of onset, and no treatment has been shown to be effective. The most important differential diagnosis is from Wilson's disease and from juvenile cases of Parkinson's disease and Huntington's chorea, which may present as a rigid parkinsonian syndrome in juveniles.

BASAL GANGLIA CALCIFICATION (Fahr's syndrome)

Some degree of basal ganglia calcification, due to the deposition of calcium within blood vessel walls, is by no means uncommon and may be visible on the skull X-ray and even more commonly on CT scanning. In the majority of patients this has no clinical significance; however, in a limited number of patients, basal ganglia calcification may be associated with rigidity and extrapyramidal disturbance, including choreic and dystonic movement with dementia and psychosis. Such disorders may be seen in hyperparathyroidism or pseudohypoparathyroidism, but there is also a group of patients in whom a familial autosomal dominant condition occurs—of calcification of basal ganglia and cerebellum without obvious disturbance of general calcium metabolism.

THE DYSTONIAS

Dystonia musculorum deformans

Dystonia is a movement disorder which is most frequently symptomatic of cerebral palsy or neurodegenerative conditions; it may also be induced by a variety of drugs (see p. 21). However, generalised and usually progressive dystonia may be seen independent of other neurological disorder in the condition of torsion dystonia (dystonia musculorum deformans). Although no consistent pathological change has been identified in this condition, it is included here because of its progressive nature.

The condition may occur as an autosomal recessive in Ashkenazic Jews, as an autosomal dominant in other populations, or perhaps most commonly in sporadic forms. The onset of symptoms is usually in the first or second decade of life, but is occasionally later in life when a more benign course is evident.

Children usually begin to develop minor movement disorders related to their limbs. They may begin to walk on their toes and to develop internal rotation and writhing of their hand and arms during walking or during specific tasks. Because these early dystonic movements seem to be related to specific activities (patients may be able to walk backwards, or to run perfectly normally whilst having great difficulty in walking), these disorders are often misdiagnosed in the early stages as being hysterical.

With the progression of the disorder the trunk may become involved, with the patient becoming bed-bound due to severe and constant dystonia, which ultimately may result in severe lordosis and scoliosis; fixed deformities of the limbs may also develop.

The drug treatment of torsion dystonia is disappointing: anticholinergic drugs, such as benzhexol, and benzodiazepines help a limited number of patients, but large doses of these agents may be necessary, the dose being built up gradually over a period of several weeks. Some patients may also benefit from carbamazepine, tetrabenazine, or dopamine antagonist drugs such as pimozide or haloperidol; however, these latter agents may have to be given in doses sufficient to induce parkinsonian side effects.

Stereotactic thalamotomy has been undertaken in a number of patients with torsion dystonia: some patients have had significant and long-lasting benefit, but the results remain unpredictable. The disorder appears to be progressive, with patients becoming chair- and bed-bound over a period of years.

Segmental dystonias

Much more common than the rare generalised torsion dystonias are the more restricted localised adult-onset dystonic disorders. Once again, no specific pathological change has been noted in patients with these syndromes, but it has been suggested that they represent a localised dystonic syndrome with occasional cases which occupy an intermediate position in the spectrum between localised and generalised dystonia.

Meige's syndrome

This cranial dystonia usually presents in adult life with blepharospasm and an oromandibular dystonia. Dystonic facial movements may be associated with abnormal posturing of the jaw, which interferes with speech and swallowing.

Spasmodic torticollis

This is the most common of the segmental dystonias. It results in the turning of the head to one side through contraction of both superficial and deep muscles of the neck; more rarely, bilateral contraction may lead to retrocollis. Initially, the movement may be episodic, but progression may occur so that fixed posturing is seen.

Writer's cramp

In this condition, the act of writing is likely to result in a progressive dystonic posturing of the hand holding the pen or pencil, with a deterioration in the legibility of the writing. This dystonic posturing is usually seen only during the act of writing and other movements of the hand are unaffected.

The treatment of these segmental dystonias is unsatisfactory. Trials of the same drugs used in generalised torsion dystonia may be of value, but their effects are minimal. Writer's cramp is rarely of such severity as to demand therapy and the simplest advice to patients may either be to learn to type, or to write with their other hand. Meige's syndrome and spasmodic torticollis are, however, more troublesome and embarrassing for sufferers, who are often desperate for effective therapy. A rare subgroup of patients are seen with onset of predominantly lower limb dystonia in early life. They respond very dramatically to treatment with L-dopa.

In the case of spasmodic torticollis, a number of surgical approaches to treatment have been undertaken: these have included ventral root section of the upper cervical roots with additional division of the spinal and accessory nerve. This operation may benefit a number of patients, but relief is often short-lived, and the procedure is not without risk and morbidity. A variety of stereotactic approaches to treatment of spasmodic torticollis have also been undertaken, with varying degrees of success. More recent approaches have included cervical cord stimulation and upper cervical dorsal root section. The effectiveness of these procedures is uncertain as longer-term follow-up of patients is not currently available. One new approach to the treatment of blepharospasm and spasmodic torticollis is local injection of a dilute solution of *Botulinum* toxin to produce a local moderate paresis: this may produce less functional disability and can be repeated when necessary; whether such local treatment could be applied to other dystonias remains to be determined.

ESSENTIAL TREMOR

This is a common and usually benign disorder. Patients have tremor affecting the hands which usually interferes with movements such as drinking from a cup; in some cases an associated tremor of the head (titubation) is seen. Patients quickly become aware that alcohol has a specific depressant effect on the tremor. A family history of tremor is evident in up to one-half of the cases. The onset of tremor may be as early as the second or third decades of life, and there may be a slow progression with the passage of time.

There may be two subtypes of essential tremor, the first of which represents an enhancement of physiological tremor and encompasses a fine, relatively fast, postural tremor of the hands at approximately 9–10 cycles per second; other patients have slower coarser tremors, sometimes associated with mild degrees of ataxia.

The tremor is often little more than a nuisance and in many patients requires no therapy. Beta-blocking drugs (propanolol) may be helpful in those patients requiring some treatment, but the benefit is rarely spectacular; primidone may also be effective against this form of tremor. Very occasionally, patients are seen with very marked disability and, on occasion, stereotactic thalamotomy may be considered in order to provide them with a usable hand and arm.

PROGRESSIVE MYOCLONUS EPILEPSY

A number of degenerative pathological states may present during adult life, with syndromes in which a prominent feature is a progressive ataxia and incoordination (largely due to action myoclonus), associated with epilepsy and degrees of dementia (progressive myoclonus epilepsy).

No specific therapy is available for these conditions: anticonvulsant drugs may help to control seizures, but these have little effect on the disabling myoclonus; benzodiazepines, such as clonazepam and nitrazepam, and valproate may be of some value. These conditions are classified in Table 15.5. Tay–Sachs and Gaucher's diseases rarely present other than in children, and will not be discussed further.

Table 15.5 Disorders causing progressive myoclonus epilepsy

Storage disorders
Tay–Sachs*
Gaucher's*
Neuronal ceroid lipofuscinosis
Lafora body disease
Sialidosis
Other miscellaneous conditions
Ramsay Hunt syndrome
Baltic myoclonus
Essential myoclonus

*Usually childhood onset.

Lafora body disease

This condition appears to be inherited as an autosomal recessive trait. The name is derived from the large basophilic cytoplasmic bodies of polysaccharide found in the dentate nuclei, brain stem and thalamic neurones. Onset is usually in late childhood or early adolescence and the first symptoms are usually of myoclonic jerks precipitated by any movement, startle, or sensory stimulus; epileptic seizures also occur. The myoclonus results in severe incoordination and ataxia, which is progressive and associated with deteriorating cognitive function. Death usually occurs before the end of the third decade.

Diagnosis is difficult during life but, on occasions, may be made on the basis of characteristic changes in liver biopsy or muscle biopsy.

Neuronal ceroid lipofuscinoses

This group of disorders of liposomal storage has a confusing variety of clinical forms. When they present in late childhood they can be characterised by the presence of action myoclonus, seizures and visual failure. Characteristic retinal changes with yellowish areas of degeneration are less frequently seen in adult than in childhood or juvenile onset cases. As the disease progresses, intellectual deterioration occurs and some patients show extrapyramidal disturbance. Death usually occurs within 10–15 years of onset. The presence of abnormal vacuoles in lymphocytes may aid diagnosis.

Sialidosis (cherry-red spot myoclonus syndrome)

This autosomal recessive condition causes ataxia, visual failure and action myoclonus, with onset in the second and third decade. Cataracts and a cherry-red spot at the macula are prominent signs.

The urine contains large amounts of sialic acid containing oligosaccharide and skin fibroblasts show sialidase deficiency.

Baltic myoclonus

Unverricht and Lundberg reported a number of pedigrees of patients presenting with action myoclonus and seizures between the ages of 6 and 12 years. The pattern of inheritance appeared to be one of an autosomal recessive trait and patients developed progressive gait ataxia, intention tremor and dysarthria with mental regression. Death occurred between 5 and 20 years after the diagnosis. The pathology in these Scandinavian cases is uncertain.

Ramsay Hunt syndrome

Ramsay Hunt described a number of patients presenting with cerebellar ataxia with associated myoclonus and occasional seizures, under the term dyssynergia cerebellaris myoclonica. Some of these patients had other signs of a relatively benign spinocerebellar degeneration. Ramsay Hunt felt that the condition was a variant of Friedreich's ataxia.

Essential myoclonus

This is a very rare and unusual condition in which families, often with an autosomal dominant pattern of inheritance, develop disability due to myoclonus without any other neurological disorder. The myoclonus is not of the classic action type, in that it does not appear to be stimulus sensitive; however, movements do exacerbate the myoclonus, which may respond preferentially to alcohol, drawing the parallel which has existed in some families between coexisting essential tremor and essential myoclonus.

TIC SYNDROMES

Tics are stereotyped (p. 21) and are rarely a major disability. However, on occasion patients have multiple tics which are disabling and embarrassing.

The most florid of such cases are often described as Gilles de la Tourette syndrome; such patients have no demonstrable neuropathology and there is considerable debate as to whether the condition is organic or psychiatric. Patients develop the condition within the first two decades of life and show multiple motor and verbal tics; the latter include grunts, sniffs and coughs as well as coprolalia (obscene speech) and echolalia. The tics are usually amenable to some degree of voluntary control and are exacerbated by stressful circumstances.

The condition tends to be chronic, but many patients are helped by haloperidol.

SPINOCEREBELLAR DEGENERATIONS

Grouped together under this term are a number of conditions characterised by the development of a progressive ataxia. The disorders are frequently familial. Although a number of classic syndromes are recognised, with the possible exception of Friedreich's ataxia it is uncommon to see cases that fit comfortably into the categories defined by these descriptions; more frequently, individual families present features unique to themselves, but which are similar between individual members of the pedigree. Underlying metabolic abnormalities have been identified in a number of conditions, but most remain poorly understood. A simplified classification is presented in Table 15.6.

HEREDITARY ATAXIAS OF METABOLIC ORIGIN

Identified metabolic abnormalities may cause either intermittent or progressive ataxic syndromes, often associated with retardation. The recognised causes are summarised in Table 15.6, but most present in infancy and childhood and are not considered further here.

Intermittent ataxias which may present in adolescence and adult life

Some partial deficiencies of enzymes involved in pyruvate metabolism can be associated with

Table 15.6 The spinocerebellar degenerations

Hereditary ataxias of known cause
Intermittent ataxias
Disorder of the urea cycle
Disorders of lactate and pyruvate metabolism
Aminoacidurias (Hartnup disease)
Progressive ataxias
Abetalipoproteinaemia
Mitochondrial cytopathy
Ataxia telangectasia
Xeroderma pigmentosa
Hereditary ataxias of unknown cause
Spinal ataxias
Friedreich's ataxia
With preserved tendon reflexes
Cerebellar ataxias
Pure cerebellar degeneration
Olivopontine cerebellar degeneration
Other less well-defined ataxic syndromes
Sporadic late-onset primary cerebellar degenerations

survival into adult life and intermittent ataxic syndromes, exacerbations often being precipitated by infection. Partial pyruvate dehydrogenase deficiency may present in this way. Some patients with pyruvate carboxylase deficiency may present the features of Leigh's disease (subacute necrotising encephalomyelopathy); this autosomal recessive trait associated with elevated pyruvate levels and metabolic acidosis usually presents in childhood with failure to thrive, hypotonicity or spasticity and often prominent brain-stem and oculomotor signs. The condition is usually fatal, but occasional cases have been reported in early adult life. In both cases blood pyruvate levels are elevated, and higher than normal during a standard glucose tolerance test.

Progressive ataxias which may present in adolescence and adult life

Abetalipoproteinaemia (Bassen–Kornzweig syndrome) is an autosomal recessive gene in which pigmentary retinal degeneration, ataxia and areflexia are associated with acanthocytes in peripheral blood, and with steatorrhoea; symptoms usually begin during the first decade. The condition may respond to treatment with vitamin E. A number of other neuronal storage diseases may cause ataxia associated with dementia (see also Table 15.5).

It has recently been recognised that some patients with mitochondrial cytopathy (p. 258) may also show evidence of cerebellar dysfunction; they have disorders of the mitochondrial respiratory chain.

Although *ataxia telangectasia* is a disorder of defective DNA repair rather than a metabolic disorder, it is discussed here. Onset is usually within the first decade of life. First signs are those of a truncal ataxia with the subsequent development of intention tremor, myoclonus and chorea; there may be impaired voluntary eye movements (oculomotor apraxia); areflexia develops together with weakness. Characteristic conjunctival and cutaneous telangectasia develop slowly with advancing age. There is evidence of immunological deficiency with a high incidence of respiratory infections, bronchiectasis and malignancy. Immunoglobulins, particularly IgA, are reduced in serum and α-fetoprotein is increased.

HEREDITARY ATAXIA OF UNKNOWN CAUSE

Spinal ataxias

Friedreich's ataxia

This is the most common hereditary ataxia with a prevalence of 1 : 50 000. It is an autosomal recessive condition; reports of autosomal dominant inheritance may well be of clinically distinct cases. Onset of symptoms is usually between between 5 and 15 years of age, although pes cavus deformities may be present before this time. Onset after the age of 20 years is rare.

The pathological changes are those of spinal degeneration, particularly affecting the posterior columns, corticospinal tracts and spinocerebellar tracts. The cerebellum and brain stem appear to be spared. Axonal degeneration and some segmental demyelination may be found in the peripheral nerves.

The clinical features are summarised in Table 15.7.

The condition is characterised by a progressive ataxia with increasing weakness of the lower

Table 15.7 Clinical features of Friedreich's ataxia (after Harding 1984)

Essential criteria	Additional criteria (present in more than two-thirds)	Other features (present in half or fewer)
Onset before 25 years	Scoliosis	Nystagmus
Ataxia of limbs and gait	Pyramidal weakness of lower limbs	Optic atrophy
Absent knee and ankle jerks	Absent upper limb reflexes	Deafness
Extensor plantars	Joint position (JPS) and vibration loss in legs	Distal wasting
Motor conduction velocity > 40 m/s	Abnormal ECG	Diabetes
Small or absent sensory nerve action potentials.	Pes cavus	
Dysarthria (within 5 years of onset)		

limbs, loss of tendon reflexes with extensor plantar responses and impaired sensation, particularly to joint position sense and vibration. Patients show evidence of pes cavus and scoliosis and ultimately evidence of cardiac dysfunction and cardiomyopathy, with death from heart failure usually some 20–25 years after the onset of symptoms. Nystagmus is present in most cases and many patients develop a scanning dysarthria characteristic of cerebellar disturbance.

Less common accompaniments are optic atrophy, deafness and disorders of ocular movement; up to one-half of the patients show wasting of the small muscles of the hand; there is a high incidence of diabetes.

Investigations in this condition are unhelpful and the diagnosis remains a clinical one. CT scans appear normal, but most patients show reduced or absent sensory nerve action potentials, and mildly reduced motor conduction velocities (more than 40 m/s).

The most likely condition to be confused with Friedreich's ataxia is the peroneal muscular atrophy syndrome in which distal wasting and weakness of lower limbs (and to a lesser degree the upper limbs) are associated with areflexia, due to hereditary motor and sensory neuropathy or distal spinal muscular atrophy. More difficult is the Roussy–Lévy variant, in which tremor and ataxia also occur, but in the latter there is an autosomal dominant inheritance.

It is of particular importance to maintain strict diagnostic criteria for Friedreich's ataxia, and not to accept 'variants'; the latter are invariably more benign. Most patients with Friedreich's ataxia will be chairbound by 25 years of age and dead by 35 years; hence, diagnostic accuracy is essential if offering over-gloomy prognoses is to be avoided.

No specific treatment is available for Friedreich's ataxia. It is, however, important to maintain mobility and to avoid contractures; in this context, tendon-lengthening operations and scoliosis surgery may warrant serious consideration.

Other spinal ataxias

A number of 'variants' on the Friedreich's ataxia theme have been reported over the years. The prime difference between these conditions and Friedreich's ataxia has been the preservation and increase of tendon reflexes in the variants. Often, the pattern of inheritance is that of an autosomal recessive, but other modes of inheritance may occur. Scoliosis, proprioceptive loss, ECG abnormalities and diabetes are rare in variant syndromes.

Primary cerebellar degeneration

In this group of conditions the predominant pathology affects cerebellum and cerebellar connections rather than spinal cord tracts. The conditions themselves are untreatable, but must be differentiated from symptomatic cerebellar degeneration seen with alcoholism, hypothyroidism, and as a non-metastatic effect of carcinoma.

Pure cerebellar degeneration

This condition was originally described by Holmes in association with hypogonadism, the syndrome being associated with his name. Patients develop a marked gait ataxia followed by incoordination of the upper limbs and dysarthria; nystagmus is

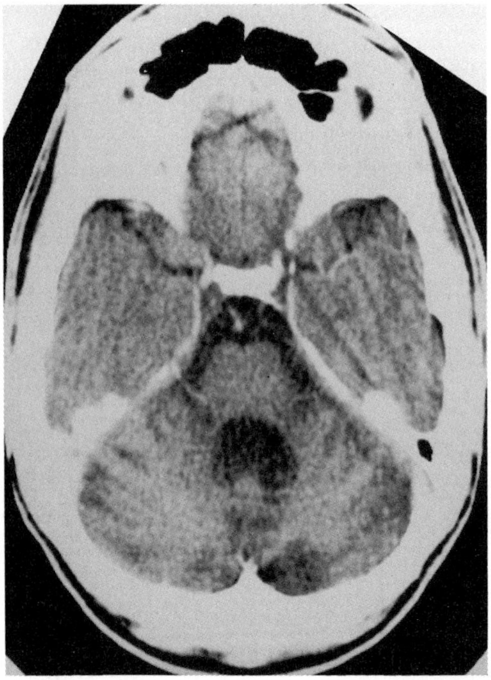

Fig. 15.5 CT scan appearances of gross selective posterior fossa atrophy in a patient with a late-onset primary cerebellar degeneration

rare. The condition may be familial or sporadic and progression is usually very slow.

Olivopontine cerebellar degeneration

In this condition there is more general atrophy of brain-stem structures than is seen in pure cerebellar degenerations, with a consequent association of other brain-stem and long-tract signs. The condition may occur either sporadically or as an autosomal dominant trait. This condition is usually more rapidly progressive, with onset usually in middle life. Patients suffer a progressive cerebellar disturbance resulting in ataxia, dysarthria and tremor. Parkinsonian features may develop, together with mild dementia, ophthalmoplegia, pyramidal tract signs and autonomic disturbance. These latter features are usually less marked than the cerebellar disturbance.

As well as these relatively pure ataxic syndromes, ataxia may occur with multisystem disorders; virtually any combination of features can occur:

1. With hypogonadism, deafness and/or dementia
2. With myoclonus (Ramsay Hunt, Baltic myoclonus)
3. With pigmentary retinal degeneration and/or deafness
4. With optic atrophy/ophthalmoplegia
5. With essential tremor.

SPORADIC LATE-ONSET CEREBELLAR DEGENERATION

Whereas much has been written concerning familial ataxia and cerebellar degeneration, it must be recognised that sporadic late-onset primary cerebellar degeneration is much more common. It is difficult to apply any unifying or satisfactory classification to these disorders.

Onset is usually after the age of 50 years and the course is relatively benign. Clinical features vary from pure cerebellar ataxia, with preserved upper-limb function, to conditions showing multisystem involvement more akin to olivoponto-cerebellar degeneration. CT scanning will exclude mass lesions, but show cerebellar or brain-stem atrophy, or both. Differentiation from secondary paraneoplastic, alcoholic or hypothyroid cerebellar degeneration is important (Ch. 18).

MOTOR SYSTEM DEGENERATIONS

HEREDITARY SPASTIC PARAPARESIS

In this condition, which is usually an autosomal dominant trait (although recessive inheritance has occasionally been documented), there is degeneration of crossed pyramidal tracts of the spinal cord which increases caudally.

Onset is very variable, but most commonly occurs in the first two decades. Clinical features are of a progressive motor disturbance due to involvement of the pyramidal tracts. The condition is slowly progressive and usually presents with increasing spasticity during walking, with preserved muscle strength; the arms and bulbar musculature are rarely involved; bladder and sphincter involvement is seen occasionally. Sensory signs are minimal or absent. Patients develop very marked degrees of spasticity, but are very often able to continue walking, with gross scissoring gaits, for many years.

The main differential diagnosis is from chronic progressive paraparesis due to demyelination. Clinically, the gross spasticity, with little loss of power and preserved walking after a long history, will usually be most helpful in differentiation. The presence of abnormal visual evoked potentials and oligoclonal bands in the c.s.f., if present, will also favour the diagnosis of demyelination.

Antispastic drugs (baclofen, dantrolene, diazepam) may be moderately beneficial in ameliorating patients' spasticity and in improving gait.

As with hereditary spinal and cerebellar ataxias, a number of reports have appeared in which an otherwise typical syndrome of hereditary spastic paraparesis has been associated with other system degenerations: these have included cerebellar signs with ocular symptoms, extrapyramidal symptoms, optic atrophy and retinal degeneration; this again emphasises the difficulty of making a precise classification of such disorders. Such complicated hereditary spastic paraplegia more frequently shows autosomal recessive inheritance.

MOTOR NEURONE DISEASE (MND)

The incidence of this condition is probably 1–2 per 100 000 population per annum. It is slightly more common in men than in women and peak onset is between the ages of 50 and 70 years, although, unfortunately, onset as early as the third decade occasionally occurs.

The aetiology of the condition remains unknown. It is of some interest that very high incidences of this condition are reported in certain areas, such as the Pacific Island of Guam. Extensive study of this population has, however, failed to define a cause for this in spite of exhaustive searches for slow virus agents and conventional viruses. A wide range of possible toxic causes of the syndrome have been explored, only to be discarded.

Clinical features

Three major types of presentation are recognised: amyotrophic lateral sclerosis, progressive muscular atrophy and progressive bulbar palsy. However, it must be realised that these particular syndromes of presentation represent a continuum of the disease and patients with an amyotrophic lateral sclerosis presentation will be likely to develop progressive bulbar palsy later in the course of the disease.

Amyotrophic lateral sclerosis (ALS)

Symptoms are usually first noted in the hands, patients becoming aware of clumsiness and weakness of grip, with some wasting of the small muscles of the hands. Very often patients begin to develop muscle cramps at this time and to become aware of muscular twitching around the shoulder girdles. The muscular wasting usually spreads to involve the muscles of the upper arms and shoulders and subsequently the muscles of the lower limbs. However, it is usually striking that tendon reflexes are not only preserved, but enhanced, and plantar responses are extensor. Sensory signs are notably absent. On occasions a presentation beginning with foot drop may occur and, very occasionally, proximal muscle weakness may be the major early symptom of the disease.

Progressive muscular atrophy

Here there is a striking absence of upper motor neurone signs and patients present with progressive wasting, usually again beginning in the small muscles of the hand. Spasticity and increased tendon reflexes are absent and the progress of the condition is usually slower than that of ALS.

Progressive bulbar palsy

In this condition, in which there is both lower motor neurone and upper motor neurone involvement of the bulbar musculature, the predominant symptoms early in the condition tend to be those of pseudobulbar palsy. Patients notice the insidious onset of difficulty in swallowing and speaking; emotional lability is common, speech becomes strained and a typical pseudobulbar facies develops, but fasciculation of the tongue is usually seen, although the jaw jerk remains brisk.

With the progress of the disease, patients presenting with ALS frequently develop progressive bulbar palsy; the reverse is not always true, as bulbar palsy carries a poor prognosis so that death may occur before patients develop significant limb dysfunction. The prognosis of motor neurone disease is extremely poor, but does show some variability: survival is usually between 2 and 5 years from diagnosis, although this may be longer in cases presenting with progressive muscular atrophy and shorter in patients with progressive bulbar palsy.

Investigation

Electrodiagnostic tests are important: in MND they usually show the presence of fibrillation, positive sharp waves and fasciculation in affected muscles (i.e. denervation); sensory nerve action potentials are normal, however, as is motor nerve conduction velocity, thus excluding neuropathic disorders.

Investigations are necessary in order to exclude a number of conditions carrying a different prognosis, some of which may be treatable. Cervical spondylotic myelopathy, cervical tumours and syringomyelia may occasionally be confused with motor neurone disease, although the absence of sensory signs would be very unusual in these conditions. However, it is wise to undertake myelography in the majority of cases presenting with ALS, to exclude these lesions and tumours of the foramen magnum. At the same time, c.s.f. should be examined to exclude changes of neurosyphilis, which could be present in patients with syphilitic amyotrophy (now an exceedingly rare condition).

In some instances CT scanning will be necessary in patients presenting with progressive bulbar palsy. The exclusion of bilateral infarction will serve to differentiate pseudobulbar palsy due to MND from that due to vascular disease, although an adequate history will usually distinguish between these two.

Confusion sometimes arises regarding patients with a previous history of acute poliomyelitis who, in later life, develop a slowly progressive weakness and wasting of muscles. This should not be diagnosed as MND, as the condition is relatively benign and probably represents a natural fall-out of lower motor neurones from a previously impoverished lower motor neurone pool.

Treatment

There is no treatment available which affects the progression of this disorder; however, patients with MND demand very active management in order to improve their independence. Some patients with marked degrees of spasticity may benefit from spasmolytic drugs, and an appropriate provision of wheelchairs and aids to feeding and dressing are necessary. One of the major problems with the progression of the disease is the development of communication difficulties because of bulbar palsy. Many patients do find the provision of microprocessor-based communication aids of enormous benefit. Families need considerable support, and distressing episodes of choking can be managed at home by an educated family with home suction equipment; in some cases, active consideration of nasogastric feeding may be necessary.

SPINAL MUSCULAR ATROPHIES (see p. 258)

This group of conditions is characterised by a progressive lower motor neurone degeneration resulting from wasting and weakness, which usually occur on a familial basis, but are not associated with upper motor neurone involvement; a wide spectrum of such diseases is now recognised.

Werdnig–Hoffman disease is a disorder of childhood, but is mentioned briefly because of its relationship to other spinal muscular atrophies. Presentation is in infancy, with a hypotonic baby frequently with feeding difficulties. Progressive weakness is apparent and tendon reflexes are absent. The disease is inherited as an autosomal recessive trait and death usually results within the first 2–3 years of life.

Kugelberg–Welander syndrome condition has historically been misdiagnosed as muscle dystrophy because of the predominance of proximal weakness. Presentation is usually in early childhood or adolescence with limb and girdle weakness. The disorder may be differentiated from the dystrophies by EMG studies, showing changes of denervation with fasciculation and fibrillation in muscles, and by muscle biopsy. Progress is usually much slower than that in MND or Werdnig–Hoffman disease.

Other spinal muscular atrophies may present typical EMG findings of denervation without evidence of motor neuropathy in subgroups of patients with otherwise typical peroneal muscular atrophy or scapuloperoneal syndromes. These cases appear to represent particularly benign and unusual spinal muscular atrophies.

The electrophysiological hallmark of all these conditions is the finding of chronic partial denervation (fasciculation and large-amplitude motor unit potentials) in the presence of normal nerve conduction.

FURTHER READING

Adams R D, Lyon G 1982 Neurology of hereditary metabolic diseases of children. McGraw-Hill, New York
Cummings J L, Benson D F 1983 Dementia: a clinical approach. Butterworths, Boston
Harding A E 1984 The hereditary ataxias and related disorders. Churchill Livingstone, Edinburgh

16

The demyelinating diseases

INTRODUCTION

The demyelinating diseases are a group of central nervous system disturbances in which the brunt of the damage is to the central nervous system myelin sheaths and in which there is relative sparing of the other nervous system elements. In addition, there is characteristically an inflammatory cell infiltrate in the blood vessels adjacent to the lesion; the distribution of the lesions is typically perivenous and there is a relative lack of Wallerian degeneration of the fibre tracts. It is evident that the diseases do not all have identical pathology, but their inclusion in a group serves to focus on the pathological change affecting myelin and thereby to begin to identify individual pathological processes which may be relevant in those diseases which do not have a proven aetiology. Some disorders which show these characteristics, such as subacute combined degeneration which is known to be due to vitamin B_{12} deficiency, and the alcohol-related diseases of central pontine myelinolysis and the Marchiafava–Bignami syndrome, are discussed in more detail in the relevant sections.

A classification of 'demyelinating disease' is shown in Table 16.1. Those diseases which have been shown to be attributable to infection, toxin, nutritional deficiency and degenerative disorder

Table 16.1 Classification of demyelinating diseases

Primary diseases of myelin
Multiple sclerosis
Devic's disease
Schilder's disease
Balo's sclerosis
'Allergic' group (perivenous encephalomyelitis)
Postviral
Postvaccinal
Antirabies immunisation
Acute haemorrhagic leucoencephalitis
Infections
Subacute sclerosing panencephalitis — SSPE (measles)
Progressive multifocal leucoencephalitis (papovavirus)
Toxic/metabolic
Carbon monoxide, postanoxic
Diphtheria toxin
Lead
Organic mercury
Triethyl tin
Oedema
Methotrexate
Nutritional
Vitamin B_{12} deficiency
Marchiafava–Bignami syndrome
Central pontine myelinolysis
Heredofamilial system degeneration
Familial spastic paraplegia
Hereditary ataxias
Leber's disease

Table 16.2 The primary diseases of myelin

Multiple sclerosis (disseminated or insular sclerosis)
Chronic relapsing encephalomyelopathic form
Acute multiple sclerosis
Neuromyelitis optica
Diffuse cerebral sclerosis
Schilder's disease
Concentric sclerosis of Balo
Acute disseminated encephalomyelitis
Following measles, chickenpox, smallpox, and rarely mumps, rubella and influenza
Following rabies or smallpox vaccination
Acute and subacute necrotising haemorrhagic encephalitis

are dealt with in other chapters. The important group included in this chapter are the primary diseases of myelin, including multiple sclerosis, Devic's disease, Schilder's disease and Balo's sclerosis, and the 'allergic' group, including postviral and postvaccinal demyelination and acute haemorrhagic leucoencephalitis (Table 16.2).

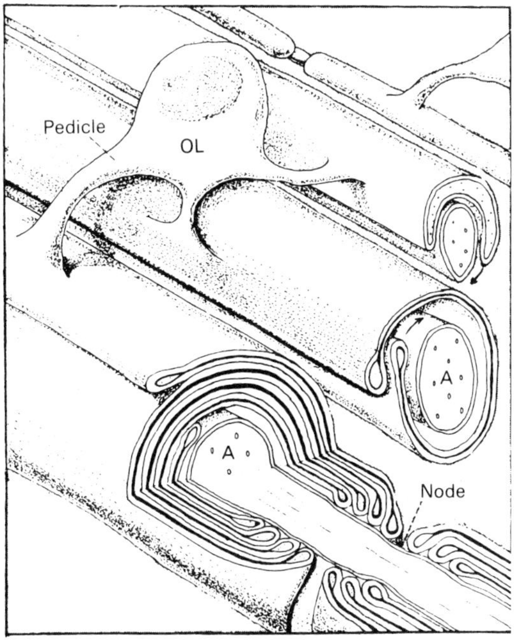

Fig. 16.1 Central nervous system myelin: the oligodendrocyte (OL) provides myelin for several axons each of which is surrounded by a spiral of extruded cell membrane.

PATHOLOGY

CENTRAL MYELIN

Myelin, the lipid-containing insulation of axons in the nervous system, is provided in the peripheral nervous system by the Schwann cell and in the central nervous system by the oligodendrogliocyte. The myelin sheath is a bilamellar extrusion of the cell membrane which spirals around the axon and increases in thickness as more membrane is produced by the cell. A single cell provides the myelin between two adjacent nodes of Ranvier; the main structural difference between the central and peripheral nervous system is that a single oligodendroglial cell is responsible for the myelin on several adjacent axons, whereas each Schwann cell provides the insulation for only a single axon (Fig. 16.1). It is believed that the axon size in the peripheral nervous system determines the thickness of its myelin sheath, but in the central nervous system there is more variation, a factor which may relate to the number of axons subserved by a single oligodendrocyte. The role of myelin is essential to the process of saltatory conduction in that it is believed that ionic flux across the internodal axon membrane is restricted by the myelin, which is therefore responsible for the development of the action potential at the node of Ranvier and thus for saltatory conduction. The loss of, or damage to, myelin, therefore will reduce conduction in the axons so affected.

Myelin is of similar composition in the peripheral and central nervous systems, consisting of high concentrations of monogalactosyl ceramide, ethanolamine phospholipid and long-chain fatty acids together with cholesterol — a mixture which resembles that of plasma membrane. The proteins are of three types: basic proteins which are held to the membrane by electrostatic bonds, like encephalitogenic protein; hydrophilic proteins which are the proteolipid apoprotein intrinsic to the membrane; and glycosylated proteins.

DEMYELINATION

The most classic form of myelin destruction is that seen in the process of Wallerian degeneration where, after disruption of the axon, the myelin sheath swells and disintegrates. This is not the same process as that seen in the demyelinating diseases, in which macrophages penetrate gaps between the myelin lamellae and release proteolytic enzymes, causing extracellular myelinolysis together with intracellular myelinolysis in these same macrophages (Figs 16.2 and 16.3). The uncertainty in the aetiology of all the demyelinating diseases is due to the questions surrounding the nature of the damage which causes the macrophages to respond in this way. Suggested underlying causes range from those involving a chronic infection of the oligodendroglial cell with a virus, a basic abnormality of the structural constitution of the myelin, damage to the myelin sheath by antibodies directed against antigens on the myelin sheath, and a secondary effect on myelin in relation to a vascular or haematological abnormality.

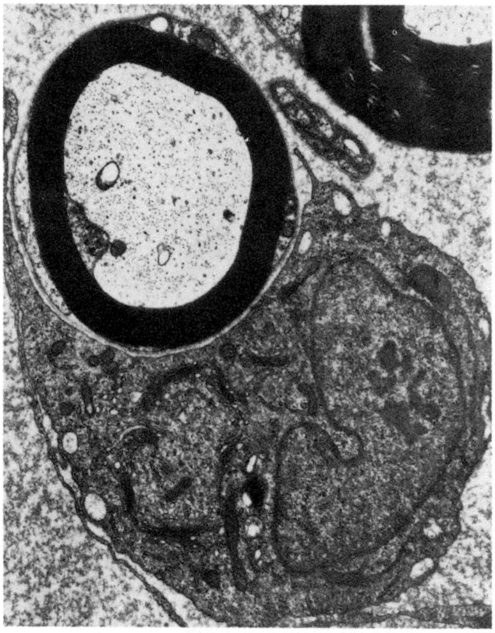

A

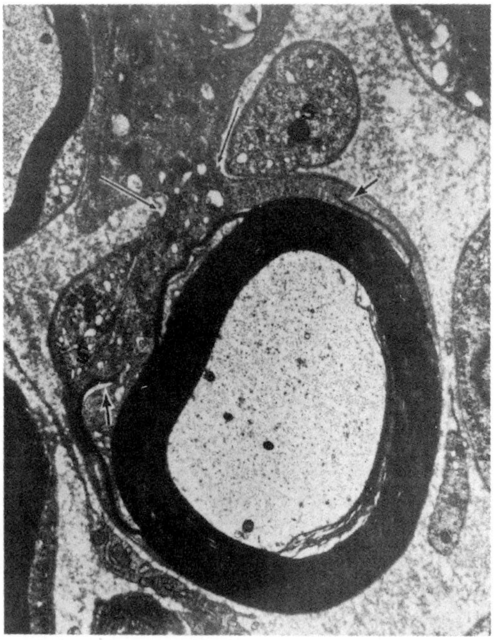

B

Fig. 16.2 **A** Electronmicrograph of a large mononuclear cell in apposition to an apparently normal nerve fibre. **B** A macrophage which has penetrated the basement membrane of the myelin and disrupted superficial myelin lamellae (arrows).

MULTIPLE SCLEROSIS

PATHOLOGY

The pathological lesions in multiple sclerosis were first described more than a century ago by Charcot. Sections of the brain and spinal cord show scattered lesions, slightly depressed below the cut surface, which stand out from the normal white matter by being pinkish-grey in colour and which appear slightly contracted. They may vary in size from a millimetre to several centimetres and they are most prominent in the periventricular regions of the white matter of the brain and in the dorsal and lateral columns of the spinal cord. They are usually found in relation to the small venules of the brain and spinal cord and, although they may appear to encroach upon grey matter, they are rarely seen on the outside of the cortex (Fig. 16.4).

Histologically, lesions vary to some extent in relation to their age. Acute lesions are perivenous and consist of loss of myelin with sparing of axis cylinders and degeneration of oligodendroglial cells. There is some neuroglial reaction and perivascular and periadventitial infiltration with mononuclear cells and lymphocytes. Older lesions show increasing degrees of gliosis with multiplication and enlargement of astrocytes, although,

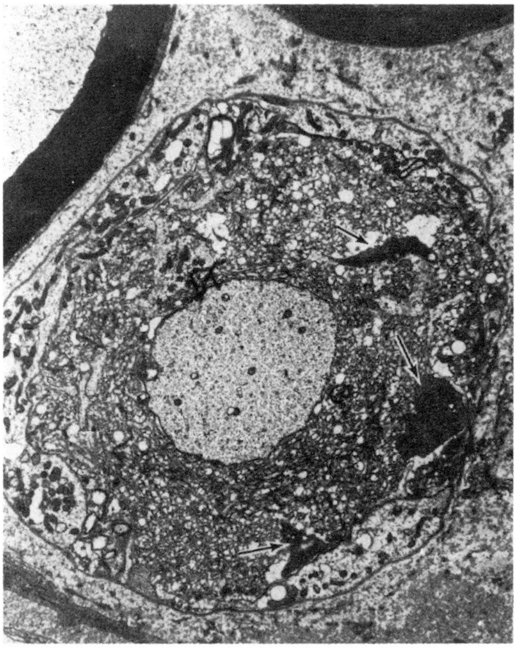

Fig. 16.3 Electronmicrograph of a nerve fibre showing complete vesicular disruption of myelin related to invading cell processes (arrows).

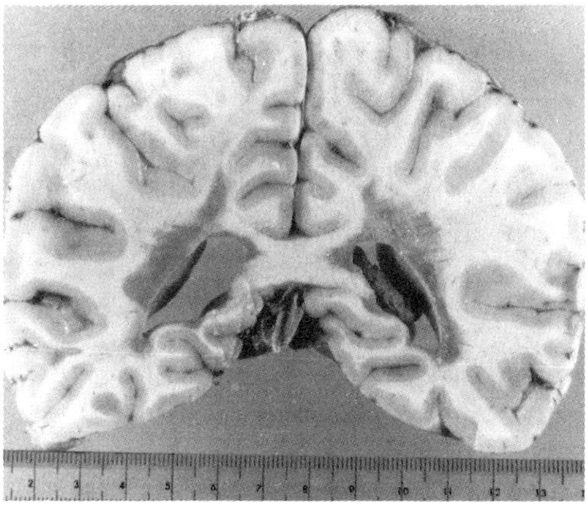

Fig. 16.4 Section of brain showing dissemination of plaques in periventricular white matter.

even at this stage, intact axis cylinders may be detected traversing the lesion. Only in the oldest lesions with loss of axis cylinders will there be evidence of damage to ascending and descending long fibre tracts. Although remyelination may be seen to occur, particularly in the earlier lesions, it is never complete and the new myelin is invariably thinner than the old.

EPIDEMIOLOGY

The aetiology of multiple sclerosis is unknown but epidemiological studies performed during the past 30 years have increasingly brought to light several factors about the incidence and the prevalence of the disease which must be taken into account in any explanation of the cause. In general, there appears to be a prevalence of less than 1 case per 100 000 in equatorial areas; less than 20 per 100 000 in the southern United States and southern Europe; and between 50 and 100 per 100 000 in the northern United States and Canada and northern Europe. There is a less pronounced variation in the incidence in the southern hemisphere and some areas, such as Japan, do not fit with the general trend, having a relatively low incidence of the disease.

This general trend of increasing incidence with increasing latitude is seen within countries, there being a lower prevalence in the southern United States and southern United Kingdom than in the north. The highest prevalence in the world is reported for Orkney and Shetland Isles with a prevalence of 140 per 100 000. Paradoxically, the most northerly race of all, the Eskimoes, do not appear to suffer from multiple sclerosis. In addition, and even within countries, blacks appear to have a lower prevalence of the disease than whites. Less substantial evidence suggests that migration from a high-risk area to a low-risk area carries with it the risk of the original area, unless the move is made before the age of approximately 15 years.

More detailed epidemiological studies within countries have also shown differences and it is suggested from studies in Norway, Switzerland and Israel that there is a relationship between the consumption of diets high in saturated fatty acids and an increased risk of multiple sclerosis. There are also examples within countries of clustering of the disease in local areas, and outbreaks suggesting either a viral or local toxic factor have been identified.

It has long been recognised that there is a familial tendency towards the development of multiple sclerosis. The risk of a first degree relative of a patient with multiple sclerosis developing the disease appears to be approximately 10 times greater than that for a member of the general population. Although no consistent genetic pattern has emerged, the concordance rate for twins is greater than that for other siblings and there has been a suggestion recently that monozygotic twins are more likely to show concordance with the disease than dizygotic twins. It has also been suggested that there is an association of the disease with certain HLA subtypes, notably the DR2 subgroup, and this may in part account for the increased familial incidence; there is, however, a low incidence of conjugal multiple sclerosis which would argue against a fact of common exposure unless this could be shown to exist early in life and have a long latency.

The incidence of multiple sclerosis in children is low, less than 1% of cases arising before the age of 15 years. The maximal age of incidence of the disease is between 25 and 35 years and, although cases have been reported to occur as late as the seventh decade, it is rare after the fifth decade. Most cases of multiple sclerosis begin between the ages of 20 and 40 years and, in a smaller group in their 50s and 60s, the disease tends to have a different pattern with a more progressive nature. Women are more likely to develop multiple sclerosis than men, the ratio being 1.7 : 1 and there is a particular risk of developing the disease or suffering an acute attack during pregnancy.

These epidemiological data suggest that, although there may be some inborn factor which makes the disease likely to occur in a certain individual, it requires an environmental factor encountered in the early years of life, which, after years of latency, causes the initial symptoms of the disease. It is suggested that this factor may be an infection and probably a virus (or several different viruses) which can exist in latent form in the oligodendroglial cell and later act as the focus for an immune assault upon this cell. However, no virus has consistently been isolated from the brain of a patient with multiple sclerosis and, to date, those suggestions of the detection of virus like particles in MS brain have proved to be unfounded. The suggestion of a chronic or latent virus infection followed by an immunological assault upon the nervous system gains credence from the fact that there have recently been reported alterations in immune cell function in patients with multiple sclerosis, most notably a decrease in the circulating T-suppressor cells in acute exacerbations of the disease. This, together with the evidence of apparently immunologically competent cells in the plaques found in the acute illness and the finding of c.n.s.-generated antibody in the cerebrospinal fluid, supports the hypothesis that, whatever the initial insult to the nervous system, the symptoms ultimately result from an autoimmune process that destroys the myelin.

CLINICAL FEATURES

The scar or plaque of multiple sclerosis is the constant and distinguishing pathological feature of the illness. The protean manifestations of the disease depend, not upon differences in the nature of the underlying lesion, but upon the site of that lesion. The predilection of the scars to occur in certain areas of the white matter results in the majority of symptoms being related to the visual system, the brain stem and the spinal cord. The typical history of the disease, encompassing acute attacks of neurological disturbance in previously fit young people, is by no means universal. The varying pattern of the disease will be described later, but neurological symptoms may develop acutely within minutes or hours in approximately one-half of the patients; in about one-third the symptoms will evolve over the space of a few days, but the remainder may show a progression of symptoms over a period of months or even years.

The classic symptoms which occur in multiple sclerosis can usefully be described in relation to the visual system, the spinal cord, the brain stem, the cerebral hemispheres and those rare symptoms which present as transient phenomena.

The visual system

Retrobulbar neuritis (p. 48)

In approximately one-quarter of patients, the initial manifestation of multiple sclerosis is retrobulbar or optic neuritis. The patient will usually describe the onset of pain in or behind the eye, particularly related to eye movement, followed in minutes to days by partial or total loss of vision in the eye. Usually only one eye is involved, although very occasionally both eyes may be affected. The vision is at first misty, with the loss of appreciation of colours, followed by blurring of vision and, ultimately complete blindness may result. Ophthalmoscopic examination of the eye may reveal no abnormalities, or the disc may look slightly injected or frankly oedematous. The presence or absence of papilloedema depends upon the siting of the plaque within the optic nerve. In those cases where the plaque lies anterior in the nerve, there may be oedema of the nerve head, but more commonly the plaque lies posteriorly within the nerve head and the optic disc may then look entirely normal—the true retrobulbar neuritis. It has been suggested that by using an ophthalmoscope with a green light it is possible to detect atrophy and loss of retinal nerve fibres in patients with retrobulbar neuritis.

It is usually possible to show an abnormality of the visual field with a central scotoma, particularly to red light, being the most common finding. In more severe cases, where vision is lost completely or where there is a marked reduction in acuity, it may be possible to demonstrate an afferent pupillary defect. It is now common practice to confirm the presence of a lesion in the optic nerve by methods involving visual evoked responses. Such tests are described in the chapter on neurological investigations and there are now well described standard figures for the number of milliseconds between stimulation and reception of the waveform, prolongation of this time from one or both eyes indicating a lesion in the relevant optic nerve.

The prognosis for optic neuritis is good: almost one-half of patients will recover normal visual acuity in the affected eye; a further one-third will achieve virtually normal vision and only a relatively small percentage will show little or no improvement. Improvement will usually begin within 10–14 days of the onset of the symptom and there remains considerable uncertainty as to whether the speed of improvement can be increased by the use of steroid therapy. Indeed, there seems little logic behind the decision to use or withold treatment with steroids in these patients—a decision which seems to depend as much upon personal prejudice of the physician concerned as upon factual information.

Some patients who have optic neuritis will never show any other manifestation of multiple sclerosis, but the proportion who go on to develop other neurological symptoms and signs appears to increase with increasing time of follow-up and is probably as high as 70–80% of patients within a 10–15 year period. There remains the dilemma as to whether a single attack of optic neuritis in fact indicates the diagnosis of multiple sclerosis in the patient or is due merely to a postinfectious episode of demyelination. Although some patients with optic neuritis achieve normal vision and the optic nerve may appear normal ophthalmoscopically, the majority will develop a degree of pallor of the optic disc over the ensuing months and years.

Recently, a condition has been described in patients who later manifest evidence of multiple sclerosis, or who had previously had evidence of optic neuritis, of a symptom in which movement of the eyes results in the patient seeing tiny flashes of light. This symptom has been called movement phosphenes and is believed to indicate irritation and inflammation in the optic nerve. It may therefore be a symptom of optic neuritis.

The differential diagnosis of optic neuritis is important and it is vital to exclude optic nerve compression by an extrinsic tumour, or a mucocele, or the presence of an intrinsic optic nerve glioma in these patients. The former two more usually cause segmental field defects and the third presents a much longer evolution of visual loss. In cases of doubt, radiological investigations, including CT scan, may be indicated. The advent of nuclear magnetic resonance scanning may make such a distinction even more accurately.

Optic atrophy

It is not uncommon, when examining patients presenting with neurological symptoms relating to other parts of the body, to find that one or both optic nerves are pale, raising the possibility of an earlier retrobulbar neuritis. There can be no doubt that patients can suffer episodes of optic neuritis without apparent symptoms and in the case of

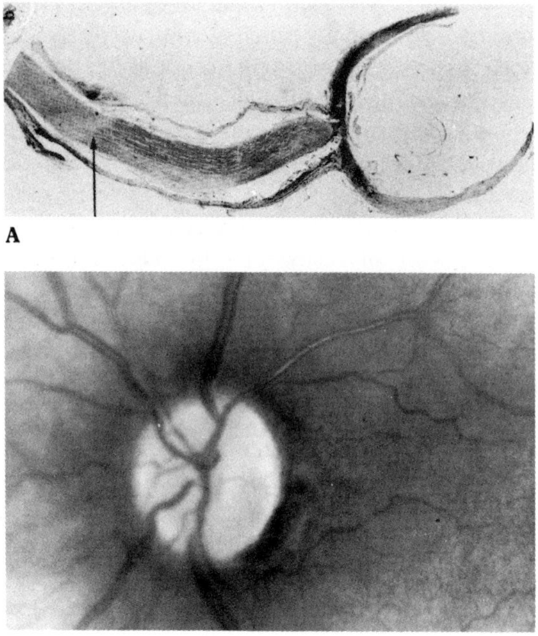

Fig. 16.5 **A** Plaque demyelination (arrowed) in an optic nerve. **B** Fundus photograph showing optic atrophy

dubious pallor of the optic disc, strong support for a lesion in the optic nerve can now be gained from the technique of visual evoked responses. The finding of optic atrophy in a young patient presenting with symptoms related to the brain stem or spinal cord strongly suggests the diagnosis of demyelinating disease, even when such patients have normal visual acuity on routine testing (Fig. 16.5).

Periphlebitis retinae

In a proportion of patients with multiple sclerosis (variously recorded as being between 5% and 20%) it is possible, on examination of the fundus, to see areas of whiteness along the sides of retinal venules. There is little pathological evidence to identify the nature of these lesions, but they appear to be areas of cellular exudation around the small venules. They are occasionally more marked in retinal diseases such as Eale's disease but, when seen asymptomatically, they raise the possibility of multiple sclerosis. They are frequently seen at some considerable distance from the optic disc and careful fundoscopy is necessary to identify them.

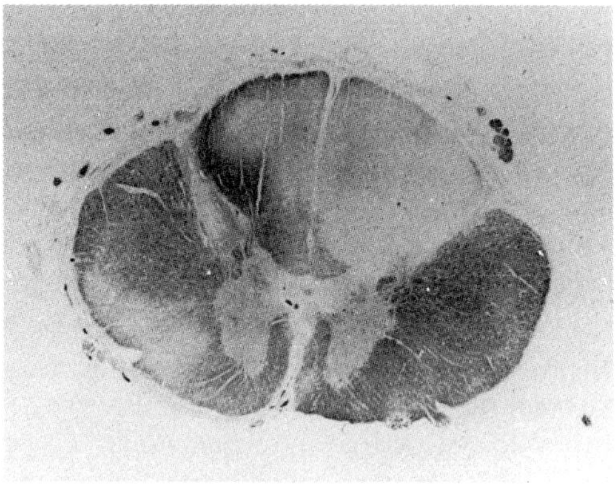

Fig. 16.6 Spinal cord lesions in multiple sclerosis

The spinal cord

The site of lesions occurring within the spinal cord will determine the site and type of symptoms presented by the patient and signs detected by the physician: lesions which occur in the cervical region are likely to cause symptoms in all four limbs; those occurring in the dorsal spine will result in symptoms confined to one or both legs. Lesions at any site may result in disturbances of bladder or bowel function, abnormalities of sweating and blood pressure control, and impotence in men.

The motor symptoms

As lesions are predominantly confined to the white matter of the spinal cord (Fig. 16.6), the most common motor symptoms developing in multiple sclerosis are those of a *spastic weakness* with increased reflexes and the development of spasms and cramps. Lesions in the cervical cord will tend to result in *tetraplegia* and, more rarely, in *hemiplegia* or *triparesis*, which is often asymmetrical; lesions in the dorsal cord will more commonly manifest as *paraparesis*. At all levels there will tend to be increased deep tendon reflexes below the level of the lesion, with alteration in the nociceptive reflexes resulting in the absence of abdominal responses and extensor plantar responses. The affected limbs show a *spastic hypertonia*, with the increase in tone being most marked in the flexors of the upper limb and the extensors of the lower limb. Weakness will follow the pattern of upper motor neurone problems, presenting with most marked weakness in the extensor muscles of the upper limb and the flexors of the lower limb. Spasms and cramps are a particular problem to the patient and development of contractures is prevented by the use of spasmolytic agents, the advice of physiotherapists and correct positioning of the limbs.

One motor symptom which is almost universal in patients with multiple sclerosis is that of fatigue; the patients will frequently notice that, although they are able to perform their daily chores relatively normally, they are aware of increasing lethargy and fatigue as the day wears on. A further problem commonly seen in these patients is that, particularly in the lower limbs, the spasticity and weakness may become more marked as they continue to exercise. In addition, as with other symptoms in multiple sclerosis, there may be a heat-related exacerbation of symptoms (Uthoff's phenomenon) in that, when the patient's core temperature is increased by drinking a hot liquid, eating or bathing in hot water, there will be an increased degree of weakness: as a result, the symptom of being able to climb into a bath but not to extricate oneself from it is not uncommonly described.

Sensory symptoms

As with motor symptoms, the disturbance of sensation may involve a single limb, both arm and leg on one side, both lower limbs, both upper limbs, three or four limbs. The rate of development of the sensory symptoms can vary considerably: in some patients the sensory loss will become apparent within hours, but in others may take weeks and even months to evolve. Depending upon whether the plaques are situated in the lateral columns or in the posterior columns, the symptoms will vary. Lesions in the lateral columns classically result in loss of sensation or numbness and occasionally pins and needles or unpleasant dysaesthetic sensations in the limbs affected. Posterior column lesions result in lack of proprioception and consequent clumsiness of the limb, which may be manifest as unsteadiness in walking, particularly in the dark, or clumsiness of the hands and a tendency to drop objects. Patients with loss of proprioception may describe band like tightness around the trunk or limb, or a feeling of swelling in the affected limb. Multiple sclerosis not uncommonly affects the posterior columns in the cervical region at their lateral limits resulting in deafferentation of the hands. Resultant symptoms of uselessness of the hands and clumsiness may be mistaken for hysterical problems in young women unless the appropriate tests are performed. Such symptoms in the hands may be referred to as the 'useless hands of Oppenheim'.

The most important result of the loss of sensation are the problems resulting from self-injury; when immobilisation and loss of sensation occur together, the patient becomes particularly susceptible to the complication of pressure sores. Such disabled patients with anaesthetic and paralysed lower limbs frequently develop painless ulcers over the sacrum, hips and heels, which may become a source of protein loss and toxin absorption, ultimately causing considerable debility and even death.

One other sensory symptom which occurs more frequently in multiple sclerosis than in any other condition is that described as Lhermitte's phenomenon, by which is meant the symptom of tingling and dysaesthesia extending down the spine and into the lower legs on neck flexion or neck movement. Although this symptom can occur with other cervical cord irritations, such as cervical cord tumour and cervical disc disease, it is most commonly seen in the context of multiple sclerosis where it may be taken to indicate the presence of a plaque in the cervical cord.

Autonomic symptoms

The most common autonomic symptoms detected in multiple sclerosis relate to the bladder and bowel, and in men, to impotence. White matter, upper motor neurone lesions affecting the autonomic supplies to the bladder and bowel, most commonly result in a spastic bladder with symptoms of frequency, urgency and precipitancy of micturition and ultimately incontinence and a spastic bowel causing constipation. Relatively rarely, patients with multiple sclerosis may develop an atonic bladder, usually with painless though occasionally with painful retention of urine and overflow incontinence. The retention of urine may occur as the result of a spastic sphincter rather than an atonic bladder and this is perhaps more frequently seen in multiple sclerosis. The problem of faecal incontinence is relatively rare in multiple sclerosis except in association with faecal impaction due to chronic constipation. Impotence in men is a relatively common symptom in multiple sclerosis and is usually part of the organic disease. Occasionally there is an additional affective component in that the depression related to other disabilities may affect potency.

The problems relating to sweating in patients with multiple sclerosis are frequently overlooked, but between 5% and 10% of such patients will show abnormalities of sweating over the trunk and lower limbs and the syndrome of intolerance to heat may occasionally arise. The potential problem of postural hypotension is uncommon because those patients liable to show such problems are usually wheelchair bound and therefore unaware of them.

Mixed syndromes

As would be expected with the diffuse nature of the disease, it is relatively rare for symptoms due to spinal cord demyelination to be confined to one system: it is much more common for the patient to have some sensory loss together with paralysis and bladder or bowel problems. In this respect, one common syndrome seen in demyelinating disease is a partial Brown-Séquard syndrome, in which multiple sclerosis affecting one half of the spinal cord results in paresis and lack of proprioception in limbs ipsilateral to the lesion, and numbness with loss of sensation in the contralateral limbs. The patient will then frequently describe the palsied limb as feeling swollen or fat and be surprised that the sensory problems appear to lie on the contralateral side.

The syndrome of posterior cord lesions is not uncommon in multiple sclerosis; that affecting solely the upper limbs has been described previously, but it is possible for deafferentation to affect both upper and lower limbs, in which case differentiation from a dorsal spinal tumour or subacute combined degeneration of the spinal cord is important; in the latter condition there will of course be reduced reflexes. Anterior spinal cord syndromes may occur in multiple sclerosis with paresis and loss of spinothalamic sensation, but relative sparing of the posterior columns. Central cord lesions are, of course, rare because this would imply problems lying within the grey matter of the cord.

Lower motor neurone problems

Although they are extremely rare, lower motor neurone symptoms including wasting, flaccid weakness and areflexia do occur in multiple sclerosis when the plaque impinges upon the region of the anterior horn cell or lies adjacent to the dorsal root entry zone. The areflexia and lower motor neurone symptoms although uncommon do not entirely exclude the possibility of the diagnosis of multiple sclerosis.

Pain

In many of the early texts about multiple sclerosis, pain was regarded as being an uncommon manifestation of the disease; it is now recognised that pain is not uncommon and may frequently be seen as the result of lesions in the spinal cord. Specific types of pain due to lesions at other sites in the nervous system will be described in the later section on transient symptoms, but those due to cord lesions include the dysaesthetic burning type of pain described in lesions of the sensory pathways, the significant and common pain due to cramps and spasms in the spastic muscles, and backache, particularly in the low lumbar spine, which may be due in part to the presence of spastic muscles at that site and in part to consequent arthritis in the spine. Very occasionally an acute spinal plaque of multiple sclerosis will cause a precisely localised pain in the spine, sometimes with radicular radiation. Such symptoms may be sufficiently acute and sufficiently severe to make the differential diagnosis from an acute disc problem, an extradural haematoma, a spinal subarachnoid haemorrhage, or epidural abscess an urgent consideration.

Brain stem

Lesions affecting the brain stem most commonly result in symptoms and signs related to eye movements, the facial muscles, articulation and balance.

Eye movement disorders

The problem of *diplopia* represents a common early complaint in multiple sclerosis. The patient will usually be able to describe a relatively acute onset of double vision in either the vertical or horizontal plane and will be able to identify the symptom as being maximal in a particular direction of gaze. Isolated sixth, third or fourth nerve palsies are rare. Routine testing of the eye movements will show the development of dysconjugate gaze in one or other direction and one of the most common findings is that due to an *internuclear ophthalmoplegia* (p. 58), where the plaque affects the median longitudinal fasciculus resulting in failure of adduction of the adducting eye together with coarse beats of nystagmus in the abducting eye: this may be seen unilaterally or bilaterally and is a classic feature of multiple sclerosis. Less commonly, the problem of *conjugate gaze paresis* may occur with the patient being entirely unable to look in one direction and yet with normal reflex eye movements in that direction of gaze. This implies a lesion either in the pontine gaze centres, or in the descending tracts from the cortex and underlying conjugate gaze paresis.

Nystagmus is a common finding in multiple sclerosis, but it is only rarely symptomatic as oscillopsia. It may be rotatory, horizontal or vertical and phasic. The unilateral nystagmus as seen in internuclear ophthalmoplegia described above is sometimes called ataxic nystagmus or Harris's sign. Pupillary abnormalities, other than afferent pupillary defects, are uncommon in multiple sclerosis, although they may occur with lesions in the midbrain.

Facial paralysis

An upper motor neurone facial palsy with sparing of frontalis is occasionally seen in hemiplegic multiple sclerosis, but should be regarded as a relative rarity. More common is a lower motor neurone facial palsy with complete involvement of one side of the face. This is believed to be due to a plaque lying at the level of the seventh nerve nucleus in the pons and may be associated with a sensory loss. The occurrence of bilateral facial palsy, though most commonly seen in sarcoidosis, may also be seen in multiple sclerosis.

Deafness and dizziness

The symptom of deafness, though reported in multiple sclerosis, is uncommon, as is that of tinnitus. Both may occur if there is bilateral damage to the ascending tracts of the auditory system. Symptoms related to dizziness are, however, among the most common of those reported in multiple sclerosis, where they may vary from a mild degree of lightheadness to a severe degree of rotational vertigo, implying the involvement of the central labyrinthine pathways. Such vertigo is usually associated with the clinical signs of nystagmus and formal vestibular function tests will be indicative of a central lesion.

Dysarthria

The most common form of dysarthria occurring in multiple sclerosis is that of a slurring, or *ataxic dysarthria*, due to lesions affecting the cerebellar connections to the brain-stem nuclei involved. Patients may frequently describe their own speech as sounding as if they are drunk; the loss of clarity in individual words and inability to make repetitive monosyllabic word sounds with regularity is classic of the abnormality.

When bilateral plaques affect the descending corticobulbar pathways a *spastic dysarthria* may also be seen in multiple sclerosis. This is usually associated with a spastic dysphonia and the high-pitched strangulated tone of the indistinctly articulated words is typical. The mixture of a spastic–ataxic dysarthria is almost pathognomonic for multiple sclerosis.

Dysphagia

Although it usually becomes evident only late in the disease, damage to the cerebellar and upper motor neurone pathways subserving the function of swallowing can result in dysphagia in the patient with multiple sclerosis. As is typical of neurological dysphagia, the problem is more marked with swallowing liquids than with solids and this is part of the syndrome of a pseudobulbar palsy.

Limb ataxia

When the cerebellar connections running to or from the cerebellar hemispheres are involved in the disease of multiple sclerosis, the symptoms appreciated by the patient are those of shakiness and clumsiness of the arms and unsteadiness of gait. The signs which may be elicited include the finding of an intention tremor on finger–nose testing and difficulty in performing rapid alternating movements of the upper limbs or the heel-knee-shin test in the lower limbs. Such problems may occur unilaterally or bilaterally. The problem may be mild and cause the patient only minimal inconvenience, but can range through a variety of disabilities up to the marked wing-beating tremor seen in patients with lesions affecting the dentato-rubral pathways, in which almost any co-ordinated movement of the upper limbs is impossible and the patients become unable to feed themselves.

Gait ataxia

When the plaques of multiple sclerosis affect the central connections to the vermis of the cerebellum, there may develop ataxia which is manifest only on walking. Initially, this results in disability in making sudden turns; later it causes the development of a wide-based gait and ultimately may be so pronounced as to prevent mobility. Early lesions may be demonstrated by asking the patient to walk heel to toe along a line drawn on the floor, by observing their performance when turning abruptly to right or left, or by asking them to walk around an object placed on the floor.

Titubation

In most patients with profound cerebellar symptoms resulting from multiple sclerosis there will be noted the sign of titubation. This consists of a persistent head-shaking movement, which occasionally may become so pronounced as to cause persistent movement of the whole of the trunk.

Mixed spastic and ataxic syndromes

Lesions in the brain stem may obviously affect not only the cerebellar pathways but also the descending long tract pathways and in this situation it is common to find a mixture of spasticity and ataxia affecting one or more limbs. It is important to remember that, whereas a minor degree of spasticity may cause the patient little inconvenience and a similar degree of ataxia may pass almost unnoticed, the combination of the two lesions can be disastrous for mobility.

Cerebral hemispheres

Although, on pathological grounds and with the new technique of magnetic resonance imaging, lesions scattered throughout the hemispheres are recognised to be common in multiple sclerosis, they are less evident clinically. As has been explained in the section on pathology, white matter lesions in the cerebral hemispheres tend to occur in the periventricular areas and many appear to be virtually asymptomatic. There are, however, certain well-recognised clinical symptoms which are seen in multiple sclerosis and which arise from the presence of plaques scattered throughout the hemispheres.

Hemiplegia

It is perhaps surprising that, with a white matter disease which can be so widespread in the central nervous system, the finding of a plaque in the posterior limb of the internal capsule is relatively uncommon. None the less, there are well-documented cases of multiple sclerosis in which there has been a true hemiplegia with involvement of the lower part of the face ipsilateral to the hemiplegia.

Dementia

Possibly the most common of the symptoms related to hemispheric plaques in multiple sclerosis is the development of mild dementia with problems in memory, seen so frequently late in the disease of multiple sclerosis and possibly the explanation for the original documentation of euphoria as a common clinical component of the patient with multiple sclerosis. In rare cases of multiple sclerosis, dementia appears to be a major part of the disease. There are well described instances in which patients with confirmed multiple sclerosis have presented with acute and progressing dementia relatively early in life and these are almost certainly due to the accumulation of numerous white matter plaques within the hemispheres, resulting in destruction of the inter-hemispheric pathways. It can well be understood how lesions adjacent to the third ventricle could account for problems with memory, which are occasionally noted late in the disease.

Epilepsy

There is no doubt that the symptom of epilepsy is more common in multiple sclerosis than in unaffected members of the population. The incidence is variously reported as between 1% and 5% of all patients with multiple sclerosis and probably occurs when a subcortical white matter plaque impinges to an extent upon the grey matter. This topic is dealt with more fully in the following section.

Dysphasia

This typically grey matter disturbance is regarded as exceptionally uncommon in multiple sclerosis. Patients have been described in whom both anterior, posterior and conduction aphasias have been associated with multiple sclerosis, but these are exceedingly rare and the occurrence of dysphasia must raise grave doubts as to the accuracy of the diagnosis.

Hemianopia

Homonymous visual field defects characterised by hemianopia are extremely uncommon in multiple sclerosis. They do occur, but the presence of the hemianopic field defect should raise doubts as to the accuracy of the diagnosis.

Transient phenomena

During the past two decades a variety of transient phenomena occurring in multiple sclerosis have been described. Although, when these occur in a patient with well-established and diagnosed multiple sclerosis, their recognition causes little difficulty, when they are the first symptom of multiple sclerosis they may cause more concern.

The epilepsies

Epileptic seizures, usually tonic-clonic due to secondary generalisation or occasionally focal in nature, are well recognised in multiple sclerosis. They probably occur in approximately 1% of patients, although some authors have recorded instances as high as 5%. They presumably reflect the presence of subcortical plaques of demyelination which impinge upon the local grey matter and result in an irritative focus. They will usually respond to adequate anticonvulsant therapy, and particularly the use of carbamazepine.

Tic douloureux

The idiopathic syndrome is virtually confined to people over the age of 50 and the occurrence of this lancinating pain in patients under this age should raise the possibility of the diagnosis being multiple sclerosis. The cause of this particular syndrome in multiple sclerosis is not well understood: it would seem likely that brain stem plaques are the cause, although lesions arising in the trigeminal nerve have occasionally been suggested. The pains will usually respond to treatment with carbamazepine, occasionally to the use of short courses of steroids. The techniques of creating lesions in the Gasserian ganglion are less likely to be effective if the underlying cause is multiple sclerosis. Occasionally the episodes of pain are more prolonged in patients with multiple sclerosis and the syndrome of tic douloureux may extend into that more usually described as atypical facial pain.

Painful tonic spasms

Episodes of acute painful spasm, usually affecting one or other of the upper limbs and causing the limb to adopt a posture of extension, together with excruciating pain are recorded in multiple sclerosis. The cause of these syndromes has been suggested to be a plaque lying across an ascending and descending pathway and allowing shorting of electrical transmission or ephaptic transmission to occur between the two separate pathways.

Kinesogenic dyskinesia

The phenomenon of sudden development of an abnormal posture in a leg or an arm on the initiation of movement has been recognised for some years and can occur as an apparently isolated syndrome. This symptom has been described in patients with multiple sclerosis and the probability is that this can be an alternative form of ephaptic transmission within the nervous system.

All of these transient phenomena may occur spontaneously during the course of the disease, but they are occasionally precipitated by intercurrent problems such as infections, a change in temperature or other external stimuli.

Temporal patterns of disease

Acute remitting and relapsing multiple sclerosis

By far the most common form of multiple sclerosis is the development in a young person over the course of many years of varying symptoms relating to differing sites in the neuraxis. Thus, the history might be expected to include an episode of retrobulbar neuritis with recovery, followed some years later by the development of paraesthesiae in one limb, then the onset of spastic weakness of both lower limbs together with some bladder disturbance, all of which symptoms show a degree of recovery; later, there is the onset of a period of ataxia, which again remits. This particular pattern occurs in approximately one-half of the patients with multiple sclerosis.

Chronic progressive disease

In the older patients, a syndrome is seen in which multiple sclerosis begins as a gradual and progressing paralysis of the lower limbs, together with disturbance of bladder and bowel function. This form of illness is most commonly seen in the fifth and sixth decade, tends not to show remissions and is usually relentlessly progressive, ultimately causing the patient to become wheelchair bound. This pattern occurs in 20–30% of patients with multiple sclerosis.

Acute fulminant multiple sclerosis

It is fortunate that only rarely (in less than 5% of patients) does the disease have a particularly fulminant course: this form is usually seen in young patients. The onset of the disease with severe ataxia and brain-stem symptoms carries a bad prognosis: the illness may not show periods of remission and the patient may rapidly become significantly disabled with dysarthria, dysphagia, dementia and total dependence, resulting in a bed-bound state.

Coma in multiple sclerosis

The occurrence of coma in multiple sclerosis is extremely uncommon and usually carries a poor prognosis. There is no doubt that lesions occurring in the dorsal brain stem may result in altered consciousness and there are documented cases of patients with multiple sclerosis lapsing into coma. Despite this, the occurrence of coma in multiple sclerosis is so rare that other causes should always be sought to explain the condition.

Benign multiple sclerosis

One of the problems bedevilling epidemiological assessment of this disease has been the difficulty in identification during life of patients suffering from multiple sclerosis. There are undoubtedly patients who have one or two minor episodes of remitting neurological illness, such as a retrobulbar neuritis followed by an episode of numbness, tingling or weakness in a single limb, both of which symptoms recover, and who then, through prolonged follow-up, show no more symptoms of disease. In addition, it has recently been shown from pathological studies that many more patients than those who are diagnosed in life can be shown at autopsy to have plaques of multiple sclerosis scattered throughout the nervous system. There therefore remains the real possibility that those patients diagnosed as having multiple sclerosis represent only the tip of the iceberg of a syndrome which is far more common in the population of northern Europe and North America. It is to be hoped that the advent of newer techniques of diagnosis, including evoked potential studies and, in particular, magnetic resonance imaging will bring to light more information about the true frequency of the disease and therefore make more valid epidemiological studies of its occurrence.

DIAGNOSIS

There is perhaps more public debate and disquiet about the diagnosis of multiple sclerosis and the notification of this diagnosis to the patient than in any other disease, apart from neoplasia. The reason is not hard to find: multiple sclerosis cannot be diagnosed with absolute certainty other than at autopsy. The clinical diagnosis is always one of probability and although, after several episodes or with a progressing illness and the necessary exclusion of other pathologies, the probability of accurate diagnosis is high, it can never be absolute. The most useful distinction for certainty of diagnosis in multiple sclerosis is that suggested by Poser et al (1984), as shown in Table 16.3. In making the diagnosis the two most important aspects are the finding of lesions scattered throughout the nervous system in different places and at different times and the exclusion of other pathological diagnoses. The physician has several methods at his disposal to identify such a diverse disease and to attempt to rule out other more definable causes.

Table 16.3 New diagnostic criteria for multiple sclerosis

Clinically definite multiple sclerosis
1. History of two attacks and clinical evidence of two separate lesions
2. History of two attacks, clinical evidence of one and paraclinical evidence of a separate lesion

Laboratory supported definite multiple sclerosis
1. History of two attacks, either clinical or paraclinical evidence of one lesion and c.s.f. oligoclonal bands
2. History of one attack, clinicial evidence of two separate lesions and c.s.f. oligoclonal bands
3. History of one attack, clinical evidence of one and paraclinical evidence of another lesion and c.s.f. oligoclonal bands

Clinically probable multiple sclerosis
1. History of two attacks and clinical evidence of one lesion
2. History of one attack and clinical evidence of two separate lesions
3. History of one attack, clinical evidence of one lesion and paraclinical evidence of a second lesion

Laboratory supported probable multiple sclerosis
1. History of two attacks and c.s.f. oligoclonal bands

N.B. Paraclinical = evidence from evoked potentials and imaging (CT or MR).

History

In few other diseases does the clinical history provide as much information for the physician as in multiple sclerosis. It is, therefore, evident that the first attack is the one most difficult to diagnose because, with a single scar in the nervous system, several other pathological conditions, such as post-viral demyelination, vascular disease, or tumour, must be considered. The history from a patient of several periods of neurological disturbance with exacerbations and remissions occurring in different parts of the nervous system would strongly support the likelihood of the diagnosis. For example, the patient who has suffered an episode of blindness in one eye some three years previously, followed by sensory disturbance in an arm and who now presents with a mild paraparesis or ataxia, is likely to have at least three lesions and therefore an increased probability of multiple sclerosis. Nevertheless, if this same patient was seen in the later years of life, then the probability of a vascular cause would still exist.

Particular care must be taken when a series of relapsing and remitting symptoms are confined to one part of the neuraxis: for example, episodes of intermittent blindness in one eye lasting for periods of days at a time, although compatible with multiple sclerosis, might be due to the presence of a mucocele in one of the paranasal sinuses. Again, episodes of intermittent cord disturbance, although raising the possibility of demyelination, might sometimes be seen in a patient with a spinal neurofibroma, meningioma, arteriovenous malformation or intervertebral disc prolapse. None the less, careful clinical history remains one of the most helpful diagnostic measures in raising the possibility of multiple sclerosis.

Examination

Similarly, the neurological examination of a patient with suspected multiple sclerosis is primarily directed toward the definition of involvement of several different sites of the nervous system. Thus, as has been alluded to previously, the finding of optic atrophy in one eye in a patient with a recent brain stem disturbance or spinal cord problem would raise the possibility of the existence of more than one lesion and therefore would increase the likelihood of the diagnosis being multiple sclerosis. In the past, much has been made of the patient who presents with symptoms in areas of the body where there are no signs and, more importantly, those who have signs where there are no symptoms. Of particular importance in this respect is the finding, on a routine neurological examination, of absent abdominal reflexes or extensor plantar responses, raising the possibility of earlier spinal disturbance. Perhaps the most common clinical findings in multiple sclerosis are those of optic pallor, internuclear ophthalmoplegia, an intention tremor, ataxia and slurring dysarthria (sometimes described as Charcot's triad), or signs of a mild and frequently asymmetrical spastic paraparesis.

When the patient's history or the examination raises the possibility of multiple sclerosis, the physician has the opportunity to pursue further investigations in an attempt to improve his confidence in the diagnosis. It should be stressed that, in a patient with mild symptoms and no or few abnormal signs, it may be pertinent to do no more than reassure the patient and continue observation, because at present there is no evidence that the definition of this disease at such a time can enable significant therapeutic measures to be undertaken to alter the future course. Nevertheless, it is this very hesitancy in making the diagnosis which creates some of the problems that so exercise lay members of society today, when they believe that information regarding a possible diagnosis of multiple sclerosis is withheld from the patient by the physician. Those tests available to help to confirm the diagnosis include the examination of the cerebral spinal fluid, the elicitation of evoked responses and magnetic resonance scanning.

Investigations (Ch. 5)

Cerebrospinal fluid (c.s.f) examination

In investigating a patient with presumed multiple sclerosis, samples should be taken for cell count, total protein, immunoglobulin, sugar and serological tests for syphilis. Ideally, synchronous blood sampling should be taken to allow proper assessment of the level of sugar and, more importantly, to allow the evaluation of the ratio between the IgG to albumin in the c.s.f. when compared with that in blood. This technique provides a reasonably simple and accurate estimation of endogenous c.s.f. production of immune globulin. In increasing numbers of laboratories now it is becoming possible to submit c.s.f. to isoelectric focusing studies that enable the identification of oligoclonal banding of immunoglobulins, which further increases the accuracy of diagnosis.

Typically, the c.s.f. in a patient with multiple sclerosis will show a mild pleocytosis containing between 5 and 50 white blood cells per cubic millimetre. Most of the cells are lymphocytes, although plasma cells and occasionally polymorphonuclear cells are described. Cellular abnormalities are more commonly found in the earlier cases of multiple sclerosis and alterations in immune globulins in the later cases. Although levels will vary from laboratory to laboratory, in most instances of multiple sclerosis the IgG will be raised above the normal 15% of the total protein in the c.s.f. and the IgG/albumin c.s.f.: IgG/albumin serum ratio will be greater than 0.6. Oligoclonal bands are discovered with a frequency of over 90% in the c.s.f. in patients with multiple sclerosis and probably represent one of the most accurate methods available today to confirm the diagnosis.

The problem with c.s.f. changes in multiple sclerosis is that the majority of diseases which may cause symptoms similar to multiple sclerosis have similar c.s.f. abnormalities. In particular, neurosyphilis, sarcoidosis and other causes of chronic meningitis or viral encephalomyelitis may have almost identical cellular and protein abnormalities.

Evoked potentials

Evoked potential studies are described in Chapter 5. Visual evoked, brain stem evoked and sensory evoked potentials all may provide information of importance in multiple sclerosis. All three methods have in common the fact that they can indicate, by the finding of delays in the speed of conduction, the presence of lesions which may not be evident clinically in the optic nerves, brain stem or sensory pathways. The finding of a lesion in one or other of these places, when taken in conjunction with the patient's recent symptoms and signs, strongly supports the possibility of multiple lesions within the nervous system and increases the probability of the diagnosis of multiple sclerosis. The accuracy of these investigations in multiple sclerosis is open to some question and the finding of abnormality in patients subjected to visual evoked responses has varied from 70% to 90%, with sensory evoked responses from 50% to 80% and with brain stem auditory evoked responses from 50% to 70%.

Magnetic resonance imaging

Although CT scanning occasionally shows areas of low density in patients with multiple sclerosis, which are taken to be the sites of plaques in the hemispheres, and which might occasionally enhance with double dose contrast techniques, it has never been adequate to confirm or refute the diagnosis. The newer technique of magnetic resonance imaging, however, shows marked signals at the sites of plaques in the cerebral hemispheres, brain stem, optic nerve and spinal cord and may ultimately become important, not only as a research tool, but in providing information as to the presence of such plaques and also the progression of silent plaques in patients with this disease. Although this equipment is not yet generally available, it will undoubtedly prove of enormous help in the diagnosis, management and study of patients with multiple sclerosis (Fig. 16.7).

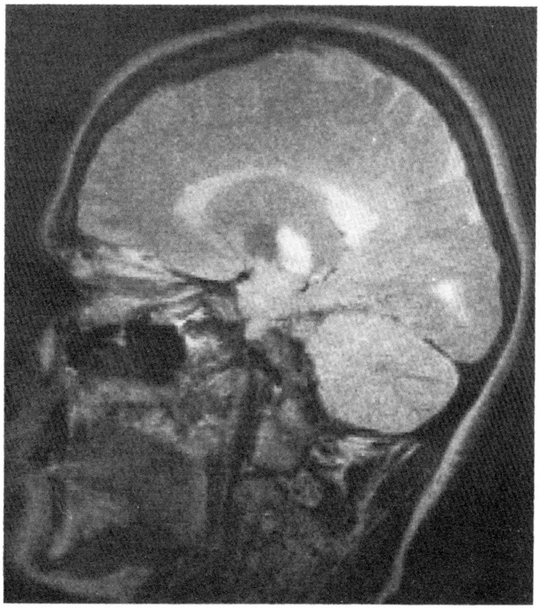

Fig. 16.7 Magnetic resonance image in multiple sclerosis.

Differential diagnosis

Since multiple sclerosis can mimic many other diseases of the central nervous system, it is inevitable that problems arise in distinguishing this disease from other conditions. Those factors which ought to be considered in the differential diagnosis will vary depending upon the presentation.

Relapses and remissions

Other diseases which might produce a picture of relapses and remissions include forms of cerebral embolic disease, in which the onset of the episode is usually more abrupt than in multiple sclerosis and a source for emboli can normally be identified, inflammatory arteritic diseases such as SLE, and chronic granulomatous conditions such as sarcoid.

Diffuse neurological involvement

The multifocal nature of multiple sclerosis may be mimicked by other conditions, causing numerous lesions within the central nervous system such as secondary tumour spread, chronic meningitis, granulomatous conditions and fungal disease.

The syndrome of chronic paraplegia

Patients who develop a progressive paraplegia may have multiple sclerosis but this illness can be mimicked by cervical spondylotic myelopathy, ischaemic myelomalacia, syringomyelia, tonsillar ectopia and many structural causes of intraspinal compression.

In each of these conditions it is important to exclude the possibility of other diseases before the diagnosis of multiple sclerosis is considered to be confirmed.

MANAGEMENT

As the cause of multiple sclerosis is not understood at present, it follows that there is not yet any preventative or curative therapy. Despite this, there are several ways in which acute exacerbations of the disease may be ameliorated, persisting symptoms alleviated and residual disability overcome with the help of the physician.

At times of acute exacerbation, there is some evidence that further deterioration may be arrested and improvement speeded by the use of steroid therapy. The most validated form of such treatment consists of a short course of intramuscular ACTH given in reducing dosage over a few weeks. Alternatively, oral prednisone or prednisolone may be used in a similar short course and recently the suggestion has been made of a short course of dexamethasone or even high-dose intravenous methyl prednisolone during acute exacerbations. It is important that the physician recognises that such medicines in general are only used in severe and disabling exacerbations and they would be unwarranted in many of the minor and purely sensory disturbances which patients may detect. The use of long-term steroid therapy in an attempt to reduce the frequency or severity of attacks is less well validated. Occasional patients will benefit from alternate-day medication with prednisone, or twice weekly injections of Depo ACTH.

There have been numerous reports of the use of cytotoxic medication in multiple sclerosis and, in some European centres, azathioprine is a commonly prescribed drug. More aggressive cytotoxic therapy with such agents as cyclosporin A, antilymphocytic globulin, together with high-dose steroid treatments, have occasionally been recommended and some authors believe that they have a beneficial effect upon the disease. The main difficulty in assessing these therapies is the unpredictable nature of the illness: it is with reluctance that one would embark upon a prolonged cytotoxic regime in a patient early in the disease who might have little in the way of further symptoms, and yet to employ such therapies in patients who have already suffered the ravages of the disease seems pointless in that it can only be directed towards stopping further attacks and will not of itself improve the damage which has already occurred.

The epidemiological finding of an increased prevalence of multiple sclerosis in populations consuming diets rich in animal fats, together with the biochemical findings of low polyunsaturated fatty acid levels in patients with the disease, has led to trials of dietary therapy and supplementation in multiple sclerosis. At best, these studies are to be regarded as inconclusive, but a simple modification of diet in consuming less animal fats, a higher concentration of vegetable fats and possible supplementation with linoleic acid and fish oil, appears to be harmless, inexpensive and to provide some evidence of reduction in frequency and severity of attacks and of improvement in overall state.

The preponderance of therapy in multiple sclerosis is directed towards symptomatic help of the patients. The painful spasms and cramps, and ultimately contractures, which may occur can be alleviated or prevented by the use of spasmolytic agents such as diazepam, baclofen and dantrolene sodium. The management of ataxic tremor is extremely difficult. There are no effective pharmacological agents though isoniazid has been suggested to be of some help and choline chloride is occasionally used. Stereotactic thalamotomy may control this tremor, but such neurosurgical approaches to the patient with multiple sclerosis may be associated with further deterioration. The management of problems with sphincter control in patients with multiple sclerosis represents one of the most important aspects of their continuing care. In terms of the bladder, it is important to understand the precise mechanism which causes the symptoms and for this reason the use of formal urodynamic assessment is indicated. In this way the relative importance of spasticity of the detrusor muscles, weakness of the detrusor, and spasticity of the sphincter muscles can be ascertained. When the detrusor muscle is spastic, agents such as imipramine, sparine or propranthelîne bromide may be used, whilst for a spastic sphincter muscle α-adrenergic blocking agents such as phenoxybenzamine may be helpful. It may occasionally be necessary to catheterise a patient, either permanently or on an intermittent basis by self-catheterisation, and the possibility of urinary diversion may be considered. Constipation will frequently need therapy with aperients and may require manual evacuation. Difficulty with potency in the male may be helped by local injections or penile implants. Pain is not uncommon as a symptom in multiple sclerosis and necessitates adequate analgesics once its cause has been ascertained. The transient phenomena occurring in multiple sclerosis will usually respond to treatment with carbamazepine: these include seizures, trigeminal neuralgia, painful tonic spasms and the rare syndrome of transient dysarthria, diplopia and disequilibrum.

In terms of coping with disability, it is important to involve other members of the medical team: for instance, the physiotherapist and occupational therapist have a large part to play in rehabilitation and should be involved in the provision of any necessary aids; such help will vary from the simple provision of a walking cane to the need for a walking frame or wheelchair and ultimately the provision of an environmental control system for the most severely disabled patients. At all stages of the disease one of the important roles of the physician is to help the patient and others involved to understand the nature of the illness and the causes of the varying symptoms. The time at which patients are advised of the diagnosis is critical. It is apparent that more information is now available in the popular press about the disease and many patients attending their physicians, or being referred to a neurologist, may already have a secret fear of the illness before they discuss matters with their doctor. This undoubtedly leads the physician towards earlier identification of the nature of the disease to the patient but, as has been explained above, for reasons of uncertainty it might be inappropriate to define the disease too clearly in the early stages when it can only be suspected. It should be recognised that certain features in the life of the patient may make it more necessary for the consultant to discuss the diagnosis with the patient and other involved parties. Obviously, impending marriage provides an indication for the discussion of the significance of earlier symptoms with the patient and the intended spouse, as would the decision in a female patient to become pregnant. Similarly, taking on additional commitments in the home or at work, possible travel abroad or emigration, may also be regarded as indications for a frank discussion of the nature of the disease. It is not possible to lay down hard and fast rules as to when and how patients should be informed of the likelihood of a diagnosis of multiple sclerosis: much will depend upon the relationship between the patient and the physician concerned, and the most important point is that sufficient time should be allowed to the patient and relatives to assimilate the information provided and to ask relevant questions of the physicians concerned.

OTHER PRIMARY DISEASES OF MYELIN

DEVIC'S DISEASE (neuromyelitis optica)

This demyelination arises with the sudden onset of bilateral visual impairment followed or preceded within days or weeks by a transverse myelitis. This particular clinical picture has been accorded the name Devic's disease, although in most cases with pathological investigation the histological appearances of the lesions are identical to that of multiple sclerosis. Although occasionally this constellation of symptoms can arise in a patient with other symptoms and signs of multiple sclerosis, it may frequently be a single episode of illness which does not recur, but which necessarily causes the patient considerable disability. There is usually little recovery from this condition and its occurrence as a monophasic illness certainly raises the possibility that it is a separate condition from the more common multiple sclerosis. It appears that such forms of the disease are more common in the Far East, where multiple sclerosis per se is a less common condition. Although the cause of Devic's disease, like that of multiple sclerosis, is unknown, the monophasic nature of the illness raises the possibility that it is a postviral syndrome. Patients are usually treated with steroids but, as is indicated above, the chances of recovery are less than in multiple sclerosis.

It is noteworthy that during the 1960s and 1970s in Japan there was an outbreak of bilateral optic neuropathy with myelopathy of slightly slower onset, which was termed subacute myelo-optic neuropathy (SMON). It was initially assumed that this condition might be related to a viral infection, but later epidemiological and toxicological studies showed that is was due to the abnormally high intake of clioquinol in the population at risk. Since the recognition of this problem, the occurrence of the disease has fallen considerably.

SCHILDER'S DISEASE

Schilder's original description in 1912 of a child of 14 dying with 'diffuse sclerosis' was complicated for some time by the subsequent use of the same term for diseases with familial occurrence, gliosis and metachromatic changes, with globoid bodies seen in the myelin in the hemispheres. There does, however, appear to be a disease that is non-familial in type and that tends to arise in children, in which there is a progressive illness involving dementia, hemianopia, cortical blindness, cortical deafness, hemiplegia, quadriplegia and pseudobulbar palsy. The c.s.f. changes frequently resemble those seen in multiple sclerosis and death usually occurs in months or years from presentation.

Such patients usually show at autopsy a large asymmetrical focus of myelin destruction involving the cerebral hemispheres, with extension across the corpus callosum. On histological examination the focus shows characteristics of multiple sclerosis and other smaller lesions may occasionally be found in the brain stem and cord. The disease can be reasonably regarded as a variant of multiple sclerosis.

Recently, the identification of a similar neurological illness in patients with Addison's disease has been recognised and, although sometimes labelled with the eponym of Addison–Schilder's disease, it is now better called adrenoleukodystrophy. It begins in the first two decades of life and is probably a sex-linked recessive disorder. Either the endocrine or the neurological abnormalities may be the first to appear and, although classically the neurological abnormalities relate to cerebral hemisphere demyelination, there are reports of spastic parapareses developing in these patients. Histologically, the myelin has degenerated rather than showing the typical picture of demyelination and the subject is further considered in the relevant section.

BALO'S SCLEROSIS

A rare pathological entity is the finding of concentric rings of demyelination and normal myelin in the cerebral hemisphere. Patients tend to present with encephalopathic symptoms and the disease, although suggesting a centrifugal spread of demyelination and raising the possibility of a toxic factor, is probably a variant of multiple sclerosis.

ALLERGIC DEMYELINATION

The syndromes described in this section have in common the pathological feature of numerous foci of demyelination scattered throughout the brain and spinal cord. These foci surround small venules within the neuraxis and, as is typical of demyelination, the axons and neuroglia are largely intact. Histologically, the lesions consist of lymphocytes and mononuclear cells cuffing the vessels and microglia within the areas of demyelination.

POSTVIRAL DEMYELINATION (acute disseminated encephalomyelitis)

This syndrome is seen most frequently following rubeola infection, although it is also seen after chickenpox, rubella and smallpox. A similar illness may be seen as a complication of mumps, but this disease is far more likely to cause a true viral meningoencephalitis.

The syndrome usually begins 2–4 days after the exanthem and typically the patient will have a recurrence of fever, confusion, convulsions, stupor and ultimately coma. More rarely, the onset is with hemiplegia or ataxia and occasionally a transverse myelitis may occur. There is a considerable variation in the severity of the illness and many patients showing episodes of confusion, headache and signs of meningeal irritation may indeed be suffering from a mild form of the disease. The c.s.f. characteristically shows a lymphocytic pleocytosis, an increased protein content and a monoclonal band of immunoglobulin on immunoelectric-focusing. The c.s.f. sugar is normal.

The important differential diagnoses are from thrombophlebitis occurring in the course of a febrile illness, toxic hepatoencephalopathy (Reye's syndrome), or hypoxic encephalopathy. Infectious mononucleosis and herpes simplex encephalitis may mimic postinfectious encephalomyelitis and, of course, the onset of seizures in a child with an exanthem may reflect no more than a febrile seizure. The frequency of this syndrome has fallen during the past two decades, probably because of the increased use of measles vaccination. The treatment is with steroids, which seem to ameliorate the disease, although the prognosis remains poor in many cases.

POSTVACCINAL ENCEPHALOMYELITIS

Perhaps the most classic example of demyelinating myeloencephalopathy following vaccination is that which follows the use of rabies vaccine. This almost certainly is due to the use of a rabbit brain homogenate and it is possible that the introduction of the newer embryo vaccines, which do not contain nerve tissue, will reduce the frequency of this disease. The syndrome rarely follows smallpox vaccination and is even more uncommon with other vaccines; in these instances the source of the vaccine does not appear to affect the frequency of the illness.

Postvaccinal encephalomyelitis usually begins abruptly with headache, drowsiness, fever and convulsion. There are frequently signs of spinal cord involvement and, in addition to hemiplegia or tetraparesis, there may be areflexia. Brain stem involvement follows and there may be stupor and coma. The c.s.f. again shows a lymphocytic pleocytosis, with an increase in protein and a normal sugar.

The mortality rate of postvaccinal encephalomyelitis is high and, even in those who recover, residual neurological signs including intellectual impairment are not uncommon. There is no known treatment for the condition and it is usual to prescribe high-dose steroids in an attempt to reduce the demyelination.

ACUTE HAEMORRHAGIC LEUCOENCEPHALITIS

This condition is rarely seen in children, but usually occurs in young adults. It is a particularly fulminant form of demyelinating disease which tends to occur within 1–2 weeks of an upper respiratory tract infection. The infection is believed to be viral in nature, although it is probable that several different viruses have the ability to generate the syndrome. The illness begins abruptly with headache, meningismus and confusion and there is usually an associated fever. Diffuse neurological symptoms can then arise, indicating hemisphere, brain stem or cord disturbance. There are frequently seizures and the development of coma. A peripheral leucocytosis is common, with a relative lymphocytosis. The c.s.f. also shows a pleocytosis, which may vary from being predominantly lymphocytic to being entirely polymorphonuclear. Occasionally, red cells are present; the protein content is increased, but the sugar level is normal.

The majority of patients die within a few days of the development of symptoms, but there are reports of some making a total recovery. The important differential diagnoses are herpes simplex encephalitis, meningitis, cerebral abscess and subdural empyema. It is usual to advise high-dose steroid treatment in the condition, although the proof of effectiveness of this therapy is lacking.

The pathological findings are of scattered purpuric lesions throughout the white matter of the hemisphere, brain stem and spinal cord and histologically there is necrosis of blood vessels with haemorrhages and inflammation in the perivascular area.

Although the precise cause of the disease is unknown, it seems probable that there is an immunological attack upon the cerebral vessels and adjacent tissue which may be due to the original presumed viral infection.

FURTHER READING

Matthews W B, Acheson E D, Batchelor J R, Weller R O (eds) 1985 McAlpine's multiple sclerosis. Churchill Livingstone, Edinburgh

Poser C M, Paty D W, McDonald W I, Schenberg L, Ebers G C (eds) 1984 The diagnosis of multiple sclerosis. Tieme-Stratton, New York

17

Neurological disease due to drugs, toxins and physical agents

INTRODUCTION

With the increasing complexity of modern life and medical treatment, iatrogenic self-induced or accidental disease is becoming increasingly common. Clinicians must be aware that chemical or physical agents may be involved in the aetiology of clinical syndromes, which may result from drug abuse, self-poisoning, therapeutics or accident.

IATROGENIC DRUG-INDUCED DISEASE

PSYCHIATRIC DISORDERS

An elaborate and convincing theory explaining the aetiology of depressive illnesses has been proposed, involving the depletion of cerebral monoamines (catecholamines and serotonin). This is based, in part, upon the finding that the antidepressant tricyclic drugs and monoamine oxidase inhibitors both possess actions which increase monoamine activity, and partly on the realisation that drugs depleting central monoamine stores may be associated with depressive illness: thus reserpine, tetrabenazine and α-methyldopa may cause depression by this mode of action.

Symptoms of *agitation* and *anxiety* frequently accompany withdrawal of sedatives such as alcohol, barbiturates and benzodiazepines (see below), or may occur as direct effects of stimulants such as amphetamines. *Hallucinatory disturbances*, too, occur in drug withdrawal syndromes but can also be caused by agents with specific dopaminergic properties: thus parkinsonian patients treated with L-dopa may have visual and auditory hallucinations and be deluded; similar changes may be seen in patients taking amphetamines and, in both cases, states almost identical to acute psychosis may arise.

A wide variety of drugs with c.n.s. actions may cause *acute confusional states* in a non-specific manner; similarly, drug overdosage may lead to coma (see below).

DRUG-INDUCED COMA

Drug-induced coma is most commonly caused by the direct effects of overdosage of centrally acting drugs taken as self-poisoning. At least 10% of acute medical admissions to hospital result from such self-poisonings, and this syndrome is particularly common between the ages of 15 and 55 years. Hypnotics, sedatives, antidepressants, analgesics and alcohol, alone or in combination, are the drugs most frequently chosen. Fortunately, the use of barbiturates in self-poisoning is decreasing and this, together with improving intensive care management, is reducing the mortality of drug-induced coma.

Although most cases of drug-induced coma are caused by the direct c.n.s. effects of the agents taken, it must be remembered that in some instances coma may develop indirectly: thus accidental hypoglycaemia due to drugs or insulin in diabetic patients may result in coma, as may delayed hepatic coma as a result of paracetamol poisoning.

Clinical features of drug-induced coma

The diagnosis of drug-induced coma is often self evident; however, certain clinical features of drug-induced coma may be helpful in diagnosis, and have important implications for the management of patients in coma generally (see p. 136). Drugs very commonly impair brain-stem ocular reflexes at an early stage: thus sedatives, barbiturates, anticonvulsants and tricyclic drugs cause early depression of oculocephalic (doll's head) and oculovestibular (caloric) reflexes; the corneal and pupillary reflexes are, however, less inhibited, and the finding of preservation of these reflexes with reduced oculocephalic and oculovestibular reflexes should always suggest the possibility of drug-induced coma. In most cases of drug-induced coma the pupils tend to be small but reacting; they may be characteristically pinpoint in opiate poisoning. Myoclonic jerking and convulsions may accompany coma due to tricyclic drugs.

Whereas in other causes of coma, depression of oculocephalic and oculovestibular reflexes suggests a poor prognosis, this does not apply to drug-induced coma: for this reason brain-stem death should never be diagnosed in patients in whom drug overdosage is suspected.

A variety of other signs may suggest drug-induced coma: these include hyperventilation in response to metabolic acidosis in salicylate poisoning, and the presence of venepuncture scars.

The prognosis of drug-induced coma is largely dependent on complications such as respiratory and cardiovascular depression, which may secondarily result in cerebral hypoxia and long-term sequelae. Where these complications can be avoided, full recovery from drug-induced coma is the rule.

DRUG-INDUCED SEIZURES

A wide spectrum of drugs may cause seizures in man, some of which are noted in Table 17.1. Two major mechanisms are involved: there may be specific c.n.s. excitatory effects, or non-selective effects resulting from very high doses of drugs often administered during self poisoning. The incidence of drug-induced convulsions is uncertain: in one series they were noted in approximately 0.1% of over 12 000 hospital inpatients, and were most commonly seen with penicillin, hypoglycaemic agents, lignocaine and phenothiazines.

High c.n.s. concentrations of drugs are important in the aetiology of seizures and particular care must be exercised when drugs are administered parenterally or intrathecally. Patients with renal or hepatic failure causing impaired drug metabolism are also at risk and, certainly, other coexisting metabolic disease may predispose patients to drug-induced seizures; patients with a previous history of epilepsy also seem to be at particular risk.

Drug-induced seizures usually take the form of tonic-clonic seizures, which may be preceded by multifocal myoclonus; they are rarely partial. When partial seizures occur, this may suggest factors other than drug-induced seizures, although occasionally patients with pre-existing cerebral disorders may have focal components of seizures due to drugs.

Table 17.1 Drugs associated with seizures

Anaesthetics	Antibiotics	Antipsychotic agents
Ether	Benzylpenicillin	Chlorpromazine
Halothane	Carbenicillin	Lithium
Ketamine	Oxacillin	
Methohexitone	Ampicillin	Radiographic contrast media
Propanidid	Cycloserine	Meglumine carbamate
Althesin	Isoniazid	Meglumine iothalamate
	Nalidixic acid	Metrizamide
Analeptics		
Nikethamide	Anticonvulsants (in overdosage)	Miscellaneous
Aminophylline	Phenobarbitone	D-Penicillamine
Amphetamines	Phenytoin	Baclofen
Ephedrine	Ethosuximide	Hyperbaric oxygen
		Folate
Anlgesics	Antidepressants	Piperazine
Cocaine	Amitryptiline	Cyclosporin
Pethidine	Imipramine	
Dextropropoxyphene	Mianserin	
	Maprotiline	
Antidysrhythmics		
Disopyramide		
Lignocaine		

A wide range of drugs have been associated with convulsions, over 70 having been reported to the Committee on the Safety of Medicines (CSM).

Antibiotics

Penicillin is a potent epileptogenic substance in animals, probably because of its GABA antagonist properties. In man, seizures may be caused by c.s.f. concentrations of over 10 units/ml, necessitating care when high-dose penicillin is administered intravenously or intrathecally. It is unwise to administer more than 10 000 units intrathecally in a single dose. Benzylpenicillin is probably the most potent antibiotic in causing seizures, followed by ampicillin and cephalothin. Isoniazid may cause seizures because of its action in antagonising the action of pyridoxine.

Psychotropic drugs

The mechanisms by which psychotropic drugs cause seizures remain uncertain, but may involve their effects on monoamine neurotransmitters. All antipsychotic drugs must be regarded as potentially epileptogenic: seizures may occur in up to 1% of patients treated with such drugs and patients with organic brain disease seem particularly susceptible; *chlorpromazine* is the drug most commonly implicated.

Overdosage with *tricyclic antidepressants* is frequently associated with myoclonus and tonic-clonic seizures; imipramine and amitriptyline have been most commonly implicated. Patients with a family history of epilepsy or organic brain disease, or those who have had previous electroconvulsive therapy, may be most at risk. Newer agents, such as mianserin and maprotiline, may also carry relatively high risks of seizures.

Anaesthetic agents

C.n.s. excitation was recognised in classic descriptions of stage I and II anaesthesia with ether; similarly, a variety of newer drugs, including ketamine, halothane, althesin and enfluorane, may have excitatory properties; patients with epilepsy appear to be particularly at risk.

Withdrawal seizures

Seizures commonly occur as part of withdrawal syndromes seen in patients abusing alcohol, barbiturates, benzodiazepines, and meprobamate. Withdrawal from alcohol causes increased excitation beginning 12–24 hours after the cessation of drinking. The EEG starts to become abnormal at this time, with overt photosensitivity lasting for up to 72 hours; during this time tonic clonic seizures and myoclonus may occur. Similar mechanisms probably occur with barbiturate withdrawal.

Radiographic contrast material

All aqueous iodinated contrast media are potentially epileptogenic. The risk of seizures is greatest following intrathecal administration for myelography or cisternography. *Dimer-X* radiculography was associated with a risk of between 0.5% and 7%. *Metrizamide* is probably safer, with only three observed convulsions during 100 000 lumbar myelograms; however, myoclonus is more frequent. The risk of seizures seems to increase when aqueous contrast media are used in the cervical region or for positive contrast cisternography. After all procedures involving the intrathecal injection of aqueous contrast the patient should be nursed sitting erect for at least eight hours.

PYRAMIDAL DISORDERS

Upper motor neurone dysfunction is very uncommon in iatrogenic drug disorders. Pyramidal signs may be apparent in drug-induced coma as they may be in many encephalopathies. There is now, however, evidence that rapid correction of hyponatraemia may be an important cause of central pontine myelinolysis (see Alcohol, p. 435) and its resultant quadriplegia.

DRUG-INDUCED EXTRAPYRAMIDAL DISORDERS

Drugs may cause a wide range of movement disorders, including tremor, chorea, dystonia and myoclonus. The most important group of drugs implicated are those which have direct actions on central dopamine receptors.

Disorders due to dopamine receptor antagonists

Five major syndromes may be associated with treatment with antipsychotic drugs. It seems likely that all drugs with dopamine receptor antagonist properties are capable of causing these syndromes, and that their potency in doing so is directly related to their antipsychotic potency.

Acute dystonias

Acute dystonias are seen in children and young adults. They appear to arise as acute idiosyncratic reactions to relatively small doses of either antipsychotics, e.g. chlorpromazine, or antiemetic drugs with dopamine receptor antagonist properties, e.g. metoclopramide. Movements most commonly affect the face, mouth and head: acute *retrocollis* or *torticollis, trismus* and *oculogyric crises* may occur; axial and limb dystonias are less commonly seen. Clinicians should suspect that drugs are implicated when such unusual movement disorders are seen in young people. In some instances drug-induced acute dystonia can be confused with tetanus!

Although attacks are self-limiting, they tend to recur when patients are rechallenged with the drug or with other drugs with similar properties. Attacks are usually responsive to intravenous anticholinergic agents, e.g. benztropine.

Drug-induced parkinsonism

A considerable proportion of patients undergoing chronic antipsychotic therapy show some features of drug-induced parkinsonism: this is manifest usually by akinesia and rigidity; tremor is rarely a prominent feature. The disorder is reversible if the offending agent can be withdrawn, but anticholinergic drugs may be of some value if this is not possible.

Akathisia

This troublesome sensation of motor restlessness and discomfort can occur in Parkinson's disease and in drug treatment with antipsychotic agents. It is perhaps most frequently seen in patients who exhibit other features of drug-induced parkinsonism.

Tardive dyskinesia

These movement disorders occur as complications of long-term antipsychotic therapy. The incidence

of colour vision as part of an acute toxicity syndrome.

Optic neuropathy

Optic neuropathy, sometimes simulating retrobulbar neuritis, may occur as a result of treatment with antituberculous drugs, e.g. ethambutol and, less commonly, rifampicin and other antibiotics, e.g. chloramphenicol. Optic neuropathy was also part of the SMON (subacute myelo-optic neuropathy) syndrome related to clioquinol therapy.

Disorders of the posterior visual pathways

The occipital cortex is at risk from hypoperfusion as one of the watershed areas: thus, patients recovering from overdosage, particularly with barbiturates, may have cortical blindness.

DRUG-INDUCED OTOTOXICITY

Many drugs posess ototoxic properties (Table 17.2). Some, when given in high dosage, may result in ionic changes within the cochlea and semicircular canals, which changes are subsequently reversible: patients with renal or hepatic failure may be particularly at risk. Other drugs, particularly antibiotics, cause irreversible degeneration of specialised receptors. Otoxicity is seen with large doses of 'loop' diuretics, causing tinnitus and sometimes persisting deafness. *Aminoglycosides*, such as streptomycin, gentamicin or tobramycin, have predominant effects on the semicircular canals, resulting in vertigo and ataxia. Neomycin and kanamycin are more likely to give rise to cochlear symptoms of deafness.

Table 17.2 Drugs associated with ototoxicity

Antibiotics	Antimalarials	Miscellaneous
Streptomycin	Chloroquine	Aspirin
Gentamycin	Quinine	Ibuprofen
Neomycin		Indomethacin
Kanamycin	Diuretics	Propanolol
Tobramycin	Frusemide	Quinidine
Vancomycin	Bumetanide	
Ampicillin	Ethacrynic acid	
Chloramphenicol		
Erythromycin		

DRUG-INDUCED CEREBELLAR DISTURBANCE

Anticonvulsant drugs, including barbiturates, phenytoin and carbamazepine, all give rise to a dose-related (and serum-level-related) ataxia, which is frequently associated with dysarthria and nystagmus. Other *sedative drugs*, including benzodiazepines and antipsychotic drugs, can cause similar changes.

Phenytoin may also cause chronic toxicity with cerebellar atrophy. Lithium can cause a chronic cerebellar syndrome persisting after intoxication. Ataxia has also been recorded with nitrofurantoin, which has a similar structure to phenytoin, and with piperazine, which is used in the treatment of threadworm infections.

It should be noted that the symptoms and signs of Wernicke's encephalopathy, whatever its cause, can be exacerbated by dextrose infusions which increase the requirements for thiamine.

DRUG-INDUCED AUTONOMIC DISTURBANCE

Symptoms of postural hvpotension and syncope may occur with a wide variety of drugs, the pharmacology of which affects function of the peripheral and central autonomic system. Anticholinesterase drugs, trinitrin, antihypertensive drugs, monoamine oxidase inhibitors and tricyclic antidepressants may all be involved.

Atropine, benzhexol and propantheline may all cause urinary retention, as may monoamine oxidase inhibitors and tricyclic antidepressants. On occasions prazosin, disopyramide and phenothiazines may predispose to urinary incontinence.

Impotence may occur with treatment with antihypertensive drugs such as clonidine, guanethidine and methyldopa.

DRUG-INDUCED NEUROPATHIES

Over 50 drugs have been proved to cause, or have been associated with, peripheral neuropathy (Table 17.3). For this reason a careful drug

Table 17.3 Drugs associated with neuropathy

	Sensory	Sensorimotor	Motor	Localised
Antibiotics	Ethionamide Chloramphenicol	Nitrofurantoin Ethambutol Isoniazid Streptomycin Ethionamide Metronidazole	Sulphonamides Dapsone Amphotericin B	Penicillin Amphotericin B
Anticonvulsants	Sulthiame	Phenytoin		
Antirheumatics		Indomethacin Phenylbutazone Penicillamine Colchicine Gold Chloroquine		
Cytotoxics	Procarbazine	Vincristine Cytarabine Chlorambucil		Mustine
Cardiovascular drugs	Propanolol	Perhexiline Hydrallazine Amiodarone Disopyramide Clofibrate		
Others	Ergotamine Methysergide	Chlorpropamide Tolbutamide Disulfiram Thalidomide Methaqualone Glutethimide	Imipramine Amitriptyline	Anticoagulants Amphetamines

history is of great importance in the diagnosis of all patients presenting with symptoms of peripheral neuropathy. The incidence with any particular drug is variable: some drugs, such as vinca alkaloids, are likely to cause neuropathy in the majority of patients treated with them; even here, however, patients with lymphoma may be more at risk than patients with non-lymphoid neoplasia; for other drugs, neuropathy may be a very rare complication. Genetic predisposition may have a role: thus, slow acetylators of isoniazid are at greater risk of peripheral neuropathy, and patients with renal or hepatic dysfunction may be at greatest risk from neuropathies caused by drugs such as nitrofurantoin and other antibiotics. Patients with underlying disorders such as diabetes, alcoholism and malabsorption, may be also more at risk from drug-induced neuropathy.

The pathology of drug-induced neuropathies that have been adequately studied is almost always that of *axonal degeneration*. Notable exceptions are perhexiline and amiodarone neuropathy, which appear to be relatively pure *demyelinating neuropathies*. Very occasionally, drugs may cause localised damage to peripheral nerves or plexus: this may occur following arterial infusions of cytoxic agents, and occasionally neuralgic amyotrophy syndromes may be seen following both immunisations and injections of penicillin.

Sensory, sensorimotor and relatively pure motor neuropathies may all be seen in association with various drugs. As Table 17.3 shows, it is rarely possible to say that specific drugs will produce specific clinical syndromes of neuropathy. However, on occasion, associations of neurological dysfunction may be helpful: thus autonomic dysfunction is particularly prominent with vincristine neuropathy; chloramphenicol neuropathy is almost always accompanied by a retrobulbar neuritis syndrome, as is the neuropathy of ethambutol.

The main importance of the recognition of drug-induced neuropathy is that it should lead to the prompt withdrawal of the responsible drug whenever clinically possible; where this is done the prognosis for recovery is excellent.

DRUG-INDUCED DISORDERS OF NEUROMUSCULAR TRANSMISSION

Although many drugs may interfere with neuromuscular transmission under experimental conditions, this is rarely of major clinical importance because of the high safety factor for transmission that exists under normal circumstances. Drug-induced disturbance of neuromuscular transmission may occur in three clinical settings:

1. A number of drugs may cause prolonged postoperative respiratory depression in patients who have been 'curarised'. This may occur with aminoglycoside antibiotics and lignocaine.
2. A presumed latent myasthenia gravis may be unmasked, or concurrent drug therapy may aggravate myasthenia.
3. Some drugs may produce a clinical syndrome of myasthenia in otherwise normal individuals.

Drugs capable of producing these three clinical problems are listed in Table 17.4.

Varying mechanisms of interference in neuromuscular transmission are important. Some drugs posessing local anaesthetic membrane activity (chloroquine, lincomycin) may inhibit transmitter release; others, such as polymyxins and procainamide, may have postsynaptic receptor blocking action; some drugs such as phenytoin, chlorpromazine and aminoglycoside antibiotics, may posess both these functions; very occasionally, drugs may cause symptoms of myasthenia by immunologically mediated mechanisms. Thus, treatment with D-penicillamine for rheumatoid arthritis, and sometimes for Wilson's disease and primary biliary cirrhosis, can lead to a syndrome of myasthenia gravis with circulating anticholinesterase receptor antibodies.

The management of drug-induced disorders of neuromuscular tranmission will depend very much upon the clinical setting. Prolonged postoperative respiratory depression may be managed with ventilatory support. In some instances intravenous administration of calcium glutamate may be helpful. Alternatively, neostigmine may be used to counter postsynaptic components of neuromuscular blockade. In D-penicillamine-induced myasthenia, a period of treatment with conventional oral anticholinesterase inhibitor drugs may be necessary.

Table 17.4 Clinical presentations of drug-induced neuromuscular blockade

	Postoperative respiratory depression	Exacerbation of existing myasthenia	Myasthenia-like syndromes
Antibiotics	Aminoglycosides Clindamycin Lincomycin	Aminoglycosides Tetracyclines	Aminoglycosides
Cardiovascular drugs	Lignocaine Quinidine	Procainamide Propranolol Quinidine	Oxyprenolol Practolol
Antirheumatic drugs	Chloroquine		Penicillamine
Psychotropic drugs	Lithium Promazine	Chlorpromazine Lithium	
Anticonvulsants		Phenytoin	Phenytoin Troxidone
Hormones		ACTH Steroids Thyroid hormones	

DRUG-INDUCED MYOPATHY

Five major clinical syndromes of drug-induced muscle disorder and the drugs associated with them are summarised in Table 17.5.

Acute rhabdomyolysis is fortunately uncommon, but results in severe muscle pain, fulminating weakness and muscle tenderness, swelling and oedema. Gross elevation of serum muscle enzymes occurs and there may be myoglobinuria and complicating renal failure. Hyperkalaemia may also occur, giving rise to cardiac dysrrhythmia.

Acute and subacute *painful proximal myopathy* is more common and presents with muscle pain, tenderness and stiffness in a proximal and symmetrical distribution. The syndrome may occur by differing mechanisms. It may result from a necrotising myopathy similar to, although less severe than, that of acute rhabdomyolysis: this syndrome is seen with clofibrate, epsilon-amino-caproic acid and emetine. An inflammatory poly-myositis may also cause this clinical syndrome, usually as part of a drug-induced SLE: D-penicillamine, hydralazine and phenytoin have been implicated in this mechanism. Finally, drug-induced hypokalaemia may occur with diuretics, liquorice and carbenoxalone; this may be distinguishable, however, in that the disorder tends to fluctuate and in some instances may produce frank periodic weakness.

Subacute or chronic *painless myopathy* is usually seen with steroid drugs, particularly fluorinated derivatives, e.g. triamcinolone and betamethasone. The incidence of this myopathy is frequently underestimated and major problems arise because of the necessity of giving some patients with polymyositis large doses of steroids over prolonged periods. Chloroquine causes a clinically similar painless myopathy but this may also cause neuropathy and electrical evidence of myotonia.

A number of drugs including chloroquine, epsilon-aminocaproic acid and some beta blockers can cause or unmask *myotonia*; however, this is rarely of clinical importance.

Focal muscle necrosis may be caused by a variety of intramuscular injections. Occasionally, localised fibrosis and contracture may result, particularly in drug addicts.

Malignant hyperpyrexia is a genetically determined syndrome in which a variety of anaesthetic agents, particularly a combination of halothane and succinylcholine, provoke a syndrome of muscle rigidity, hyperpyrexia and sweating. The syndrome can occur in patients with Duchenne dystrophy, myotonia congenita and central core myopathy. However, its major clinical importance is its occurrence as an autosomal dominant susceptibility in patients who are otherwise clinically normal or have only a very mild asymptomatic myopathy.

DRUG ABUSE SYNDROMES

There is an increasing prevalence of drug abuse in modern society. Drugs which are abused share a number of common properties: they usually have direct c.n.s. effects, which show the development of tolerance, habituation and physical addiction. The recognition of drug-abuse syndromes is important in two main clinical contexts: drug abuse should be considered first in patients presenting with unexplained episodes of altered consciousness or behaviour; secondly, patients

Table 17.5 Drug-induced myopathy

Acute rhabdomyolysis	Acute/subacute painful myopathy			Subacute/chronic painless myopathy	Focal necrosis/fibrosis	Malignant hyperpyrexia
	Necrotising	*Hypokalaemic*	*Inflammatory*			
Alcohol Heroin Barbiturates Phencyclidine Epsilon-amino caproic acid	Clofibrate Epsilon-amino caproic acid Emetine Vincristine Beta-blockers	Diuretics Liquorice Carbenoxalone Amphotericin B	D-Penicillamine Hydrallazine Procainamide Phenytoin	Corticosteroids Chloroquine	Antibiotics Opiates Chlorpromazine	Inhalational anaesthetics (particularly halothane + succinyl choline

who are chronic drug abusers are at risk of a number of unusual neurological complications.

ALCOHOL

A classification of alcoholic neurological syndromes is presented in Table 17.6 and also discussed in Chapter 18.

Acute alcoholic intoxication

The acute administration of alcohol has a number of generalised effects including tachycardia, a rise in blood pressure, vasodilatation, sweating and diuresis. In the relatively naive subject blood levels up to 50 mg/100 ml result in euphoria and mild incoordination; at approximately 100 mg/100 ml ataxia and dysarthria become evident; at 200 mg/100 ml frank confusion may be present, and by approximately 300 mg/100 ml individuals become stuporose and subsequently may, at higher concentrations, exhibit deep anaesthesia and respiratory depression. However, chronic users of alcohol will tolerate much higher blood levels of alcohol with fewer neurological effects.

Alcohol-withdrawal syndrome

The three major neurological components—tremor, confusional state (often associated with hallucination) and seizures—are usually associated, but may occur independently. They are also usually accompanied by some systemic disturbances, including vasodilatation, tachycardia, anorexia, nausea and vomiting.

Tremor is of a relatively rapid frequency, and tends to be present throughout movement, but is suppressed when the patient lies quietly. It does not have any specific intention element. The tremor usually reaches a peak 24–36 hours after the cessation of drinking and is promptly aborted by further alcohol; however, with continued abstinence the tremor usually resolves over a period of 7–10 days.

A variety of *hallucinations* are described as part of the withdrawal syndrome: they may be visual, auditory or occasionally tactile. It is doubtful whether the often-described animal or insect hallucinations are in any way specific to the alcohol-withdrawal syndrome.

Withdrawal seizures most commonly occur between 24 and 48 hours after the cessation of drinking. During this period the EEG develops generalised paroxysmal discharges and becomes abnormally photosensitive. Seizures are of a tonic-clonic type and status may occur. It is important to suspect alcohol withdrawal in young and middle-aged adults developing apparently primary tonic-clonic seizures.

When all these features are present a highly characteristic syndrome of *delirium tremens* results: this consists of severe autonomic overactivity with dilated pupils, pyrexia, tachycardia and sweating with tremor, restlessness and acute delirium with frank hallucinosis. The syndrome is frequently seen in patients admitted to hospital as a result of injuries or acute infections. The treatment consists of full investigation and treatment of any associated disorders, e.g. pneumonia, the maintenance of adequate hydration, high-dose multivitamin therapy, and an adequate sedation produced by an anticonvulsant agent, e.g. diazepam or chlormethiazole.

Table 17.6 Neurological complications of alcoholism

Acute intoxication
Withdrawal syndrome
Nutritional complications
Wernicke–Korsakoff syndrome
Neuropathy
Tobacco–alcohol amblyopia
Hepatic complications
Acute hepatic encephalopathy
Chronic portosystemic encephalopathy
Miscellaneous
Cerebellar degeneration
Dementia/brain atrophy
Central pontine myelinolysis
Marchiafava–Bignami syndrome

Nutritional disorders secondary to alcoholism

(see p. 469)

Wernicke's encephalopathy due to thiamine deficiency is the most striking neurological syndrome of nutritional origin associated with alcoholism. The syndrome, comprising a clinical triad of ataxia, oculomotor palsies and a confusional state, is fully described in Chapter 18.

Alcoholic neuropathy is similar in most respects to that of beri-beri, and probably shares a similar nutritional basis. It is a symmetrical sensorimotor axonal neuropathy, but varies in severity from being virtually asymptomatic, through mainly sensory neuropathies, which are painful and often accompanied by burning dysaesthesiae and hyperpathia, to more acute syndromes in which there is considerable motor weakness affecting proximal as well as distal muscles. Recovery occurs slowly with multiple vitamin therapy, and is again variable in its completeness.

Optic atrophy is occasionally seen in alcoholics. It is similar to nutritional amblyopia seen in Second World War prisoners in the Far East. Deficiencies of a variety of B group vitamins may be involved in both these syndromes, and tobacco smoke may exacerbate this by chronic cyanide poisoning. 'Tobacco–alcohol' amblyopia may thus have multiple causes.

Other syndromes associated with alcoholism

A number of other neurological syndromes have been found to be particularly prevalent in alcoholics.

There is a higher-than-expected incidence of presenile and senile *dementia* in alcoholic patients; this is associated with a demonstrable atrophy on CT scanning, which to some degree may be reversible. The mechanisms producing dementia are poorly understood, and the dementia of alcoholism has no specific features to differentiate it from other causes of dementia.

Alcoholic cerebellar degeneration evolves subacutely or chronically in predominantly male alcoholics. It is characterised by truncal and gait ataxia: there is incoordination of the lower limbs with relatively little involvement of the upper limbs; nystagmus and dysarthria are rare. The relationship of this syndrome to Wernicke's encephalopathy is debatable. Although some patients with the condition do improve with thiamine therapy, and the clinical features of the ataxia may be indistinguishable from that of Wernicke's encephalopathy, pathologically Purkinje cell loss may be prominent, differentiating this from Wernicke's. The precise aetiology remains uncertain.

Central pontine myelinolysis is rare and almost always seen with chronic alcoholism. It may, however, occur in disseminated malignant disease, severe bacterial infection, and renal and hepatic failure.

It is an acute syndrome, with the development of quadriplegia and pseudobulbar palsy, sometimes with associated abnormalities of eye movements. Some patients show a locked-in syndrome. Pathologically, there is a gross demyelinating lesion of the ventral pons. Some cases have been associated with gross hyponatraemia, or may even be caused by rapid correction of hyponatraemia. The prognosis for this condition is extremely poor and survival is rare; treatment with thiamine or other high-dose vitamins does not appear to influence the outcome.

Marchiafava–Bignami syndrome is a pathological diagnosis, originally described in Italian chianti drinkers, and is characterised by demyelinating lesions in the corpus callosum. No specific neurological syndrome can be related to this, the majority of patients presenting with a dementia, sometimes with fits, with progressive decline to stupor and coma.

Alcoholic myopathy may present with acute painful proximal wasting and weakness, particularly of the lower limbs. Some of this group of patients do appear to have primary muscle damage and may even show a fulminant rhabdomyolysis; however, other subjects with less severe symptoms can show evidence of acute denervation of proximal muscles, suggesting a neuropathic origin of their symptoms.

BARBITURATE ABUSE

Acute barbiturate intoxication represents one of the most dangerous forms of self poisoning. Following ingestion of high doses of barbiturates there may be marked respiratory depression and hypotension, as well as signs of intoxication ranging through cerebellar disturbance, nystagmus and diplopia to coma.

Chronic barbiturate intoxication is becoming less common. Because of the rapid development of tolerance, increasing doses of barbiturates must be ingested in order to achieve an anxiolytic effect. Sudden withdrawal results in disturbances which can closely mimic delirium tremens: for this reason, withdrawal from barbiturate drugs should always be undertaken in a gradual stepwise fashion.

OPIATE ABUSE

Acute opiate intoxication results in varying degrees of depression of consciousness, usually with respiratory depression with a low respiratory rate and low tidal volume. Bradycardia and hypothermia are common and the pupils are characteristically pinpoint. Many of these effects can be reversed rapidly by the intravenous administration of naloxone, a specific opiate antagonist. However, the drug may have to be used with caution in opiate addicts because it may precipitate a typical acute withdrawal syndrome, consisting of confusion, delirium, tremor and seizures, with associated profound autonomic overactivity (salivation, piloerection, tachycardia, lability of blood pressure and vomiting).

As opiate addicts commonly use an intravenous route of administration, a wide variety of neurological syndromes are seen (Table 17.7). Many of these complications may be related to the inadvertent injection of impurities, leading to a *drug-induced arteritis*: the most commonly seen are acute transverse myelitis, acute brachial and lumbosacral plexus neuropathies (very similar to neuralgic amyotrophy), acute mononeuropathies or mononeuritis multiplex; an acute rhabdomyolysis syndrome may also be seen.

Table 17.7 Neurological complications of opiate abuse

Acute intoxication
Withdrawal syndrome
Transverse myelitis
Cranial nerve disorders
Nerve deafness
Quinine amblyopia
Peripheral nerve lesions
Painful plexus syndromes
Traumatic/atraumatic mononeuropathy
Acute/subacute diffuse neuropathy
Muscle disorders
Acute rhabdomyolysis
Chronic myopathy
Complications of infection
Cerebral abscess
Mycotic aneurysm
Tuberculous meningitis/tuberculoma

TOXINS

A wide variety of industrial chemicals may have toxic effects on the central and peripheral nervous system. Symptoms may develop because of accidental industrial exposure, or because of abuse or, very occasionally, as a result of self poisoning.

ORGANIC CHEMICALS

Organophosphates

Widely used as insecticides, plasticisers and in lubricants, organophosphates share a common property of being acetylcholine esterase inhibitors.

Acute intoxication leads to muscarinic effects with pupillary constriction, rhinorrhoea and bronchial constriction due to local absorption by inhalation. Bradycardia and hypotension may occur. The neurological effects initially result in involuntary twitching, fasciculation and cramp. Nicotinic effects can cause weakness, and paralysis may occur because of depolarisation block. C.n.s. effects include restlessness, tremor and confusion, sometimes with ataxia; convulsions may occur. These acute effects of organophosphates may be counteracted by the use of atropine and by the use of specific anticholinesterase reactivators.

Patients surviving acute intoxication may develop axonal neuropathy. The compound most commonly implicated is triorthocresyl phosphate. This degreasing agent has caused epidemics of a mainly motor neuropathy due to accidental contamination of cooking oil.

Organochlorines

Organochlorines have become widely used as insecticides. DDT is the original compound in this group, but a host of derivative compounds are used and possess similar neurotoxic properties. They may be absorbed by cutaneous, respiratory and GI routes. They produce a syndrome of tremor, myoclonus, opsoclonus and seizures; in addition there may be mental change with anxiety, irritability and ataxia. They do not appear to cause neuropathy.

A variety of hexocarbon *solvents* used in the production of glues and paint thinners are neurotoxic. These include *n*-hexane and toluene, but these are rarely used alone and are usually mixed with other solvents for industrial use. Neurotoxicity due to industrial exposure is rare, but these compounds are increasingly abused for their euphoriant and intoxicating affects in glue sniffing.

The most commonly reported problem is one of a slowly progressive axonal sensorimotor neuropathy. On occasions more fulminant cases may show more profound motor disturbance and weakness; such cases may develop subacutely and present a picture with slowed motor conduction and demyelinating neuropathy which may closely mimic the Guillain–Barré syndrome. Chronic exposure may result in mental change, tremor, ataxia and seizures.

Sensorimotor neuropathies may also be seen following exposure to acrylamide and carbon disulphide. The latter compound may also produce central effects with mood change and psychotic disturbance.

HEAVY METAL TOXICITY

Many heavy metals are neurotoxic. The diagnosis of toxicity can be confirmed by estimation of serum and urine concentrations, but analysis of hair and nail clippings may be of particular value, because the metals become concentrated therein.

Lead

Organic and inorganic lead may cause acute, subacute or chronic central or peripheral neurotoxicity. Children appear to be particularly at risk from lead encephalopathy. This leads to delayed psychomotor development, lethargy, ataxia and seizures. Severe cases may also exhibit headache and papilloedema, possibly due to raised intracranial pressure secondary to brain swelling.

The peripheral neuropathy of lead toxicity is a pure motor neuropathy which most commonly causes wrist drop and foot drop. Associated systemic disturbances of lead poisoning include anaemia, renal disease and increased radiological bone density, particularly of the skull. Lead toxicity may be treated with chelating agents, e.g. diamine tetracetate.

Mercury

The neurotoxicity of mercury differs, depending on whether exposure is to organic mercurial compounds or to inorganic mercury. The most severe disturbances are seen with methyl mercury compounds, which cause a subacute syndrome (Minamata disease). After a latent period, symptoms start with paraesthesiae, visual field restriction, severe cerebellar disturbance and deafness.

A more chronic syndrome is due to toxicity with inorganic mercury, which represents a largely historical occupational disorder of miners, hatters and workers in thermometer factories. There is mental change, of gradual onset and sometimes with frank hallucinations, which becomes associated with tremor of the hands, eyelid and tongue. Subsequently, frank cerebellar intention tremor may become evident, with titubation (hatter's shakes) and, in severe cases, a wide variety of severe involuntary movement disorders may occur. There may be evidence of optic neuropathy with constricted visual fields.

Arsenic

Arsenical poisoning may arise from accidental contamination of foodstuffs and beverages. Intake usually results in nausea and vomiting. Mees' lines (pigment lines across the nail bed) appear on the nails subsequently, and there may be hyperkeratosis of the feet and palms. Patients may develop acute, subacute or chronic neuropathy, depending on the dosage and time course of exposure. Neuropathy is symmetrical and sensorimotor, although in more acute cases there may be clinical changes similar to a Guillain–Barré syndrome.

Manganese

Manganese poisoning is a largely occupational disease of those involved in mining and smelting. It causes central neurotoxicity, with the early development of mental change with agitation and psychotic behaviour. Patients become emotionally labile and may develop marked extrapyramidal disturbance with increasing rigidity, involuntary movement disorders, dysarthria and tremor. In addition to treatment with chelating agents, the parkinsonian features of manganese poisoning may be responsive to L-dopa.

Thallium

Thallium salts have been used in rodent control and in cosmetic agents. Ingestion of large doses cause major gastrointestinal symptoms, which are followed after a brief latent period by the development of a painful neuropathy. Cranial nerves may be involved and an optic neuritis can occur. Central effects are less prominent with occasional choreic movements, confusion and psychosis. Mees' lines may appear on the nails, as in arsenic intoxication. The diagnosis of thallium intoxication is particularly suggested by loss of head and body hair.

BIOLOGICAL TOXINS

A number of toxins produced by plants, fungi, snakes, shellfish and fish all have important neuropharmacological properties. The resultant syndromes are rare but are summarised in Table 17.8.

The mechanisms of toxicity vary, some producing encephalopathy, others autonomic disturbance and some interference with nerve conduction and neuromuscular transmission.

Management is largely directed to supportive measures, particularly ventilation in patients with muscular paralysis. Specific treatments are mentioned in Table 17.8.

Table 17.8 Biological toxins

Syndrome	Causative agent	Clinical factors	Treatment
Ergotism	Rye fungus	Gangrene Convulsions and myoclonus Areflexia and ataxia	
Mushroom poisoning	*Amanita muscaria*	Parasympathetic stimulation Sweating, bradycardia, low BP Seizures, tremor, delirium	Atropine
	Amanita phalloides	Confusion, seizures, coma Cardiovascular collapse	
Lathyrism	Chickpea and common vetch	Pain and paraesthesiae Lower limb weakness Spastic paraparesis	
Snake poisoning	Viperidae	Haemorrhagic complications Rare ptosis and ophthalmoplegia	Antivenom
	Elapidae (cobras, etc)	Haemorrhagic complications Coma & seizures Neuromuscular blockade	Antivenom
Shellfish poisoning	Mussels, clams, etc. (saxitoxin)	Paralysis (blocking of muscle action potentials and nerve conduction)	
Fish poisoning	Puffer fish (tetrodotoxin)	Paraesthesiae Pallor, sweating, low BP Bulbar paralysis Areflexia	

NEUROLOGICAL DISEASE DUE TO PHYSICAL AGENTS

RADIATION

Radiotherapy may be complicated by a number of neurological disturbances: these are related to total dose and the period over which this is given. Early symptoms are common and may relate to localised swelling and oedema: for this reason, high-dose steroids are frequently employed where the brain or spinal cord are involved. More troublesome are symptoms arising from delayed necrosis, which particularly affects white matter, and the occurrence of which may simulate tumour recurrence.

Cerebral hemisphere delayed necrosis may occur after treatment of primary or secondary cerebral tumours and, in the past, following scalp irradiation; the latent period may vary from 6 months to several years. The upper limit of the tolerated dose for cerebral fields is probably of the order of 4000 ± 1000 rad fractionated over a period of 30–35 days. The tolerance in children may be lower by a factor of about 75%. Initial symptoms are commonly focal seizures followed by a progressive and localised disturbance, including hemianopia, aphasia and hemiparesis. Frequently there are signs and symptoms of a mass lesion which may prompt surgical exploration to exclude tumour recurrence. Fields which involve the pituitary and hypophyseal regions may occasionally cause acute disturbances, including pituitary apoplexy. A late complication of pituitary irradiation may be arterial damage leading to carotid stroke syndromes.

The *brain stem* seems particularly at risk from delayed radionecrosis. This disorder has been documented following irradiation for carcinomas of the middle ear, nasopharynx and carotid regions. Symptoms frequently develop earlier than those following hemisphere irradiation, with a latent period of 2–6 months. The progression of the disorder is usually rapid and the prognosis bleak.

The *spinal cord* is at particular risk from delayed radionecrosis and may be involved in the field of radiotherapy for a wide variety of tumours, including lymphoma and bronchogenic carcinoma. Latency between treatment and the development of symptoms may be between 6 months and 4 years. Early symptoms are usually sensory with paraesthesiae, pain and occasionally Lhermitte's phenomenon. Progress is usually relentless, with developing motor weakness and loss of sphincter control. It seems that patients receiving a dose to the spinal cord of more than 2500 rad are at risk, especially when the dose is given over a period of less than 14 days.

Brachial and lumbosacral plexus disorders may also follow radiotherapy, the latent period being from 6 months up to several years. Higher doses of 5000–6000 rad are usually implicated. Symptoms begin with pain and sensory loss in an appropriate distribution, with the subsequent development of motor disturbance. This syndrome is often confused with tumour recurrence, and difficulty in investigating lumbar and brachial plexus regions usually prolongs this confusion.

ELECTRICAL INJURY

Electrical injury may occur either from lightning stroke, or as a result of domestic or industrial accidents. Such exposure is often fatal, but surviving subjects may suffer from a number of neurological problems. Their nature will largely be determined by the pathway taken by the electrical current; in addition, electrical injury is also particularly liable to cause psychological and psychiatric disturbance.

With *lightning stroke*, the point of entry is usually at the head. This often results in instantaneous death, with severe cerebral damage. Those surviving frequently have a prolonged period of coma, with subsequent periods of confusion. A variety of permanent deficits have been noted: these include intellectual disturbance and psychosis, extrapyramidal features and, more rarely, hemipareses or aphasia. Hydrocephalus may occur as a late complication, as frequently these injuries are complicated by subarachnoid haemorrhage.

Entry of lightning at points other than the head is rare: when it occurs there may still be transient loss of consciousness, even when the head does not lie on the direct pathway of the electrical current. There is often immediate brief sensory and motor paralysis, and vasomotor disturbances affecting various parts of the body are a marked feature. A rare later complication is bilateral progressive lower motor neurone disturbance, which appears to reflect anterior horn cell damage.

Accidents involving domestic or industrial electrical supplies usually involve passage of electricity from one limb to another via the trunk. The major danger is one of cardiological involvement and ventricular fibrillation: survivors may therefore exhibit typical hypoxic cerebral damage. With low-tension currents (up to 1000 volts) loss of consciousness is rare, but immediate vasomotor effects are prominent. Sometimes late cord damage may be apparent when the passage of current is from arm to arm through the cervical cord. Severe peripheral nerve and spinal cord damage may occur if these structures are involved in the local passage of high-tension current.

HYPERBARIC AND HYPOBARIC DISORDERS

Changes in the ambient atmospheric pressure may result in changes in the volume of the gas-filled cavities of the body (chest, sinuses and middle ear) and in changes in the saturation of the blood with varying gases: such changes have important neurological consequences.

Medical problems of divers

Breathing pure oxygen at depth can rapidly lead to oxygen toxicity, and exposure to 2 atmospheres of pure oxygen will result in convulsions: a nitrogen/oxygen mixture is therefore used at depths of up to approximately 100 feet. However, at greater depths, increasing partial pressure of nitrogen can result in a state of narcosis which may lead to unconsciousness at depths of approximately 300 feet.

The most common problems of diving result from decompression. Ascent from only moderate depths during breath-holding can lead to an expansion of air within the chest, with subsequent pneumothorax, air embolism and subcutaneous or mediastinal emphysema. Air embolism can result in immediate death, loss of consciousness, or apparent stroke. Such accidents demand that the patient be placed in a steep head-down tilt and immediately recompressed. Other forms of barotrauma include round-window rupture, which may result in sudden deafness, tinnitus and dizziness, or rupture of the tympanic membrane with or without haemorrhage into the middle ear.

The other major hazard of diving is *decompression sickness* (the 'bends'). This occurs on rapid decompression and results in small gas bubbles appearing in the blood. In its mildest form it gives rise to symptoms of fatigue or drowsiness, itching of the skin and cutaneous mottling. These mild symptoms may be associated with other more serious ones: in type 1 decompression sickness there is severe pain in the limbs (usually the arms); type 2 decompression sickness includes all symptoms other than simple pain. Functional disturbance of the spinal cord may produce paraesthesiae, paralysis of the lower limbs and, occasionally, quadraparesis; the cerebral circulation, however, does not seem to be greatly affected: nevertheless, vascular disturbances of the inner ear may lead to vertigo and unsteadiness (the 'staggers'). Occasionally, blurring of vision or blindness may occur.

The major arm of treatment for decompression sickness is recompression. Steroids may be of some value in patients with overt spinal cord symptoms.

Hypobaric disorders

Acute exposure to higher altitudes may cause all the effects of barotrauma and decompression sickness seen in divers ascending from depths. Explosive decompression in aircraft at height may cause cerebral as well as spinal cord disturbance. More subtle symptoms are seen in acute mountain sickness when those accustomed to sea-level atmospheric pressure are exposed to a high-altitude environment: subjects experience fatigue, nausea and headache, which may be complicated by pulmonary and cerebral oedema. Most of these symptoms are reversible by increasing the amount of inspired oxygen.

NEUROLOGICAL COMPLICATIONS OF SURGERY AND ANAESTHESIA

A short classification of the wide variety of complications of surgery and anaesthesia is presented in Table 17.9.

Inevitably, it is possible to produce almost any kind of neurological damage accidentally during surgery: thus the median or ulnar nerve may be damaged during surgery to the wrist; paraplegia may follow aortic surgery, due to vascular damage to the cord and cauda equina; lumbar spinal manipulation can result in saddle anaesthesia and retention of urine, and cervical spinal manipulation can result in spastic quadraparesis or vertebral vascular disturbance.

Particular care must always be taken in the positioning of patients, because of a possibility of pressure palsies. The brachial plexus and peripheral nerves of the upper limbs are most at risk, but improper positioning in 'stirrups' can result in lateral popliteal palsy.

ENT surgery can result in dural penetration with c.s.f. fistula and subsequent infection. Particularly high risks of neurological disturbance inevitably follow neurosurgery itself, cerebrovascular surgery (for intracranial aneurysm or carotid endarterectomy), and cardiac surgery involving the use of bypass procedures.

A number of less direct complications of surgery will be recognised: these include psychiatric disturbances following mastectomy and hysterectomy and neurological complications of endocrine ablative surgery; gastrectomy has been associated with a number of neurological complications, including neuropathy and subacute combined degeneration due to vitamin B_{12} deficiency; portacaval anastomosis, by giving rise to shunting, can cause both acute and chronic encephalopathies.

The most tragic of anaesthetic complications is cerebral hypoxia, which may complicate even the most trivial of procedures. Spinal anaesthesia, when performed electively or inadvertently during attempted epidural procedures, may be complicated by paraparesis or cauda equina syndromes.

Table 17.9 Neurological complications of surgery

Surgical
Direct trauma (peripheral/c.n.s.
Vascular complications
Aneurysm surgery
Carotid endarterectomy
Cardiac bypass
Aortic reconstruction
Complications of positioning/manipulation
Anaesthetic
Cerebral hypoxia
Drug complications
Complications of spinal anaesthesia
Late complications
Psychiatric (postmastectomy)
Endocrine ablation
Deficiency states (postgastrectomy)
Metabolic (portocaval anastomosis)

FURTHER READING

Argov Z, Mastaglia F L 1979 Disorders of neuromuscular transmission caused by drugs. New England Journal of Medicine 301: 409–413

Argov Z, Mastaglia F L 1979 Drug induced peripheral neuropathies. British Medical Journal 1: 663–666

Blain P G, Lane R J M 1983 Drugs and muscle. Adverse Drug Reactions and Accidental Poisoning Review 2: 1–24

Cartlidge N E F 1981 Drug-induced coma. Advances Drug Reaction Bulletin no 88, p 320–323

Chadwick D 1983 Drug-induced convulsions. In: Capildeo R, Rose F C (eds) Recent progress in epilepsy. Pitman Press, London, p 151–159

18

The neurology of systemic disease

INTRODUCTION

A classification of the disorders to be considered in this chapter is presented in Table 18.1. The common theme of these disorders is that they are the sort of neurological problems that are often seen on medical wards and they share a common pattern in that there is multifocal or diffuse involvement of the nervous system including the cerebral hemispheres, the brain stem, the cerebellum, the spinal cord, the peripheral nerves and muscle.

Table 18.1 The neurology of systemic disease: a classification

Organ failure/disordered function
Cardiovascular
Respiratory
Gastrointestinal
Skin
Bony
Haematological
Endocrine
Renal
Specific pathological processes
Malignant disease
Collagen vascular disease
Deficiency disorders
The neurological complications of pregnancy

Examples of the clinical syndromes that cross the barriers of these various disorders include 'the acute confusional state' and 'peripheral neuropathy'. The differential diagnosis of these would include many of the conditions to be considered in this chapter.

These disorders may be separated into two groups:

1. Disorders due to organ failure or disordered function
2. Disorders due to a specific pathological entity or a specific pathological process.

ORGAN FAILURE OR DISORDERED FUNCTION

CARDIOVASCULAR DISORDERS

The importance of the blood supply to the brain and the requirements of the brain for oxygen and other nutrients is discussed in Chapter 11. Impairment of blood supply to the brain may occur as a result of cardiovascular disorders and the clinical phenomenology which results depends on the following factors:

1. Focal ischaemia to the brain usually results from localised obstruction to one individual artery. Occasionally, either as a result of anomalies of the circle of Willis, or as a result of extensive extracranial vascular disease, focal ischaemia in the brain may occur as a result of generalised cerebral hypoperfusion.
2. Anomalies of the circle of Willis are common and this may affect the clinical patterns resulting from cerebral hypoperfusion: for example, in almost one-third of all brains the major blood supply to one or both posterior cerebral arteries is derived from the internal carotid artery without a major collateral circulation from the primary source, the basilar artery.
3. Although the brain is completely dependent upon the cardiovascular activity, there are intrinsic mechanisms for regulating delivery and utilisation of oxygen for cerebral function—so-called autoregulation.
4. The border zones—these are the areas of the cerebral hemispheres between the areas of supply of the major cerebral surface arteries. An extensive literature has built up concerning the neuropathological consequences of hypotension and the concept of 'border zone' infarction and 'watershed' infarction. In patients who die as a result of cerebral hypoperfusion, the pathological involvement of the cerebral cortex is often greatest in the parieto-occipital regions, these being the border zones between the anterior, middle and posterior cerebral arteries.

In relation to the conditions that are now to be considered, the neurological problems affecting the cerebral hemispheres can be regarded as occurring either on the basis of generalised cerebral hypoperfusion, with the provisos above, or on the basis of localised vascular obstruction resulting in focal ischaemia

Table 18.2 lists a classification of cardiovascular disorders and their effects on the nervous system.

Table 18.2 Cardiovascular disorders and the nervous system

Congenital heart disease
Generalised anoxia
Cerebral embolism
Cerebral abscess
Cerebral venous thrombosis
Valvular heart disease
Cerebral embolism
Intermittent cerebral hypoperfusion
Ischaemic heart disease
Cerebral hypoperfusion
Cerebral embolism
The neuropsychiatric sequelae of cardiac arrest
Hypotension and cardiac arrhythmia
Subacute bacterial endocarditis
Cerebral embolism
Mycotic aneurysm
Cardiac myoxma
Loeffler's endocarditis
The neuropsychiatric sequelae of open heart surgery
The neurological sequelae of aortic aneurysms and their treatment

Congenital heart disease

Congenital heart disease is defined as being present from the time of birth. It is by far the most common form of cardiac abnormality of childhood and the majority of the disorders considered in this section are disorders seen only in children.

Patients with congenital heart disease have a wide variety of neurological problems. As many as 25% of children with congenital heart disease may develop signs or symptoms of neurological disorder and the pattern of the neurological disorders varies considerably, depending on the underlying cardiac abnormality.

In a young child the low cardiac output resulting from severe heart disease may be associated with apparent delayed motor development. It is important to recognise that this is not in most instances due to primary c.n.s. damage: speech, which usually develops at a normal age, is a much more valid indicator of cerebral function.

Anoxia

Anoxic spells and syncope commonly occur in children with congenital heart disease; they usually are associated with the severe forms of heart disease and correlate strongly with the presence of hypoxia and anaemia. Anoxic convulsions may occur and the greater the degree of cyanosis, the greater the likelihood of seizures. It is important to remember that seizures in children with congenital heart disease may occur from other causes, such as cerebral abscess or cerebral infarction.

Cerebral infarction

For some considerable time it has been recognised that children with congenital heart disease may suffer cerebral infarction and this most commonly occurs in children under the age of 20 months. Infarction may occur on the basis of cerebral arterial thrombosis, cerebral venous thrombosis or cerebral embolism. Cerebral thrombosis usually results from the increased viscosity of the blood secondary to the polycythaemia associated with cyanotic heart disease; a rarer cause is bacterial endocarditis with rupture of a mycotic aneurysm. Strokes within the first few years are commonly associated with residual neurological deficits and are not infrequently followed by seizures. Twenty per cent of those suffering a hemiplegia in early life will have subsequent mental retardation.

Cerebral abscess

Cerebral abscess is a common neurological complication of congenital heart disease and is particularly important to recognise because it is potentially treatable. It is more frequently associated with cyanotic heart disease as a result of the right-to-left shunt. Abscesses are excessively rare in patients under the age of 2 years; after this age they probably are associated with the development of teeth and the presence of secondary gingival infections. Abscesses are usually single, large, and may occur in any portion of the cerebral hemispheres. The presenting signs are those of abscesses generally, but it is important to emphasise that focal signs developing in a patient with congenital heart disease should be assumed to be due to a brain abscess until proved otherwise. The absence of fever does not exclude the diagnosis. Investigation and treatment are as described in Chapter 12.

Miscellaneous disorders

Mental deficiency. A higher proportion of mental deficiency is seen in patients with congenital heart disease than in the normal population. This usually results from the neurological complications, such as cerebral infarction, but generalised cerebral hypoperfusion may result in a degree of intellectual impairment.

Headaches. Headaches are a frequent complaint in patients with congenital heart disease, occurring in as many as 10% above the age of 2 years. Although many of these are benign and related to changes in cerebral blood flow (producing migraine-like headaches), it is important to emphasise that the recent onset of headaches in a patient with congenital heart disease should alert the clinician to exclude such causes as a cerebral abscess, meningitis or a subarachnoid haemorrhage.

Valvular heart disease

Cerebral embolism

A relationship between systemic embolism and valvular heart disease, alone or in conjunction with atrial fibrillation, is so well known that stroke registries have used the presence of these features as major criteria in deciding whether an ischaemic stroke was of embolic origin. There remains, however, considerable controversy concerning the incidence of cerebral embolism in patients with uncomplicated valvular heart disease. It is now clearly established that once a single episode of embolism has occurred, there is a significant risk of recurrence; furthermore, the presence of atrial fibrillation increases the risk of cerebral embolism quite significantly. Compared with atrial fibrillation, most other arrhythmias seem to carry a smaller risk of embolism.

It has become common clinical practice in the last 25 years to give anticoagulant therapy in many cases of valvular heart disease in the hope of reducing the incidence of embolic complications; there is general agreement that, once one episode of cerebral embolism has occurred, then anticoagulants should be given prophylactically. The major difficulty is in deciding which patients with valvular heart disease should be given anticoagulants prophylactically to prevent their first episode of embolism. There appears to be general agreement that patients with rheumatic valvular heart disease and atrial fibrillation should receive prophylactic long-term anticoagulants. Their role in non-rheumatic valvular disease is controversial.

Intermittent cerebral hypoperfusion

This most commonly is seen in patients with aortic stenosis resulting in exertional syncope. It is thought to be due to a fixed cardiac output, which is unable to keep up the demands imposed by exertion, resulting in cerebral ischaemia. It is usually taken as an indication for surgical treatment.

Ischaemic heart disease

Unfortunately and increasingly one of the commonest neurological sequelae of ischaemic heart disease is that resulting from a cardiac arrest. Prompt resuscitation following cardiac arrest in a patient with ischaemic heart disease will usually prevent serious neurological damage; however, particularly in the United States, patients suffering out-of-hospital cardiac arrests are resuscitated either after a delay or inefficiently, and this results in ischaemic brain damage. Brain death is often the consequence. Lesser degrees of brain damage resulting in irrecoverable brain function are less well delineated and are under active study at present in an attempt to allow prediction of such an outcome. The persistent vegetative state is one of the many terms used to describe patients who suffer such extensive ischaemic damage to the cerebral cortex yet have preservation of function of the brain stem. These patients may recover consciousness, as evidenced by eye opening, yet do not recover awareness (see p. 130). A variety of other clinical syndromes may be seen, presumably depending on anomalies of the cerebral circulation and the length of the ischaemic period. Border zone infarction resulting in a biparieto-occipital syndrome is not uncommonly encountered. The natural history of these sequelae and the recovery curves have not yet been fully established.

Cerebral embolism

Mural thrombi following myocardial infarction are not uncommon and these may embolise to the brain, even in the absence of cardiac dysrhythmia. Currently it is not felt that this risk is of sufficient magnitude to justify routine prophylactic anticoagulation of patients after myocardial infarction. Unfortunately, it is not possible to identify high-risk patients for this complication but, once embolism has occurred, anticoagulants are generally recommended.

Other causes of cerebral embolism are discussed in the chapter on cerebrovascular diseases. Increasingly, however, it has become recognised that cerebral emboli of cardiac origin are more common than was previously thought.

Hypotension and cardiac arrhythmia

The effects of cerebral hypoperfusion occurring as a result of these cardiac disturbances do not differ from those of any other form of hypoperfusion. They are included here simply to emphasise the need to consider these when faced with a patient with unexplained syncope.

Bacterial endocarditis

The incidence of cerebral symptoms in patients with bacterial endocarditis ranges from 10% to 50%, but evidence of emboli at autopsy is considerably higher as many produce no signs or symptoms. In as many as 20% of patients, cerebral embolism is the presenting feature of the disorder.

At least four clinical and pathological pictures can be distinguished:

1. Focal areas of cerebral infarction caused by embolic occlusion of large arteries constitute one of the most typical clinical pictures.
2. Some patients have multiple small, often microscopic, areas of cerebral infarction (the so-called flea-bitten brain) producing a clinical

picture of diffuse encephalopathy with alterations in mentation and consciousness.

3. Embolic blockage of meningeal vessels by small infected emboli may produce meningitis or multiple cerebral abscesses.

4. The impaction of an infected embolus in some vessels produces local arteritis in the cerebral arterial wall, resulting in mycotic aneurysm formation. These may often be multiple and may rupture, producing the clinical picture of a subarachnoid or intracerebral haemorrhage.

Any patient who presents with a subarachnoid haemorrhage, an acute cerebral infarct, or acute encephalopathy for no apparent reason, with heart murmurs, fever or anaemia should be considered as a possible case of bacterial endocarditis.

Cardiac myoxma

Cardiac myxoma is the most common of the primary heart tumours and it is the only one that frequently involves the nervous system. The clinical manifestations may occur as a result of obstruction to blood flow, embolisation or constitutional effects; a broad spectrum of signs and symptoms may result. Most myxomas, which are friable and usually have a pedicle, arise from or near the fossa ovalis in the right atrium or the septum primum of the left atrium; this location allows the tumour to obstruct blood flow or to shed part of itself into the bloodstream as an embolus.

Blood flow obstruction of either the mitral or tricuspid valve may lead to syncope or even sudden death. Embolic effects are the most likely mechanism that will bring the patient to the neurologist's attention and these occur in 50% of left atrial myxomas. Neurological involvement can take a number of different forms, the most common being either transient ischaemic attacks or ischaemic infarction. Occasionally multiple cerebral aneurysms can be formed and cerebral haemorrhage may occur. Seizures may result from epileptogenic foci secondary to cerebral infarcts. Multiple cerebral emboli sometimes may present as a progressive neurological problem with dementia.

A cardiac myxoma should be suspected in any patient with unexplained cerebral emboli and in patients with the findings of mitral stenosis without atrial fibrillation. The most definitive and helpful diagnostic procedure is echocardiography.

Loeffler's endocarditis

Eosinophilic fibroplastic endocarditis was described by Loeffler in 1936. The clinical features of the condition are those of cardiac failure occurring in association with profound eosinophilia. There are often systemic symptoms of fever and joint pains. The neurological complications take a variety of forms and most commonly result from multifocal areas of cerebral infarction. The aetiology of the condition is unknown and there is no specific treatment.

CHEST DISORDERS AND THE NERVOUS SYSTEM

A classification of these is presented in Table 18.3.

Respiratory encephalopathy

The more effective treatment of chronic lung disease has resulted in more prolonged survival of

Table 18.3 Chest disorders and the nervous system

Respiratory encephalopathy
Mental changes
Personality change
Memory impairment
Somnolence
Confusion
Coma
Neurological changes
Headache
Motor abnormalities
Sensory abnormalities
Ocular changes
Chemosis
Papilloedema
Benign intracranial hypertension
The Pickwickian syndrome
Miscellaneous
Electroencephalographic changes
Changes in the cerebrospinal fluid
Infections
For example, association between bronchiectasis and cerebral abscess
Tumours
Direct involvement
Metastatic spread to nervous system
Involvement as a result of paraneoplastic syndrome

patients with respiratory insufficiency, a greater number of whom now reach a stage where they develop the neurological complications. The majority of these result from chronic hypoxia and/or hypercapnia—so-called respiratory encephalopathy, the clinical features of which are listed in Table 18.3.

Apart from headache, mental disturbance is undoubtedly the common manifestation of this syndrome and early changes are those of tiredness, apathy, irritability, or depression. Inversion of normal sleep rhythm with nocturnal insomnia may occur and this usually precedes disorders of consciousness. Hypersomnia is characteristic of the Pickwickian syndrome (see below). As the respiratory failure gets steadily worse, disorders of consciousness appear with confusion, disorientation, delirium and finally coma. Muscular weakness, tremors, myoclonus, convulsions and asterixis may all occur. The headache has many of the clinical features of the headache of raised intracranial pressure; it is thought to result from the vasodilator effect of carbon dioxide on the cerebral blood vessels, which may increase intracranial pressure and eventually result in papilloedema. One of the hallmarks of papilloedema in this situation is that it is associated with preserved venous pulsation. A raised P_aCO_2 in arterial blood is a constant finding in patients with chronic respiratory encephalopathy and papilloedema.

The treatment of respiratory encephalopathy is the treatment of the respiratory failure. Occasionally, such simple measures as weight loss and stopping smoking are sufficient to produce improvement. In patients with marked polycythaemia and a high haematocrit, therapeutic venesection may be of benefit.

The cardiorespiratory syndrome of obesity
(Pickwickian syndrome)

The clinical picture of this syndrome is that of an obese individual who has symptoms of dyspnoea, somnolence and periodic respiration and signs of oedema, hepatomegaly, jugular congestion and cyanosis. The most marked clinical peculiarity is the sleep disorder, and diurnal somnolence is striking, intense and intractable. The patient may fall asleep while recounting his history or in the middle of a meal. Intermittent obstruction of the upper respiratory tract during sleep has been shown to be an additional factor of significance in these obese subjects and any evidence of upper respiratory tract obstruction should lead to appropriate treatment. The basic treatment of the condition is weight loss.

THE NEUROLOGICAL COMPLICATIONS OF GASTROINTESTINAL DISORDERS

A classification of these disorders is listed in Table 18.4.

The neurological complications of liver disease

All progressive liver diseases ultimately cause severe cerebral dysfunction, with disorders of mentation, motor functioning and consciousness. The importance of these in clinical practice is that an early diagnosis may lead to appropriate treatment, with resolution of the neurological manifestations.

The syndrome of hepatic encephalopathy consists of:

1. Personality change and impaired mental function
2. Motor abnormalities including asterixis, tremor, bilateral pyramidal signs and extensor posturing
3. Alterations in consciousness, delirium, stupor and coma
4. Focal and generalised seizures
5. Characteristic changes in the brain stem reflexes

Table 18.4 The neurological complication of gastrointestinal tract disorders

The neurological complications of liver disease
Bilirubin encephalopathy
Pancreatic encephalopathy

The neurological complications of bowel disturbances
  Malabsorption syndrome
  Whipple's disease
  Inflammatory bowel disorders

Genetically determined disorders with neurological and gastrointestinal tract abnormalities

6. A fairly consistent constellation of laboratory abnormalities.

The course of hepatic encephalopathy is fluctuating and unpredictable and depends on the underlying liver disease. A number of definite subtypes of the disorder may be recognised:

1. Acute hepatic coma
2. Subacute or chronic hepatic encephalopathy
3. Intermittent stupor with portosystemic shunts
4. Acquired hepatocerebral degeneration.

Pathophysiology

Failure of liver cell function invariably induces cerebral insufficiency, but despite many years of study the precise cause for this has not yet been established. The liver, of course, has many chemical functions, including detoxifying potential neurotoxic substances absorbed from the gut and supplying the nervous system with substrates for oxidation (glucose) and biosynthesis (amino acids and fatty acids).

Acute hepatic necrosis, as occurs in viral hepatitis, may lead to coma within a matter of hours of development of the first neurological symptoms. Reye's syndrome is acute encephalopathy accompanying fatty degeneration of the liver and is associated with clinical neurological changes similar to those of hepatic coma. There is considerable debate as to whether the liver and brain disorders are independent manifestations of a common pathogen such as a virus.

Pathology

In acute hepatic failure resulting in coma, there typically is gross cerebral oedema with rostrocaudal herniation. There are often few gross or microscopic signs. Changes in the glial cells, however, are common in chronic hepatic failure with encephalopathy, particularly an increase in the size and number of the protoplasmic astrocytes.

In patients with a more protracted course, more severe microscopic abnormalities may develop with time producing the clinical picture of so-called acquired hepatocerebral degeneration. In such cases a patchy spongy degeneration is seen in the deep layers of the cerebral cortex and the subcortical white matter, particularly in the parieto-occipital region and basal ganglia. Patients with chronic liver disease may also develop spinal cord demyelination and occasional cases of segmental demyelination of the peripheral nerves have been described.

Clinical syndromes

Acute liver failure (fulminant hepatic failure). Cerebral symptoms invariably are associated with fulminant liver failure, the mortality of which approaches 100%. The cause of the liver damage appears to be unimportant in the pathogenesis of the neurological symptoms. In the early stages, nervousness and restlessness are common and later are followed by confusion, delirium and coma. Increasing muscle tone becomes a feature by the time the patient is in coma and multifocal myoclonus may be seen as may epileptic seizures. Typically, by the time the patient is in coma there is a characteristic pattern of signs in that there is flexion or extension posturing of the limbs, yet preservation of the brain-stem reflexes, such as the pupil reflexes, corneal reflexes and reflex eye movements.

Encephalopathy with subacute or chronic liver failure. Severe chronic liver disease produces a fairly consistent clinical neurological picture. A fluctuating course is the rule and characteristic features include changes in cognitive and mental function and abnormalities of skeletal muscle control, eventually leading on to coma. Involuntary movements are prominent and include an irregular tremor and asterixis: the latter consists of an irregular, coarse quick and characteristic flexion/extension movement of the outstretched hand at the wrist and metacarpophalangeal joints. Subacute or chronic liver sclerosis combines the abnormalites of hepatocellular disease and vascular bypass. Surgical portocaval shunt, without pre-existing disease of the liver, may also cause encephalopathy, suggesting that toxins are an important cause of the neurological problems.

Chronic hepatocerebral degeneration. This syndrome blends in closely with the intermittent encephalopathy described above, but the major difference is that signs of a chronic motor disturbance are superimposed upon the other signs of hepatic coma. This is the least common form of hepatic encephalopathy and usually such patients have evidence of portocaval shunting, which in many cases may have been performed surgically to overcome portal hypertension. Mental changes are common, with dementia a prominent feature. The motor abnormalities are usually striking and include tremor, extrapyramidal rigidity, facial dyskinesia, chorea and dystonia. Bilateral pyramidal tract signs are present in some patients with extensor plantar responses, increased tone and brisk reflexes.

Electroencephalography

The EEG is abnormal in all patients with the neurological manifestations of liver disease and the abnormality may precede any clinical signs. Typically, there is symmetrical slowing initially over the frontal areas, and in precoma large (4–5 per second) triphasic waves arise bilaterally in the frontal and central regions. Terminally, delta discharges predominate. The EEG changes in hepatic encephalopathy are not diagnostic, but are typical of a 'metabolic encephalopathy'.

Prognosis

Hepatic coma carries a poor prognosis, which depends largely on the underlying liver disease: fulminant hepatic failure with coma has an almost 100% mortality; coma in a patient with chronic liver disease has a better prognosis, with a survival of 50%.

Other neurological complications

Very occasionally, in patients with chronic progressive hepatic failure, the spinal cord seems to be selectively involved, with myelopathy, comprising demyelination in the corticospinal pathways. Other neurological complications include peripheral neuropathy and myopathy. A problem in such patients is to differentiate the complications attributable to the liver disease from the complications caused by associated disorders such as alcoholism.

Bilirubin encephalopathy (kernicterus)

This condition has now virtually disappeared as a result of the development of passive immunisation of rhesus negative mothers with anti-Rh gammaglobulin. The clinical syndrome resulted from high levels of unconjugated bilirubin in the serum crossing the blood–brain barrier and damaging the brain tissue, with a predilection for the basal ganglia. The condition has virtually been eliminated from newborn infants, although premature infants may still be at risk.

Pancreatic encephalopathy

Acute pancreatitis is an uncommon disease, but it presents acutely with abdominal pain and vomiting. It may be accompanied by a number of biochemical changes, which alone or in combination may result in confusion, stupor or even coma. There are now a number of recorded cases of patients who developed progressive neurological deficits including seizures, focal neurological signs and coma and in whom, at autopsy, extensive demyelination has been found in the cerebral hemispheres: this is thought to result from the released pancreatic enzyme lipase in the bloodstream.

THE NEUROLOGICAL COMPLICATIONS OF CHRONIC BOWEL DISTURBANCE

These almost invariably result from malabsorption and are due to deficiency disorders. These are dealt with in a later section.

Whipple's disease

This is a rare disease characterised by the accumulation of a polysaccharide protein complex in intestinal and mesenteric lymph nodes. Clinically, the disorder presents in middle-aged males, most typically with signs of a gastrointestinal disturbance and malabsorption in combination with polyarthritis and lymphadenopathy. Central nervous system manifestations are occasionally described, with progressive dementia, myoclonus and seizures. Treatment is by a broad spectrum antibiotic, but the prognosis is poor.

Inflammatory bowel disorders

There are a variety of systemic complications of the inflammatory bowel disorders, such as ulcerative colitis and Crohn's disease. Evidence of systemic vasculitis is occasionally seen and this may affect the nervous system, producing cerebral involvement with multifocal or localised areas of infarction: in addition, both these disorders may be complicated by the development of cerebral venous thrombosis. Epileptic fits appear to have a higher incidence in these disorders, although the cause of this is unknown.

DERMATOLOGICAL DISORDERS AND THE NERVOUS SYSTEM

Disorders of the skin and the nervous system may be associated in a number of ways:

1. Genetically determined disorders with skin and central nervous system manifestations (the neurocutaneous syndromes)—Table 18.5.

2. A disorder of the nervous system giving rise to skin manifestations, for example, trophic ulceration in polyneuropathy or tabes dorsalis, herpes zoster.

3. Skin disease giving rise to a disorder of the nervous system, for example, infection of the skin with spread to the brain.

4. Skin and central nervous system abnormalities occurring independently as a result of a common underlying disorder, for example, sarcoidosis, pellagra, syphilis, leprosy, etc.

The common neurocutaneous disorders are tuberose sclerosis, neurofibromatosis (Fig. 18.1), Sturge–Weber syndrome, telangiectasia–ataxia, hereditary haemorrhagic telangiectasia and the von–Hippel–Lindau syndrome.

A number of other dermatological conditions of uncertain aetiology, some of which may be genetically determined, may be associated with neurological abnormalities.

Table 18.5 Neurocutaneous syndromes

Name	Neurological manifestations	Cutaneous manifestations
Tuberous sclerosis	Epilepsy, mental retardation	Facial adenomas, subungual fibromas, shagreen patch
Neurofibromatosis	Intracranial, intraspinal and peripheral nerve neurofibromas Intracranial meningiomas Any intracranial tumour	Café au lait patches, cutaneous neurofibromas
Sturge–Weber syndrome	Mental retardation, epilepsy, ipsilateral cerebral cortex calcification	Facial port wine haemangioma
Ataxia telangiectasia	Progressive cerebellar ataxia and myoclonus	Telangiectasia of conjunctiva and face
Hereditary haemorrhagic telangiectasia	Intracranial angiomas	Cutaneous and mucous membrane telangiectasia

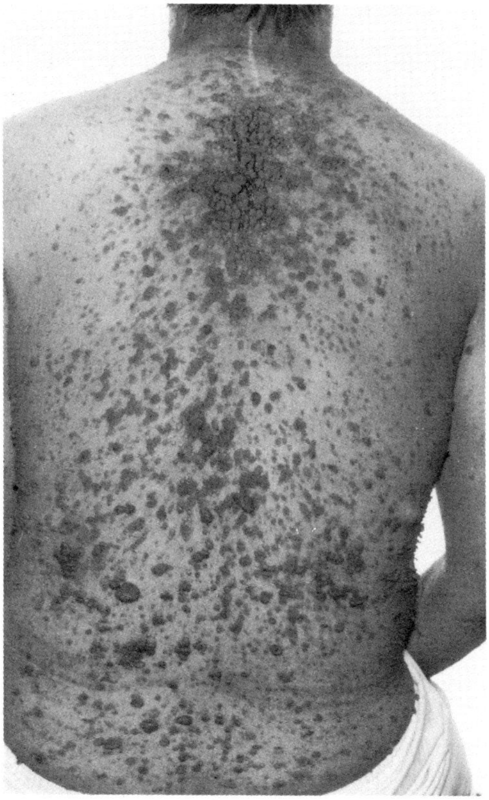

Fig. 18.1 Back view of male with neurofibromatosis showing typical cutaneous lesions.

Melkerson–Rosenthal syndrome

Recurrent or chronic facial oedema with relapsing facial palsies and lingua plicata.

Pseudoxanthoma elasticum

Skin abnormalities, angioid streaks in the retina, premature arteriosclerosis with cerebral infarction.

Xeroderma pigmentosum

Abnormal skin with cutaneous photosensitivity associated with mental retardation and in some instances progressive cerebrospinal degeneration.

Angiokeratoma corporis diffusum
(Andersen–Fabry's disease)

Multisystem involvement, with changes in the small arteries, multiple small vascular lesions in the skin, often cramping or girdle pains in the limbs, premature stroke.

NEUROLOGICAL COMPLICATIONS OF BONY DISEASE

This section does not include the neurological complications of bone tumours, infections of bone or the arthropathies. Developmental abnormalities such as achondroplasia, and congenital abnormalities of the spine such as spinal dysraphism are dealt with in Chapter 9.

Neurological involvement secondary to disorders of bone may result from:

1. Involvement of the skull
2. Involvement of the spine
3. Involvement of the long bones.

Paget's disease

Paget's disease appears in approximately 3–4% of the population over the age of 40, with an incidence of almost 10% in the ninth decade. The basic cause is uncertain, but there is excessive resorption of bone accompanied by active, disorganised and excessive proliferation of coarse new bone, resulting in thickening of the bone cortex. The pelvis, femur, spine, tibia and skull are especially involved.

Skull involvement (Fig. 18.2)

Over 50% of patients with Paget's disease have involvement of the skull, but only one-third of these reach the fully developed deformity and enlarged skull state. Headache is a common complaint and narrowing of the foramina of exit of cranial nerves by bone overgrowth may produce cranial nerve palsies, the commonest of which is deafness. The abnormally soft quality of the bone of the skull in this disease may result in remoulding of the base, producing basilar impression; this in turn may produce symptoms and signs of brain stem and upper spinal cord compression.

Spinal involvement

The vertebral bodies are commonly affected in Paget's disease and this may produce spinal cord compression. This most commonly occurs in either the dorsal or lumbar regions, but any level may be involved.

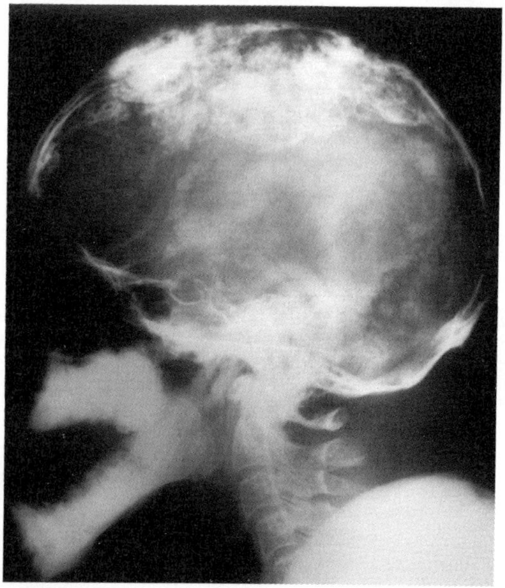

Fig. 18.2 Lateral skull radiograph showing Paget's disease of the vault.

Peripheral nerve involvement

Involvement of the long bones may result in entrapment neuropathies, the most common being entrapment of the median nerve in the carpal tunnel.

Treatment

Treatment of Paget's disease has advanced considerably in recent years with the introduction of calcitonin, disodium etidronates and mithramycin. Occasionally, patients with spinal involvement will require decompressive surgery followed by appropriate drug treatment. Osteogenic sarcomas may sometimes develop in Paget's disease: a biopsy is necessary to make this diagnosis, treatment thereafter being radiotherapy and chemotherapy.

Osteopetrosis

This is a rare disorder associated with increased sclerosis of the skeleton. Bone involvement produces a clinical picture similar to that seen in Paget's disease, with optic atrophy a frequent additional finding. Treatment is primarily palliative.

Fluorosis

Chronic poisoning with fluoride salts (usually in drinking water) may produce extensive sclerosis and thickening of bone; this may occur both in the vertebral column and the skull. Involvement of the vertebral column may be associated with spinal cord compression or radicular involvement. Involvement of the skull is rarely so gross as to produce neurological deficit.

Osteoporosis

This is a common disorder, being found at autopsy in as many as one-quarter of patients over the age of 50 years. As many as 30% of patients over 50 years old may show a degree of osteoporosis on radiological examination, and 5% of these have spinal compression-fracture. Spinal deformity, backache and vertebral compression are the common presentations, but spinal cord compression as a result of osteoporosis is exceptional.

Osteomalacia

Osteomalacia is attributable to demineralisation of bone as a result of inadequate available calcium and phosphorus and the serum calcium is often low. The clinical picture in infancy is that of rickets, with bony deformity, muscular weakness and pain. In adults, pain is a prominent feature and there is often an associated muscular weakness resulting in gait disturbance. Although skeletal abnormalities are common, involvement of the central nervous system from the bony changes is exceptional.

NEUROLOGICAL COMPLICATIONS OF HAEMATOLOGICAL DISORDERS

Table 18.6 lists a classification of these disorders.

General neurological features of anaemia

Patients with anaemia may complain of a variety of symptoms, including tiredness, fatiguability, faintness, dizziness and headache. Symptoms do not correlate well with the level of haemoglobin concentration and occasionally patients remain asymptomatic with haemoglobin levels of 6 g/dl or lower. The variation in symptoms depends on many factors and one is the state of the cerebral vessels themselves. Patients with cerebrovascular disease may develop symptoms of a transient cerebral ischaemia during a period of anaemia.

A variety of ocular abnormalities may be seen in anaemia: the most obvious is some impairment of the reddish colour of the fundus and decolor-

Table 18.6 Haematological disorders and the nervous system

The anaemias
Neurological complications of iron deficiency anaemia
Neurological complications of megaloblastic anaemia—folic acid deficiency, B_{12} deficiency (pernicious anaemia)
Neurological complications of sickle cell disease and the forms of haemolytic anaemia
The haemorrhagic disorders
The hyperviscosity syndromes
The leukaemias
The lymphoproliferative disorders including the lymphomas

ation of the optic disc. Small spindle-shaped haemorrhages may be seen and these may be surrounded by cotton wool exudates; they do not occur when the haemoglobin level is greater than 50% of normal. A minor degree of oedema of the optic disc may be seen and the retinal vessels may appear wider than normal.

The neurological features of the megaloblastic anaemias and of folic acid and vitamin B_{12} deficiency are considered in the section dealing with the deficiency disorders.

The haemolytic anaemias

A number of possible mechanisms may operate in the production of neurological complications associated with the haemolytic anaemias (Table 18.7). Firstly, there may be the non-specific features of anaemia itself: most haemolytic states are characterised by episodes of acute haemolysis and non-specific symptoms may be particularly prominent at this stage; second, neurological complications may be produced by vascular obstruction caused by the sickle cells in the sickle-cell anaemias, or by microaggregates as in cold agglutinin disease; third, the poorly understood activation of the coagulation system in paroxysmal nocturnal haemoglobinuria may cause thrombotic complications in both peripheral and central nervous systems; finally, increased levels of unconjugated bilirubin, which is a feature of all haemolytic states, may produce the well-known syndrome of bilirubin encephalopathy in neonates.

Sickle-cell anaemia

This is an inherited disorder characterised by the presence of an abnormal haemoglobin in the red cells. It is important clinically to differentiate the homozygous state from the heterozygous state as sickle-cell crises occur in the former. Neurological complications are common, occurring in as many as one-quarter of such patients:

1. Thrombosis and infarction:
   a. small vessel
   b. large vessel
2. Intracranial haemorrhage
3. Infection—meningitis
4. Fat embolism.

The basic cause of the neurological complication is sludging, particularly in the microcirculation. This results from a number of factors, the most obvious of which is the presence of numerous rigid deformed sickle cells. The commonest neurological manifestations are hemiplegia, coma, convulsions and visual disturbances; damage to the spinal cord, brain stem, cranial nerves and peripheral nerves occurs much less commonly. Occasional instances of cerebral haemorrhage are encountered.

Table 18.7 Mechanisms of neurological complications in haemolytic anaemia

Common to all haemolytic anaemias
Anaemia
Jaundice (billirubin encephalopathy)
Specific disorders
Sickle cell disease and its variants
Paroxysmal nocturnal haemoglobinuria

The haemorrhagic disorders

The excessive bleeding which occurs in disease with altered coagulation may occasionally involve the nervous system and is a not uncommon cause of death in such patients. The bleeding may occur in the intracranial cavity, around the spinal cord, in the nerve roots or in the peripheral nerves or plexuses.

The haemophilias

This group of disorders can be broadly defined as haemorrhagic diatheses characterised by impairment of the first stage of coagulation. Unlike acquired coagulation defects, where the bleeding tendencies may be multiple, the defect in this group of conditions is usually solitary. One of the most feared neurological complications of haemophilia is intracranial haemorrhage, which most commonly occurs in children. In almost one-half of such patients, the bleeding follows a head injury and may be primarily intracerebral or into the subdural or subarachnoid spaces. The prognosis in such cases used to be poor, but with better management of the underlying bleeding disorder it is now possible to operate on some patients and to enable them to survive.

Bleeding around the spinal cord is the least frequent type of neurological complication in haemophilia. Bleeding may be over the surface of the cord or within the substance of the cord itself.

Compression of a peripheral nerve by bleeding in haemophilia is not uncommon. The bleeding may involve any of the peripheral nerves, but most commonly either the sciatic or femoral nerves are involved. More rarely, bleeding around the cranial nerves may produce abnormalities and the commonest of these is bleeding into the facial canal.

Thrombocytopenia and other purpuras

In these conditions, haemorrhage within and around the brain is not infrequent and, as in haemophilia, intracerebral bleeding in thrombocytopenia can be in the form of numerous small punctate haemorrhages (brain purpura). Larger intracerebral haemorrhages may occur but subarachnoid bleeding and subdural haematomas are less common. Spinal cord and peripheral nerve haemorrhage in thrombocytopenia are rare.

One particular syndrome associated with thrombocytopenia is thrombotic thrombocytopenic purpura (thrombotic microangiopathy). Neurological involvement occurs in 90% of patients with this condition and often the neurological problems are the presenting features. Pathologically, there is evidence of multiple small vessel occlusions with multiple areas of infarction. The clinical picture produced is that of an organic mental syndrome with focal signs such as hemiparesis and aphasia and ultimately seizures and coma.

Disseminated intravascular coagulation is now recognised as a fairly common acquired haemorrhagic thrombotic syndrome which occurs as a result of the presence of thrombin in the systemic circulation; it occurs in a variety of systemic states, including disseminated infections. It presents clinically with a picture of bleeding at multiple sites and neurological involvement results from bleeding into the central nervous system and multiple microthrombi.

Hypoprothrombinaemia

This is a common cause of clinical bleeding, very often as a complication of therapeutic anticoagulant therapy. The pattern of the haemorrhages is similar to that seen in haemophilia, with haemorrhage occurring intracranially, intraspinally and into the peripheral nerves.

The hyperviscosity syndromes

Hyperviscosity may occur in a variety of haematological disorders:

1. Polycythaemia
2. Leukaemia
3. Thrombocytosis
4. Sickle cell anaemia
5. Macroglobulinaemia
6. Cryoglobulinaemia
7. Myeloma.

The clinical features result from sludging of blood in the cerebral vessels with multiple areas of infarction and occasionally haemorrhage. The commonest cause of this is an increase in the red cell mass (polycythaemia). It has been shown in polycythaemia that there is a significant reduction in cerebral blood flow as soon as the haematocrit begins to rise above 50%.

Common symptoms of the sludging disorders are headache, lethargy and dizziness. Focal areas of infarction may produce visual symptoms, hemiparesis, aphasia and brain stem abnormalities; transient ischaemic attacks in either the carotid or vertebrobasilar territories also occur; less common are thrombotic episodes involving venous sinuses. In some patients with polycythaemia there may be progressive symptoms suggesting an intracerebral neoplasm; less common complications are chorea and spinal cord infarction. Papilloedema may develop as a result of intracranial venous stasis or of local venous stasis in the eye. Another rare hyperviscosity syndrome is that seen in essential thrombocythaemia; this presents in a manner similar to that in the other hyperviscosity syndromes.

The leukaemias

Neurological complications in leukaemia may result from a variety of different processes:

1. Intracranial haemorrhage
2. Leukaemic infiltration
3. Infections
4. Paraneoplastic syndromes, e.g. progressive multifocal leucoencephalopathy
5. Effects of treatment
6. Hyperviscosity syndromes.

Before the introduction of prophylactic nervous system radiotherapy, the incidence of central nervous system involvement in children with acute non-lymphoblastic leukaemia was about 25%, compared with a 56% incidence in lymphoblastic leukaemia. The recognition of this in the early 1970s prompted the adoption of various prophylactic measures, including craniospinal irradiation.

Clinical features

Meningeal leukaemia. The commonest symptoms of this are nausea, vomiting and headache. Cranial or spinal root involvement may produce appropriate signs and there may be confusion, ataxia, seizures or focal deficit. Papilloedema is a common sign and neck stiffness is a common finding. The diagnosis is confirmed by finding leukaemia cells in the cerebrospinal fluid.

Localised deposits. Any part of the central nervous system may be invaded by leukaemia deposits, many of which may be asymptomatic and discovered only at autopsy.

Chloromas. Chloromas are solid tumours of non-lymphatic leukaemias and they are most common in the cranial and facial bones. Commonly these present with proptosis; they may involve cranial nerves or extend intracranially, producing raised intracranial pressure.

The other complications of the leukaemias are dealt with in the appropriate sections of other chapters.

The lymphoproliferative disorders and the lymphomas

Myeloma

The nervous system is commonly involved in myeloma and at least three categories of complications may be recognised:

1. Compression of the spinal cord, cauda equina or nerve roots
2. Cranial nerve or intracranial involvement
3. Peripheral neuropathy.

Involvement of the spinal cord, cauda equina or nerve roots. The spinal vertebrae are commonly infiltrated with myeloma cells which may extend to produce spinal cord or root compression; this most commonly occurs in either the dorsal or lumbar regions.

Cranial nerves and intracranial involvement. Involvement of the intracranial cavity is rare, but involvement of the skull with secondary involvement of the cranial nerves is more common.

The cranial nerves most frequently involved are the second, third, fourth and sixth. Occasionally meningeal infiltration may occur in myeloma and this may involve spinal nerve roots.

Peripheral neuropathy. Peripheral neuropathy in myeloma may occur based on a number of different mechanisms and may be seen not only in multiple myeloma but also in patients with a solitary myeloma. Mechanisms include:

1. Paraneoplastic neuropathy
2. Ischaemic neuropathy due to amyloid or paraprotein deposition in the vasa nervorum.

Lymphomas

Because of the changing nomenclature and classification of lymphomas, an estimate of the incidence of central nervous system involvement is difficult to obtain. Involvement of the nervous system may occur as a presenting feature or more commonly as a manifestation of relapse. At least four main varieties of neurological complications may occur:

1. Meningeal involvement
2. Cranial nerve involvement
3. Spinal cord compression

4. Parenchymal central nervous system involvement.

Indirect effects may be noted as with the other haematological malignancies.

The clinical patterns are similar to those seen in the leukaemias; overall neurological involvement is more common in non-Hodgkin's lymphomas than in Hodgkin's disease itself.

ENDOCRINE DISORDERS

Apart from the syndromes considered below, disorders of the endocrine glands and neurological abnormalities may be linked in a number of different clinical syndromes. There are, for example, the syndromes of multiple endocrine adenomatoses, a number of which have neurological abnormalities. There are also neurological disorders which have associated endocrine abnormalities: obvious examples are those of myotonic dystrophy and Friedreich's ataxia and their association with diabetes mellitus. The classification in Table 18.8 lists those endocrine disorders which are associated with neurological complications.

Table 18.8 Endocrine disorders and the nervous system

Pituitary
Excess
Cushing's syndrome
Acromegaly
Hypopituitarism
Adrenal
Excess:
Conn's syndrome
Cushing's syndrome
Phaeochromocytoma
Deficiency
Addison's disease
Hypoaldosteronism
Other
Adrenogenital syndrome
Adrenoleucodystrophy
Thyroid
Hyperthyroidism
Myxoedema
Dysthyroid eye disease
Parathyroid
Hyperparathyroidism
Hypoparathyroidism
Pseudohypoparathyroidism
Pancreas
Hypoglycaemia
Diabetes mellitus
Disorders of salt and water metabolism
Hyponatraemia
Hypernatraemia
Hypomagnesaemia
Hypermagnesaemia

Pituitary disorders

Acromegaly

Apart from the neurological complications of the pituitary adenomas that occur in acromegaly, a number of secondary complications may be seen. The commonest are those resulting from bony overgrowth, resulting in entrapment neuropathies such as a carpal tunnel syndrome. Muscular weakness with atrophy of the muscles has been recognised for many years and it has now been clearly established that patients with acromegaly suffer from a myopathy; a variety of personality changes may occur, including depression, anxiety and apathy; diabetes may develop with its associated neurological complications (see below).

Hypopituitarism

Pituitary failure may in turn produce the symptoms of adrenal failure and of thyroid failure (see below). Aesthenia and muscle weakness are perhaps the commonest symptoms and others include hypothermia, hypoglycaemia, water intoxication, dehydration, sodium depletion and hypotension.

Adrenal disorders

Cushing's syndrome

The commonest neurological complication is muscular weakness due to myopathy. Personality changes may occur and as many as one-quarter of the patients become psychotic. Rarer complications are polyneuropathy and convulsions related to the electrolyte changes.

Phaeochromocytoma

A common symptom in such patients is headache related to the high blood pressure. In some instances the hypertension may be so marked as to produce hypertensive cerebral haemorrhage or subarachnoid haemorrhage and these characteristically are precipitated by exertion.

Primary aldosteronism (Conn's syndrome)

Characteristically, this syndrome is associated with hypertension and hypokalaemia. Muscle weakness due to the metabolic abnormality may be present, as may headaches due to the hypertension. Paraesthesiae and tetany-like symptoms may result from the metabolic alkalosis.

Addison's disease

Adrenal failure produces a characteristic clinical pattern, the commonest symptoms being those of fatigue and weakness; personality changes are common and psychotic reactions may occur. The general weakness in part may be due to a myopathy. Acute adrenal insufficiency presents with profound weakness, shock, headache, vomiting, confusion and, ultimately if untreated, may result in convulsions, coma and even death. Occasionally in Addison's disease there may develop a clinical picture of raised intracranial pressure with papilloedema. Signs of a spinal cord disturbance resulting even in paraplegia occasionally occur, as may contractures in the lower limb muscles; many of these changes are thought to be due to associated electrolyte abnormalities.

Hypoaldosteronism

Cases of pure aldosterone deficiency are rare, but in those cases that have been described there is quite marked muscle weakness secondary to low potassium levels. Syncope is common, due to the associated hypertension.

Thyroid disease

Hyperthyroidism

The neurological manifestations are listed in Table 18.9.

Cerebral. Personality changes are common in hyperthyroidism, varying from a degree of anxiety to hyperexcitability, restlessness and gross agitation.

Table 18.9 The neurological manifestations of hyperthyroidism

Cerebral
Personality changes
Pyramidal tract weakness
EEG changes
Convulsions
Tremor
Chorea
Muscle
Ophthalmoplegia
Thyrotoxic myopathy
Periodic paralysis
Myasthenia gravis
Nerve
Peripheral neuropathy
Optic neuropathy

In a thyroid crisis there may be extreme agitation with frenzy, confusion, hyperpyrexia, fits and eventually collapse. In occasional cases there may be pyramidal tract signs with hyperactive reflexes, ankle clonus and extensor plantar responses. Half the patients may show EEG changes, although these are usually only minimal. The thyrotoxic tremor, which is one of the hallmarks of the condition, appears to be simply an exaggerated physiological tremor; in some instances more gross involuntary movements (such as chorea) may develop.

Muscle. The ophthalmoplegia of hyperthyroidism is considered below (under dysthyroid eye disease) but a number of the ocular manifestations are separate and attributable to sympathetic overactivity. The lid retraction of thyrotoxicosis may be abolished by guanethidine eye drops.

Muscle weakness in thyrotoxicosis occurs in as many as two-thirds of the patients and occasionally this may cause quite acute bulbar weakness. The hallmark of the myopathy is that it is associated with preservation or even briskness of the tendon reflexes. There is evidence to suggest that sympathetic overactivity, at least in part, is the cause of the muscle weakness, as this often responds to treatment with beta adrenergic blocking agents.

Periodic paralysis (the hypokalaemic form) is an uncommon, but well recognised, complication of thyrotoxicosis, particularly in those patients of Chinese origin. The relationship between thyrotoxicosis and myasthenia gravis is well recognised, although only 1% of patients with hyperthyroidism develop this complication.

Nerve. A peripheral neuropathy has been described in a few patients with thyrotoxicosis, as has an optic neuropathy similar to retrobulbar neuritis and not related to the other thyroid eye problems.

Hypothyroidism

The thyroid plays an important part in the development of the nervous system and hypothyroidism in the developing child produces quite striking abnormalities, the most important of which is mental retardation; deafness and spasticity are other common complications.

In the adult, mental symptoms are common and these include poor memory, lack of concentration and apathy. Myxoedema is an important and not-to-be-missed cause of dementia. In such patients the EEG usually reveals low voltage, slow rhythms and, in some cases, the patients may lapse into coma. It is important to be aware that the c.s.f. protein is frequently raised in hypothyroidism.

Impairment of hearing, headaches and hoarseness of voice are other common symptoms and a variety of muscular syndromes may occur; patients often feel weak and clinical evidence of a myopathy may be seen in at least 50%. The tendon reflexes characteristically show a slow relaxation, and myoedema and rarely myotonia may be demonstrated. In children a specific form of myopathy is seen, with muscle hypertrophy. Although there are rare cases described of a symmetrical peripheral neuropathy, symptoms of a carpal tunnel syndrome occur frequently.

Patients with myxoedema often complain of difficulty in walking and one well-recognised cause of this is cerebellar ataxia. This is a rare complication of myxoedema, but all patients presenting with cerebellar ataxia should have thyroid function tests to exclude it as a cause. In severe cases dysarthria may be present, but nystagmus is unusual.

Dysthyroid eye disease

Ocular changes in thyrotoxicosis are common, but it is now recognised that a similar pattern of eye abnormalities may occur in patients who do not show thyroid overactivity. The aetiology of these eye changes is uncertain, but there is increasing evidence to suggest that they are due to a disorder of the immune system. The same pattern of changes may be seen in a patient who is thyrotoxic or who is euthyroid, and the eye abnormalities may be either bilateral and symmetrical or unilateral.

The most common abnormalities are lid retraction and weakness of the superior rectus muscle. Lid retraction is a manifestation of sympathetic overactivity, but the extraocular muscle weakness is a separate problem and attributable to an intrinsic abnormality of the extraocular muscles. In more severe cases all the extraocular muscles are involved and these become oedematous and may be associated with gross proptosis.

In severe cases (malignant exophthalmos) there is marked bilateral proptosis with chemosis. Before effective treatment, patients with this condition used to go blind because of traction damage to the optic nerves; treatment with high-dose prednisone and immunosuppressive drugs produces significant improvement.

In a patient without either clinical or biochemical evidence of thyroid dysfunction, the diagnosis of dysthyroid eye disease may present problems. The diagnosis should always be entertained in any patient presenting with unilateral proptosis with or without lid retraction or extraocular muscle weakness. The diagnosis may occasionally be suggested on a CT scan, as this often shows swelling of the extraocular muscles. Recently, specific autoantibodies have been demonstrated in such cases.

Parathyroid disorders

Calcium has an important role in the excitation and transmission of nerve impulses and in muscular contraction: not surprisingly, therefore, disorders of calcium metabolism are associated with a variety of neurological problems.

Hyperparathyroidism (hypercalcaemia)

Mental changes are common and include insomnia, depression and confusional states. These usually clear as the serum calcium returns to normal, but a sudden fall in the serum calcium—such as that seen following removal of a parathyroid adenoma—may precipitate mental changes such as an acute psychosis. Headache and sleep disturbances may occur and there is an increased risk of stroke in the hypercalcaemic patient. The bony manifestations may produce intracranial manifestations, such as erosion of the sella.

The hypercalcaemic crisis presents with drowsiness, weakness and increasing confusion and without rapid treatment there is a high mortality rate. In such patients the electroencephalogram shows bilateral slowing and occasionally the c.s.f. protein is raised. A variety of other rarer manifestations may be seen, such as basal ganglia dysfunction, cerebellar ataxia and spinal cord dysfunction. Muscle weakness attributable to a specific myopathy occurs and the muscle weakness characteristically is associated with cramps, pain on movement and exaggerated tendon reflexes.

Hypoparathyroidism (hypocalcaemia)

As with hyperactivity of the parathyroid glands, underactivity may produce manifestations attributable to involvement at all levels of the neuraxis, the commonest of which are tetany and convulsions. As many as one-quarter of the patients show evidence of mental abnormality, including psychoses, confusion and delirium. These changes and convulsions are particularly common in patients who experience sudden hypocalcaemia. Basal ganglia calcification may develop and result in extrapyramidal motor abnormalities, including chorea, dystonia and a parkinsonian syndrome. In some patients, raised intracranial pressure with papilloedema develops, although the mechanism for this is uncertain. Muscle weakness may occur and, more rarely, signs of a spinal cord disturbance or a peripheral neuropathy may be seen.

Pseudohypoparathyroidism

This is defined as a form of parathyroid hormone resistance and patients often show a variety of somatic defects, such as short stature. The end biochemical result is the same as that in hypoparathyroidism, with a similar pattern of neurological abnormalities. Subnormal intelligence, however, occurs in two-thirds of these patients.

Pancreatic disorders

Hypoglycaemia

In older infants, children and adults, hypoglycaemia is defined as a blood glucose concentration of less than 40 mg per 100 ml associated with suggestive signs and symptoms. Blood sugar levels less than 30 mg per 100 ml in full-term infants and less than 20 mg per 100 ml in premature and small-for-age infants define hypoglycaemia in neonates, although some experts feel that the higher value should apply to all age groups.

Clinical features. There are many causes of hypoglycaemia and the symptoms are numerous: these vary depending on age and the rapidity of onset of the hypoglycaemia. Acute hypoglycaemia is typically associated with symptoms of sweating, weakness, tachycardia, nervousness and hunger; general symptoms of malaise and anxiety may accompany the former symptoms and, with very low blood sugar levels, psychosis, seizures and coma may develop. In subacute hypoglycaemia the symptoms of autonomic activity are absent and lethargy and somnolence may gradually develop. Chronic hypoglycaemia, although rare, is characterised by insidious personality changes, defective memory and abnormal behaviour.

In man, the commonest situation in which hypoglycaemia occurs is in the diabetic who is either on insulin or taking a long-acting hypoglycaemic agent. Usually such diabetics soon begin to recognise the symptoms of their 'hypos' and are able to take avoiding action. Occasionally, however, the hypoglycaemia may occur through the night and manifest itself only as a nocturnal convulsion. In patients with diabetic autonomic neuropathy the symptoms of hypoglycaemia may be less evident.

The other important hypoglycaemic syndrome in adults is the syndrome of spontaneous hypoglycaemia caused by a pancreatic islet cell tumour. Hypoglycaemia in this context may produce a variety of symptoms and may be misdiagnosed in the early stages as a psychiatric disorder, transient cerebral ischaemia, or even epilepsy. The diagnosis should always be considered in any patient presenting with an intermittent personality change or behavioural abnormality. One of the peculiarities of hypoglycaemia is that it may present with focal signs or symptoms, such as monoparesis, hemiparesis, aphasia or visual field defect. In infancy and childhood, convulsions are the most common presenting signs and any child presenting for the first time with an epileptic fit should have an urgent blood sugar estimation. The risk of permanent neurological damage resulting from hypoglycaemia is especially high during the first few months of life and it is important not to miss the diagnosis. Similarly, unexplained coma in a child (or in an adult) warrants blood sugar estimation as a matter of urgency.

The diagnosis of hypoglycaemia may readily be made by estimation of the blood sugar, although occasionally such cases are diagnosed following a lumbar puncture, when the c.s.f. sugar is shown to be exceedingly low. In any patient suspected of having this condition, a 48-hour fast should be undertaken with regular blood sugar and insulin estimations being made.

Diabetes mellitus

A whole variety of neurological complications may occur in diabetes mellitus, the most obvious of which are those resulting from hyperglycaemia leading to either diabetic ketoacidosis or to hyperosmolar non-ketotic diabetic coma. The neurological complications of diabetes mellitus are listed below and to this list may be added the complications caused by premature atherosclerosis, which is so common in diabetics:

1. Symmetrical peripheral neuropathy
2. Asymmetrical neuropathy (mononeuritis multiplex)
3. Radioculopathy
4. Autonomic neuropathy
5. Cranial neuropathy
6. Retinopathy
7. Myelopathy
8. Myopathy
9. Teratogenicity.

Peripheral neuropathy A peripheral neuropathy sufficiently severe to cause obvious symptoms or signs occurs in as many as 10% of diabetics, and nerve conduction abnormalities are found in a higher proportion of such patients. The neuropathy is often mild and may be suspected only on the finding of asymptomatic vibration sensory loss at the ankles in association with absence of the ankle jerks. More severe forms of symmetrical motor and sensory polyneuropathy do occur and these usually indicate the need for more stringent control of the diabetes. There is now good evidence to suggest that the better the diabetic control, the less the chance of developing a diabetic neuropathy. It is perhaps worth noting at this point that the c.s.f. protein is often raised in diabetes mellitus, with or without peripheral neuropathy. Pathologically, the peripheral nerves in diabetic neuropathy show evidence of patchy segmental demyelination.

Mononeuritis multiplex in diabetes differs in many respects from the symmetrical polyneuropathy. The syndrome is commonly ushered in with pain and the predominant symptoms are motor rather than sensory. The femoral nerve appears to be the most frequently involved (so-called diabetic amyotrophy), but any other of the peripheral nerves may be affected, including the intercostal nerves, resulting in the clinical picture termed diabetic truncal neuropathy. The clinical course is that of a rapid or abrupt onset followed by spontaneous improvement. Strict control of the diabetes is occasionally required in order to achieve the improvement. It is generally felt that these mononeuropathies are a result of occlusion of the vasa nervorum, secondary either to damage to the small vessels via the diabetes or to premature arteriosclerosis.

Radiculopathy. Occasionally the nerve roots. rather than the nerves themselves may be affected in diabetes and, as with the mononeuropathy, the outstanding symptom is usually pain. Occasionally the thoracic or lumbar roots may be affected, producing a characteristic girdle pain and sensory loss; infarction of the nerve root is thought to be the cause.

Autonomic neuropathy. In some patients with diabetic peripheral neuropathy there is selective and extensive involvement of the autonomic ganglia producing an autonomic neuropathy. This may cause a pseudo–Argyll–Robertson pupil, but most commonly shows itself as loss of sweating over the extremities with occasionally trophic ulceration. The autonomic neuropathy may affect the gastrointestinal system, most commonly resulting in bowel disturbances with constipation intermixed with diarrhoea. Involvement of the cardiovascular system may result in orthostatic hypotension, and involvement of the genitourinary tract may give rise to bladder disturbances and, in men, impotence. The latter occurs in as many as 25% of diabetic males between the ages of 30 and 35 and in 75% of those between the ages of 60 and 65.

There have been few studies of the pathology of diabetic autonomic neuropathy, but those that have been made have shown abnormalities in the autonomic ganglia.

Cranial neuropathy. Mononeuropathies of the cranial nerves may occur in diabetes and the most common is that affecting the third nerve: this is often painless and the pupil is usually spared. The cause is thought to be arteriosclerosis of the vasa nervorum. Occasionally the sixth cranial nerve may be involved and Bell's palsy may also occur.

Diabetic retinopathy. Diabetic retinopathy occurs in two-thirds of all patients with long-standing diabetes and presents a wide variety of abnormalities with, ultimately, visual loss.

Diabetic myelopathy. The evidence for this condition is somewhat inconclusive, although a number of pathological studies suggest that microinfarction may occur in the spinal cord as a complication of the arteriosclerosis accelerated by diabetes. It has been suggested that similar areas of infarction may occur in diabetics in the brain and in muscle.

DISORDERS OF SALT AND WATER METABOLISM

Hyponatraemia and hypernatraemia

Homeostatic maintenance of sodium concentrations within certain limits is critical for proper functioning of excitable cells and neurological symptoms commonly occur with either hyponatraemia or hypernatraemia. These effects, however, are difficult to dissociate from the effects of simultaneously altered osmolality.

Hyponatraemia

In most instances hyponatraemia indicates a reduced plasma osmotic pressure due either to excessive sodium loss or to water retention. The development of neurological symptoms depends on the rapidity of fall of the serum sodium rather than on its absolute level. The signs include those of a metabolic encephalopathy, including weakness, lethargy, restlessness, confusion, stupor and coma; muscle twitches, tremor and asterixis may be striking features. Nausea, vomiting and headache are common and are thought to be due to the raised intracranial pressure which develops; papilloedema may be seen. In chronic cases the intracranial pressure is normal. Hyponatraemia predisposes to convulsions and these may be either generalised or focal. The brains of patients dying of hyponatraemia usually show cerebral oedema. The treatment is the removal or correction of the underlying cause and rigid water restriction.

Hypernatraemia

Thirst is almost always present in alert patients with hypernatraemia who do not have abnormalities of thirst mechanisms. Signs of dehydration are usually present and some patients will show some evidence of circulatory collapse. Alteration of consciousness with delirium and coma may occur and increased muscle tone, rigidity and seizures are not infrequent. Muscle twitching and myoclonic jerking is particularly common in children and muscle weakness may be a feature in some cases. Pathologically, there is evidence of widespread vascular damage with intracranial and subarachnoid bleeding and often evidence of cortical venous thrombosis and haemorrhagic infarction. These changes are particularly prevalent in children. The treatment of hypernatraemia is rehydration, but it is occasionally at this stage that the seizures develop.

Abnormalities of potassium metabolism

There are a number of highly efficient mechanisms in the central nervous system for maintaining potassium haemeostasis in the face of changes in the serum levels and there are no clearly recognised central nervous system manifestations of either hypo- or hyperkalaemia. Either of these, however, may produce peripheral nervous system manifestations, most notably muscle weakness. The cardiac effects of changes in serum potassium will usually be more obvious than the neurological effects.

Disorders of magnesium metabolism

Magnesium deficiency

The symptoms of magnesium deficiency mimic those of calcium deficiency, yet occur much less commonly. Any patient with symptoms of neuromuscular hyperexcitability who has a normal serum calcium should be screened to exclude magnesium deficiency.

Magnesium overload

This is excessively rare and clinical signs occur only when the magnesium level is increased two- or threefold.

Drowsiness, hyporeflexia and muscle weakness may occur and the weakness may progress to respiratory paralysis. Magnesium overload is usually iatrogenic.

NEUROLOGICAL COMPLICATIONS OF RENAL FAILURE

The treatment of renal failure has dramatically changed the evolution of its clinical manifestations. New neurological syndromes have been defined as a consequence both of increased longevity and of the complications of treatment, and some syndromes are now no longer seen (Table 18.10).

Table 18.10 Neurological complications of renal failure

Effects of uraemia
Encephalopathy
Seizures
Myoclonus
Peripheral neuropathy
Myopathy
Effects of treatment
Dialysis
Dialysis disequilibrium syndrome
Dialysis dementia
Subdural haematoma
Transplantation (immunosuppression)
Infections
Lymphomas
Others
Wernicke–Korsakoff syndrome
Central Pontine myelinolysis
Drug sensitivity
e.g. aminoglycosides

Uraemic encephalopathy

Alterations of alertness and awareness are early signs: patients may be apathetic, with poor concentration. Obtundation and coma may become apparent as the metabolic abnormality becomes more marked. Occasionally, frank hallucinations with agitation may be present, producing the clinical picture of delirium; dysarthria may accompany these features.

Asterixis is a sensitive and early indication of uraemic encephalopathy despite its occurrence in many other metabolic abnormalities; tremulousness may occur, as may multifocal myoclonus. Tetany, as evinced by carpopedal spasms, may accompany the myoclonus.

Motor abnormalities in the form of clumsiness and unsteadiness occur at an early stage and primitive reflexes develop. In profound uraemia, extensor posturing may be seen and occasionally there are focal signs such as hemiparesis. Convulsions are usually a late manifestation of chronic renal failure and they may be generalised or focal. Epilepsia partialis continua may occur without generalised seizures.

The electroencephalogram often shows slow background activity with an excess of theta or delta waves. In patients with seizures, foci of spike activity may be seen and, as the uraemic state progresses, the electroencephalogram becomes gradually slower.

Signs of meningeal irritation with neck stiffness occasionally occur in patients with uraemia and a proportion of these patients show pleocytosis in the c.s.f., which also commonly contains an increased level of protein.

A variety of neuropathological changes may be found in patients with fatal uraemic encephalopathy, but many of the changes described are non-specific and not necessarily related to the uraemic state. Cerebral oedema does not result from uraemia.

The uraemic patient is susceptible to the toxic effects of a variety of drugs because of his inability to excrete them: these therefore may influence the clinical picture and produce specific abnormalities: for example, dystonic reactions may occur with only small doses of phenothiazines.

The neurological effects of uraemia are similar to those of other toxic-metabolic disorders affecting the nervous system. The clinical features of uraemic encephalopathy do not correlate precisely with any single biochemical abnormality, but are related more to the rate of development of the biochemical disturbance; profound encephalopathy is thus more common in acute than in chronic renal failure.

Uraemic neuropathy

Peripheral neuropathy occurs in at least two-thirds of patients who are about to begin dialysis for chronic failure and is usually a distal symmetrical mixed sensorimotor polyneuropathy. The rates of progression of the neuropathy are quite variable, although it follows a more rapid course in men than in women. Occasionally such patients have symptoms of the 'restless legs' syndrome, preceding the development of the peripheral neuropathy. Another early manifestation is that of burning feet, similar to that encountered in alcoholics, and muscle cramps are also common. In some patients a fulminant course occurs, with rapidly developing flaccid quadriplegia. Effective treatment by haemodialysis will usually either stabilise or improve the neuropathy, and most patients who undergo a successful renal transplant have complete resolution of their symptoms.

Even in asymptomatic patients with uraemia, evidence of a peripheral neuropathy can be found on nerve conduction studies. Pathologically, the neuropathy appears to be a primary axonal degeneration with secondary demyelination. The observation that uraemic neuropathy improves with dialysis has led to the conclusion that it results from the accumulation of a dialysable metabolite, but this has not been identified.

Neurological complications of dialysis

The dialysis disequilibrium syndrome

This syndrome is usually only seen in its most florid form following rapid dialysis in the early stages of a dialysis programme. It begins with headache, nausea and muscle cramps and then is followed by agitation, delirium, coma and convulsions. Headache alone is a very common symptom in patients undergoing dialysis and the commonest variety of this is a migrainous type of headache.

The evidence suggests that the cause of this syndrome is shifts of water into the brain, producing features similar to those of water intoxication. Less rapid dialysis usually will prevent the syndrome developing.

Subdural haematoma

Patients on haemodialysis are frequently given anticoagulant treatment, and subdural haematoma is a well-recognised complication. In the early stages the symptoms often occur only in relation to dialysis, but eventually they become persistent.

Wernicke's encephalopathy

Thiamine is a water-soluble vitamin which may pass through the dialysis membranes with ease, thus bringing about deficiency of the vitamin in patients undergoing regular dialysis. Wernicke's encephalopathy is, however, a rare complication of dialysis and may be prevented by good nutritional advice.

Central pontine myelinolysis

This rare syndrome occasionally occurs in patients who are undergoing regular dialysis and usually is associated with hyponatraemia.

Progressive dialysis dementia

Until a few years ago this condition was one of the commonest causes of death in patients undergoing regular haemodialysis. It is a progressive encephalopathy characterised by disturbances of speech, dementia, involuntary movements, seizures, and eventually death. In the early stages the symptoms appear during dialysis and remit during the ensuing 4–12 hours; eventually, however, the clinical features become gradually progressive and death occurs within a matter of a few months to a year. There is now very good evidence to suggest that the condition is attributable to aluminium intoxication; deionising the dialysate of aluminium has led to the virtual disappearance of the disorder.

Neurological complications of renal transplantation

Brain tumours

The risk that lymphoma will develop after a renal transplant is about 35 times greater than normal, derived almost entirely from an increased incidence of reticulum cell sarcoma. At least half of these tumours involve the central nervous system and in over one-third the brain alone is affected.

Infections of the nervous system

The immunosuppressed state which accompanies renal transplantation predisposes to unusual infections. These include mycotic infections of the blood and brain, of which aspergillosis and candidiasis are the most common; toxoplasmosis, herpes simplex and cytomegalovirus infections of the brain also occur.

SPECIFIC PATHOLOGICAL PROCESSES

THE NEUROLOGICAL EFFECTS OF MALIGNANT DISEASE

Apart from direct spread to the nervous system, malignant disease may produce a number of remote effects via a series of differing mechanisms. These include:

1. Haematological abnormalities such as excessive bleeding secondary to marrow involvement or thrombotic microangiography.
2. Cardiological abnormalities such as marantic endocarditis with emboli to the brain.
3. The effects of cachexia and malnutrition on the nervous system.
4. Opportunistic infections resulting from diminished resistance.
5. C.n.s. disturbances resulting from endocrine and metabolic disturbances, for example, hypercalcaemia and dilutional hyponatraemia.
6. The complications of treatment of malignant disease, for example of radiotherapy and chemotherapy.
7. A group of disorders of uncertain aetiology (the so-called paraneoplastic syndromes).

The last few years have seen an increasing recognition of the idiopathic paraneoplastic syndromes which may occur in association with malignant disease. Some general points concerning these syndromes should be noted:

1. They may occur in association with almost any malignant disease, but are chiefly seen in the common malignancies such as carcinoma of the breast or lung.
2. These neurological syndromes may precede the obvious clinical development of the malignancy, or may occur in a patient who is known to have a malignant disease.
3. In some instances the evolution of the neurological problem is influenced by treatment of the underlying malignancy. Complete resolution of one of these neurological syndromes subsequent to 'cure' of the underlying malignancy is, however, exceptional.
4. With certain exceptions the aetiology of the syndromes is unknown, but there is increasing evidence that some may have an immunological basis and others be due to opportunistic infection.

The paraneoplastic syndromes may be conveniently divided into three groups: the encephalopathies, the myelopathies and the neuromyopathies.

The paraneoplastic encephalopathies

Progressive multifocal leucoencephalopathy (p. 319)

This demyelinating disease is seen usually in patients with reticuloses and may also follow immunosuppressive therapy, suggesting the release of a latent virus infection due to altered immunological competence. Pathologically, there are eosinophilic intranuclear inclusions in the oligodendroglia and a papovavirus (SV 40) has been isolated. The patient presents with epileptic fits, dementia and focal neurological signs; the condition usually progresses rapidly to death.

Dementia

Impairment of mental faculties is a common feature in a variety of malignant diseases; its neuropathological basis has been poorly documented.

Encephalomyelitis

Some patients with malignancies show evidence of damage at varying levels within the nervous system and at autopsy there are signs of an inflammatory process affecting the brain, brain stem, spinal cord, posterior root ganglia and nerve roots. The inflammatory reaction consists of perivascular cuffing by lymphocytes, with associated damage to, and loss of, neurones. Some patients may present with features of multifocal involvement of the neuroaxis, but two clinical syndromes are worthy of mention.

Limbic encephalitis is the term applied to subacute encephalitis occurring in patients with malignancy who show with features of a memory disturbance; seizures may occur and dementia usually is the end result. Pathologically, the brunt of the inflammatory process is borne by the hippocampal formation.

Subacute brain stem encephalitis may occur, with predominant involvement of the medulla. Symptoms of vertigo, vomiting, nystagmus and ataxia predominate, although occasionally the clinical picture may be one of progressive bulbar palsy. One other variant of this syndrome which has been recognised is that of *opsoclonic cerebellopathy*, in which cerebellar signs and opsoclonus are prominent features.

In this group of diseases pleocytosis is often found in the c.s.f. and the clinical syndromes usually progress rapidly, leading to death within one or two years.

Cortical cerebellar degeneration

This is one of the more common encephalopathies, with a very characteristic clinical and pathological pattern. Clinically the picture is one of acute or subacute progressive cerebellar disturbance, which, in some instances, may progress to the full-blown picture within a month. Prominent symptoms are ataxia of the limbs and gait, dysarthria and vertigo; nystagmus occurs in approximately one-half of the patients. Macroscopically the cerebellum appears normal, but microscopic examination shows a striking loss of Purkinje cells. In a typical case the diagnosis is so obvious that a careful screening of the patients for an underlying malignancy is mandatory. The prognosis is poor and there is no beneficial treatment.

Central pontine myelinolysis

This syndrome occurs in a variety of different situations, usually being associated with cachexia and a low serum sodium.

Remote effects of cancer on the spinal cord

There is some confusion in the literature concerning an association between spinal cord disorders and malignant disease: the suggested association between motor neurone disease and malignant disease has yet to be substantiated. The one clearly defined syndrome that does appear to be associated with malignant disease is the syndrome of *subacute necrotising myelopathy*: this is a rare clinical syndrome of unknown aetiology which presents with a rapidly ascending spinal cord disturbance, with an ascending paraplegia usually progressing over days or weeks; pathologically, there is massive and extensive necrosis of the cord with microscopic cavitation.

The carcinomatous neuromyopathies

Subacute sensory neuropathy

This is a very characteristic clinical syndrome presenting with a painful sensory neuropathy developing over weeks or months. Pathologically there is degeneration of neurones in the dorsal root ganglia and the dorsal columns, with a lymphocytic infiltration.

Sensorimotor polyneuropathy

Subacute or chronic mixed peripheral neuropathy may occur in patients with malignant disease, and there are no particular characteristic features to suggest the diagnosis of an underlying malignancy. Occasionally a more rapidly developing form of polyneuropathy may occur, resembling the Guillain–Barré syndrome.

Myasthenia gravis

This characteristic clinical syndrome is occasionally associated with a tumour of the thymus.

The myasthenic syndrome (Eaton–Lambert syndrome)

This syndrome most typically occurs in patients with oat cell bronchogenic carcinoma. It is characterised by fatiguable muscle weakness and the EMG shows typical changes (see p. 251).

Myopathy

Non-specific proximal weakness is common in patients with malignant disease and in many instances this is attributable to a degree of myopathy. A syndrome indistinguishable on pathological or clinical grounds from polymyositis occurs in some patients with visceral malignancies and 20% of all patients with polymyositis have an underlying tumour. There may be skin manifestations, producing the clinical picture of dermatomyositis.

Investigations

The wide clinical pattern of syndromes described above covers many conditions that present to the neurologist or physician and it may be questioned how far such patients should be investigated in looking for an underlying malignancy: for example, to what extent should a patient presenting with a mixed peripheral neuropathy be investigated when a malignant disease is only one of the possible causes? In general this is usually a matter of the physician's personal choice, but there is no doubt that certain clinical syndromes justify intensive investigation: these include the syndrome of subacute cerebellar degeneration, subacute sensory neuropathy, polymyositis in men over 40 years of age, and the Eaton–Lambert syndrome.

THE COLLAGEN VASCULAR DISORDERS
(Connective tissue disease)

These diseases are somewhat arbitrarily included together as disorders which have several common histological features, some common clinical features, and other features which suggest that they may have an immunological basis. The disorders are listed below and many of them are considered in other chapters:

1. Systemic lupus erythematosus
2. Polyarteritis nodosa
3. Giant cell arteritis
4. Thrombotic thrombocytopenia purpura
5. Dermatomyositis
6. Scleroderma/systemic sclerosis
7. Rheumatoid arthritis
8. Ankylosing spondylitis
9. Granulomatous arteritis
10. Polymyalgia rheumatica
11. Wegener's granulomatosis
12. The aortic arch arteritis
13. Rheumatic fever
14. Sjögren's syndrome.

Systemic lupus erythematosis (SLE)

At least 25% of patients with SLE will show neurological complications, the most frequent manifestations of which are seizures or a psychosis. Pathologically, the neurological complications are caused by the vasculitis, and recurrent disseminated lesions may occur at various levels within the nervous system: these may result in focal neurological deficits such as hemiplegia, a variety of brain stem signs, transverse myelitis, mononeuritis multiplex and polymyositis—these syndromes often occurring in combination. Rarer neurological complications are subarachnoid haemorrhages and cerebral embolism from the non-bacterial endocarditis (Libman–Sacks endocarditis), which is occasionally associated with SLE. In such cases the cerebrospinal fluid often shows a raised protein level pleocytosis and antiDNA antibodies. Central nervous system involvement is an indication for treatment with corticosteroids and/or immunosuppressive agents.

Polyarteritis nodosa

The vasculitis associated with this condition may produce a pattern of abnormalities similar to that of SLE and the neurological complications may be the presenting feature; mononeuritis multiplex is the most common of these. Cerebral symptoms are less common than in SLE and, occasionally, a spinal cord syndrome may occur.

Wegener's granulomatosis

This rare condition usually affects the peripheral nervous system, producing mononeuritis multiplex. The granulomatous angiitis, which is the hallmark of this condition, very occasionally may affect the central nervous system.

Rheumatoid arthritis

Rheumatoid arthritis is a disease which is not limited to the joints, although joint involvement affecting the spinal column produces the commonest neurological complications: these are spinal cord compression in the cervical cord resulting either from atlantoaxial subluxation or from subaxial disease affecting the cervical vertebrae; this occurs in as many as one-third of patients. Involvement of the lower spine less commonly produces compression of the cauda equina. The connective tissue changes of rheumatoid arthritis often involve peripheral nerves, to produce mononeuritis, the most common form of which is the carpal tunnel syndrome. In some patients with rheumatoid arthritis, necrotising arteritis develops, which produces a very striking mononeuritis multiplex; the prognosis for this is poor and, paradoxically, treatment with corticosteroids appears to have a deleterious effect. Involvement of the central nervous system by a vasculitic process is a rare complication of rheumatoid arthritis; laryngeal paralysis may appear, with involvement of the cricoarytenoid joint.

Ankylosing spondylitis

The spinal involvement of ankylosing spondylosis may sometimes produce spinal cord compression, which usually occurs in the lumbar region, leading to compression of the cauda equina. Involvement at the level of the atlantoaxial joint may produce atlantoaxial subluxation, and cervical spine involvement occasionally produces distortion of the vertebral artery, resulting in brain stem ischaemia.

Polymyalgia rheumatica

This is a not uncommon disorder of patients in the older age groups, characterised by aching muscles and stiffness; muscle weakness is not a feature and the sedimentation rate is usually markedly elevated. Some of these patients may subsequently develop cranial arteritis. The syndrome responds dramatically to prednisone and is usually self-limiting.

INFLAMMATORY DISORDERS OF UNCERTAIN AETIOLOGY

Sarcoidosis

Sarcoidosis is a systemic granulomatous disease of uncertain aetiology with involvement of multiple organs of the body, the nervous system being involved in as many as 5% of cases. Pathologically, the involvement takes one of three forms:

1. Diffuse granulomatous leptomeningeal infiltration
2. Diffuse perivascular infiltration
3. Granulomatous mass.

In the meningeal form, cranial nerve palsies and hypothalamic or pituitary disorders are common. The most usually involved cranial nerve is the seventh, which may be affected bilaterally. Spinal cord or root involvement is less usual and involvement of the peripheral nerves is rare. Skeletal muscle involvement with myopathy occurs quite commonly, although this is often asymptomatic and discovered only on muscle biopsy. Diffuse perivascular involvement of the brain is uncommon, but has a bad prognosis. Local tumour masses may be intracerebral or intraspinal and may mimic a neoplasm. Progressive multifocal leucoencephalopathy is a rare complication of sarcoidosis. Hypercalcaemia of sarcoidosis occasionally may affect the nervous system.

Behçet's disease

This is a chronic relapsing disease characterised by iritis, aphthous ulcers of the mouth or genitals, and involvement of a variety of other organs including skin, joints, heart and central nervous system. Thrombophlebitis is a common accompaniment. Neurological manifestations occur in 10–20% of cases: in some instances this takes the form of aseptic meningitis, but there may be involvement of the central nervous system with a picture akin to that of ascending or transverse myelitis, an encephalitic-type illness with delirium, convulsions and stupor, or a progressive syndrome attributable to brain stem involvement. There may be sudden neurological deficits simulating strokes. A syndrome mimicking benign intracranial hypertension is sometimes seen, possibly due to cerebral venous thrombosis.

Reiter's disease

This presents with the triad of urethritis, conjunctivitis and arthritis. Neurological involvement is rare, the most common complication being distal polyneuropathy or mononeuritis multiplex. Central nervous system involvement in the form of a meningoencephalitis has been described.

Uveomeningoencephalitis

This rare syndrome is characterised by the combination of uveitis and relapsing meningoencephalitis: in its fullblown form these are accompanied by deafness and depigmentation of the skin and hair; this particular combination is characterised as the Vogt–Koyangi–Harada syndrome. The aetiology is uncertain, but it is possible that some of the abortive cases are simply manifestations of a viral disease. These cases often enter the differential diagnosis of meningitis of uncertain aetiology.

THE DEFICIENCY DISORDERS

Introduction

Worldwide these disorders usually arise from a primary nutritional deficiency resulting from inadequate intake. Other causes are listed in Table 18.11: in the western hemisphere, alcoholism is one of the common causes.

Protein-calorie malnutrition

Worldwide this, unfortunately, is an all-too-prevalent condition and during fetal life maternal starvation may produce a variety of effects. The child at birth has a lower birth weight and a smaller head size than average and, if the malnutrition continues during the first year or so after birth, then permanent mental retardation may result. Such deprivation in the second and third years of life probably does not produce a similar effect.

A diet lacking predominantly protein results in the fairly specific clinical pathological picture of kwashiorkor. Neurological manifestations include mental changes, such as apathy and retardation, and the EEGs in these children show very striking abnormalities with slower than expected wave forms. When such children are treated they often develop a mixed combination of physical signs such as tremors, hyper-reflexia and myoclonus. If treated early enough, complete recovery may occur, although in some cases mental retardation may be a permanent after-effect.

Table 18.11 Causes of deficiency disorders

Failure of input
Starvation
Failure of absorption
Malabsorption syndromes
Impairment of metabolism
Liver failure
Drug interaction
Increased use
e.g. folate and pregnancy

Vitamin deficiency disorders

Vitamin A

Deficiency of vitamin A in adults and children produces night blindness at an early stage, followed by keratinisation of the cornea which may lead to permanent damage to the eye. Deficiency in infants may be associated with mental retardation, hydrocephalus, and facial palsy. Vitamin A intoxication (for example, following vitamin tablet abuse or eating polar bear's livers) produces cerebral oedema resulting in headaches and papilloedema. The clinical picture simulates that of benign intracranial hypertension.

Vitamin B_1 (thiamine) deficiency

Thiamine deficiency produces characteristic systemic symptoms, such as anorexia, within as short a period as three months. The neurological complications are:

1. Peripheral neuropathy
2. Amblyopia
3. The Wernicke–Korsakoff syndrome.

Peripheral neuropathy Thiamine deficiency as a result of nutritional deprivation produces beri beri, which is the combination of polyneuropathy and myocardial dilatation due to cardiac muscle failure. The neuropathy is usually distal, symmetrical and ascending, beginning with paraesthesiae in the feet and often accompanied by pain. In some cases, motor involvement predominates and, in others, sensory involvement; the neuropathy is axonal in nature. Strachan's syndrome includes the triad of sensory ataxia, atrophy of the optic nerve and nerve deafness, and is thought to be due to nutritional deprivation resulting in thiamine deficiency. In infants, cerebral symptoms predominate with cerebral oedema, apathy, rigidity and convulsions.

Amblyopia. Thiamine deficiency may produce progressive impairment of function of the optic nerves characterised by visual failure, progressive optic atrophy and central scotomas.

Wernicke–Korsakoff syndrome. The original descriptions of these conditions were quite separate, Wernicke's disease being characterised by nystagmus, abnormalities of eye movement, ataxia of gait and confusion and Korsakoff's psychosis being characterised by a unique mental disorder in which retentive memory is predominantly affected. It is now recognised that it is rare for the disorders to occur separately and, as they both result from thiamine deficiency in the adult, they are usually considered together, as the Wernicke–Korsakoff syndrome.

This disorder occurs most frequently in alcoholics between the ages of 30 and 70 years. It, occasionally, is first seen following an episode of delirium tremens but may present in isolation. Early symptoms are those of ataxia, ocular disturbances or confusion; some impairment of consciousness is common but frank coma is rare. A global confusional state associated with lethargy and drowsiness is the most common combination. Ocular abnormalities are common including nystagmus, paralysis of individual extraocular muscles, conjugate gaze palsies and pupillary abnormalities and ptosis. Ataxia of gait and limb ataxia with dysarthria may occur and usually such patients have signs of associated peripheral neuropathy. Tachycardia is common. In the acute stages there is no response to caloric testing and this is thought to result from vestibular paresis.

Without treatment, patients with this syndrome die and it is important that they are given high doses of thiamine at an early stage. After such treatment there may be a dramatic improvement in the ocular signs, but the confusion will usually persist for some time. As the confusion clears it is usually possible to detect the amnestic component of the Korsakoff psychosis, which may be very gross, such that the patient may forget the examiner's name within a few minutes of learning it; confabulation is a prominent feature. Complete recovery of the memory defect occurs in only a small proportion of patients, although improvement may continue for up to 3–6 months. In patients who die in the acute stages, the brain shows characteristic features with haemorrhagic lesions affecting the mamillary bodies, the brain stem, the thalamus and the hypothalamus.

Nicotinic acid and nicotinamide deficiency (pellagra)

This is characterised by the combination of dermatitis, glossitis, stomatitis, gastroenteritis, proctitis and neurological complications, of which peripheral neuropathy is the most common. In the full-blown picture of pellagra, a psychosis develops which may be followed by stupor and coma. Seizures may occur and at this stage, parkinsonian rigidity is often a striking feature.

Pyridoxine (vitamin B_6) deficiency

In infants, pyridoxine deficiency may present as seizures which respond dramatically to replacement therapy. These occur in two separate syndromes: vitamin B_6 deficiency resulting in seizures and vitamin B_6 'dependent' seizures. Vitamin B_6 is important in the metabolism of GABA and decreased GABA levels may be the cause of the seizures.

In adults, vitamin B_6 deficiency most commonly is seen in patients who are being treated with isoniazid for tuberculosis. This shows itself as a peripheral neuropathy and patients being treated with isoniazid should routinely be given pyridoxine. Rarely, a psychosis may occur.

Folic acid

There is considerable debate as to whether folic acid deficiency may affect the nervous system. The inter-relationship between epanutin and folic acid has been studied at great length and is considered in the section on epilepsy. There is some evidence to suggest that a pure folic acid deficiency may be associated with peripheral neuropathy and even mental changes, but this is disputed. Some patients with a picture of subacute combined degeneration of the spinal cord have also been reported with folate deficiency only.

Vitamin B_{12} deficiency (subacute combined degeneration of the spinal cord)

This most commonly occurs as pernicious anaemia: the neurological complications may occur before the anaemia is discovered, or may accompany the anaemia. Pathologically there is demyelination in the white matter of the spinal cord, usually in the dorsal columns. The lateral columns are often similarly affected; the anterolateral or spinothalamic columns less often affected. Peripheral nerves similarly show an abnormality. In severe cases there is evidence of demyelination in the white matter of the cerebral hemispheres and involvement of the optic nerves.

Clinically, sensory symptoms are among the earliest to develop, often starting with dysaesthesia in the hands, which then spreads proximally and becomes followed by proprioceptive loss in the hands and feet. Positive symptoms, such as tight bands around the hands, feet and trunk, and Lhermitte's phenomenon are common. Motor disturbances in the form of weakness may occasionally be early symptoms and, as the condition progresses, are invariable. Autonomic disturbances such as involvement of bladder and bowel function are rare. Visual loss attributable to optic nerve involvement and mental changes occur in severe cases and may, in some instances, be the presenting feature. The combination of peripheral nerve and dorsal column involvement with corticospinal tract involvement, produces in the legs, a very characteristic finding of absent reflexes with extensor plantar responses.

The prognosis is directly related to the length of time the neurological symptoms have been present. The diagnosis should be borne in mind in all patients presenting with peripheral neuropathy, myelopathy of uncertain aetiology, and dementia.

Deficiencies of other vitamins

Vitamin C deficiency rarely produces nervous system manifestations in adults, but it may be associated with a bleeding tendency, resulting in a subdural haematoma; this is much more common when the deficiency occurs in infancy. Abnormalities of vitamin D metabolism produce disturbances of calcium metabolism and are dealt with elsewhere. Vitamin K deficiency results in a haemorrhagic diathesis (see above). For many years it has been suggested that vitamin E deficiency produces a number of neurological abnormalities, but this has always been disputed. A recent suggestion has been made that vitamin E deficiency is the cause of the cerebellar ataxia which occurs in some forms of malabsorption syndrome. There is no doubt that there are a number of neurological manifestations which occur in malabsorption syndromes, such as coeliac disease, and which have yet to be defined as being caused by specific deficiency disorders.

Mineral depletion syndromes and the trace elements

Deficiencies of minerals such as sodium and calcium are considered in the endocrine section. For many years there has been interest in the question of trace element deficiency and neurological disorders. So far, it has not been possible to define a specific role for trace element deficiency in producing neurological abnormalities.

THE NEUROLOGY OF PREGNANCY

A variety of neurological problems may be seen in pregnancy. In some, the association is merely that of coincidence, but in the majority considered here the conditions are either caused or aggravated by the pregnancy. We have made no attempt to classify disorders by aetiology. There are at least three possible mechanisms whereby neurological conditions may occur in pregnancy:

1. Conditions occurring as a direct result of the physical, physiological, or pathological changes occurring in pregnancy
2. Conditions merely aggravated by the physical or physiological changes during pregnancy
3. Conditions resulting from procedures or therapy given during the pregnancy or at the time of birth.

In this section we have adopted a disease-orientated classification (Table 18.12).

Table 18.12 Neurological complications of pregnancy

Eclampsia
Vascular disorders
Hypertension
Cerebral venous thrombosis
Arterial occlusive disease
Rare forms of cerebral infarction
Intracranial haemorrhage
Caroticocavernous fistula
Neuropathies
Muscle disorder
Infections
Tetanus
Multiple sclerosis
Tumours
Headache
Epilepsy
Psychoses
Rare disorders
Chorea gravidarum

ECLAMPSIA

Though one of the best recognised, this is fortunately one of the rarest disorders to be seen in pregnancy, although there is considerable variation in the incidence in different parts of the world. The term is defined as epileptic seizures and/or other neurological deficits occurring as a result of the toxaemia of pregnancy. The onset of the seizures may occur during the last trimester of pregnancy, during labour, and rarely is seen more than 24 hours after delivery.

The convulsions are usually preceded by premonitory signs and symptoms such as headache and there is invariably hypertension, albuminuria and oedema. The neurological features are similar to hypertensive encephalopathy, although the blood pressure may not be so markedly raised. Visual symptoms are common, occurring either on the basis of gross retinal changes or as a result of occipital lobe ischaemia; other symptoms of focal cerebral ischaemia may occur. Recovery usually occurs, although occasionally there may be persisting deficits and death may result from intracranial haemorrhage or uncontrolled status epilepticus. Treatment should be directed to the control of blood pressure.

VASCULAR DISORDERS

Hypertension

Hypertension in pregnancy may be a manifestation of toxaemia, but may in some instances be due to those causes which occur in non-pregnant females. It is particularly important that there is satisfactory control of the hypertension, which may predispose to accelerated toxaemia and even to eclampsia. Persisting hypertension post-partum may occur and be associated with the usual neurological problems.

Cerebral venous thrombosis

This produces a well-recognised syndrome which occurs after delivery, usually within the first three weeks post partum. The clinical features are those of a rapidly progressive focal neurological deficit accompanied by focal or generalised convulsions. The neurological deficit may progress and be associated with symptoms and signs of raised intracranial pressure; in such cases the prognosis is poor (p. 290).

The cause is uncertain; in some instances it may be due to the hormonal changes occurring at this time predisposing to in situ thrombosis; in some it is thought that pelvic vein clots are carried by the paravertebral venous plexus to the cranium.

Arterial occlusions

These occur in pregnancy and may affect either the cerebral blood vessels or the spinal vessels. The causes are uncertain and there is some debate as to whether the incidence of such disorders is any more common during pregnancy.

Rarer forms of stroke

Air embolism and amniotic fluid embolism are rarer causes of cerebral ischaemia and are thought to result from air or amniotic fluid entering the systemic circulation and reaching the brain. Both usually occur either during labour or shortly thereafter.

Intracranial haemorrhage (p. 282, p. 286)

Subarachnoid haemorrhage may occur in pregnancy, due either to ruptured intracranial aneurysm or bleeding from an arteriovenous malformation. Bleeding most commonly occurs during the third trimester or during delivery. Any patient known to have an aneurysm or arteriovenous malformation is at risk of bleed during the pregnancy and delivery should usually be by elective caesarian section.

Caroticocavernous fistula

This rare condition may develop following delivery and in women childbirth is one of the commonest causes.

NEUROPATHIES (Ch. 10)

A variety of different pathological mechanisms may damage the cranial and peripheral nerves during pregnancy, although in some the prognosis is uncertain. Such mechanisms are:

1. Due to physiological changes of pregnancy, e.g. water retention (carpal tunnel syndrome).
2. Mechanical, e.g. traction during labour (obdurator nerve palsy).
3. Vitamin deficiency (thiamine deficiency—rare).

Only common conditions are discussed here.

Bell's palsy

This appears to be not uncommon in pregnancy and is usually seen in the second trimester. The increased risk during pregnancy is thought to be due to a tendency of the facial nerve to swell as a result of the physiological changes of pregnancy. Prognosis is good.

Peripheral mononeuropathies

Of these the most common is carpal tunnel syndrome and this usually responds to symptomatic treatment. Resolution in the puerperium is almost invariable.

Pressure palsies during pregnancy

These may occur as a result of damage to the lumbosacral plexus during delivery, or as a result of inappropriate positioning of one of the lower limbs during anaesthesia for either a vaginal delivery or caesarian section. Prognosis is universally good.

LUMBAR DISC DISEASE

There has been debate for many years regarding the risk of lumbar disc prolapse during pregnancy. Low back pain and leg pain during pregnancy is common and often has been attributed to lumbar disc prolapse. In many such cases the pain is probably due to compression of the lumbosacral plexus. Rest is the treatment of choice.

MUSCLE DISORDERS

There is little definite evidence that any muscular disorder is either aggravated or precipitated during pregnancy. There is some suggestion that relapses of myasthenia gravis may occur during pregnancy, but the association is by no means clear cut. What is true for all the neuromuscular disorders is that they may complicate the delivery and the patient may be fatigued during the pregnancy. In view of the risk of neonatal myasthenia specific care needs to be taken of mother and infant at the time of delivery in myasthenia gravis.

INFECTIONS

A variety of infections may occur during pregnancy and affect the nervous system. In many the association is merely coincidental; one exception to this is tetanus resulting from pelvic infection during the puerperium, and this most commonly results from inadequate technique in the context of criminal abortion.

CHOREA GRAVIDARUM

It has long been known that an acute form of chorea may occur during pregnancy and its relationship to poststreptococcal chorea (Sydenham's chorea) is uncertain. Most attacks occur in the first pregnancy and there is a tendency to recurrence. In most patients symptoms begin in the first two trimesters of pregnancy.

MULTIPLE SCLEROSIS (Ch. 16)

Although the first symptoms of multiple sclerosis may develop during pregnancy the evidence suggests that the risk of relapse during pregnancy is reduced. It is rare for severely affected patients with multiple sclerosis to become pregnant and, hence, it is uncommon for difficulties with labour to ensue, because of physical incapacity.

TUMOURS

Cerebral tumours (Ch. 13)

It is rare for intracranial tumours to develop during pregnancy, but there is a well-recognised association between pregnancy and the development of symptoms of cerebral tumours as a result of swelling of the tumours; this association is recognised most particularly for pituitary tumours and for intracranial meningiomas. When symptoms develop early in the pregnancy, appropriate surgical treatment will need to be given; if the symptoms develop towards the end of the pregnancy elective caesarian section should be undertaken and the tumour then should be treated on its own merits.

Spinal tumours

These may similarly enlarge during pregnancy with the development of symptoms of spinal cord compression. In most instances surgical treatment will need to be undertaken.

BENIGN INTRACRANIAL HYPERTENSION

This condition may develop for the first time during pregnancy and treatment with repeated lumbar punctures may have practical difficulties. The condition usually resolves following delivery.

HEADACHE AND MIGRAINE

The development of headache during pregnancy is unusual, but occasional tension headaches may develop for the first time and usually emotional factors may be incriminated.

The haemodynamic changes of pregnancy may in some women induce vascular headaches akin to a typical migraine.

The headaches of migraine (p. 194) usually get better during pregnancy. Occasionally, in the third trimester the vasospastic symptoms of migraine may develop for the first time or become more prominent and this may be particularly frightening in someone who has never previously suffered such symptoms. The diagnosis can be made on clinical grounds and prognosis is good.

EPILEPSY (Ch. 7)

Four separate components should be considered:

1. The effect of epilepsy on pregnancy
2. The effect of the pregnancy on epilepsy
3. The effect of the drugs on the fetus
4. Breast feeding.

See page 178 for discussion of epilepsy and pregnancy.

PSYCHOSES ASSOCIATED WITH PREGNANCY

These are prone to develop during the puerperium, but may occur at any stage of pregnancy. So-called puerperal psychosis may take many forms, but most commonly is a manifestation of agitated depression.

DISORDERS PREVIOUSLY RECORDED AS OCCURRING IN PREGNANCY (now rare)

Modern medical practice has seen the virtual disappearance of a variety of disorders which previously used to be seen in pregnancy, but which are now virtually unheard of: these include damage due to the inappropriate administration of drugs, damage from poorly managed general anaesthetics, damage from poorly managed spinal anaesthetics, and damage from abortifacients. Similarly, vitamin deficiencies due to malnutrition during pregnancy are now extremely rare in the civilised world.

FURTHER READING

Aita J A 1964 Neurologic manifestations of general diseases. C C Thomas, Springfield, Illinois

Spillane J D 1947 Nutritional disorders of the nervous system. Williams & Wilkins, Baltimore

Vinken P J, Bruyn G W 1979 Neurological manifestations of systemic disease. In: Handbook of clinical neurology, vols 38, 39. North Holland Publishing Company

19

Functional and psychiatric disorders

INTRODUCTION

This chapter is concerned with the wide variety of disorders that straddle the boundaries between the specialties of neurology and psychiatry. Among the most common are symptoms simulating neurological disorders, which occur as a manifestation of a psychosomatic illness: tension headache falls into this category. The differentiation of organic neurological disturbances from functional disorders is often difficult and in some instances (as will be seen below) may be made only after prolonged and intensive investigation: in other words, the diagnosis of a functional disorder can often be made only after organic disorders have been excluded.

Organic psychiatric disorders, on the other hand, tend to have certain clinical features in common, which allow them to be distinguished on clinical grounds from non-organic mental illnesses. However, certain organic disorders such as confusion may occur as the manifestation of widely differing pathologies. Such disorders as confusion and dementia, therefore, are not a diagnosis, they are merely a symptom and an underlying cause should always be sought.

The symptoms that may be common to both organic disorder of the brain and functional disorders of the mind make the diagnosis of these extremely difficult; indeed psychiatry is often regarded as one of the most difficult specialties and was termed by the late Henry Miller 'neurology without physical signs'.

One group of disorders that merits discussion are those neurological abnormalities that present with symptoms suggesting a psychiatric disturbance, e.g. a patient with a frontal tumour presenting with personality change. Another group of disorders comprises psychiatric illnesses presenting to the neurologist, e.g. a patient with retarded depression simulating the dementia of Alzheimer's disease; finally, there are those neurological illnesses often complicated by a psychiatric disturbance, e.g. the patient with mild multiple sclerosis who has a gross functional overlay resulting in apparent paraplegia.

DISTURBANCES OF DIFFERING NEUROLOGICAL FUNCTIONS

CONSCIOUSNESS

Organic disturbances of consciousness are considered in Chapter 6. As mentioned there, stupor and coma rarely occur, either as a psychosomatic manifestation or as a manifestation of psychiatric illness. Stupor may occur in severe depression, as a manifestation of hysteria, or as a manifestation of catatonic schizophrenia; it may be differentiated from organic stupor by the normality of the EEG. Frank coma is rarely seen on a non-organic basis and when it does occur it is usually a manifestation of hysteria. Nystagmus to caloric stimulation (see p. 134) indicates that a coma is non-organic.

Periodic disturbances of consciousness are much more commonly seen in psychiatric illnesses. Blackouts are a not uncommon manifestation of depression, and fainting is often emotionally determined or precipitated by emotional disturbances. Neurotic vasodepressor fainting is usually accompanied by fear and anxiety and often has many features of associated hyperventilation. Hysterical fainting conversely occurs without anxiety.

One of the most difficult clinical syndromes is that of simulated seizures. Clinically it may be impossible to differentiate genuine from simulated seizures and the electroencephalogram is of considerable value in this situation. An epileptic fit associated with total loss of consciousness will usually be associated with an abnormality of the EEG at the time of the seizure and thereafter with a persisting abnormality for some hours. A normal EEG at the time of an apparent seizure or a normal EEG performed within a matter of an hour or so of an apparent tonic-clonic seizure exclude seizure discharge as the cause of the apparent loss of consciousness. Occasionally it is necessary to undertake ambulatory EEG monitoring in these cases.

Although it is rare in simulated seizures for the individual to bite his tongue or to become incontinent, minor degrees of bruising are not uncommon.

Mistaking genuine seizures for a non-organic disturbance occasionally occurs and is usually due either to a lack of basic knowledge or to a lack of information concerning the episode. Akinetic seizures in young people, or drop attacks in old people, may be mistaken for functional disturbances; similarly, the strange behaviour of postictal confusion may be readily mistaken for a psychiatric disturbance, as may postseizure automatisms.

The acutely disturbed behaviour of a patient who has become hypomanic, or who is in the excitable phase of a schizophrenic psychosis may readily be mistaken for an acute confusional episode and vice versa. The middle-aged person who suddenly develops garbled speech is more likely to have a Wernicke's aphasia than a confusional state or a psychiatric disturbance (see below).

INTEGRATIVE CORTICAL FUNCTION
(agnosia, aphasia and apraxia)

The organic causes of these are dealt with in Chapter 6. Disturbances of body image may occur in a variety of psychiatric disturbances: hysterics, for example, may complain that their body feels peculiar, distorted and out of shape. Similar symptoms are offered in schizophrenia, where there may be complaints that one half of the body feels distorted or larger than it should be. This type of body image disturbances, when attributed to organic disturbances, may be mistaken as functional, or as symptoms of a psychiatric illness.

Aphasia may be confused with a variety of psychiatric disturbances. The speech of a patient with Wernicke's aphasia may be mistaken for the schizophrenic 'word salad'. It also may be mistaken for an acute confusional state, or even thought to be a functional disturbance. Inability to get a word out, or difficulty with naming, are common symptoms in functional disorders and must be differentiated from a genuine aphasia. Even more gross examples are occasionally encountered, such as total inability to speak, produced by a patient in an attempt to claim compensation following a head injury (see below).

THE CRANIAL NERVES

Taste and smell—olfactory nerve

Although organic anosmia may in some people produce little in the way of symptoms, it may in others be associated with a profound disability. This appears to be more common in women, or in those in whom the sense of smell is important (for example wine connoisseurs). In such people loss of the sense of smell might have a quite devastating effect and depression is a common associated psychological disturbance.

Psychosomatic smell disturbances occur in a number of clinical syndromes. In hysteria, anosmia may be unilateral or bilateral whereas in malingering it is usually bilateral. In organic anosmia the perception of irritating odours through trigeminal pathways persists, whereas failure to react to irritating odours occurs in hysteria and in simulation. The ageusia which may accompany anosmia can be psychogenic, however, even if the anosmia is a result of confirmed organic pathology.

In addition to psychogenic anosmia there are subjective smell experiences that present problems of differential diagnosis. The olfactory hallucinations which occur in some people with temporal lobe epilepsy are very characteristic. Similar hallucinations may be experienced by patients with a variety of psychological disturbances and these are often rather more vague and continuous. A few very disturbed patients may complain that they can smell their body odour and in some instances this is a monosymptomatic psychosis. Parosmia and parageusia may occur as a complication of olfactory nerve damage and this is most commonly seen in damage following a head injury. It is easy to mistake this for a psychogenic disorder.

Vision—optic nerve

Visual disturbances are common psychogenic complaints. The common abnormalities include photophobia resulting in blepharospasm, convergence spasm, or spasm of accommodation, concentric contraction of the visual fields, micropsia, loss of vision, and amblyopia.

Photophobia is quite common: not infrequently, patients with headaches wear dark glasses in the mistaken belief that their headaches will be improved. Transient or continued blurring of vision is often seen after head injuries and such patients may show spasm of accommodation or have abnormal visual fields with concentric constriction or even spiral fields. Occasionally even a hemianopia may be simulated, although this is uncommon. The differentiation of simulated visual loss from organic disturbances may sometimes be difficult. The preservation of pupillary reactions in a blind patient does not necessarily mean that the visual loss is simulated, as such a pattern can be seen in cortical blindness. The preservation of optokinetic responses in an apparently blind patient, however, indicates that the visual loss is simulated. Visual evoked responses are often helpful in making this differentiation, but it should be noted that visual evoked responses may vary depending on the patient's attention and it is possible to alter these responses voluntarily by failing to concentrate on the visual stimulus. Genuine visual impairment is not uncommonly accompanied in the early stages by anxiety and in the later stages by depression. Genuine visual hallucinations may have an organic structural basis but, more commonly, are due to a diffuse organic or metabolic cerebral disturbance.

Double vision and other disorders of ocular motility—oculomotor nerves

Patients with a blepharospasm often complain that they are unable to open their eyes, simulating weakness of the levator palpebrae superioris. In fact, the spasm is caused by contraction of the orbicularis oculi. Psychogenic ocular muscle spasms with squint are not uncommon, as are complaints of monocular diplopia.

Any normal individual may readily break binocular vision and, when tired, may experience transient diplopia; this is a common symptom in neurotics. Total inability to move the eyes is rare as an organic disturbance in isolation, although theoretically it could occur in profound myasthenia gravis. In the absence of other signs, however, it is likely to be psychogenic in nature.

Hysterical nystagmus or voluntary nystagmus are uncommon but may pose diagnostic difficulties. Typically, the nystagmus is very fine and is brought on only by intense gaze.

One organic disorder that affects the extraocular muscles and that is sometimes mistakenly misdiagnosed as a functional disturbance is myasthenia gravis. The initial complaints may be vague and signs in the early stages may be difficult to elicit. Evident fatiguability of the extraocular muscles or of levator palpebrae superioris is one of the useful diagnostic clues, as is the response to intravenous edrophonium.

Facial disorders—trigeminal and facial nerves

Psychogenic sensory loss in the face in isolation is uncommon. However, an intermittent tingling in the face as a psychogenic symptom is seen not infrequently and usually occurs as part of the hyperventilation anxiety syndrome as a sensation of tingling in the lips and tongue. Psychogenic facial and dental pain are not uncommon. The aetiology of atypical facial pain remains uncertain, but there is a strong body of evidence to suggest that it is simply a variant of chronic tension headache and, in most instances, a manifestation of a psychoneurosis or of a depressive illness. Like most other forms of facial pain it is often misdiagnosed in the early stages as trigeminal neuralgia.

Psychogenic disturbances of the trigeminal musculature are uncommon. Trismus or tonic spasm of the muscles may occur in hysteria. Genuine weakness of the jaw muscles, attributable to a disorder such as myasthenia gravis and resulting in inability to close the jaw, may initially be mistaken for a psychogenic disorder; the associated signs of weakness of other muscles should allow the diagnosis subsequently to be made, however.

The commonest psychogenic facial nerve disorder is blepharospasm. Although this disorder may be a manifestation of an underlying organic disorder, such as Meiges syndrome, it usually occurs as a functional disorder and in some cases is a manifestation of frank hysteria. On the other hand, hemifacial spasm (which in some instances is misdiagnosed as a functional disturbance) is almost invariably organic. Psychogenic facial weakness is uncommon, but a genuine total unilateral facial weakness may, because of its cosmetic effects, be associated with quite pronounced psychiatric symptoms such as depression.

Tics are common at all ages, but are most common in children. Although it is clear that some occur as a result of an organic c.n.s. disturbance, many are simple habit spasms and some are frankly hysterical in origin.

Disorders of hearing and balance—eighth cranial nerve

Psychogenic auditory disorders are not uncommon and often, in the hysteric with unilateral symptoms, there is accompanying unilateral deafness. Psychogenic deafness may be either partial or complete, unilateral or bilateral. The introduction of compensation for industrial deafness has been associated with an increased incidence of psychogenic hearing impairment, which can usually be detected by careful audiometry. Total psychogenic deafness is uncommon, but may occur in hysteria. Tinnitus is a common psychogenic symptom.

Organic deafness not infrequently is associated with some psychological reactions. The deaf child particularly is subject to considerable emotional stress and deafness is more responsible than blindness for secondary mental inadequacy.

Psychogenic vestibular disturbances are extremely common: dizziness is a symptom common to neurotic patients and patients with depression. Although complaints of dizziness often are vague, dramatic vertigo occasionally is a symptom, particularly in patients with phobic anxiety where the vertigo develops in the appropriate phobia-producing situation. Patients with organic vertigo not infrequently become depressed and this may complicate the clinical picture, as is the case with post-traumatic vestibular damage.

Swallowing and speaking

Psychogenic disturbances affecting vocalisation and swallowing are fairly common: disorders of vocalisation include mutism, stuttering, hoarseness and hypervocalisation. Psychogenic dysphonia is readily differentated from organic dysphonia by the persistence of the patient's ability to cough. Spastic dysphonia is a characteristic disorder of speech which usually is accompanied by spastic dysarthria and due to bilateral corticobulbar damage: isolated spastic dysphonia may occasionally be due to organic disturbances but most commonly occurs as a functional disorder: it may be recognised as such by its abolition after exercise when the patient is short of breath.

The commonest psychosomatic swallowing disturbance is globus hystericus. This is a common complaint in emotionally disturbed people and is described as a sensation of a tight feeling or a lump in the throat, resulting in difficulty in swallowing. Characteristically, the difficulty in swallowing is for liquids, solids and even the patient's own saliva.

The eleventh cranial nerve

The only possible psychosomatic disorder affecting the eleventh cranial nerve is that of spasmodic torticollis. There is considerable debate in the literature as to whether this is an organic neurological disturbance or a psychosomatic disorder, but there is no doubt that, in many patients, psychosomatic features are prominent.

The tongue

Psychosomatic disorders of the tongue are rare. Occasionally in a gross hysteric there will be hysterical spasm of the tongue, and unilateral inability to move the tongue may be seen in a simulated hemiplegia. The psychosomatic nature of this may be recognised by the fact that the patient is unable to move the tongue to the paralysed side, which is of course the opposite of what might be expected.

SENSATION

In Chapter 2 we have referred to the difficulty of evaluating sensory disorders because of their subjective nature. Psychogenic sensory disorders are among those most commonly encountered: of these the most frequent are the sensory disturbances that, to many of us, are normal everyday occurrences, but to the neurotic appear to assume special significance. These sensory disturbances include the numbness that occasionally occurs during sleep following nerve pressure, the transient numbness encountered on accidentally injuring a peripheral nerve, and the numbness or tingling produced by hyperventilation.

Psychogenic sensory loss may usually readily be differentiated from organic sensory disturbances and the following are pointers to such a diagnosis:

1. Sensory loss that does not conform to an anatomical pattern, e.g. sensory loss including the whole of one limb
2. Total anaesthesia—on an organic basis this is exceedingly uncommon
3. Sensory loss of one particular area with a preserved segment within that area
4. Sensory loss discovered on examination as an incidental finding in the absence of sensory symptoms.

A variety of positive psychogenic sensory symptoms may be encountered and of these the most common is psychogenic pain. Untold varieties of this symptom may present and many of them are dealt with in the appropriate sections of this chapter.

Genuine pain is often accompanied by psychological symptoms of which the most common is depression. It may be difficult in this situation to assess the contribution to symptomatology of the pain itself and of the depression and often both require treatment. One of the commonest clinical syndromes where this combination coexists is the syndrome of postherpetic neuralgia.

Occasionally, genuine sensory symptoms may be mistakenly diagnosed as non-organic. Patients with posterior column loss in the hands may have little in the way of sensory symptoms and may predominantly complain of inability to use the hands. Power may appear normal and the lack of motor signs may in some instances lead the inexperienced to misdiagnose the case as being non-organic.

MOTOR FUNCTION

In the early stages, a variety of organic motor disturbances may be mistakenly diagnosed as functional. Parkinsonism may be difficult to diagnose and the general slowing up of the patient may suggest a depressive illness. The reverse is also true, in that depression may be misdiagnosed as parkinsonism because of slowness of volitional movement.

Psychogenic motor disturbances present with a variety of symptoms. These include obsessive preoccupation with muscle disease, ready fatiguability, muscle ache, poorly sustained motor activity, tremor, weakness, disturbances of gait and a variety of abnormalities of posture and involuntary movements.

Although the diagnosis of psychogenic motor disturbances can usually readily be made, it is important to emphasise that, in some instances, a degree of genuine muscle weakness may be accompanied by a degree of functional overlay. This combination may pose considerable diagnostic difficulties.

Preoccupation with muscle disease may occur as one manifestation of hypochondriasis. It may also occur as part of the atlas syndrome: this is a condition of middle-aged men who complain of feeling weak yet who show no evidence of an organic disturbance and the symptoms are felt to be a psychoneurotic reaction to the changes of middle age. Fatiguability, muscle ache and poorly sustained motor activity are not infrequent psychogenic disturbances and in some instances these symptoms follow an organic neurological disturbance that has resolved. Muscle ache involving the paraspinal muscles of the neck or lumbar spine merges into the difficult problem of neck ache and backache. Very often these symptoms occur in the context of an injury where the factor of compensation looms in the background.

Benign muscle cramps and fasciculation are occasionally brought to the attention of the medical profession by the neurotic individual who becomes preoccupied by what is a normal phenomenon. Benign nocturnal myoclonus also falls into a similar category.

Weakness

Psychogenic muscle weakness may resemble paralysis due to organic disease, although this resemblance is not usually exact. Gross hysterical weakness may, in some instances, be accompanied by muscle wasting and trophic changes in the skin, but this is exceptional. No changes in the tendon reflexes are seen. In gross hysteria there may be bizarre postures such as camptocormia, which consists of flexion of the body at the waist; this is often accompanied by a complaint of severe back pain. Similar posturing in the limbs may be seen, not only in hysteria but also in catatonic schizophrenia.

The pattern of psychogenic muscle weakness is often bizarre. For example, the patient may claim to be unable to walk, yet have perfectly normal strength when tested on the bed lying down. This is often called astasia–abasia. Similarly, the limb which enables the patient to undress himself may on formal testing appear grossly weak.

Involuntary movements

Psychogenic involuntary movements include tics, tremors and a whole variety of bizarre disorders of movement and posture. Psychogenic tremor has many of the features of so-called essential tremor, but is usually characterised by a marked variability. One specific disorder of motor function, which may in some instances have a psychogenic basis, is writer's cramp. Early and focal dystonias are sometimes mistaken for psychogenic disorders, both in adults and in children, and there is some evidence to suggest that writer's cramp might be an early focal dystonia in some cases.

Gait

Psychogenic disturbances in gait are quite varied. It is in this situation that there is commonly found a degree of functional overlay, particularly in old people. Genuine symptoms of dizziness in old people are often accompanied by bizarre disorders of gait. Patients with severe retarded depression often move slowly and have difficulty in walking, because of lack of volition. As mentioned previously, these gaits bear a superficial resemblance to parkinsonism.

In some instances, organic motor disorders may be accompanied by psychological symptoms. The patient with hemiplegic stroke is often depressed, which may retard his rehabilitation. On the other hand, a patient with pseudobulbar palsy and hemiplegia might resemble a depressive patient, but in many instances the outward show of emotion is not accompanied by an inward disturbance. One particular organic gait disturbance is sometimes thought to be functional in nature, at least in the initial stages: this is the so-called apraxia of gait, which is usually a manifestation of a medial frontal lobe disturbance. In the early stages it may not be accompanied by any other neurological manifestations and the bizarre nature of the gait may readily lead to a diagnosis of a psychogenic disorder.

THE AUTONOMIC NERVOUS SYSTEM

Psychogenic disorders of the autonomic nervous system are common and many of these are considered in Chapter 4. The most frequently encountered of these is psychogenic impotence.

Cranial nerve autonomic disturbances

Psychogenic disturbances are rare. Neurotic patients occasionally complain of either excessive salivation or of dryness of the mouth, but this is uncommon. Patients with blepharospasm often complain of dryness of the eyes and in some instances genuine lacrimal gland dysfunction may be demonstrable. Occasionally, usually in paramedical or nursing staff, pupillary abnormalities are simulated. The most common abnormality is that of a dilated pupil, induced by the judicious use of eyedrops containing atropine-like substances.

Sweating

Although genuine hyperhydrosis does occur as an organic syndrome, many patients who complain of excessive sweating have no demonstrable abnormality and it probably is a psychoneurotic symptom. A complaint of decreased sweating is rarely, if ever, psychogenic in nature.

Vasomotor function

The interplay between organic and psychiatric factors in disordered vasomotor function is considered in the section concerned with syncope. There is a close association between anxiety and certain forms of syncope, such as vasovagal syncope; in many instances such attacks are precipitated by anxiety-provoking situations, such as an impending visit to the dentist.

Bowel, bladder and sexual function

An almost universal obsession with bowel function is one manifestation of a national neurosis. Disordered bowel function, usually constipation but also diarrhoea, is common in all forms of psychiatric illness. Disorders of bladder function are less common: however, particularly in women, complaints of disordered bladder function may occur in psychoneurotic illnesses. Of these, the rarest is psychogenic incontinence and there should be some hesitation in making this diagnosis. Psychogenic retention of urine is more common and this is almost invariably painful. Impotence is commonly psychogenic, whereas failure of ejaculation is commonly organic and due to loss of sympathetic supply to the sexual organs. One common psychogenic symptom is failure to achieve a satisfactory orgasm despite normal erection and ejaculation. Disorders of sexual function are considered in Chapter 4.

PSYCHOSOMATIC NEUROLOGICAL SYNDROMES

These are discussed within the context of a clinical classification.

BRAIN TUMOURS

Not infrequently, the neurologist encounters hypochondrial or neurotic patients who are preoccupied with the fear that they have a brain tumour. Usually such patients are suffering from chronic tension headache and often they have been subjected to a variety of unnecessary investigations. Fear of a brain tumour is so common that it is worth asking any patient presenting with headache whether such a thought has crossed his mind and then specifically providing reassurance that such a diagnosis is not correct. Unfortunately, there is now an increasing tendency amongst patients to demand the reassurance of a CT scan that they do not have a cerebral tumour.

There is ample support for the concept that premorbid personality determines to a significant degree the emotional and mental changes that occur in patients with brain tumours and there are no mental symptoms that are specific for brain tumours. There is no doubt that psychoneurotic symptoms, in the absence of any specific symptoms, may be an early feature in a patient with a brain tumour, but occasionally genuine symptoms, such as those resulting from a non-dominant parietal tumour, may be mistaken for neurotic symptoms.

Changes in personality are among the most common symptoms occurring as a result of a brain tumour and these usually occur in frontal or temporal lobe tumours. In frontal tumours changes in attention and concentration are often early symptoms and the clinical picture may be readily confused with depression. The vivid hallucinations experienced by some patients with temporal lobe tumours may occasionally lead to a mistaken diagnosis of a schizophreniform psychotic illness and in dominant temporal lobe tumours the florid speech abnormalities may bear a superficial resemblance to the schizophrenic word salad. Diencephalic tumours readily produce stupor, often in the absence of other localising signs. This must be differentiated from psychiatric stupor and, in such instances, the electroencephalogram will usually show a very striking abnormality.

HEAD INJURY

A patient with a head injury and associated brain damage often shows a variety of psychological disturbances: these include organic disturbances of memory and intellectual function, change in personality, and occasionally frank psychotic reactions. This range of disorders in general relates to the severity of the injury and the degree of underlying damage.

The opposite is true for the post-traumatic neuroses and these, the postconcussional syndrome, and the roles of compensation and frank malingering, are dealt with in Chapter 14.

INFECTIONS OF THE NERVOUS SYSTEM

As with any organic cerebral process, psychological symptoms may occur as presenting manifestations of infections of the nervous system. This is uncommon in brain abscess or in meningitis, but is not infrequent in certain forms of encephalitis, particularly subacute encephalitis. In such cases subtle changes in personality and lack of drive may be early symptoms and these may be mistaken for a psychoneurosis, depression or a frank psychotic illness. Herpes simplex encephalitis is one particular infection that may show psychotic features in the early stages.

A variety of personality and other mental changes may be after-effects of encephalitis and of meningitis. In some instances, neurotic reactions may follow complete physical recovery from these illnesses and it may be difficult to differentiate these from the effects of organic damage.

One particular syndrome associated with psychosomatic symptoms is that known as the Royal Free disease, or benign myalgic encephalomyelitis. There is considerable debate as to the nature of this illness and many authors regard it as a form of epidemic hysteria. There is no doubt that some neurotic individuals are only too happy to be labelled as suffering from the condition and, indeed, a society has now been formed to support patients claiming to suffer from this condition.

Frank simulation of meningitis occasionally occurs, with occasional examples of patients simulating meningitis on numerous occasions, qualifying the individual as an example of Munchausen's syndrome.

A variety of other viral illnesses, notably infectious mononucleosis, may be associated with, or followed by, psychosomatic neurological symptoms. Such symptoms not uncommonly develop in students and often become prominent prior to the examinations. They are attributed to the effects of a viral illness, although they are often no more than a manifestation of a psychoneurosis or even frank malingering. Postinfluenzal depression is probably a genuine entity and in some instances responds to appropriate treatment.

CEREBROVASCULAR DISEASE

There is some evidence to suggest that certain forms of stroke may be precipitated by stress: patients' relatives often describe a stroke sufferer as having been under considerable stress at the time the episode occurred. Patients who have suffered a stroke not infrequently become depressed and this often complicates and inhibits rehabilitation. In the acute stages of stroke, psychological manifestations occasionally are very prominent. Miller Fisher has referred to the so-called 'angry stroke' which occurs when the area of damage is predominantly in the right temporal lobe. Similar manifestations are not uncommon in patients who are aphasic as a result of stroke; these symptoms are probably simply an expression of frustration.

Patients occasionally simulate strokes. Frank examples are rare, but patients who have suffered genuine transient ischaemic attacks occasionally subsequently develop similar symptoms that are not genuine.

MIGRAINE

Psychological factors are common in migraine. The placebo response in migraine is such that, in most trials, 60% of patients receiving a placebo show an improvement in their symptoms. Migraine is commonly precipitated by stress, anxiety or depression and one of the most common causes of frequent migraine headaches is a psychological disturbance.

EPILEPSY

Frank simulation of epilepsy is uncommon and usually is seen only in those within the first three decades of life. In the same age group, however, not infrequently there is seen the problem of the patient with genuine epilepsy who has, in addition, non-genuine fits. This appears to be more common in women and is also seen in those of limited intelligence.

The interrelationships between psychological disturbances and epilepsy are complex and, as we shall see, psychiatric and psychological disturbances are common in patients who have epilepsy. Perhaps of more practical importance is the influence of psychological disturbances on the epileptic. There is now considerable evidence to support the view that psychological factors may precipitate epileptic fits and make epilepsy worse. In some instances the relationship is simply because psychological disturbance has resulted in poor treatment compliance; however, clinical experience indicates that patients undergoing periods of psychological stress resulting in anxiety and depression commonly have frequent seizures at these periods. This should always be borne in mind when dealing with a patient whose epilepsy is difficult to control.

A number of complex and inter-related factors are responsible for the psychological and psychiatric problems seen in patients with epilepsy. These include:

1. The effect of drugs
2. The effect of associated brain damage, e.g. secondary to birth trauma
3. The effect of the stigma of epilepsy
4. The effect of the epileptic fits themselves.

Of these, perhaps the most underrated is the effect of the stigma of epilepsy. There is no doubt that in the general population epileptics are regarded as being 'different' and the stigma is emphasised in a situation where an epileptic has problems in his job, or problems because of loss of a driving licence. It is not altogether surprising that an individual who has a disorder characterised by sudden falls to the ground and abnormal behaviour becomes anxious or depressed. Whatever the cause, such problems are common in epileptics and have been estimated as occurring in as many as 20–50% of sufferers. They are found in both adults and children and may occur in both mild and severe forms of epilepsy.

Personality disorders

Much has been written about the so-called epileptic personality. One of the main prejudices that has surrounded epilepsy and coloured public opinion is the idea that the sufferer is in some way fundamentally changed by the epilepsy; epileptics are said to be untrustworthy, disruptive in the community and prone to sudden aggressive behaviour.

It is now clear from community surveys that only a small proportion of patients with epilepsy suffer from personality difficulties of any great degree. Similarly, there is no broad pattern of personality abnormality distinctive for epilepsy. It remains a matter of controversy whether or not certain traits may characterise certain types of epilepsy. There is some presumptive evidence to suggest that there is a special association between temporal lobe epilepsy and personality disorder, but this as yet lacks a firm scientific foundation. The personality disorders that do occur may result from psychosocial effects, the effect of brain damage, the effect of seizures and the effect of drugs.

Sexual disorders may occur in epilepsy, particularly in temporal lobe epilepsy. These include hypersexuality or hyposexuality, and perversions of sexual interest and outlet. Occasionally, disordered sexual activity may accompany or follow a temporal lobe seizure.

Neurosis

This is the most common type of abnormality seen in epileptics, accounting for half the psychological problems that are encountered. The form which the neurotic disability takes has little that is distinctive for epilepsy and the characteristics depend principally on patterns of premorbid personality. Depression and anxiety are the most frequent; obsessive–compulsive disorders are uncommon. Fear of attacks often approaches the degree of a phobia and occasionally specific phobias, such as agoraphobia, may precipitate a fit.

Psychoses

The epileptic psychoses are of particular interest as they provide an opportunity for exploring relationships between cerebral dysfunction and mental disorders. Transient schizophrenia-like episodes may occur in epilepsy and, in temporal lobe epilepsy, may be a manifestation of a subclinical seizure discharge. A chronic schizophrenia-like psychosis is occasionally seen in patients with temporal lobe epilepsy; the patients have usually suffered from epilepsy for many years and the early signs are those of a change in personality.

Depression

Depression occurs in as many as one-third of patients with epilepsy and in one-half of these the depression is endogenous in type. The high incidence of depression in patients with epilepsy almost certainly accounts for the high suicide rate in the epileptic population. The incidence is at least twice that of the general population, or five times greater when the figures are corrected for age.

Treatment of epilepsy may lead to an improvement in the psychiatric complications, although this is not always so; in general these require treatment in their own right.

DEGENERATIVE DISEASE

Alzheimer's disease and other dementing disorders

As with any diffuse cerebral process, dementia in the early stages may present a picture that may be confused with a psychiatric disturbance. The subtle change in personality, or the slight impairment of memory, may be confused with a psychoneurotic illness, and lack of volitional drive may suggest depression. Similarly, the slowness of mental processes in severe depression may readily be mistaken for an early dementia. In various forms of psychoneurosis, complaint of impairment of memory is common and this must be differentiated from the organic loss of memory of an early dementing process. In general, the patient with lack of memory due to dementia rarely complains of this spontaneously, because loss of insight is usually an early feature.

Occasionally, gross examples of simulation of dementia may be encountered, the so-called Ganser syndrome. The diagnosis is usually suggested by the bizarre responses given by the patient in response to simple questions. The following are examples of some of the responses from one of Ganser's original cases:

'In what City are we?
'In Berlin in Russia.'
'What are you doing here?'
'We wanted to go hunting and we unhitched our horses'.
'How many noses do you have?'
'I don't know'.
'Have you any nose at all?'
'I do not know if I have a nose'.
'Have you eyes?'
'I have no eyes.'
'How many fingers do you have?'
'Eleven'.

The clue to the diagnosis is not the approximate nature of the answers, but the absurdness. In most instances, patients with the Ganser syndrome are thought to be malingering.

Parkinson's disease

The subtle nature of the initial symptoms in Parkinson's disease may often lead to a misdiagnosis of a functional disorder. Psychological disturbances in parkinsonism are common and as many as 20% of patients eventually go on to show some degree of intellectual impairment, which is often apparent first as intermittent confusion triggered by therapy.

It is now well established that there is an association between parkinsonism and depression which is often reactive in nature. This may develop at any stage of the disease and does not appear to relate to the degree of disability. In most instances it merits treatment and shows a reasonable response. Personality changes may develop, the most common of which is irritability. Euphoria is rare.

One other aspect of parkinsonism that deserves mention is its occasional precipitation by a particular psychological stress. There are now many clear-cut documented examples of the onset of parkinsonian tremor following a particularly stressful situation. The tremor may persist unchanged for many years to be followed by the frank onset of parkinsonism in later life.

Motor neurone disease

Considering the seriousness of this disorder, the majority of patients show remarkably little psychiatric disturbance. Depression may occur, but is not particularly common and the most obvious psychomotor abnormality is emotional lability resulting from pseudobulbar palsy. Since the turn of the century there have been claims that occasional patients with motor neurone disease go on to develop dementia, but this is extremely rare.

MULTIPLE SCLEROSIS

It is now well recognised that organic mental changes, intellectual impairment in particular, are fairly common in multiple sclerosis and result from demyelination of the cerebral white matter. Patients who have died of multiple sclerosis are often found to have enlargement of the ventricular system caused by widespread intracerebral demyelination. Euphoria is often stressed as being one of the early manifestations of this intellectual change. In general, these changes usually occur in the patient with severe multiple sclerosis and they are often combined with other signs of cerebral white matter demyelination, such as gross cerebellar incoordination. In some patients cerebral manifestations appear at an early stage and may simulate an encephalitis-like illness or even a tumour.

A variety of affective changes are common in multiple sclerosis, with depression and euphoria being equally common. Depression tends to occur in the early stages of the disease, whereas euphoria is more common in the later stages. The author has seen two examples of patients who had suffered their first attack of presumed multiple sclerosis and who, when told the presumptive diagnosis, committed suicide. Although a decision about when to tell the patient the diagnosis is always difficult, and no fixed rules can be given, the shattering effect that the diagnosis has upon an otherwise normal individual should lead to caution in dealing with such patients.

Personality changes in multiple sclerosis result either from the mood changes or from the intellectual impairment and there is no evidence to suggest that a specific personality disorder exists. Similarly, psychotic illnesses in multiple sclerosis do not follow a specific pattern.

There is now a considerable amount of clinical information to suggest that disorders of the emotions may affect the progress of the disease. Many patients complain that they suffer exacerbations when under stress or when emotionally disturbed; in general, such observations should suggest that social and psychological support has a role in the management of the patient with multiple sclerosis.

One of the most intriguing features of multiple sclerosis is the relationship of the disease to hysteria. It is a frequent observation in patients with multiple sclerosis that some take to a wheelchair at an early stage when, in practical terms, their neurological deficit is slight. Such patients appear to simulate the most severe manifestations of the disease: in some instances this is conscious simulation and in others, unconscious; in some it is simply a matter of a degree of functional overlay. Gross hysterical simulation of a paraplegia, or other more profound deficits, does occur and probably accounts for those occasional cases in which multiple sclerosis is cured by faith healing or other forms of alternative medicine.

MUSCULAR DISORDERS

Psychological disturbances are not particularly common in the muscular disorders although as incapacity increases depression may become a prominent feature. The generalised weakness of a psychoneurotic illness may have to be differentiated from a genuine muscular disorder, and gross examples of simulation of a myopathic pattern of muscular weakness may occasionally be encountered. Myotonic dystrophy is one particular muscle disease where there is clear evidence of central nervous system involvement. Psychiatric abnormalities occur in a high proportion of patients, one of the most common being impairment of intellectual function. Personality abnormalities and social deterioration are fairly common, yet many of the patients face their physical and social decline with equanimity.

Myasthenia gravis

This has attracted the attention of psychiatrists on several grounds: emotional factors may precipitate the onset in some cases and have a significant role in aggravating the symptoms; the psychological make-up of patients with myasthenia is thought in some instances to be abnormal. Finally, the disease may pose important problems in differential diagnosis. Without question it is one of the disorders most commonly misdiagnosed in the early stages and often it is misdiagnosed as a psychosomatic disorder. This because the fatiguability, or muscle weakness, which is the hallmark of myasthenia gravis, is a prominent symptom in a variety of psychoneurotic illnesses.

It has been estimated that as many as one-third of patients with myasthenia gravis have some emotional disturbance preceding the onset of symptoms and as many as 50% of patients with the disease complain that their symptoms are exacerbated by an upset of their emotions. It has been suggested that the emotional reaction of an individual to his disease is an important factor in determining prognosis: those with significant emotional and psychiatric problems have twice the mortality rate of those without.

Patients with functional weakness occasionally are misdiagnosed as having myasthenia gravis and started on treatment with anticholinesterase drugs. Occasionally, such patients become dependent on these drugs and this may pose considerable diagnostic and practical problems. Examples where myasthenia gravis is misdiagnosed as a functional disorder are equally common.

Periodic paralysis

One other disorder which may readily be mistaken for a functional disturbance is periodic paralysis. For some reason, the profound muscle paralysis in this condition rarely affects either the bulbar muscles or the muscles concerned with respiration, and this may lead to a mistaken diagnosis of hysteria.

PERIPHERAL NERVE DISORDERS

Apart from depression, psychological disturbances in peripheral nerve disorders are uncommon. The combination of striking psychological symptoms and a peripheral neuropathy should alert the clinician to one of a number of diagnostic possibilities.

One obvious diagnosis to consider is that of acute intermittent porphyria. The prominent psychological symptoms in these cases often leads to a mistaken diagnosis of hysteria and the muscular weakness which develops as a result of the peripheral neuropathy may be labelled as hysterical. The mental disturbances include emotional behaviour, depression, restlessness and occasionally even violence. Emotional lability is common, with histrionic behaviour. Occasionally, psychotic symptoms resembling schizophrenia may develop. The development of psychological symptoms often leads to the patients being given sedative drugs, many of which may make porphyria worse and precipitate neurological complications, such as epileptic fits or the peripheral neuropathy.

A combination of confusion and peripheral neuropathy suggests a number of possibilities, including pernicious anaemia, drug-induced peripheral neuropathy, alcoholism, or one of the paraneoplastic syndromes.

STRESS AND NEUROLOGICAL DISORDERS

References have already been made to the precipitation of symptoms in a variety of disorders by stress. Epileptic seizures, exacerbations of multiple sclerosis and the onset of symptoms in myasthenia gravis may all follow stress. The precipitation of similar problems may also occur with the onset of certain psychiatric illnesses, notably depression. In such cases, symptoms may improve with treatment of the underlying depression. In some instances this relationship is less clear: for example, patients often attribute the onset of a stroke to stress or overwork, although probably no such clear relationship exists.

MALINGERING, HYSTERIA AND SIMULATION

It is in consideration of this topic that there is a diversity of opinion between psychiatrists and neurologists. There is a body of thought that regards malingering as the frank and deliberate simulation of disease and hysteria as an unconscious simulation. In fact, the differentiation is remarkably difficult and it is preferable to use the term 'simulation' to encompass all forms of fraud relating to matters of health. This includes the simulation of disease or disability which is not present; the much commoner gross exaggeration of minor disability (the functional overlay); and the conscious and deliberate attribution, for personal advantage, of a disability to an injury or accident that did not, in fact, cause it. Frank malingering is probably quite rare and is seen in its most gross form as the Munchausen syndrome. Patients with this syndrome seem to have a pathological desire for regular medical attention and often simulate quite major disabilities in order to be admitted to hospital for further investigation. Some patients, indeed, undergo repeated surgical procedures and travel from hospital to hospital in a nationwide search for attention.

In the neurological field, one of the commonest situations where these problems arise is in the context of the post-traumatic syndrome, and this is particularly common after head injury. Such cases almost invariably occur in the context of a compensation issue and it has been pointed out on numerous occasions in the literature that such symptoms do not develop in patients with sporting injuries, where there is seldom any question of compensation. The late Henry Miller commented that the differentiation of the differing degrees of simulation, and in particular the differentiation of conscious from unconscious simulation in this context, is always difficult. He tended to take the pragmatic view that to attempt this differentiation in the payment of compensation was illogical: 'To compensate a man financially because he is stated to be deceiving himself as well as trying to deceive others is strange equity and stranger logic'.

What can be stated with some certainty is that there should always be hesitation about making the diagnosis of a simulated deficit of whatever degree. Minor degrees of functional overlays are exceedingly common and many examples are quoted above. Grosser degrees are less common, and often in such patients there eventually turns out to be at least a degree of underlying organic illness. It has been said on many occasions that you should 'beware the hysteric'.

FURTHER READING

Lishman W A 1981 Organic psychiatry. Blackwell Scientific Publications, Oxford

Index